MANAGEMENT OF DIABETES MELLITUS
Perspectives of Care Across the Life Span

MANAGEMENT OF DIABETES MELLITUS
Perspectives of Care Across the Life Span

Edited by

DEBRA HAIRE-JOSHU, MSEd, MSN, PhD, RN
Director, Diabetes Education Center
Diabetes Research and Training Center
Washington University School of Medicine
St. Louis, Missouri

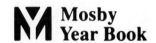

**Mosby
Year Book**

St. Louis   Baltimore   Boston   Chicago   London   Philadelphia   Sydney   Toronto

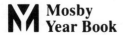
Mosby
Year Book
Dedicated to Publishing Excellence

Editors: Don Ladig, Terry Van Schaik
Developmental Editor: Jeanne Rowland
Project Manager: Gayle May Morris
Project Editor: Donna L. Walls
Designer: Susan Lane

Printed in the United States of America.

Mosby–Year Book, Inc.
11830 Westline Industrial Drive
St. Louis, Missouri, 63146

Library of Congress Cataloging-in-Publication Data

Management of diabetes mellitus : perspectives of care across the lifespan /
  edited by Debra Haire-Joshu.
     p.   cm.
  Includes index.
  ISBN 0-8016-2429-0
  1. Diabetes.   I. Haire-Joshu, Debra.
  [DNLM: 1. Diabetes Mellitus.   WK 810 M266]
  RC660.M333 1992
  616.4′62—dc20
  DNLM/DLC   91-36708
  for Library of Congress   CIP

93 94 95 96   CL/CD/VH   9 8 7 6 5 4 3 2

Contributors

Wendy Auslander, PhD
Assistant Professor of Social Work
George Warren Brown School of Social Work
Washington University
St. Louis, Missouri

Christine Beebe, MS, RD, CDE
Diabetes Program Manager
St. James Hospital & Health Centers
Chicago Heights, Illinois

R. Keith Campbell, RPh, FAPP, CDE
Associate Dean and Professor of Pharmacy
College of Pharmacy
Washington State University
Pullman, Washington

William Coleman, DPM
Podiatrist
Department of Endocrinology
Ochsner Clinic
New Orleans, Louisiana

Denis Daneman, MB, BCh, FRCP(C)
Associate Professor of Pediatrics
University of Toronto
Staff Endocrinologist
The Hospital for Sick Children
Toronto, Canada

Gail D'Eramo-Melkus, EdD, RN
Assistant Professor and Director
Nurse Practitioner Program
Yale University School of Nursing
New Haven, Connecticut

James A. Fain, PhD, RN
Associate Professor and Chairperson
Non-Nurse College Graduate Division
Yale University School of Nursing
New Haven, Connecticut

Marcia Frank, MHSc, RN
Diabetes Nurse Educator
The Hospital for Sick Children
Toronto, Canada

Marion J. Franz, MS, RD, CDE
Director of Nutrition and Publications
International Diabetes Center
Minneapolis, Minnesota

Martha Mitchell Funnell, MS, RN, CDE
Associate Director for Administration
University Hospitals
Ann Arbor, Michigan

Douglas A. Greene, MD
Professor of Internal Medicine
University of Michigan
Ann Arbor, Michigan

Debra Haire-Joshu, MSEd, MSN, PhD, RN
Director, Diabetes Education Center
Diabetes Research and Training Center
Washington University School of Medicine
St. Louis, Missouri

Joan Heins, MA, RD, CDE
Project Manager
Diabetes Research and Training Center
Washington University School of Medicine
St. Louis, Missouri

Douglas N. Henry, MD
Fellow, Pediatric Endocrinology
University of Michigan School of Medicine
Ann Arbor, Michigan

William H. Herman, MD
Chief, Epidemiology and Statistics Branch
Division of Diabetes Translation
Centers for Disease Control
Atlanta, Georgia

Priscilla Hollander, MD
Diabetologist
International Diabetes Center
Minneapolis, Minnesota

Cheryl Houston, MS, RD
Research Coordinator
Center for Health Behavior Research
Washington University School of Medicine
St. Louis, Missouri

Jennifer H. Merritt, MS, RN
Clinical Nurse Specialist
Turner Geriatric Clinic
University Hospitals
Ann Arbor, Michigan

Sharon L. Pontious, PhD, RN
Director
Jewish Hospital School of Nursing;
Research Associate Professor
Washington University School of Medicine
St. Louis, Missouri

Robert E. Ratner, MD
Associate Professor of Medicine
Director of the Diabetes Center
Division of Endocrinology
George Washington University School of
    Medicine
Washington, DC

Barbara Schreiner, MN, RN, CDE
Diabetes Nurse Specialist
Assistant Director, Children's Diabetes
    Management Center
Department of Pediatrics
University of Texas Medical Branch
Galveston, Texas

Barbara Tesno, MSN, RN
Patient Care Manager
St. Louis Children's Hospital
St. Louis, Missouri

John White, RPh, PharmD
Assistant Professor, Pharmacy Practice
Washington State University-Spokane
Spokane, Washington

Neil H. White, MD
Associate Professor of Pediatrics
Division of Pediatric Endocrinology
    and Metabolism
Washington University Diabetes Research
    and Training Center
Washington University School of Medicine
St. Louis, Missouri

Frank Vinicor, MD
Director, Division of Diabetes Translation
Division of Diabetes Study
Centers for Disease Control
Atlanta, Georgia

Consultants

Jean Betschart, MN, RN, CDE
Diabetes Educator
President Elect-AADE
Children's Hospital of Pittsburgh
Pittsburgh, Pennsylvania

Jeanne Bubb, MSW, ACSW
Behavioral Scientist, Diabetes Control and
    Complications Trial
Washington University School of Medicine
St. Louis, Missouri

Gregory A. Casalenuovo, MSN, RN,
    CCRN, CS
Clinical Specialist, Diabetes
Methodist Medical Center
Oak Ridge, Tennessee

Sandy Cook, PhD
Research Associate (Assistant Professor)
Center for Research in Medical Education and
    Health Care
Department of Medicine
The University of Chicago
Chicago, Illinois

Edwin B. Fisher, Jr, PhD
Associate Professor of Psychology
Director, Center for Health Behavior Research
Washington University School of Medicine
St. Louis, Missouri

Karen Flavin, RN, CDE
Chief Clinical Coordinator
Islet Transplant Center
Washington University School of Medicine
St. Louis, Missouri

Marianne Gergely, BSN, RN, CDE
Diabetes Education Project Manager
Indiana University Diabetes Research and
    Training Center
Indianapolis, Indiana

Claudia Graham, PhD, CDE
Exercise Physiologist
Diabetes Management and Research Center
Los Angeles, California

Patricia Granuci, MSN, RN, CPNP, CDE
Diabetes Program Coordinator
Eisenhower Medical Center
Rancho Mirage, California

Deborah L. Gray, MSN, RN, CPNP, CDE
Pediatric Clinical Nurse Specialist
Indiana University Diabetes Research and
    Training Center
Indianapolis, Indiana

Diana W. Guthrie, PhD, RN, CDE, FAAN
Professor
University of Kansas School of Medicine at
    Wichita
Wichita, Kansas

Linda B. Haas, MN, RN, CDE
Clinical Nurse Specialist, Endocrinology
Seattle Department of Veteran's Affairs
    Medical Center
Seattle, Washington

Lynn Heggen, MSN, RN, CDE
Diabetes Clinical Specialist
Private Practice
Des Moines, Iowa

Patricia DeConti Johnson, MSN, RN,
    CDE
Clinical Nurse Specialist, Pediatric Diabetes
University of Michigan Diabetes Research and
    Training Center
Ann Arbor, Michigan

Monica Joyce, BS, RD, CDE
Diabetes Educator and Nutritionist
Office of Dr. Gerald W. Sobel
Chicago, Illinois

Ben R. Leedle, Jr, MS, CDE
Program Director
Diabetes Treatment Center
Roper Hospital
Charleston, South Carolina

Lucy Levandoski, PA-C
Trial Coordinator, Diabetes Control and
  Complications Trial
Washington University School of Medicine
St. Louis, Missouri

Wylie L. McNabb, EdD
Assistant Professor
Director, Center for Research in Medical
  Education and Health Care
Department of Medicine
The University of Chicago
Chicago, Illinois

Patricia S. Moore, MSN, RN, CDE
Outreach Research Associate
Indiana University Diabetes Research and
  Training Center
Indianapolis, Indiana

Darlene J. Paduano, MSN, RN, CS,
  CDE, CETN
Director, Diabetes Nursing Practice
The Diabetes Center
University Hospital at Stony Brook
Stony Brook, New York

Joyce Green Pastors, MS, RD, CDE
Diabetes Nutrition Specialist
University of Virginia Diabetes Center
Charlottesville, Virginia

Julio V. Santiago, MD
Diabetologist
Professor of Pediatrics
Director, Diabetes Research and Training
  Center
Washington University School of Medicine
St. Louis, Missouri

Condit Steil, PharmD, CDE
President, Crystal Care Corporation
Ashland, Kentucky

*To **Joel, Corrie, Erin,** and as always, **Eric***

Preface

Various excellent books currently available address comprehensive components of diabetes care and management from the perspective and role of a specific discipline, and specialty books provide detailed information regarding a single aspect of diabetes. A major goal of *Diabetes Management: Perspectives of Care Across the Lifespan,* is to provide a *general* foundation of diabetes knowledge pertinent to health care providers from various disciplines. There are 3 assumptions which have been made regarding the development of this text.

The first of these assumptions is that diabetes represents a model of chronic disease care in which effective management requires the interaction of various professional disciplines. As such, the focus of care among nurses, dietitians, and physicians, for example, reflects a view unique to the body of knowledge of that particular discipline. Optimal diabetes management requires that the unique contributions of these disciplines be additive in order that model diabetes care be implemented. The content of this book was developed following input from experts representing various health care disciplines. The specific chapter content reflects the expertise of these specific disciplines, but also highlights the common theme across professions of the need for preventive education via active collaboration between the individual with diabetes and the health care team.

A second assumption is that diabetes is a disease that affects each person uniquely. Individualizing diabetes care requires an understanding of the differences that emerge not only because of physical changes in growth but as well in the emotional/psychologic changes in development. This book addresses issues related to diabetes management as it affects the individual across various times in life and is valuable to the health care providers who care for individuals and families with diabetes over long periods.

Finally, a major assumption of this book is that education is an ongoing component in the practice of any health professional who cares for individuals with diabetes. The importance of diabetes education is addressed throughout the book. Variations in the teaching/learning process as is affected by changes in growth and development, and issues related to evaluation and accountability of practice, are recurrent themes that bear continual emphasis.

The Organization of the Text

The text is divided into two main parts, the first of which provides a clinical overview of the components of diabetes care and management. Specific sections provide a foundation of knowledge regarding the therapeutic regimen, progressive complications of diabetes, and special considerations of management, including acute manifestations of diabetes as well as pregnancy. Since entire books have been written on each of these topics, our purpose was to provide the reader with an overview of the respective topics in relation to state-of-the art diabetes care, as well as resources for additional in-depth information.

The second part of the text refers to diabetes management across the lifespan. This section begins with an introduction to diabetes care as it mirrors social, family, and community perspectives. Within this framework, diabetes as it affects the developing human being is discussed. The subsequent chapters discuss normal aspects of growth and development and then address the effect of diabetes on these individuals.

The final section of the book refers to diabetes education, a common and recurring theme throughout this text. The final chapters make the assumption that diabetes education is a critical component of any practice, and that such education needs to be conducted within the context of accountability and evaluation. Strategies for encouraging behavior change, as well as issues related to evaluation from a programmatic as well as educator's perspective, are provided.

Finally, the appendices of this book include a resource list for additional materials related to education and support of the individual with diabetes and his or her family. This substantial list will prove to be of great benefit to those health care providers who view diabetes as affecting the individual in all facets of life.

About the Contributors

A major strength of this book lies in the expertise of the individual contributors of each chapter. These health care providers are noted experts in diabetes, who have authored their chapters within the context of their professional backgrounds. The contributors believe that each discipline provides an expertise that needs to be collaboratively incorporated if state-of-the-art diabetes care is to be effectively implemented. Dietitians, educators, nurses, social workers, physicians, and psychologists were involved in the planning, writing, and reviewing of this text. The rationale for this approach was so that the unique perspectives of each group could be incorporated into the text. The perspectives of the contributors vary depending upon their background and training. Inevitably however, this diversity provides the reader with a broad picture of diabetes care.

A guiding principle in the editing of this text was that the content be clear, concise, and accurate, but also sensitive to the individual contributor's perspective of the issues of paramount importance to the subject at hand. As such in several chapters, resources are provided for more traditional information, with content highlighting current issues such as the public health implications of diabetes.

Finally, a general effort has been made to be consistent in terminology. However, the reader will note some terms have been used interchangeably, such as glycated and glycosylated hemoglobin. The varied use of such terms is commonplace and reflects not only the current terminology common in the field today, but the preferences of the contributors.

About the Audience

This book was written for health care providers from a variety of disciplines who are interested in providing diabetes care via two avenues. The first avenue is clinical practice. This book will be a useful and utilized resource to health care professionals interested in specializing in diabetes care and education. In particular, those whose interests include attaining certification as a diabetes educator, as well as those who seek recognition of their diabetes programs, will find the content of this book broad enough to serve as a useful addition to their library.

Secondly, this book is designed for those health care providers who are concerned with professional education. Many faculty members are charged with educating the generalist health care provider regarding diabetes amidst finite constraints of time allotted for such material. This book is meant to be a resource to those faculty members by providing an overview of clinical aspects of management, while addressing diabetes as it affects the individual and family at all ages.

Acknowledgements

I would like to acknowledge the assistance of several people without whose help I could not have seen this book to fruition. First, I want to recognize the assistance and support of Julio V. Santiago, MD, and Edwin B. Fisher, Jr., PhD, of the Diabetes Research and Training Center at Washington University School of Medicine. They have provided consistent encouragement, expertise, and support for activities designed to promote professional education and expert care of the individual with diabetes, a paramount theme within this environment. In addition, their support of my work on this book was available across all levels and roles, including development, consultation, and review.

I am especially grateful to the contributors, whose efforts and expertise are represented in this book. Without them, none of this would have been possible. In the midst of their already frenetic schedules, these individuals have endured deadlines, telephone calls, and heavy correspondence regarding the schedule and content of the book. They have done so with amazing patience and good humor, for which I am grateful.

The reviewers as well donated their time and efforts to this text, and in doing so, were able to ensure the focus, accuracy, and completeness of material. Reviewers are often the unsung heroes in any publication process, but without them, the product would suffer.

I am also grateful for having had the opportunity to work with Jeanne Rowland, Don Ladig, and Terry Van Schaik of Mosby, who have always been helpful, patient, and a pleasure to work with. And finally, the support services, patience, and organizational capabilities of Cherie Hill and Beth Gruber in the preparation of materials for this book were invaluable. As with any outcome, this one represented the team efforts of numerous talented people.

Debra Haire-Joshu

Contents

SECTION III · SPECIAL CONSIDERATIONS, 249

PART TWO   DIABETES MANAGEMENT ACROSS THE LIFE SPAN

SECTION IV · INDIVIDUALIZING DIABETES CARE, 355

SECTION V · DIABETES EDUCATION

APPENDIX

MANAGEMENT OF DIABETES MELLITUS
Perspectives of Care Across the Life Span

PART ONE

COMPONENTS OF DIABETES CARE

CHAPTER **1**

Overview of Diabetes Mellitus

ROBERT E. RATNER

INTRODUCTION

Diabetes has long been a clinical model for general medicine. The primary defect in fuel metabolism results in widespread, multiorgan complications that ultimately encompass virtually every system of the body and every specialty of medicine. To know diabetes—it has been said—is to know medicine and health care. Although from a clinical standpoint this may be true, our increasing knowledge of the pathophysiology of the syndrome, together with the mechanisms of long-term complications, has placed diabetes research at the frontier of immunology and molecular biology. In addition, implementation of clinical care for the individual with diabetes is now serving as the paradigm for a chronic-disease model of health care delivery. Nowhere else in health care is the individual with a disorder more incorporated into his or her own clinical care plan. Involving the individual in his or her health care is the first step toward implementing preventive medicine and is revolutionizing the concept of health care delivery. In essence, the individual with diabetes is becoming his or her own primary health care provider. Thus the evolution of diabetes care and research places diabetes at the forefront of both scientific and social advances in the health care sciences.

The objectives of this chapter are to encourage the reader to:

Know the groups at risk for the development of diabetes; understand the impact of diabetes care on health care delivery and financing; know the diagnostic criteria for diabetes mellitus; know the difference beween the various forms of diabetes mellitus; understand the stages of development of insulin-dependent diabetes mellitus and the implications for early intervention; understand the mechanisms by which non–insulin-dependent diabetes mellitus occurs and the risk factors for its development; be aware of the available technologies for measuring glycated hemoglobin and of their limitations and clinical utility; be aware of the available systems for self-monitoring of blood glucose levels and the importance of appropriate instruction in the proper operation and use of the data the sys-

3

tems provide; understand the interrelationhips among the various health care providers involved in the team approach to diabetes care; know the legal restrictions and liability concerns involved in diabetes education; and understand the health care financing ramifications of diabetes education and the implications for the chronic care model.

EPIDEMIOLOGY AND DEMOGRAPHICS

Diabetes mellitus is a clinical syndrome characterized by inappropriate hyperglycemia caused by a relative or absolute deficiency of insulin or by a resistance to the action of insulin. It is the most common endocrine disorder, affecting approximately 12 million individuals in the United States, and perhaps as many as 200 million worldwide. Perhaps more importantly, individuals with diabetes are disproportionate users of the health care system. Approximately 3% of all outpatient physician visits involve a diagnosis of diabetes.[11] The individual with diabetes sees a physician an average of three times per year. In addition, the rate of hospitalization for individuals with diabetes is twice that of age-matched controls. Once hospitalized, individuals with diabetes also have disproportionately long hospital stays—almost 2 days longer than those of patients without diabetes, but with similar disorders.[57] In total, direct costs of illness for diabetes mellitus range from $9.6 to $13.7 billion per year.[11,12] This total is considerably higher on a proportional basis than that found for other diseases. As an example, direct medical costs account for 43% of total costs for diabetes, as compared with only 22% for cancer, 27% for circulatory disease, and 11% for musculoskeletal diseases.[30]

These costs must be borne by society in general. However, those within our society who are least capable of paying are those most commonly affected. Non–insulin-dependent diabetes mellitus (NIDDM, or type II), which is discussed in detail in a later section, accounts for approximately 90% of diabetes in the United States and increases significantly with age. According to the Second National Health & Nutritional Examination Survey (NHANES II), 18% of Americans aged 65 to 74 have diabetes.[41] Perhaps most alarming is that half of this population was undiagnosed before this broad-based screening study. Subsequent studies have substantiated this high prevalence of diabetes in the elderly, with a systematic increase in prevalence at each decade over the sixth.[64] This becomes a major public health concern with the progressive aging of our population and anticipates a future epidemic of diabetes. Although some have argued that carbohydrate intolerance is a natural consequence of aging, it still requires intervention because of the short-term disabilities and acute complications as well as the potential for exacerbation of macrovascular disease.[48] Underlying defects in carbohydrate handling include delays in glucose-induced insulin secretion, impaired insulin-mediated glucose uptake, and defective intracellular glucose transport.[27] As will be seen in the following section, these mimic the defects noted in type II diabetes. The high prevalence of diabetes in the elderly population also raises questions about specific educational needs. Cognitive abilities, physical constraints, and social and financial status must be considered in the context of modifying lifelong health beliefs and practices.[19]

In addition, minority populations have significantly higher relative rates of NIDDM when compared with an age-matched white population—specifically, diabetes is 2 times more common in blacks, 2½ times more common in Hispanics, and 5 times more common in Native Americans.[25,65] Black Americans have suffered from a progressive increase in the prevalence, morbidity, and mortality associated with diabetes since the turn of the century.[47] Although obesity certainly contributes to these increased risks, black Americans are more likely to have diabetes even when adiposity and socio-economic status are controlled.[44] Some authors have suggested a specific form of diabetes selectively affecting blacks that mimics maturity-onset diabetes of the young.[64,65] Educational techniques again must be adapted to the specific social, financial, and educational context of these minority populations.[33]

DIAGNOSIS AND CLASSIFICATION

Any efforts—either social or medical—to improve the care and prognosis of individuals with diabetes require precise definitions and classifications of diabetes. Although not ideal, the National Diabetes Data Group (NDDG) classification has provided a framework for both diagnosis and classification.[42] The accompanying box gives three independent criteria for diagnosing diabetes mellitus. Any one of these criteria is sufficient to establish a firm diagnosis pending further classification in type. For patients presenting with classic signs and symptoms of diabetes—including polydipsia, polyuria, and unexplained weight loss—random serum glucose determinations in excess of 200 mg/dL (11 mmol/L) is sufficient to make the diagnosis. In those individuals who are asymptomatic, fasting plasma glucose determinations must be performed. In this circumstance, fasting glucose levels in excess of 140 mg/dL (7.7 mmol/L) on two occasions are necessary to meet diagnostic criteria. In those unusual circumstances in which fasting glucose is normal and yet there is a high index of suspicion that diabetes exists (i.e., family history or other risk factor, or clinical signs suggestive of long-term diabetic complications), then and only then is a glucose tolerance test necessary. In the nonpregnant adult, this test is a standardized 75-gram liquid glucose challenge extending for a 2-hour period. This test should be limited to

---

_____ **CRITERIA FOR DIAGNOSIS OF DIABETES MELLITUS** _____

These are diagnostic criteria for diabetes mellitus in the nonpregnant adult. Any one of the following is sufficient to make the diagnosis.
1. A random plasma glucose level >200 mg/dL together with classic signs and symptoms, including polydipsia, polyuria, polyphagia, and weight loss.
2. A fasting plasma glucose level >140 mg/dL on two measurements, independent of symptoms.
3. A fasting plasma glucose level <140 mg/dL, but an abnormal response to two 75-gram oral glucose tolerance tests as manifested by a 2-hour plasma glucose >200 mg/dL with an intervening value >200 mg/dL.

those individuals who are ambulatory with no intercurrent illness, and it should be performed after a 3-day diet consisting of at least 150 grams of carbohydrate and only in the morning following an overnight fast. Criteria to establish diagnosis of diabetes include a 2-hour postglucose load of serum glucose in excess of 200 mg/dL with 1 intervening value also in excess of 200 mg/dL. In general, the glucose tolerance test is rarely necessary to identify individuals with diabetes and is most valuable in proving that an individual at risk does not have the disorder.

Diagnostic criteria for diabetes in the pregnant woman remain quite controversial. The NDDG accepted diagnostic criteria originally established by O'Sullivan and Mahan[45] in 1964, and these modified criteria continue to be used for diagnosis. Current recommendations include screening all pregnant, nondiabetic women for gestational diabetes (see Chapter 9). This involves a 50-gram glucose challenge test typically performed between weeks 24 and 28 of gestation as an initial screen for identification of patients at risk. Definitive diagnosis of gestational diabetes involves a 100-gram liquid glucose challenge followed over a 3-hour period. Diagnostic criteria require that 2 values—including baseline, 1-hour, 2-hour, and 3-hour values—exceed the modified O'Sullivan limits of:

Fasting—105 mg%
1 hour—190 mg%
2 hours—165 mg%
3 hours—145 mg%

Gestational diabetes is defined as the diabetic condition that initially manifests during pregnancy.[5] Some authors have suggested that a substantial percentage of gestational diabetes is in fact only the identification of preexisting carbohydrate intolerance because of increased surveillance.[24] Although this may very well be true in a large percentage of individuals, the subsequent normalization of carbohydrate tolerance postpartum would suggest that impaired glucose handling is an acquired defect inherent in the pregnant state. The occurrence of gestational diabetes, however, remains a significant risk factor for the ultimate development of diabetes mellitus outside of gestation, with 50% developing diabetes within 20 years of the affected pregnancy.[45]

Once the diagnosis of diabetes is established by NDDG criteria, it is imperative to subsequently classify this syndrome into specific disorders. Although rather primitive, the NDDG classification does serve as a model for differentiation. The historic classification of juvenile-onset versus adult-onset diabetes eroded with the realization that both forms of diabetes may occur in any age group. The newer classification is an attempt to define the specific diseases according to etiologic mechanism. The disorder previously described as juvenile-onset diabetes is now more appropriately described as insulin-dependent diabetes mellitus (IDDM), or type I diabetes. Adult-onset diabetes mellitus is now more appropriately described as non–insulin-dependent diabetes.

Two major problems emerge from this diagnostic classification system. First, the terms IDDM and NIDDM tend to suggest that the disease classification depends on whether insulin is used in the treatment. This, in fact, is not the case. Approximately 50% of all individuals with diabetes currently being treated with insulin have NIDDM, or type II diabetes.[38] This remains a major stumbling block in the effective education of health professionals and patients as to appropriate classification and prognosis of the disorder. Second, the descriptions of type I and type II disease in no way suggest the etiologic mechanism underlying the disorder. It is a firm belief and hope that future efforts to standardize diagnoses and classification will establish designations relevant to the pathophysiology of any given disorder rather than to descriptive terms of therapy. From a social standpoint, the societal limitations and activities of an individual with diabetes are now predominantly decided on the basis of whether the individual is using insulin in his or her therapeutic management. This is most inappropriate because individuals with type I diabetes have a markedly different response to insulin therapy and a unique prognosis as compared with insulin-treated, non–insulin-dependent individuals (see Appendix C, "Comparison of IDDM and NIDDM")

The NDDG classification also calls for the identification of other forms of diabetes, particularly secondary forms of the disease. These may include diabetes occurring as a complication of (1) pancreatic disease or surgery; (2) complications of endocrine disorders such as acromegaly, pheochromocytoma, or Cushing's syndrome; and (3) complications of pharmacologic therapy such as glucocorticoids, streptozotocin, or pentamidine. These are potentially reversible forms of diabetes with no genetic linkage. The historic description of borderline, or chemical, diabetes has now been eliminated. To remove the stigma of a diagnosis including the term "diabetes," this status is now defined as impaired glucose tolerance. These individuals may be diagnosed only by glucose tolerance testing and are classified by the findings of a 2-hour post-glucose–load serum glucose of less than 200 mg/dL with 1 intervening value in excess of 200 mg/dL. Approximately a third of these individuals will subsequently develop carbohydrate intolerance, meeting criteria for diabetes mellitus. Also, these individuals remain at risk for the development of severe macrovascular complications.[42]

Pathogenesis and Pathophysiology: IDDM

Our current understanding of the pathogenesis of the different forms of diabetes should serve as a framework for the development of nomenclature more descriptive of the etiology. For example, it is known that type I, or IDDM, is the result of an autoimmune attack on the beta cell.[17] Thus the ultimate designation of IDDM as autoimmune diabetes would be far more descriptive and better understood than either insulin-dependent, or type I, diabetes mellitus. But putting these problems with nomenclature aside, IDDM is characterized by the abrupt onset of clinical signs and symptoms associated with marked hyperglycemia and the strong propensity to the development of ketoacidosis. Now classic studies performed at the Joslin Clinic have demonstrated pathologic and biochemical changes as long as 9 years before the clinical onset of disease.[58] Type I diabetes may now be broken down into five stages of development (see box on p. 8).

It has long been known that there is a genetic propensity for the occurrence of IDDM. The risk of IDDM in the general population ranges from 1 in 400 to 1 in 1000. That risk is substantially increased in the offspring of individuals with diabetes to approximately 1 in 20 to 1 in 50.[51] Subsequent studies examining the genetics of IDDM have

---

____ PATHOPHYSIOLOGIC STAGES IN THE DEVELOPMENT OF IDDM ____

Stage 1 Genetic predisposition
Stage 2 Environmental trigger
Stage 3 Active autoimmunity
Stage 4 Progressive beta-cell dysfunction
Stage 5 Overt diabetes mellitus

---

focused on the histocompatibility locus, or HLA system, on the sixth chromosome. Early studies of class I antigens within the HLA system reveal a markedly elevated relative risk of developing IDDM in those individuals found to be positive for B8 and Bw15.[43] Analyses of this sort do not identify the specific locus resulting in the disease, but rather identify a linkage disequilibrium at that area. Subsequent analyses of class II antigens found the B8 and Bw15 association to be in linkage disequilibrium with DR3 and DR4. Positivity at DR3 and DR4 loci confers a higher degree of relative risk than does positivity B8 or Bw15, suggesting that DR3 and DR4 are more important for the genetic predisposition to the disorder (see Table 1-1).

In one population, 95% of individuals with IDDM were found to have either DR3 or DR4 HLA markers.[18] More recent studies have suggested even more specific HLA loci. In particular, DQ3.2 markedly increases the relative risk of diabetes, whereas the codon for aspartic acid at the 57 position of the DQ beta peptide conveys a negative correlation with IDDM.[7,40,56] The inverse, aspartic-acid–negative DQ beta alleles, were found in virtually all patients with IDDM. In addition to the presence of aspartic acid at codon 57 of the DQ beta chain, dominant protection also appears to be confirmed by the presence of the antigen DQw1.2.[7] Regardless of the aspartic acid status of codon 57, this DQw1.2 allele was sufficient to protect the individual from subsequent development of IDDM. Thus our understanding of the genetics of IDDM is leading to the identification of markers of susceptibility for this disorder.

However, it is abundantly clear that not all individuals at genetic risk for IDDM ultimately develop it. Epidemiologic surveys reveal that 40% of Caucasian individuals express the DR3 or DR4 haplotype, but despite this high prevalence, fewer than 1% ultimately develop diabetes.[18] Further convincing evidence that genetics are not sufficient for the development of the disease is the finding of a 50% discordance rate of IDDM between identical twins.[61] This would suggest that specific alleles within the class II antigens of the histocompatibility complex on chromosome 6 are necessary but not sufficient conditions for the development of IDDM. In particular, some trigger is necessary for the expression of this genetic propensity.

Environmental triggers for the development of IDDM have long been suspected. Epidemiologic studies have suggested that the incidence of IDDM is increased in both the spring and fall and is coincidental with epidemics of various viral disorders.[20] Older studies relating apparent epidemic outbreaks of IDDM in populations previously affected by

Table 1-1　Genetic Risk for the Development of IDDM

HLA haplotype	Relative risk
Bw15	2.1
B8	3.1
Bw15/B8	9.8
DR3	3.8
DR4	4.4
Dw4	6.2
Dw10	7.0
DQ3.2	5.9
Dw4/DQ3.2	12.1
DR3/Dw4,DQ3.2	38.0

Adapted from Sheehy MJ, et al: A diabetes-susceptible HLA haplotype is best defined by a combination of HLA-DR and DQ alleles, J Clin Invest 83:830-835, 1989.

outbreaks of mumps provide strong circumstantial evidence. The finding of activated T cells and active autoimmunity in as many as a third of individuals suffering from congenital rubella syndrome further supports a viral etiology.[49] The finding of a beta-cell cytotropic Coxsackie B virus in a young child dying of ketoacidosis when presenting with IDDM was the first apparent demonstration of direct viral attack on the beta cells.[66] Although this direct viral hypothesis remains controversial, it is quite evident that several viruses appear to trigger the subsequent immunologic response in genetically predisposed individuals who develop diabetes. The dilemma in identifying specific triggers involves the apparently long latency period between the triggering of active autoimmunity and the subsequent clinical development of diabetes mellitus. Thus it is extremely difficult to identify which insult over the past 7 to 10 years may have been the actual trigger of the disease process. More likely is the possibility that a wide variety of viral agents may trigger expression of the genetic predisposition to the disease.

Regardless of the trigger, early IDDM is first identified by the appearance of active autoimmunity directed against the beta cells of the pancreas and their products. Various immunologic markers occur in individuals before the development of carbohydrate intolerance and diabetes. These immunologic markers include the presence of Ia-positive activated T cells,[28] the presence of complement-fixing anti-islet cell antibodies,[8] a description of a 64,000 M_r islet-cell antigen,[6] and the recent identification of antibody-mediated inhibition of glucose uptake by islet cells.[29] In addition to basic immunologic dysfunction and direct immunologic attack on the beta cell, there also appears to be an immunologic attack on insulin, the product of the beta cell.[46] Thus a substantial proportion of individuals with early IDDM will also be found to have anti-insulin antibodies despite never being exposed to exogenous insulin administration.

The combination of autoimmune attack on the beta cell and insulin by insulin autoantibodies progressively diminishes the effective circulating insulin level. Before the clinical onset of diabetes mellitus, intravenous (IV) glucose tolerance testing demonstrates a progressive fall in first-phase insulin secretion in those individuals with positive immunologic markers.[59] More than 50% of individuals with positive islet cell antibodies but normal glucose tolerance tests have first-phase insulin secretion falling within the tenth percentile of the normal population.[36] To date, most of these individuals have subsequently developed overt diabetes mellitus.

It is not until greater than 90% of the secretory capacity of the beta cell mass has been destroyed that the patient will ultimately manifest hyperglycemia and symptoms consistent with the diagnosis of diabetes mellitus. Thus the clinical onset may be abrupt, but the pathophysiologic insult is a slow, progressive phenomenon. At any time during this progressive fall in beta cell function, overt diabetes may be precipitated either by acute illness or by stress increasing the insulin demand beyond the reserve of the damaged islet cell mass. Hyperglycemia will ensue until such time as the acute illness or stress is resolved; then the patient may revert to a compensated state for a variable time period in which the beta cell mass is sufficient to maintain normoglycemia. This has been referred to as the "honeymoon period" and is a variable period of noninsulin dependency following acute decompensation (see Chapter 8). It is now apparent that continued beta cell destruction occurs and these patients ultimately require insulin within 3 to 12 months and then, apparently, permanently have diabetes.

The identification of these multiple stages of development of IDDM has provided a provocative framework for potential interventions for prevention and cure. The identification of HLA markers may allow recognition of populations at risk at the time of birth. Further delineation of environmental triggers may allow the development of specific vaccines for prevention. If prevention of the trigger is ineffective, the identification of active autoimmunity by the measurement of anti-islet cell antibodies may serve as a marker for those individuals destined to ultimately develop diabetes. As we develop more specific immunosuppressive therapy with fewer side effects, intervention at this prediabetic phase may become practical. Early evidence using cyclosporin A would suggest that suppressing the immunologic attack on the beta cell may be effective in preventing the disorder.[9] At the present time, immunosuppressive therapies remain too nonspecific and have too many side effects to be practical for therapeutic intervention in those individuals who are at risk but not yet diagnosed as having diabetes mellitus.

Finally, our understanding of the basic autoimmune pathogenesis of IDDM sheds great light on the potential use of transplantation as a modality of ultimate therapy for individuals with IDDM. It is quite apparent that the simple transplantation of islet cells will be insufficient for curing individuals with IDDM. The subsequent anamnestic immunologic response seen following pancreas transplantation between HLA-identical twins reveals the underlying nature of the disorder and the likelihood of the immunologic attack simply destroying subsequent islet cell transplants.[60] Future considerations may include the use of either HLA nonidentical islet cell tissue, transplantation of islet cells into immunologically privileged sites, or the combined use of immunosuppressive therapy with islet cell or pancreas transplantation. Finally, the identification of a prediabetic state together with specific immunosuppressive therapy may provide the best opportunity for preventing the disease; it would require extensive educational intervention for the recognition of those individuals at risk.[37]

Pathogenesis and Pathophysiology: NIDDM

Type II, or NIDDM, diabetes is a very distinct disorder as compared with IDDM. NIDDM classically develops in an older patient population and may or may not require the use of therapeutic insulin. NIDDM is a heterogeneous disorder, characterized by variable plasma insulin levels associated with hyperglycemia and peripheral insulin resistance. Heredity plays a major role in its transmission. Although there is no recognized HLA linkage, the offspring of a patient with type II diabetes has a 15% chance of developing NIDDM and a 30% risk of developing impaired glucose tolerance.[51] In addition, there is a greater than 90% concordance rate between monozygotic twins if one has type II diabetes, suggesting the primacy of the genetic defect in this form of disease.[61] From a clinical standpoint, approximately 75% of patients with NIDDM are obese. Clinical studies would suggest that obesity allows for increased expression of the genetic propensity.

Multiple theories exist to explain the defects observed in NIDDM.[15,35,62] It is an opinion that NIDDM will ultimately be broken down into several specific defects, which may include (1) primary beta cell dysfunction, (2) rare insulin-receptor abnormalities, and (3) specific postreceptor defects, which may include altered glucose transporter function or specific enzymatic defects modulating intracellular insulin activity. At the present time, however, clinical observations would suggest several phenomena at work in NIDDM.

Limitation in beta cell response to hyperglycemia appears to be a cornerstone of the pathophysiology of NIDDM. Regardless of the degree of peripheral insulin resistance, if the islet cells have an unlimited capacity to secrete insulin, then sufficient insulin should be available to overcome any degree of resistance. However, it is apparent that the beta cell is unable to respond appropriately to a hyperglycemic challenge. Morphologic studies have revealed an approximate 50% reduction in beta cell mass in individuals with NIDDM as compared with controls, particularly when the degree of obesity is also taken into account.[32] No evidence of autoimmune insulitis is found within these beta cells, but the expected degree of hypertrophy and hyperfunction caused by chronic hyperglycemia is distinctly absent.

This concept has been referred to as glucose toxicity. In essence, it has been found that beta cells chronically exposed to hyperglycemia become progressively less efficient in responding to subsequent glucose challenges. This is a reversible phenomenon in which normalization of ambient glucose produces a dramatic improvement in insulin secretory response to a fixed glucose challenge.[35] Not only is the secretory capacity of the beta cell altered in NIDDM, but the ratio of proinsulin to insulin is also substantially increased.[54] As a result, the biologically active form of insulin is further reduced by this altered secretory process.

A second hallmark of NIDDM is the presence of resistance to the biologic activity of insulin noted in both the liver and peripheral tissues.[53] The capability of insulin to suppress hepatic glucose production at the level of the liver has been well documented in individuals with NIDDM. In the fasting state, circulating blood glucose is maintained by hepatic glucose production via glycogenolysis and gluconeogenesis. Insulin suppresses these processes in a sharp dose-response fashion. Those with NIDDM have a substantial shift to the right of these curves, with a decrease in both the sensitivity and response of the system.[39] Thus, regardless of circulating insulin levels, individuals with NIDDM have a continued hepatic glucose production that increases circulating glucose levels. Ordinarily this would not result in circulating hyperglycemia unless the periphery—specifically muscle and fat—were unable to compensate with increased glucose uptake. Similar studies using a euglycemic hyperinsulinemic clamp show both decreased sensitivity and response in peripheral glucose disposal in individuals with NIDDM as compared with nondiabetic controls.[16] Thus the pathogenesis of NIDDM appears to be a heterogeneous mixture of altered beta cell function and insulin secretion together with diminished insulin effects at the level of the liver and periphery.

The mechanism by which the peripheral insulin resistance occurs is not entirely clear. Early suggestions of impaired insulin receptor function have not been borne out. Although rare individuals have been identified to have altered insulin-receptor structure and function, in the vast majority of individuals with NIDDM, insulin binding to its receptor, insulin-receptor number, and insulin-receptor activity appear to be entirely normal. Ongoing studies suggest that the defect may be distal to the insulin receptor and may involve translocation of glucose transporter molecules to the cell membrane or specific insulin-stimulated enzyme processes within the cell.[22] Further delineation of the pathophysiologic mechanisms underlying NIDDM and subclassification according to the specific defect should allow for a more refined definition of the disease as well as more directed therapeutic approaches. For example, individuals with predominant beta cell defects may universally require intervention with insulin to overcome the absolute deficiency in beta cell insulin secretion. In distinction, those individuals with predominant peripheral insulin resistance may respond more efficiently to interventions that improve insulin response at the target tissue. Direct inhibition of hepatic glucose production would tend to lower fasting blood glucose levels and reduce the effects of glucose toxicity on the beta cell, thus allowing for more efficient insulin response to a subsequent meal. Likewise, an increase in non–insulin-mediated glucose disposal in the periphery (e.g., by exercise) will lower circulating glucose levels independent of beta cell function.

CLINICAL CHEMISTRY ASSESSMENT

Diabetes management has historically been a hospital-based system, necessitating frequent visits for venipuncture to measure serum glucose and electrolytes and to determine appropriate pharmacologic intervention. Two laboratory components have become standards of care by providing both immediate and longer term information regarding blood glucose control.

Self-monitoring of blood glucose (SMBG) technology allows for the more realistic management of glycemia on an outpatient basis and facilitates implementing intensive insulin regimens. The growth in the use of this technology has been consumer driven. Physicians were initially quite skeptical of the utility and acceptability of whole blood testing of glucose on a daily basis. The presumed pain, inconvenience, and expense were all believed to be impediments to widespread clinical use. It very quickly became apparent that individuals with diabetes sought precise information concerning ambient glucose levels and accepted the minor discomfort, annoyance, and cost in exchange for improved sense of well-being and control. Various technologies rapidly became available, using dry reagents in either a colorimetric or an ion exchange methodology. It is almost impossible to provide a comprehensive listing of available systems since new meters are entering the marketplace at an astounding rate. Nonetheless, an attempt to provide an abridged listing is found in Table 1-2. The diabetes educator is best prepared to evaluate the accuracy, precision, and applicability of any given monitoring system for a particular patient. Matching monitors to the needs and technical capabilities of the individual is imperative to ensure proper use of SMBG technology.

Innumerable manuscripts can be cited to validate the precision and accuracy of various systems. User variability remains the major stumbling block in the proper operation and use of SMBG technology.[49,50] These findings underscore the critical importance of diabetes education in the use of particular monitors and the interpretation and application

Table 1-2   Commonly Available Systems for Self-Monitoring of Blood Glucose

Product	Manufacturer
Visual	
Chemstrips bG	Boehringer-Mannheim
Monitors with internal memory	
Accuchek II	Boehringer-Mannheim
Accuchek III	
Accuchek Easy	
Tracer II	
One-Touch 2	Lifescan
Glucometer 3	Miles Laboratories
Glucometer M+	
Monitors downloading to computer-based data managers	
Merlin	Boehringer-Mannheim
Accuchek II, III, and Easy	
One-Touch 2	
Homer	Diva Medical Systems
Romeo	
Glucofacts	Miles Laboratories
Glucometer M+	
One-Touch 2	
Monitors using no-wipe technology	
Accuchek Easy	Boehringer-Mannheim
One-Touch 2	Lifescan
Exactech	Medisense
Companion	
Pen 2	

of the data provided. Despite the potential pitfalls in the clinical implementation of SMBG technology, methodologies exist for assessing clinical accuracy, and the critical importance of the information provided makes SMBG an indispensable adjunct to patient care.[2,13]

Glycated hemoglobin determinations are an additional clinical laboratory assessment that have become invaluable in both research and clinical care. This measurement is predicated on the nonenzymatic, irreversible binding of glucose to the amino terminus of the beta chain of hemoglobin. This reaction depends solely on the ambient glucose concentration during the iife of the red cell and serves to both reflect past glucose control and model the cellular effects of hyperglycemia.[21] The implications of advanced glycosylation end products is beyond the scope of this chapter, but excellent reviews are available in the recent literature.[10] The more relevant application of glycated hemoglobin is the assessment of long-term glycemic control. At a clinical level, it allows the health care givers to validate the results of SMBG and reinforce the means of achieving glycemic control. From the research perspective, it is an indispensable parameter in relating glycemic control and long-term diabetic complications.[23] Recent studies suggest that glycated hemoglobin results can be used as a very effective educational and motivational tool to improve overall diabetes control.[34]

Multiple methodologies with varying normative values exist for measuring glycated hemoglobin. As a result, comparisons between laboratories are hazardous at best and probably inaccurate. Characteristics of the assay that are critical to interpretation include (l) whether the assay measures hemoglobin A_{1c} (Hb A_{1c}) or total hemoglobin A_1 (Hb A_1), (2) the ability to separate the labile from the stable fraction of glycated hemoglobin, (3) the temperature dependence of the system, and (4) the degree of interference by hemoglobin F.[31] A compilation of assay characteristics is shown in Table 1-3.

THE ROLE OF THE HEALTH CARE TEAM IN DIABETES MANAGEMENT

Despite rapid advances in medical research exploring the outer limits of molecular biology and immunology, pharmacologic intervention in individuals with diabetes has remained virtually unchanged over the last 20 years. Our interventions with diet, exercise, sulfonylureas, and insulin are different only in degree from those used in the 1950s. The

Table 1-3   Characteristics of Glycated Hemoglobin Assays

Method	Measures	C.V. (%)	Interferences
HPLC (ion exchange)	A_{1c} + labile A_{1c}	3%	Hemoglobin F
Minicolumn (ion exchange)	A_1 + labile A_1	2-16%	Hemoglobin F
Minicolumn (affinity)	Total A_1	1-3%	None
Electrophoresis	A_1 + labile A_1	4-10%	Hemoglobin F
Colorimetric	Total A_1	4-18%	None

Adapted from King ME: Glycosylated hemoglobin. In Kaplan LA and Pesce AJ: Clinical chemistry: theory, analysis, and correlation, ed 2, St. Louis, Mosby–Year Book, 1989.

greatest advance in clinical care since the discovery of insulin has been the development and improvement of SMBG techniques. Not only has SMBG allowed for improved glycemic control, but it has also revolutionized the approach to clinical care. Although Elliott Joslin had advocated diabetes education in the 1920s, it was not until SMBG technology was introduced into clinical care that the individual with diabetes was integrated into the therapeutic decision-making process. It is now apparent that a well-educated individual with diabetes is far more capable of caring for his or her diabetes than are the most expert health delivery systems. To allow for optimal use of this remarkable tool, a health care team encompassing the physician, nurse educator, nutritionist, exercise physiologist, pharmacist, and psychosocial professionals must interact with the patient for beneficial outcomes. Diabetes is now the prototypical model for integration of individuals into their own health care. This will become the cornerstone for preventive measures in a chronic disease health care model.

With integration of the individual with diabetes into the health care delivery team, individualized goals of therapy may be determined. Establishing goals depends on the individual's ability to learn and his or her psychosocial environment as well as on determination of specific outcome variables. Applying education techniques to various populations is described in far greater detail in subsequent chapters of this text; however, it is the responsibility of the members of the health care team to work directly with the individual with diabetes to determine both the goals and the approaches to diabetes therapy (see Appendix D, "Sample Diabetes Care Protocol").

Added patient responsibility demands that education and psychologic support be provided as an integral part of health care delivery. Diabetes education is now firmly entrenched as the cornerstone of diabetes care. As such, members of the health care team function as an integrated unit to meet the specific ongoing needs of the individual with diabetes. These needs may change over time, with emphasis being directed sequentially from survival skills, to the effects of diet, to psychologic support, to pharmacologic intervention, to foot care, and ultimately to coping with chronic complications. Depending on the specific needs of the patient, various members of the health care team may play the dominant interventional role.

Client needs change through the lifespan, as considerations such as growth and development change to issues of pregnancy or management of chronic complications. The health care team undertakes continuous needs assessment to determine educational goals and the most appropriate techniques with which to achieve them. Concerns of reading level, social support systems, and financial ramifications must all be weighed in the determination of the most appropriate educational approach to the individual client at any particular time.

LEGAL RAMIFICATIONS OF DIABETES EDUCATION

The introduction of the health care delivery team together with increased patient responsibilities for self-care has introduced both a unique medical model and potential legal ramifications. Two practical issues become readily apparent: first, are the nonphysician members of the treatment team practicing medicine without appropriate licensure and, second, with whom does the civil liability for such practice reside? The first issue pertains to criminal activity independent of the quality of care. The second is a civil concern that addresses negligence in the performance of a duty. To date, there have been no legal challenges to the expanding role of diabetes educators in health care management of individuals with diabetes.[52]

The practice of medicine has traditionally been limited to individuals holding doctorates of medicine or osteopathy. However, the definition of the practice of medicine has remained fluid throughout the years, and with the expansion of responsibilities, it is quite apparent that more and more activities are falling within the purview of other health professionals. Ultimately, the limits of activities of health professionals are delineated by their state's licensure requirements, and criminal practice would be defined as activities specifically requiring a specialized degree. For example, licensure within a state may limit the parenteral administration of pharmacologic agents to either physicians or nurses; therefore nutritionists and exercise physiologists may not administer an insulin injection to an individual with diabetes. However, it is unclear whether or not the recommendation of insulin adjustments with alterations in eating patterns or exercise would also be precluded by these restrictions. With the growth of diabetes team intervention, it is probable that those members of the team not *traditionally* allowed to administer pharmacologic agents may be allowed to make such recommendations according to an established protocol. This view has been supported in the courts to a limited extent.[55]

The second issue, civil liability for negligent performance, is a more difficult problem. Clearly, anyone can be sued for virtually any reason. Typically, those named in malpractice cases are those who are able to pay the most. Perhaps rapport and communication with the patient is the best recommendation for avoiding malpractice litigation, but once a suit is filed, identification of those liable for negligent performance of duty and standards of care are the critical issues.

Precedent teaches that nonphysician health professionals may be held independently liable for negligent practice independent of the actions of the responsible physician.[14] If a diabetes educator acting within the scope of his or her responsibilities performs in a negligent manner, then liability for the negligence should be borne by the educator directly; this is of particular importance as diabetes educators become independent providers of health care outside of the hospital or physician's office. Because of this, diabetes educators may be held independently liable for negligent acts stemming from improper instruction in insulin administration or adjustment, poor implementation or understanding of the prescribed therapy, or negligent assessment of patient comprehension of instruction.

To best provide service and avoid litigation, members of a diabetes treatment team should first ensure that both their program and their individual educators are recognized and certified by the American Diabetes Association (ADA) and the National Certification Board for Diabetes Educators, respectively. This will serve to identify the expanded responsibilities of the team members, together with their specialty expertise. The responsibilities of each person should be viewed as legal requirements. Depending on the expertise of the educators, written outlines of procedure and content of instruction should be centrally developed and categorically implemented. These programs should adhere to the ADA Standards of Medical Care.[4]

Educators must ensure sufficient patient comprehension of instructions in self-care techniques to carry out therapy both safely and effectively. In addition, there is a continuing responsibility to reassess the effectiveness of instruction and to thoroughly document all information concerning the patient's therapy. Although litigation may be brought against the diabetes care team for any number of reasons, thoughtful attention to the national practice standards may serve as a potent defense to claims of negligent patient care.

IMPACT OF TEAM CARE ON HEALTH CARE DELIVERY AND FINANCING

The emphasis on team management and patient education has made the individual with diabetes an active participant in the health care process. As such, we may be less likely to use the passive health care delivery inherent in a hospital situation. In general, patients sick enough to require hospitalization are not in a situation conducive to learning anything more than survival skills. On the other hand, outpatient diabetes education may provide sufficient care to preclude the necessity for routine hospitalization of individuals with diabetes for problems such as initiation of insulin management, difficulties with uncontrolled diabetes, and prevention of chronic complications.[3] As a result, the ultimate costs of health care delivery should be reduced substantially. To the extent that expenditures for hospitalization account for approximately two-thirds of the direct costs of diabetes, a reliance on outpatient education and management should be expected to substantially reduce both the frequency of hospitalization as well as the duration of hospital stays—and consequent health care costs.[63]

The reliance on diabetes education as a primary modality of therapy will force us to reevaluate our means of health care reimbursement and financing. By defining diabetes education as diabetes care, direct third-party reimbursement for such services would be logical. This may, however, require an entire restructuring of health care financing within the United States to move away from the acute care model with its emphasis on palliative and sometimes curative procedures, toward a chronic care model of prevention of disease and complications. The recent introduction of the Resource-Based Relative Value Scale[26] is a move in this direction, and the recent conference on Financing the Care of Diabetes in the 1990s[1] demonstrates continued efforts to provide health care coverage for long-term diabetes care, including diabetes education.

SUMMARY

In sum, our exploration of the pathophysiology of type I diabetes has taken us to the frontiers of genetics, immunology, and immunomodulation. Exploration of type II diabetes is at the forefront of molecular biology and physiology. Implementing diabetes education and a health care team directed towards patient involvement in self-care and prevention of complications is a model for a revolution in health care delivery and financing within the

United States. At all levels—research, education and clinical care—diabetes intervention is progressing rapidly and is at the forefront of its respective disciplines.

REFERENCES

1. American Diabetes Association: Conference summary: financing the care of diabetes mellitus in the 1990s, Diabetes Care 13:1021-1023, 1990.
2. American Diabetes Association: Consensus statement: self monitoring of blood glucose, Diabetes Care 13(suppl 1):41-46, 1990.
3. American Diabetes Association: Hospital admission guidelines for diabetes mellitus, Diabetes Care 13:1118-1119, 1990.
4. American Diabetes Association: Standards of medical care for patients with diabetes mellitus, Diabetes Care 12:365-368, 1989.
5. American Diabetes Association, Freinkel N, ed: Summary and recommendations of the second international workshop-conference on gestational diabetes mellitus, Diabetes 34(suppl 2):123-126, 1985.
6. Baekkeskov S and others: Antibodies to a 64,000 Mr human islet cell antigen precede the clinical onset of insulin-dependent diabetes, J Clin Invest 79:926-934, 1987.
7. Baisch JM and others: Analysis of HLADQ genotypes and susceptibility in insulin-dependent diabetes mellitus, N Engl J Med 322:1836-1841, 1990.
8. Bottazzo GF and others: Complement-fixing islet-cell antibodies in type I diabetes: possible monitors of active beta-cell damage, Lancet 1:668-672, 1980.
9. Bougneres PF and others: Factors associated with early remission of type I diabetes in children treated with cyclosporine, N Engl J Med 318:663-670, 1988.
10. Brownlee M, Vlassara H, and Cerami A: Advanced glycosylation end products in tissue and the biochemical basis of complications, N Engl J Med 318:1315-1321, 1988.
11. Carter Center of Emory University: Closing the gap: the problem of diabetes in the United States, Diabetes Care 8:391-406, 1985.
12. Center for Economic Studies in Medicine, Pracon Inc: Direct and indirect costs of diabetes in the United States in 1987, Alexandria, Va., 1988, American Diabetes Association.
13. Clarke WL and others: Evaluating clinical accuracy of systems for self-monitoring of blood glucose, Diabetes Care 10:622-628, 1987.
14. *Darling v Charleston Community Memorial Hospital*, 33 Ill 2d 326, 211 NE 2d 253, cert denied 383 US 946, 1965.
15. DeFronzo RA: The triumvirate: beta-cell, muscle, liver: a collusion responsible for NIDDM, Diabetes 37:667-687, 1988.
16. DeFronzo RA, Ferrannini E, Koivisto V: New concepts in the pathogenesis and treatment of non-insulin dependent diabetes mellitus, Am J Med 74 (suppl 1A):52-81, 1983.
17. Eisenbarth GS, Connelly J, Soeldner JS: The "natural" history of type I diabetes, Diabetes Metab Rev 3:873-891, 1987.
18. Eisenbarth GS and Kahn CR: Etiology and pathogenesis of diabetes mellitus. In Becker KL, ed: Principles and practice of endocrinology and metabolism, Philadelphia, 1990, JB Lippincott Co.
19. Funnell MM: Role of diabetes educator for older adults, Diabetes Care 13(suppl. 2):60-65, 1990.
20. Gamble DR and Taylor KW: Seasonal incidence of diabetes mellitus, Br J Med iii:631-633, 1969.
21. Garlick RL and others: Characterization of glycosylated hemoglobins: relevance to monitoring of diabetic control and analysis of other proteins, J Clin Invest 71:1062-1072, 1983.
22. Garvey W and others: Role of glucose transporters in cellular insulin resistance of type II non-insulin dependent diabetes mellitus, J Clin Invest 81:1528-1538, 1988.
23. Goldstein DE and others: Feasibility of centralized measurements of glycated hemoglobin in the diabetes control and complications trial: a multicenter study, Clin Chem 33:2267-2271, 1987.
24. Harris MI: Gestational diabetes may represent discovery of preexisting glucose intolerance, Diabetes Care 11:402-411, 1988.
25. Harris MI and others: Prevalence of diabetes and impaired glucose tolerance and plasma glucose levels in the US population aged 20-74 years, Diabetes 36:523-534, 1987.
26. Hsiao WC and others: Results and policy implications of the resource-based relative-value study, N Engl J Med 319:881-888, 1988.
27. Jackson RA: Mechanisms of age-related glucose intolerance, Diabetes Care 13(Suppl. 2):9-19, 1990.

28. Jackson RA and others: Increased circulating Ia-antigen–bearing T cells in type I diabetes mellitus, N Engl J Med 306:785-788, 1982.

29. Johnson JH and others: Inhibition of glucose transport into rat islet cells by immunoglobulins from patients with new-onset insulin-dependent diabetes mellitus, N Engl J Med 322:653-659, 1990.

30. Jonsson B: Diabetes—the cost of illness and the cost of control, Acta Med Scand 671:19-27, 1983.

31. King ME: Glycosylated hemoglobin. In Kaplan LA, and Pesce AJ, eds: Clinical chemistry: theory, analysis, and correlation, ed 2, St Louis, 1989, Mosby–Year Book, Inc.

32. Kloppel G and others: Islet pathology and the pathogenesis of type 1 and type 2 diabetes mellitus revisited, Surv Synth Pathol Res 4:110-125, 1985.

33. Kuminyika SK and Ewart CK: Theoretical and baseline considerations for diet and weight control of diabetes among blacks, Diabetes Care 13(suppl 4):1154-1162, 1990.

34. Larsen ML, Horder M, and Mogensen EF: Effect of long-term monitoring of glycosylated hemoglobin levels in insulin-dependent diabetes mellitus, N Engl J Med 323:1021-1025, 1990.

35. Leahy JL: Natural history of beta-cell dysfunction in NIDDM, Diabetes Care 13:992-1010, 1990.

36. MacLaren NK: How, when and why to predict IDDM, Diabetes 37:1591-1594, 1988.

37. Marks JB and Skyler JS: Immunotherapy of type I diabetes mellitus, J Clin Endocrinol Metab 72:3-9, 1991.

38. Martin DB and Quint AR: Therapy for diabetes. In National Diabetes Data Group, ed: Diabetes in America, NIH Publ No 85-1468, Washington, DC, 1985, US Government Printing Office.

39. Mitrakou A and others: Contribution of abnormal muscle and liver glucose metabolism to postprandial hyperglycemia in NIDDM, Diabetes 39:1381-1390, 1990.

40. Morel PA and others: Aspartic acid at position 57 of the HLA-DQB gene protects against type I diabetes: a family study, Proc Natl Acad Sci USA 85:8111-8115, 1988.

41. National Center for Health Statistics: The second national health and nutrition examination survey, 1976-1980. Vital and Health Statistics Ser 10, No 15, DHHS-PHS Publ 81-1317, Hyattsville, Md, 1981, US Government Printing Office.

42. National Diabetes Data Group: Classification and diagnosis of diabetes mellitus and other categories of glucose intolerance, Diabetes 28:1039-1057, 1979.

43. Nerup J, Mandrup-Poulsen T, and Molvig J. The HLA-IDDM association: implications for etiology and pathogenesis of IDDM, Diabetes Metab Rev 3:779-802, 1987.

44. O'Brien TR and others: Are racial differences in the prevalence of diabetes in adults explained by differences in obesity? JAMA 262:1485-1488, 1989.

45. O'Sullivan JB and Mahan CM: Criteria for the oral glucose tolerance test in pregnancy, Diabetes 13:278-285, 1964.

46. Palmer JP and others: Insulin antibodies in insulin-dependent diabetics before insulin treatment, Science 222:1337-1339, 1983.

47. Pi-Sunyer FX: Obesity and diabetes in blacks, Diabetes Care 13(suppl 4):1144-1149, 1990.

48. Porte D and Kahn SE: What geriatricians should know about diabetes mellitus, Diabetes Care 13(suppl 2):47-54, 1990.

49. Rabinowe SL and others: Congenital rubella: monoclonal antibody-defined T cell abnormalities in young adults, Am J Med 81:779-782, 1986.

50. Rachlin JA, Meadows SK, and Kelly RT: User errors in blood glucose monitoring, Diabetes 39(suppl 1):225A, 1990.

51. Raffel LJ and Rotter JI: The genetics of diabetes, Clin Diabetes 3:49-54, 1985.

52. Ratner RE and El-Gamassey ER: Legal aspects of the team approach to diabetes treatment, Diabetes Educ 16:113-116, 1990.

53. Reaven GM: Role of insulin resistance in human disease, Diabetes 37:1595-1607, 1988.

54. Saad MF and others: Disproportionately elevated proinsulin in Pima Indians with non-insulin dependent diabetes mellitus, J Clin Endocrinol Metab 70:1247-1253, 1990.

55. *Sermchief v Gonzales,* 660 SW 2d 683, 684, Mo banc 2 1983.

56. Sheehy MJ and others: A diabetes-susceptible HLA haplotype is best defined by a combination of HLA-DR and DQ alleles, J Clin Invest 83:830-835, 1989.

57. Sinnock P: Hospital utilization for diabetes. In National Diabetes Data Group, ed: Diabetes in America, NIH Publ No 85-1468, Washington, DC, 1985, US Government Printing Office.

58. Srikanta S and others: Islet-cell antibodies and beta-cell function in monozygotic triplets and twins initially discordant for type I diabetes, N Engl J Med 308:322-325, 1983.

59. Srikanta S and others: Type I diabetes mellitus in monozygotic twins: chronic progressive beta-cell dysfunction, Ann Intern Med 99:320-326, 1983.
60. Sutherland DER and others: Twin-to-twin pancreas transplantation: reversal and reenactment of the pathogenesis of type I diabetes, Trans Assoc Am Physicians 97:80-87, 1984.
61. Tattersall RB and Pyke DA: Diabetes in identical twins, Lancet 2:1120-1125, 1972.
62. Warram JH and others: Slow glucose removal rate and hyperinsulinemia precede the development of type II diabetes in the offspring of diabetic patients, Ann Intern Med 113:909-915, 1990.
63. Weinberger M: Hospitalizations for patients with diabetes mellitus: changing perspectives, Mayo Clin Proc 65:1268-1271, 1990.
64. Wingard DL and others: Community-based study of prevalence of NIDDM in older adults, Diabetes Care 13(suppl 2):3-8, 1990.
65. Winter WE and others: Maturity-onset diabetes of youth in black Americans, N Engl J Med 316:285-291, 1987.
66. Yoon JW and others: Isolation of a virus from the pancreas of a child with diabetic ketoacidosis, N Engl J Med 300:1173-1179, 1979.

CHAPTER 2

Nutritional Management of Diabetes Mellitus

JOAN M. HEINS AND CHRISTINE A. BEEBE

Food is more than a source of nutrition. Food holds cultural significance, binds social customs, and satisfies individual senses of taste, smell, and appetite. While diets are prescribed as nutrients to meet metabolic requirements, they are consumed as food selected in kitchens, restaurants, vending machines, and diverse social settings. Adherence to a prescribed diet requires knowledge of correct food choices but is strongly influenced by societal demands and personal preferences.

In addition to promoting overall good health, diets prescribed for diabetes have the added challenge of overcoming an abnormal metabolic response to food. Size, composition, and timing of meals must be designed to maximize insulin efficiency and promote as near normal energy metabolism as is possible. While diet is recognized clinically as the cornerstone of diabetes therapy, individuals with diabetes say that dietary compliance is the most difficult part of their treatment regimen. Because of the physiologic ramifications, psychosocial implications, and the magnitude of information, the dietary prescription in diabetes cannot be communicated in a preprinted diet pamphlet. Dietary regimens must be developed in consultation with the patient to incorporate nutrient and metabolic needs in meal patterns that meet the individual's lifestyle and personal goals.

On completion of this chapter, the reader will be able to: outline recommendations for carbohydrate, protein, and fat composition of diets prescribed for diabetes; differentiate strategies for meal planning for IDDM, NIDDM, and pregnancies complicated by diabetes; state reasons that the meal plan, education, and counseling must be individualized for nutritional management of diabetes; identify potential adjustments in diet that can be made, based upon self-monitoring of blood glucose (SMBG) values, to improve glycemic control; calculate individual caloric requirements; discuss use of caloric and noncaloric sweeteners; describe the role of obesity in NIDDM and strategies for weight management; list four or more options in nutrition teaching

Table 2-1 Food and Nutrition Board, National Academy of Sciences–National

Designed for the maintenance of good nutrition of practically all healthy people in the United States.

Category	Age (years) or condition	Weight† (kg)	Weight† (lb)	Height† (cm)	Height† (in)	Protein (g)	Fat-soluble Vitamins Vita- min A (µg RE)‡	Vita- min D (µg)§	Vita- min E (mg α-TE)‖	Vita- min K (µg)
Infants	0.0-0.5	6	13	60	24	13	375	7.5	3	5
	0.5-1.0	9	20	71	28	14	375	10	4	10
Children	1-3	13	29	90	35	16	400	10	6	15
	4-6	20	44	112	44	24	500	10	7	20
	7-10	28	62	132	52	28	700	10	7	30
Males	11-14	45	99	157	62	45	1,000	10	10	45
	15-18	66	145	176	69	59	1,000	10	10	65
	19-24	72	160	177	70	58	1,000	10	10	70
	25-50	79	174	176	70	63	1,000	5	10	80
	51 +	77	170	173	68	63	1,000	5	10	80
Females	11-14	46	101	157	62	46	800	10	8	45
	15-18	55	120	163	64	44	800	10	8	55
	19-24	58	128	164	65	46	800	10	8	60
	25-50	63	138	163	64	50	800	5	8	65
	51 +	65	143	160	63	50	800	5	8	65
Pregnant						60	800	10	10	65
Lactating	1st 6 months					65	1,300	10	12	65
	2nd 6 months					62	1,200	10	11	65

*The allowances, expressed as average daily intakes over time, are intended to provide for individual
Diets should be based on a variety of common foods in order to provide other nutrients for which human
†Weights and heights of Reference Adults are actual medians for the U.S. population of the designated age,
Hamill and others (1979). The use of these figures does not imply that the height-to-weight ratios are ideal.
‡Retinol equivalents. 1 retinol equivalent = 1 µg retinol or 6 µg β-carotene.
§As cholecalciferol. 10 µg cholecalciferol = 400 IU of vitamin D.
‖α-Tocopherol equivalents. 1 mg d-α tocopherol = 1 α-TE.
¶1 NE (niacin equivalent) is equal to 1 mg of niacin or 60 mg of dietary tryptophan.

materials available for instructing individuals with diabetes; summarize strategies for nutritional management during illness; evaluate role and responsibilities of patient, dietitian, and other members of the health care team in nutritional management of diabetes.

DIETARY RECOMMENDATIONS

Nutritional requirements for individuals with diabetes are fundamentally the same as those for healthy individuals without diabetes.[4] While restoration of optimal blood glucose and lipid levels is a primary goal,[2] diet therapy starts with principles of good nutrition and adds modifications to accommodate abnormalities of glucose metabolism. These two ob-

Research Council Recommended Dietary Allowances,* Revised 1989

Water-soluble vitamins							Minerals						
Vita-min C (mg)	Thia-min (mg)	Ribo-flavin (mg)	Niacin (mg 91)	Vita-min B_6 (mg)	Fo-late (µg)	Vita-min B_{12} (µg)	Cal-cium (mg)	Phos-phorus (mg)	Mag-nesium (mg)	Iron (mg)	Zinc (mg)	Iodine (µg)	Sele-nium (µg)
30	0.3	0.4	5	0.3	25	0.3	400	300	40	6	5	40	10
35	0.4	0.5	6	0.6	35	0.5	600	500	60	10	5	50	15
40	0.7	0.8	9	1.0	50	0.7	800	800	80	10	10	70	20
45	0.9	1.1	12	1.1	75	1.0	800	800	120	10	10	90	20
45	1.0	1.2	13	1.4	100	1.4	800	800	170	10	10	120	30
50	1.3	1.5	17	1.7	150	2.0	1200	1200	270	12	15	150	40
60	1.5	1.8	20	2.0	200	2.0	1200	1200	400	12	15	150	50
60	1.5	1.7	19	2.0	200	2.0	1200	1200	350	10	15	150	70
60	1.5	1.7	19	2.0	200	2.0	800	800	350	10	15	150	70
60	1.2	1.4	15	2.0	200	2.0	800	800	350	10	15	150	70
50	1.1	1.3	15	1.4	150	2.0	1200	1200	280	15	12	150	45
60	1.1	1.3	15	1.5	180	2.0	1200	1200	300	15	12	150	50
60	1.1	1.3	15	1.6	180	2.0	1200	1200	280	15	12	150	55
60	1.1	1.3	15	1.6	180	2.0	800	800	280	15	12	150	55
60	1.0	1.2	13	1.6	180	2.0	800	800	280	10	12	150	55
70	1.5	1.6	17	2.2	400	2.2	1200	1200	320	30	15	175	65
95	1.6	1.8	20	2.1	280	2.6	1200	1200	355	15	19	200	75
90	1.6	1.7	20	2.1	260	2.6	1200	1200	340	15	16	200	75

variations among most normal persons as they live in the United States under usual environmental stresses.
requirements have been less well defined.
as reported by NHANES II. The median weights and heights of those under 19 years of age were taken from

jectives are incorporated into dietary meal plans to assure adequate nutrient intake while achieving normoglycemia. Recognizing the dual roles of diet therapy for diabetes provides insight into the processes involved in developing individual meal plans and an understanding of why specific foods are encouraged or restricted.

Guidelines For Good Nutrition

Several approaches to defining good nutrition have gained wide acceptance in the United States. The Recommended Dietary Allowances (RDAs) are a quantitative method developed by the Food and Nutrition Board of the National Research Council (Table 2-1). The RDAs are defined as "the levels of intake of essential nutrients that, on the basis of scientific knowledge, are judged by the Food and Nutrition Board to be adequate to meet the known nutrient needs of practically all healthy persons."[44] The RDAs should not be interpreted as minimal or optimal standards but as guidelines for adequate levels of essential nutrients that should be consumed as part of a normal diet. As nutrients required for growth, development, and maintenance of a healthy body vary across the life span and to some degree by gender, the RDAs are defined for females and males in age groupings that reflect major stages of development. Specific nutrient requirements will vary by body size, energy requirements, and health status. Currently, the RDAs do not define upper limits of nutrient intake—a change that may be included in future editions.

The *basic four food groups* is a nutrition education method designed to translate the RDAs into practical information for the average person. Foods with comparable nutrient content are grouped together into four categories: milk, meat, fruits and vegetables, and grain. Recommended serving sizes are adjusted so that each food within a group provides similar nutrients. Calories, however, are not necessarily the same. Recommendations are given on the minimum number of servings from each group needed to meet nutrient requirements at various stages of the life span. The concept of the *basic four food groups* has been incorporated into a variety of teaching tools including materials developed by the National Dairy Council.

A widely used definition of good nutrition, the *Dietary Guidelines For Americans,* is a qualitative approach published by the U.S. Department of Agriculture and the U.S. Department of Health and Human Services. The *Guidelines* are designed to give simple, positive information about eating a nutritious diet. The third edition of the guidelines, published in 1990, includes suggestions on the number of servings from five food groups that will provide a nutritious daily diet (Fig. 2-1). The *Guidelines* provided the structure for recommendations in a 1989 consensus report, "The Healthy American Diet," developed by eight health organizations including the American Cancer Society, American Diabetes Association, and American Heart Association. The report considers total nutrition needs as well as prevention and control of cancer, diabetes, heart and blood vessel disease, and stroke. The consensus in the report underscores the fact that recommendations for preventive and therapeutic nutrition have common messages and lends credibility to the slogan, "A diabetic diet is really just a healthy diet that is good for everyone."

Nutritional Recommendations for Individuals with Diabetes

Recommended dietary modifications have been changed throughout the history of diabetes to reflect new knowledge of the underlying disease processes and advances in treatment modalities. The American Diabetes Association (ADA) published their first nutritional recommendations in 1950 as precalculated meal plans that accompanied the newly introduced *Exchange Diet.*[24] The 40% carbohydrate, 20% protein, and 40% fat distribution of calories used in these meal plans became the standard dietary prescription for diabetes. In 1971, emerging information on the effect of diet on blood glucose and cholesterol levels prompted the ADA to publish a special report: Principles of Nutrition and Dietary Recommendations for Individuals with Diabetes [3] which, when updated in 1979, provided specific recommendations to liberalize the carbohydrate content of the diet to 50% to 60% of calories and to restrict saturated and polyunsaturated fats each to 10% of total calories.[4] The 1979 update also stressed that every person with diabetes should have the opportunity to meet with a diet counselor to set personal goals and plan an individu-

Dietary guidelines

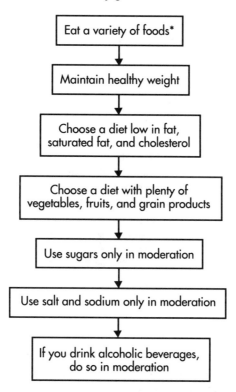

If you drink alcoholic beverages, do so in moderation

*A daily food guide

Food group	Suggested servings
Meat, poultry, fish, dried beans, or eggs	2 to 3 servings (daily total approximately 6 oz)
Milk and dairy products	2 to 3 servings
Grain products	6 to 11 servings
Vegetables	3 to 5 servings
Fruit	2 to 4 servings

Fig. 2-1   Dietary guidelines. (Adapted from Dietary Guidelines for Americans, ed 3, 1990, US Department of Agriculture.)

alized diet. Preprinted handout diets were discouraged and the ADA discontinued publication of their series of precalculated *Exchange Diets*. In 1986, an ADA position statement: Nutritional Recommendations and Principles for Individuals with Diabetes Mellitus,[2] updated the 1979 guidelines to reflect new information in the field of nutrition for diabetes and in approaches to nutrition education. The 1986 Recommendations, which are summarized in Table 2-2, include specific information on a variety of nutrients and on

Table 2-2   Nutrient Recommendations for Adults with Diabetes Mellitus

Nutrient	Recommended daily intake
Calories (kcal)	Rx to achieve and maintain reasonable weight
Carbohydrate	Up to 55-60% of total kcal
Protein	0.8 g/kg of body weight*
Fat	<30% of total kcal with:
	PUS = 6-8%†
	S = <10%
	MS = 12-14%
Cholesterol	<300 mg
Fiber	40 g or 25 g/1000 kcal
Sodium	1000 mg/1000 kcal up to 3000 mg
Vitamins and minerals	Sufficient to meet recommended requirements
Alcohol	If used—moderation (1 to 2 equivalents/1 or 2 times/week)‡

Adapted from American Diabetes Association: Nutritional Recommendations and Principles for Individuals with Diabetes Mellitus: 1986 (Position Statement), Diabetes Care 10:126-32, 1987.
*The Recommended Dietary Allowance for adults; requirements vary for children, pregnant and lactating women, the aged, and those with special medical conditions. Patients with incipient renal failure may require less protein.
†PUS = Polyunsaturated, S = Saturated, MS = Monounsaturated.
‡One equivalent is equal to the amount of alcohol in 1½ ounces of distilled liquor, 4 ounces of wine or a 12-ounce beer.

diet planning for insulin-dependent diabetes mellitus (IDDM) and non–insulin-dependent diabetes mellitus (NIDDM). They serve as the current standards for nutritional management of diabetes. Emerging information, however, will continue to demand frequent updates. Moreover, it is important to note that the recommendations are offered as guidelines to advise but not direct patient therapy. Each diet planned for a person with diabetes must be modified to reflect individual physiologic, educational and socioeconomic needs. Consideration of the metabolic processes of carbohydrate, protein, and fat and an awareness of other nutritional issues guides modification of these guidelines to meet individual needs.

Carbohydrate

Carbohydrates are naturally occurring compounds constructed of carbon, hydrogen, and oxygen and are found in a variety of forms in food. Simple carbohydrates (i.e., sugars) include monosaccharides such as glucose, fructose, and galactose, and disaccharides such as sucrose and lactose. Sucrose (table sugar) is composed of glucose and fructose, whereas lactose (milk sugar) is made up of glucose and galactose. Complex carbohydrates (starches) contain a large number of glucose molecules in either straight chains (amylose) or branched chains (amylopectin).

Metabolism of carbohydrates   Digestion of carbohydrates begins in the mouth, continues in the stomach, and is completed in the small intestine where the end product monosaccharides are absorbed into the portal blood.[10] The concentration of blood glucose achieved and the rate at which it rises depends on the amount of carbohydrate consumed and factors, such as the fat, protein, and fiber content of the meal, that effect how quickly food is digested and absorbed.[79] The normal pancreas senses rising glucose levels and releases insulin in comparable amounts.

The liver plays a key role in glucose homeostasis. Nearly 60% of ingested glucose is taken up by the liver, where it is converted to glycogen and stored.[52] Some glucose is taken up by muscle tissue, converted to glycogen, and stored. The amount of glucose stored as glycogen in the muscle will depend upon the amount already stored. If exercise has recently occurred and muscle glycogen stores are low, then glucose uptake and conversion to glycogen is rapid. Excess glucose not stored as glycogen is converted to fat and stored in adipose tissue. This process is facilitated by lipoprotein lipase—an insulin-sensitive enzyme.

The assumption that molecular structures of carbohydrates (complex versus simple) defined the rate of digestion and predicted glycemic response supported the belief that starches were digested and absorbed slowly because they needed to be broken down into individual glucose molecules. Thus, starches were the preferred carbohydrate in the diabetic meal plan. Simple sugars were to be avoided because they digested rapidly. In the 1970s, this concept was challenged when Crapo and colleagues[36] found wide variations in glucose responses to four starchy foods, selected for their similarity in macronutrient content. Subsequent studies demonstrated that the chemical distinction of complex versus simple did not differentiate the rate of carbohydrate metabolism nor did it predict subsequent physiologic response of blood glucose.[61,62]

Recommended amount in diet   The ADA recommendations for carbohydrates in the diet include:

- The amount of carbohydrate should be *liberalized,* ideally to 55% to 60% of total calories, and *individualized*. The optimum level of carbohydrate depends on the impact on blood glucose and lipid levels.
- Foods containing unrefined carbohydrate with fiber should replace highly refined carbohydrates whenever acceptable to the patient.
- Sucrose and other refined sugars, in modest amounts, may be included in the diet for some individuals, contingent on metabolic control and body weight.[2]

These recommendations are to be adjusted to accommodate individual tolerances, eating patterns, and personal preferences.

Glycemic index   Attempts to reclassify carbohydrates by their impact on blood glucose led to development of the "glycemic index" by Jenkins and colleagues in 1981.[62] Their initial classification, developed from data on normal individuals and later subjects with diabetes used glucose as the standard for comparing the rise in blood sugar that could be expected from ingestion of a particular food. Some common starchy foods, such as cornflakes and potatoes, were found to raise blood glucose quickly and to a greater degree than sucrose (table sugar), whereas others, including oatmeal and spaghetti, showed much lower effects.[62] Because it has more routine application, white bread was substituted for glucose as the reference standard using the following formula[60]:

$$\frac{\text{incremental blood glucose area after food}}{\text{corresponding area after equicarbohydrate portion of white bread}} \times 100$$

Table 2-3   Glycemic Index: Values for Selected Foods

Mean glycemic index (GI) values of foods adjusted proportionately so that GI of white bread = 100.

Food	GI
Glucose	138
Russet potato, baked	128
Honey	126
Instant potatoes	118
Cornflakes	115
White bread	100
Sucrose	89
Porridge oats	87
Banana	84
New potato, boiled	80
Sweet corn	80
Polished brown rice, boiled 15 minutes	79
Potato chips	77
All bran	74
Parboiled brown rice, boiled 25 minutes	65
Green peas, frozen	65
Spaghetti, boiled 15 minutes	61
Orange	59
Ice cream	52
Whole milk	49
Skim milk	46
Kidney beans	45
Red lentils	37
Fructose	31

GI values from Jenkins DJA, Wolever TMS, & Jenkins AL: Starchy food and glycemic index, Diabetes Care, 11:149-159, 1988.
*Mean GI values from studies using normal, NIDDM, or IDDM subjects.

Table 2-3 shows food values determined by this formula based on data from multiple studies.[61] The somewhat moderate glycemic effect of sucrose (GI = 89) may be explained by the rankings of its component monosaccharides (i.e., the high value of glucose [GI = 138] is offset by the low score of fructose [GI = 31]).

The utility of the glycemic index is still uncertain. Clinical application is limited by differences in individual response, by loss of predictive effect when foods are combined as mixed meals, and by lack of agreement in studies conducted at different centers.[61] SMBG can help individuals measure their own glycemic response to different carbohydrate foods and meal combinations.[14] Multiple factors, however, influence a food's effect on blood glucose. Variety, ripeness, form, method of processing, and cooking methods can alter the impact of a single food. Coingested fat, protein, liquid, and salt influence the glycemic response as does the rate at which the meal is consumed.[34] It is important to recognize that the nutrient value of a food is independent of its glycemic effect. Table sugar may produce a lower rise in blood glucose than potatoes, but it lacks the essential vitamins and minerals provided by the potatoes. Decisions on foods must be made on the basis of contribution to overall nutrition, as well as on the impact on glucose homeostasis.[5]

Dietary fiber   Dietary fibers are predominantly nonstarch carbohydrate polysaccharides and lignin that are not digested within the human small intestine. Although not digested and absorbed, fibers play an important role in human nutrition. Dietary fibers increase satiety, alter transit time through the gastrointestinal (GI) tract, increase colonic bulking, and bind or absorb organic materials. Fibers that are water insoluble (e.g., cellulose) seem to have their greatest effect in the lower GI track. As a fecal bulking agent they appear to improve bowel regularity, decrease constipation and diverticular disease, and may bind and dilute carcinogens, thus reducing the risk of colon cancer.[9,95] Water-soluble fibers (e.g., pectins, gums) effect the upper GI track by delaying stomach emptying and by altering transit and absorption of digestible carbohydrates in the small intestine.[95,96] Soluble fibers appear to have a beneficial influence on lipid and glucose levels; however, mechanisms of action and optimum therapeutic amounts are not clearly established.[98] For patients with NIDDM, soluble fiber may improve postprandial glucose responses.[15] In IDDM the effect is less clear but is demonstrated by a decrement in the circadian glucose profile.[96] Recommendations for intake of dietary fiber currently are not differentiated by water solubility.[2]

An individual can easily increase fiber intake by selecting fiber-rich choices of foods they commonly consume. For example, switching from white to whole grain bread, from cornflakes to 40% bran flakes, and from orange juice to orange slices provides three to four times more dietary fiber per serving. The 1986 edition of the *Exchange Lists for Meal Planning,* published by the American Dietetic Association and the American Diabetes Association, provides average dietary fiber values for food groups. In the starch/bread exchange list, average fiber values per serving are 3 to 4 g for starchy vegetables and legumes, 2 g for whole grain cereals and breads, and 1 g or less for other starch-bread foods. The vegetable list offers 3 g fiber per serving when raw and 2 g if cooked or canned. Fiber values for the fruit list range from 3 g/serving for dried, 2 g/serving for fresh, canned, or frozen, to less than 1 g for fruit juices.[7] In addition, foods offering 3 g or more of dietary fiber are individually highlighted.

Fiber supplements are marketed commercially. For fiber supplementation to show a beneficial effect, however, a high total carbohydrate intake (>50% of calories) is required.[2] In general, use of high-fiber foods versus fiber supplements is the recommended approach to increase fiber in the diet.[9,96]

While most individuals with diabetes can increase the fiber content of their diets without side effects, some general guidelines are important. A gradual increase in consumption of high-fiber foods and an increase in fluid intake should be recommended to avoid discomfort. For some diabetic individuals on insulin therapy, a high-fiber diet can reduce blood glucose levels to a point where less insulin is required. As fiber intake is increased, careful SMBG can guide reduction of the insulin dose and prevent hypoglycemia.

Sugars   Although sugars occur naturally in fruits and vegetables (glucose, fructose, and sucrose) and in milk (lactose), these sources generally are not included in evaluations of sugar in the diet. It is sugars used as sweeteners that are targeted in recommendations on consumption. For all individuals, the nutritionally "empty" (i.e., low nutrient) calories of sugar should be of concern. For people with diabetes, the effect of sugars on blood glucose is an additional consideration. Research continues to demonstrate that small amounts of sugars, incorporated into meals, cause no alteration in glycemic control in well-insulinized diabetic individuals.[13,14,29,75,100] Allowing sugar in the diet for diabetes is not new. The original version of the *Exchange Lists* included sugar-containing options such as angel cake, ice cream, and graham crackers. The Family Cookbook Series, introduced in 1980 by The American Diabetes Association and The American Dietetic Association, contains recipes using limited amounts of sugar. The 1986 ADA recommendations do not include limits on the amount of sugar that can be added to the diet.[2] Up to 5% of total carbohydrates has been suggested as an acceptable level for sucrose used as an added sweetener.[8,77] For an 1800 calorie diet with 55% or 990 calories as carbohydrate (CHO), 5% equals 50 calories (12.5 g CHO). One teaspoon of table sugar contains 16 calories (4 g CHO). The average intake of sucrose in the United States has been estimated at 41 g (¼ cup) a day.[8]

Protein

Metabolism of protein   Metabolism of protein to amino acids begins in the stomach and continues through the lumen and brush border of the small intestine. Once absorbed into the blood stream, amino acids circulate through the portal vein to the liver and then to the rest of the body. Entry of amino acids into muscle cells is facilitated by insulin released from the pancreas. Certain amino acids are known to stimulate insulin secretion, whereas others stimulate the secretion of glucagon.

Amino acids are used for muscle protein synthesis as well as the production of enzymes, hormones, and other constituents of cells. Any amino acids consumed in excess of those required to build tissue will be converted to carbohydrate or lipids and used for energy. As much as 50% to 58% of protein ingested may be metabolized to glucose. This gluconeogenic tendency of many of the amino acids has led some diabetologists to conclude that protein should be considered when counting the total amount of glucose available from a given food or meal. Others surmise that the presence of protein-rich foods stabilizes blood glucose levels by providing substrate for gluconeogenesis after carbohydrate itself has been absorbed and metabolized.

Since protein breakdown and synthesis is occurring continuously and concurrently, it is not clear whether amino acids ingested at the most recent meal are specifically earmarked for gluconeogenesis following that meal. In reality, amino acids are not truly stored in the body but circulate and turn over constantly. As much as 300 to 400 g of protein/day are recycled through synthesis and breakdown.[74] This represents three to five times the amount of protein consumed by an average 70 kg adult. More research is needed before we can conclude that protein has a lasting and significant effect on blood glucose in a mixed meal.

Nine of the twenty amino acids found in the diet are considered essential in that they cannot be made by the body. Protein requirements are based on meeting the need for these nine amino acids. Animal protein is considered to be of higher biologic value than vegetable protein since all of the essential amino acids are present. Yet vegetable proteins can be combined to provide all of the essential amino acids.

Recommended amount in diet   The current ADA recommendation for protein is 0.8 g/kg/day for adults[2] (see Table 2-2). This is the same as the RDA for protein.[44] In the past, protein was specified as a percentage of calories (i.e., 12% to 20%.) The most recent guideline (1986) avoids this, allowing more flexibility in intake and promoting a lower intake that may be healthier for most individuals.

Younger children require greater amounts of protein to promote normal growth and development. Infants require approximately 1.6 to 2.2 g/kg/day, 1.1 to 1.2 g/kg/day are required by children ages 1 to 6, and approximately 1.0 g/kg/day is required by children through ages 7 to 14.[44] Adolescent males require 0.9 g/kg/day to age 18. Requirements for females in this age group are the same as those for adults.

Pregnant and lactating women have increased protein needs to promote fetal development and milk production. The RDA is increased 0 to 15 g/day for these women.[44]

Elderly patients may also have increased protein needs. The rate of protein synthesis decreases with age requiring more protein to originate from the diet. Thus at least 12% to 14% of calories should come from protein in the person over 51 years old.[47] This represents an intake of 0.8 to 1.0 g/kg/day. Even higher levels of protein may be necessary following periods of undernutrition or increased protein loss such as after surgery or prolonged illness.[56]

As a rule, most experts agree that the majority of Americans consume too much protein. It is not uncommon for an adult American male to consume 100 to 150 g/day or as much as 17% to 29% of total calories. Frequently the person with diabetes will have a rather high protein intake for various reasons. Most clinicians are well aware of the diabetic diet history that includes eggs, cheese, or peanut butter at every breakfast or snack. Whether the original intent was to diminish the blood glucose response or satisfy the "meat group" requirement, the current trend is to decrease these high-fat protein sources.

Modifying protein intake   If the average reference male (77 kg) were to reduce intake to the ADA recommendation, protein intake would be approximately 62 g/day or 12% of calories. While this represents a dramatic drop from the average intake, some investigators suggest that at least working toward that level may be judicious.[21] Initially the trend to reduce protein intake was part of the effort to reduce fat intake and reduce incidence of cardiovascular disease in diabetes. Many high-protein foods are indeed major sources of saturated fat and cholesterol. More recently, considerable evidence is accumulating that suggests that low-protein diets may maintain renal function and reduce proteinuria in patients with renal insufficiency.[80] It is thought that the maladaptive increase in blood flow and filtration rates seen in chronic renal failure can be lowered with reduced protein intakes. If this turns out to be true for persons with diabetes, low-protein diets could prevent or delay the onset of renal damage and chronic renal failure. Several studies conducted in patients with diabetes have found a reduction in proteinuria to occur during protein restrictions of 40 to 60 g/day.[28,41] Interestingly, plasma albumin actually increases during protein restriction in nephrotic patients.[41] This data represents the reverse of past dietary intervention for these patients where it was once thought that protein intake should be increased to compensate for protein lost in the urine.

Individuals who accept this data as valid are faced with the question of when in the course of diabetes as a disease should one begin restricting protein intake. Could we prolong or prevent the development of renal complications in diabetes by restricting intake to the RDA at diagnosis, or should we wait until proteinuria occurs? New technology has made it possible to detect micro amounts of protein in the urine. Early detection of proteinuria could lead to earlier therapeutic intervention with drug and/or diet therapy. Is this early enough? The answer requires more research.

In the meantime, a gradual reduction of protein intake is most realistic (1 to 1.5 g/kg/day), since many patients are not willing to comply with the more severe restrictions of the RDA level. If intake could be kept reasonable at diagnosis and gradually reduced towards the RDA throughout the life span, the restriction may be better accepted and the patient's renal status improved. Food preferences and habits, age, and other medical conditions should be considered when determining a reasonable protein level in the diet. Vegetables, grains, cereals, and milk provide a considerable amount of the daily protein intake. Limiting intake to the RDA or lower (0.6 to 0.8 g/kg) may be reserved for individuals with nephropathy. Such a restriction limits protein intake from animal sources to less than 4 ounces/day.

Fat

Dietary fat or lipid can be divided into three classes: triglyceride, cholesterol, and phospholipid. Triglyceride, which is composed of three fatty acids attached to a 3-carbon glycerol molecule, is the body's primary storage form of energy in adipose tissue cells. Cholesterol functions as a component of cellular membranes and as a precursor for bile acids and steroid hormones. Phospholipids are major membrane-forming molecules that have both hydrophobic (i.e., water-hating) and hydrophilic (i.e., water-loving) amphipathic properties that make them useful in transporting other lipid molecules.

Metabolism of fat   Fat is digested predominantly in the intestine to its component parts. Before fat can be absorbed across the intestinal wall it must first be combined with proteins to form chylomicrons. These chylomicrons then carry fat into lymph and from there to the blood.

Chylomicrons are one of several lipoproteins that function as transport vehicles for fats. Because of the hydrophobic nature of fat it must be combined with protein to be soluble in the aqueous blood system. Lipoproteins consist of a combination of triglyceride, cholesterol, phospholipids, and apoproteins (Fig. 2-2). Phospholipid surrounds a core layer of cholesterol, cholesterol esters, and triglyceride. Phospholipids serve to suspend fat by having the hydrophobic ends facing toward the fat and the hydrophilic ends facing outward toward blood. Apoproteins are present on the surface of the particle to strengthen its structure, guide the lipoprotein particle to its receptor, and serve as cofactors for enzymes involved in cholesterol and triglyceride metabolism.

Lipoproteins are classified by their density. Each class of lipoprotein varies in the

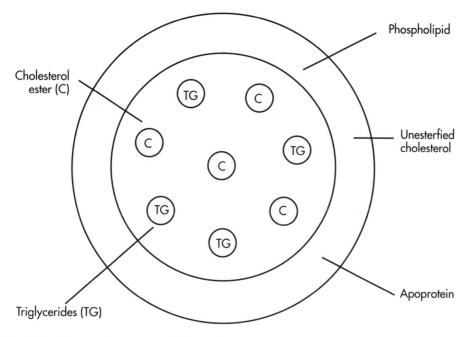

Fig. 2-2   Lipoprotein structure. (Adapted from Erkelens DW: Diabetes mellitus, Indianapolis, 1987, Eli Lilly.)

amount of triglyceride, cholesterol, phopholipid, and protein present (Fig. 2-3). Chylomicrons are the least dense lipoprotein because they are made up almost entirely of exogenous triglyceride.

More than 90% of chylomicrons are taken up by the liver where they are catabolized to free fatty acids (FFA), glycerol, cholesterol, and phospholipids. Before these products re-enter the blood stream they are recombined into very low–density lipoproteins (VLDL). The major component of VLDL is triglyceride as nearly 65% of the VLDL particle is endogenous triglyceride. The rate of VLDL production and secretion by the liver is influenced by factors such as the diet, degree of obesity, glucagon, and insulin levels. Insulin stimulates VLDL production by the liver; thus the hyperinsulinemia found so often in obesity and NIDDM can cause an overproduction of VLDL and hypertriglyceridemia.[40,102] Excessive caloric consumption, regardless of the source, increases the level of FFA in the blood and increases hepatic production of VLDL. Hypertriglyceridemia is a hallmark of the obese patient with NIDDM.

The VLDL particle is normally catabolized to low-density lipoprotein (LDL) through an intermediate known as intermediate-density lipoprotein (IDL). LDL transports cholesterol from the liver to peripheral tissues. The LDL particle is nearly 43% cholesterol; the remainder of the particle is phospholipid and protein. Measurement of serum LDL cholesterol is generally described as "bad cholesterol" because it represents the majority of circulating cholesterol. Normally, LDL particles are taken up and metabolized by recep-

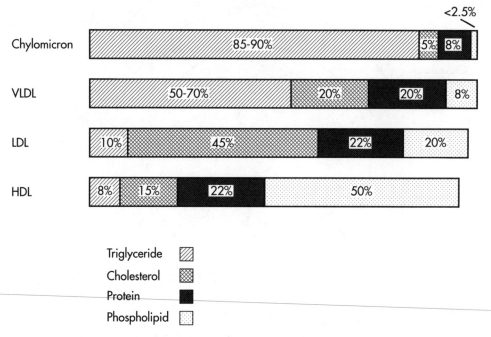

Fig. 2-3   Approximate content of plasma lipoproteins. (Adapted from Silver EN: Heart disease, ed 2, New York, 1987, Miller Publishing Co.)

tor-mediated pathways on the liver and the peripheral tissues. These receptors, located on the surface of cells, recognize and bind the apoproteins attached to LDL particles. More than 30% of daily LDL production is metabolized this way.[25,51]

Hypercholesterolemia occurs in diabetes, although to a much lesser extent than hypertriglyceridemia. The cause of elevated cholesterol in diabetes may be hypertriglyceridemia, since LDL is derived from VLDL, but is also thought to result from altered receptor pathways.[40,85,89] It appears that LDL particles may be glycosylated during poor diabetes control.[101] This glycosylation interferes with LDL uptake, and cholesterol accumulates in the blood stream.

High-density lipoprotein (HDL) is often referred to as the "good cholesterol" because of its primary function in transporting cholesterol from peripheral tissues back to the liver where it is metabolized. HDL cholesterol is composed primarily of protein and phospholipid, with less than 18% of the particle containing cholesterol. Studies have found an inverse relationship between HDL concentration and atherosclerosis. It has been observed that HDL levels may be low in many individuals with diabetes but are increased with improvements in glycemic control.[17,63] Since HDL is inversely related to triglyceride levels, it is not unusual to find low HDL levels in NIDDM patients.

Recommended amount in diet   A desire to reduce the atherogenic potential in diabetes has prompted the American Diabetes Association to recommend a dietary fat intake for adults that is no more than 30% of total calories and a cholesterol intake of less than

300 mg/day (see Table 2-2). This is identical to the recommendations of the American Heart Association and the American Cancer Institute. Epidemiologic data clearly associate elevated serum cholesterol levels with increased risk of cardiovascular disease. The Lipid Research Clinics Coronary Prevention Trial has indicated that for every 1% reduction in serum cholesterol there is an estimated 2% reduction in risk for a cardiovascular event.[68] Metabolic studies suggest that diet influences serum cholesterol levels.[31] Controlling fat intake and obesity are two important dietary interventions that can have an effect on serum lipid levels.

Cholesterol   There is no dietary requirement for cholesterol since cholesterol is made by the liver, intestinal cells, and several other tissues. In fact, the majority of plasma cholesterol is derived from endogenous sources. Cholesterol entering through the diet comes only from foods of animal origin. Approximately 40% of this is absorbed, and the rest is excreted. The concern is that excess cholesterol from the diet will be stored in tissues such as the coronary arteries. Connor and Connor have found that consuming dietary cholesterol in excess of 100 mg/day can produce a rapid rise in plasma cholesterol.[31] It is currently estimated that the average American diet contains nearly 400 to 500 mg/day.

Reducing dietary cholesterol by 100 mg/day is estimated to reduce plasma levels by 7 mg/dL.[31] Individuals with large cholesterol intakes are most likely to benefit from dietary cholesterol restriction. Egg yolks remain one of the largest sources of cholesterol in the diet, containing approximately 200 mg/yolk. Current recommendations suggest that egg yolk consumption be kept to three to four per week. Liver, kidney, and brains contain large amounts of cholesterol (up to 1500 mg/serving) but are consumed less frequently than eggs. They should be severely limited in a low-cholesterol diet. A common misconception is that beef and pork contain more cholesterol than chicken or turkey. In reality each contains about 75 mg in a 3 ounce serving. Poultry however, contains less total fat and much less saturated fat than either beef or pork.

Total fat intake   The total amount of fat consumed daily can have an impact on serum lipid levels since the quantity of chylomicrons circulating in the blood stream is directly proportional to the amount of fat consumed. A large increase in triglycerides can serve as a precursor to atherogenic particles such as LDL cholesterol. The average American consumes approximately 40% of his/her diet as fat. Reducing fat to 20% to 30% of calories decreases chylomicron production and reduces atherogenic risk.

In addition to its lipemic effects, dietary fat may have an impact on the development and maintenance of obesity. Fat provides 9 cal/g, more than twice the amount of calories provided by either protein or carbohydrate. Although protein and carbohydrate must be altered by the body to be stored as fat in the adipocyte, dietary fat requires little alteration. As a result, the body is more efficient at transforming dietary fat to body fat. In fact, the body utilizes 23% of energy to convert every gram of carbohydrate to fat, but only 3% of energy for every gram of fat converted to fat.[91] Thus, by controlling total fat intake, fewer calories may be converted to fat. It has been shown that as much as 200 to 300 more calories/day are required for weight maintenance in subjects consuming diets that contain 20% of calories as fat.[39]

Saturated fat   Not only is reducing the total amount of fat important in reducing car-

Table 2-4   Fatty Acid Composition of Selected Fats (Percentage of Total Lipid)*

Type of fat	Saturated fat (SFA)	MUFA	PUFA
Animal			
Beef†	39	44	4
Butter	66	30	4
Chicken	28	36	21
Lamb†	33	42	7
Pork†	34	45	12
Turkey	29	41	26
Veal†	24	31	9
Vegetable			
Canola	7	55	33
Coconut	86	6	2
Corn	13	25	62
Olive	14	72	9
Palm	49	37	9
Peanut	19	46	30
Safflower	9	12	74
Soybean	15	23	58

*Pennington, Bowes & Church's: food values of portions commonly used, ed 15, Philadelphia, 1989, J.B. Lippincott Co.
†Source: National Livestock and Meat Board-Food and Nutrition News, 59:2, 1989.

diovascular risk, so is modifying the type of fat consumed. Saturated fat has been shown to be highly atherogenic and has an even greater impact on serum cholesterol than does cholesterol intake itself. Saturated fatty acids increase chylomicrons and LDL cholesterol concentration. The American Diabetes Association agrees with the American Heart Association in reducing saturated fat intake to less than 10% of calories. It is estimated that the American diet may contain as much as 17% to 20% as saturated fat.

Nearly all saturated fat comes from animal sources. Saturated fats by nature have all carbon atoms in the fatty acid chain saturated with hydrogen. As a result, these fats are generally solid at room temperature. Several plant fats are also saturated and have represented a major portion of fat consumed in the American diet. Coconut and palm oil, for example, are highly saturated and have been routinely used in commercial baked products because of their stability and long shelf life as well as their low price. Recent concern over their atherogenicity has prompted many baked good and snack manufacturers to replace them with less saturated fats such as soy, cottonseed, and corn oils. Table 2-4 shows the fatty acid composition of common fats consumed in the American diet.

Monounsaturated fat   The recommendation for monounsaturated fat (MUFA) is 10% to 14% of total calories. Traditionally MUFAs were thought to have a neutral effect on plasma cholesterol levels. Recent research suggests that they may not be as innocuous as once thought. Studies with normal subjects [53,72] and patients with hyperlipidemia[48] have found that substituting MUFAs for saturated fatty acids in the diet reduced LDL cholesterol without reducing HDL cholesterol (a criticism of high polyunsaturated fat diets is that they lower HDL as well as LDL cholesterol). This data is controversial, however, as the effect on maintaining HDL levels appears variable.

One of the major lipid problems in NIDDM is hypertriglyceridemia. Several studies have shown that hypertriglyceridemia in NIDDM is exaggerated by high carbohydrate diets regardless of the carbohydrate source (i.e., complex or simple).[33,48,71] Garg and associates suggest that partial replacement of complex carbohydrates with monounsaturated fats may improve the hypertriglyceridemia of NIDDM without raising LDL cholesterol or compromising diabetes control.[48] Ginsberg and others[49] demonstrated that a diet containing 38% fat—predominantly from MUFA (18%)—had the same effect on lipid values as an American Heart Association step-one diet. These data have sparked considerable controversy about the recommendation of a high-carbohydrate diet for individuals with diabetes, particularly for those with NIDDM.

As the controversy continues, the clinician is faced with a decision every time an obese patient with NIDDM and hypertriglyceridemia is present. The choice to use a 60% carbohydrate diet with 25% of calories as fat, or a 45% carbohydrate diet with 40% fat (predominantly MUFAs) is going to be affected by the patient's current intake, food preferences, and ability to make changes. If the patient's fat intake is around 40%, all effort should be made to reduce intake toward the recommended 30%. Sometimes a gradual reduction is necessary to allow the patient to comply with the diet. In this case, a higher level of fat (i.e., 35%) may be incorporated with a greater emphasis on MUFA food sources with an eventual reduction in total fat intake.

The major sources of MUFA in the diet are peanut, canola, and olive oils (see Table 2-4). Interestingly, poultry, beef, lamb, and pork each contain 40% to 45% of fatty acids from the monounsaturated variety. Thus, there is no reason why the recommended 10% to 14% of calories from MUFAs cannot be at least partially met by consuming lean varieties of meat. In general, patients can increase the MUFA content of their diet by substituting olive or canola oil in salads and cooking. Very little research has been performed with peanut oil as the major source of MUFA; thus few assumptions can be made concerning the therapeutic effects of its use.

Polyunsaturated fat   Polyunsaturated fatty acids (PUFAs) are predominantly found in plant sources but are also found in marine life. The most common PUFAs are linoleic, linolenic, and arachidonic. PUFAs can be divided into two types, omega 6 or omega 3 fatty acids, meaning they have a double bond on either the sixth carbon or the third from the methyl end of the fatty acid chain. PUFAs maintain the function and integrity of cells and are precursors to prostaglandin synthesis. Since the body does not synthesize polyunsaturated fatty acids, they are considered essential.

Studies have shown that polyunsaturated fatty acids lower plasma cholesterol levels, particularly LDL cholesterol. This clearly can have a beneficial effect to the person with diabetes who has a four to six times greater cardiovascular risk than the general population. The recommendation is that 6% to 8% of total calories come from PUFAs. The ratio of polyunsaturated to saturated fat in the diet (P/S ratio) is aimed at 1.0. Thus an equal amount of PUFAs to SFAs would be ideal as opposed to the ratio of 0.5 or less that is typical of the American diet.

Because of the nature of their chemical structure (i.e., containing more than one double bond), PUFAs are liquid at room temperature. These oils are often hydrogenated, however. Hydrogen is added to some of the double bonds to harden the oil into the form used in stick and tub margarines. This process reduces the polyunsaturated properties of these oils, including their hypocholesterolemic effect. Thus the softer tub varieties of margarine or the liquid oil itself are better dietary choices.

The major source of omega 3 fatty acids is fish oils. Eicosapentaenoic acid (EPA) and docosahexanoic acid (DHA) are the major fatty acids in this class. Epidemiologic studies suggest that these omega 3 fish oils may be beneficial to individuals with NIDDM because of their ability to reduce serum triglycerides.[65,85] Clinical trials with supplementation of omega 3 fatty acids are inconclusive, however, as large doses of fish oil are needed to produce an effect. Recent studies in individuals with diabetes have found that supplementation with large amounts of fish oil can elevate blood glucose levels and increase insulin requirements.[50,57]

Fish oil capsules purchased at health food stores are not regulated by the Food and Drug Administration and therefore may contain variable amounts of fish oil. Some even contain cholesterol. Currently, dietary supplementation with fish oil capsules is not generally recommended. The practice of consuming a tablespoon of cod liver oil daily also is discouraged because of the high vitamin A content and the high caloric value. Elderly individuals are most vulnerable to such claims and practices. Instead, patients should be encouraged to consume about 6 to 8 ounces of fish per week. Usually this is done by choosing two to three fish meals per week. Although salmon, mackerel, and herring are the best sources of omega 3 fatty acids, all fish should be encouraged because of its low fat content and proportion of polyunsaturated fatty acids. Previous limitations on shellfish consumption are no longer enforced because they too are sources of omega 3 fatty acids (albeit low levels) and have very low levels of saturated fat.

Sweeteners

Advice on the use of sweeteners by persons with diabetes has varied over the years as new information and new products become available. The term *sweeteners* includes naturally occurring nutritive compounds that contribute calories to the diet (e.g., sucrose, fructose, sorbitol) and chemically manufactured nonnutritive products that provide negligible or no calories.

Caloric sweeteners   Sucrose, fructose and sugar alcohols (sorbitol and mannitol) are naturally occurring nutrients that contribute 4 calories per gram to the diet.

Sucrose (cane sugar), the most widely used of the three, provides the standard for measuring sweetness, and it enhances the color, texture, and stability of manufactured and baked products. Aside from calories, sucrose provides little nutrition and has the greatest effect on blood glucose among the commonly used caloric sweeteners. Sucrose is not prohibited in a diet for diabetes; however, careful consideration must be given to the amount and manner in which it is consumed.[2,5] Taken in liquid form on an empty stomach, it can be quickly metabolized and can contribute to a rapid increase in blood glucose. To be used appropriately by a person with diabetes, it should be incorporated into the preparation of the food (e.g., emulsified, baked) and consumed as part of a meal.[78] Suggested limits for intake have been set at 10% to 15% of total calories for healthy individuals and up to 5% of carbohydrate for the diabetic individual.[8]

Fructose is a sugar found primarily in fruits and honey. It is available in a crystalline form, which is 100% fructose, or as high-fructose corn syrup, which contains from 10% to 57% glucose. While fructose has been rated 1.5 times sweeter than sucrose, this advantage may be lost in baking. Calorie-conscious consumers may find they need less fructose than sucrose to sweeten cold foods or beverages. Fructose produces a lower rise in blood sugar than sucrose in nondiabetic individuals and in diabetic individuals who have adequate available insulin.[12,34,87] The effect of fructose on triglycerides, however, is less clear. For individuals with persistent hypertriglyceridemia, use of fructose as a sweetener should be carefully evaluated and monitored.[35] No dietary limits have been recommended for fructose ingestion; however, the caloric contribution must be considered. A daily intake of more than 75 g/day has been shown to cause osmotic diarrhea.[8]

Sorbitol, manitol, and xylitol are polyalcohols that are found naturally in a variety of plants or are produced commercially from monosaccharides. Although less sweet than sucrose, they have the advantage of producing a lower glycemic effect because of slow absorption and metabolism to fructose. The sugar alcohols are frequently used as sweeteners in the manufacturing of "dietetic" products such as candies and cookies but generally are not available for home use. Calories in the manufactured products are often equivalent to sucrose-sweetened products; therefore for weight-loss diets the sugar alcohols offer little advantage other than glycemic effect. Some individuals consuming dietetic products sweetened with sorbitol experience flatulence and diarrhea. To avoid these potential side effects, patients should be advised to limit foods containing sorbitol to portions containing 20 kcal or less.[8]

Noncaloric sweeteners   Saccharin is a white powder synthesized from toluene that is up to 400 times sweeter than sucrose. The oldest of the nonnutritive sweeteners, it was initially marketed to the food canning industry as an economic alternative to sugar. Saccharin gained wider use during wartime sugar shortages. Saccharin can be used in cooking but does not act as a sugar in providing texture or color. Many people complain that it leaves a bitter aftertaste. When the FDA banned cyclamates in 1970, saccharin was the only nonnutritive sweetener approved for use in the United States. In 1977, an FDA ban on saccharin was proposed following a study showing a high incidence of bladder cancer in rats fed very large quantities in relationship to their body weight.[73] The relative risk to humans was debated by the scientific community, and Congress responded with a moratorium on the ban to allow time for further study. This moratorium routinely has been extended each time it expired. Suggested limits for saccharin intake are given in a 1955 GRAS (Generally Recognized as Safe) list published by the FDA. Recommended limits are: 500 mg/day in children and 1000 mg/day for a 70 kg adult.[8] While saccharin contains no calories, it may be packaged with a nutritive compound. The product Sweet and Low, for example, includes dextrose, which provides 4 calories per packet.

Aspartame is an amino acid compound that contains 4 calories/g. Because it is approximately 200 times sweeter than sucrose, the amount used as a substitute for table sugar is calorically insignificant. Aspartame is marketed under the brand name NutraSweet and as the table top sweetener, Equal. Equal includes a nutritive buffer that provides 4 calories/teaspoon. High consumer satisfaction has made it one of the most popular low-calorie sweeteners. Although it is stable in dry foods, when combined with liquids or subjected to high temperatures, aspartame can be degraded. Because it decomposes with heat, aspartame is not an appropriate sweetener to use in cooking. Monsanto Chemical Company petitioned the FDA in 1989 to use an encapsulated form of aspartame in baked products; approval currently is pending. Aspartame does not effect blood glucose control in diabetes; however, there are questions on safety that are applicable to the general population including people with diabetes. The normal metabolic breakdown of aspartame yields aspartic acid, phenylalanine; and methanol. Phenylalanine is restricted in diets of people with phenylketonuria; therefore aspartame consumption is contraindicated. About 10% by weight of aspartame is converted to methanol, an amount that is less than levels naturally occurring in many common fruits and vegetables.[87] Various side effects have been attributed to aspartame ingestion. In 1984 the Centers for Disease Control investigated 512 reports and concluded that the data did not provide evidence of serious, adverse consequences to health, but that some individuals may be unusually sensitive to aspartame.[8] The FDA has established the acceptable daily intake (ADI) of aspartame at 50 mg/kg/day.[8]

Acesulfame potassium (K), a synthetic sweetener that received FDA approval in 1988, is marketed by Hoechst under the name, Sunnette. Acesulfame-K is 130 to 200 times sweeter than sugar and has a synergistic effect with other sweeteners that increases this value. For example, when combined in a 1→1 ratio with aspartame, the mixture can be four to six times sweeter. It is heat stable and therefore suitable for baking. Acesulfame-K resembles saccharin in chemical structure. Some people say that it leaves a saccharin-like aftertaste when used in large concentrations. After FDA approval, the safety of acesulfame-K was contested by a consumer affairs group who claimed a study showed tumor formation in rats fed large amounts of the compound. The FDA reviewed the study data and found the tumors were not related to acesulfame-K consumption.[18,97] Acesulfame-K is packaged for retail sale as a table top sweetener under the label Sweet One. Each packet contains 1 gram of dextrose, which contributes 4 calories. The ADI for acesulfame-K is 15 mg/kg/day.[97]

Sucralose, a noncaloric sweetener derived from sucrose, is rated 600 times sweeter than table sugar. It is not metabolized by the body and therefore yields no calories and has no effect on blood glucose. Sucralose is stable in a wide range of foods, is acceptable for baking, and has a synergistic effect when combined with other sweeteners. Application for FDA approval was filed by McNeil Specialty Products Company in 1987 and is expected by 1992. For retail market packaging, Sucralose will be combined with a maltodextrin to provide volume so that it can be measured like table sugar. The maltodextrin contributes 4 calories/teaspoon.

Alitame is a protein consisting of the amino acids L-aspartic acid, d-alanine and a new amine (2,2,3,3-tetramethylthietanyl amine).[18,97] It is 2000 times sweeter than sucrose; therefore calories are negligible. Alitame also has a synergistic effect with other sweeteners. It is stable at high temperatures except in an acidic condition when it can give an "off" taste. Approval by FDA, petitioned by The Pfizer Company in 1986, is still pending.

Cyclamate, a derivative of cyclohexylsulfamic acid, is only 30 times sweeter than sucrose but is stable in heat and cold, has a long shelf life, and leaves almost no aftertaste. It was used in the United States from 1950 until 1970 when it was banned based on evidence of bladder tumors in rats. The carcinogenic effect may be related to the conversion of cyclamates to cyclohexylamine by rats and some humans.[30] Not all humans convert cyclamates, however, and cyclamate use is not banned in some countries, including Canada. Application for reapproval by the FDA was submitted by Abbot Laboratories in 1984. A National Academy of Sciences committee reviewed cyclamate at the FDA's request and concluded that cyclamate alone is not a carcinogen but may be a cocarcinogen in that it may enhance the effect of other cancer-causing substances.[18,30,97] The FDA has no policy for cocarcinogens; therefore reapproval of cyclamates may be delayed for an extended period of time.[18]

Considerations for use of sweeteners   Two important points must be emphasized in discussing the use of sweeteners by individuals with diabetes. First, caloric sweeteners, used as a taste additive, must be substituted for, not added to, other carbohydrate in the diet. This is required to minimize the effect on blood glucose and to assure that unrecognized calories are not being consumed. Second, noncaloric sweeteners, while not contributing calories of their own, may be associated with caloric nutrients either in the packaging (e.g., dextrose or lactose buffers in table top sweeteners) or in the food product they are sweetening. Terms on labels such as "sugar-free" or "dietetic" often lead people to ignore calories contributed by other ingredients in the product which may exacerbate blood glucose along with promoting undesirable weight gain.

The increasing number of sweeteners available to consumers offers individuals the opportunity to use a variety of products in their diet. Selections can be made based upon the advantages of a sweetener in enhancing a particular food (e.g., baked product, canned beverage, etc.). New products offer the synergistic quality that, when combined with other sweetening agents, provides more sweetness for less sweetener. The advantages of diverse intake and synergistic effect are that amounts ingested of any one sweetener are reduced and overall consumption of sweeteners can be moderated.

Use of sweeteners by children must be evaluated by body weight and maturation. The American Academy of Pediatrics 1985 Diabetes Task Force report included the following guidelines on use of sweeteners: (1) fructose and sorbitol may be used *in limited amounts*; (2) use of cyclamate and saccharin by children with IDDM should be limited pending further review; (3) aspartame is a satisfactory nonnutritive sweetener; and (4) use of combinations of artificial sweeteners is reasonable to limit risks with any one sweetener. The report said that guidelines on use of simple sugars (sucrose and fructose) must wait for studies of the glycemic effect that are conducted in children.[37]

Use of sweeteners by pregnant women is often questioned. No evidence of fetal distress has been found for any of the products currently approved by the FDA. Saccharin does cross the placenta, and, although there is no demonstrated effect on the fetus, avoiding heavy use appears prudent.[8] Many pregnant women choose to avoid consuming sweeteners during their pregnancy. For pregnant women seeking guidelines, use of a variety of sweeteners, in moderation, can be advised.

Alcohol

While use of alcoholic beverages by individuals with diabetes is not encouraged, it is not prohibited. Cautions on the use of alcohol, made for reasons of safety and health, apply to people independent of diabetes status. For the person with diabetes, alcohol consumption has an added risk of potentiating medication or exercise-induced hypoglycemia. Moderate alcohol intake can enhance the glucose-lowering effect of exogenous insulin and oral hypoglycemic agents.[45] Alcohol inhibits hepatic gluconeogenesis, a source of glucose that can be critical in the fasted state or for replenishing glycogen stores after exercise.[45]

A major concern for persons with diabetes is the similarity of signs of hypoglycemia and of intoxication. Symptoms of a severe insulin reaction may be ignored by observers who could offer assistance but believe they are dealing with an inebriated individual. Two of the first-generation oral hypoglycemic agents, chlorporpamide and, to a lesser extent, tolbutamide, may interact with alcohol and cause side effects (headache, flushing, and nausea.) The reactions have not been observed with the second-generation sulfonylureas.[7] Guidelines for alcohol consumption demand moderation: if alcohol is used, not more than two drinks should be consumed at one time. The American Diabetes Association recommends that consumption be limited to once or twice a week.[2]

Some alcoholic beverages, such as liqueurs, sweet wines, wine coolers, and sweet mixes contain large amounts of carbohydrate and should be avoided. Regular beer also contains carbohydrate, about as much as a slice of bread. Light beer offers the advantage of less carbohydrate, alcohol, and calories and is the recommended option. Table 2-5 provides information on the alcohol, carbohydrate, and calorie content of common alcoholic beverages.

The way that alcohol should be incorporated into the meal plan varies by type of diabetes. For IDDM, alcohol should be consumed with a meal and added to the daily food intake. No food should be omitted because alcohol does not require insulin for metabolism and eating less would augment the potential hypoglycemic effect.[2] For NIDDM, the similarity of alcohol to fat in calories (7 kcal/g in alcohol; 9 kcal/g in fat) and in metabolic pathway suggests substituting alcohol for fat in the diet for diabetes. A drink the size of one alcohol equivalent equals 2 fat exchanges (90 calories).[2] For individuals with IDDM and NIDDM who are overweight, the high calorie/low nutrition characteristics of alcohol advise avoidance during weight loss programs.

Sodium

The general American diet contains excessive amounts of sodium, contributed largely by processed foods. The association of sodium and hypertension is the major concern of

Table 2-5 Composition of Alcoholic Beverages and Mixes

Beverage	Serving (oz)*	Alcohol (g)	Carbohydrates (g)	Calories
Beer				
Regular	12	13	13	150
Light	12	11	5	100
Near beer	12	1.5	12	60
Distilled spirits				
80 proof (gin, rum, vodka, rye, whiskey, scotch)	1.5	14	Trace	100
Dry brandy, cognac	1	11	Trace	75
Table wine				
Dry white	4	11	Trace	80
Red or rose	4	12	2	85
Sweet wine	4	12	5	105
Light wine	4	6	1	50
Wine cooler	12	13	30	215
Dealcoholized wines	4	Trace	6-7	25-35
Sparkling wines				
Champagne	4	12	4	100
Sweet kosher wine	4	12	12	132
Appetizer/dessert wines				
Sherry	2	9	2	74
(Sweet sherry, port, muscatel)	2	9	7	90
Cordials, liquers	1.5	13	18	160
Vermouth				
Dry	3	13	4	105
Sweet	3	13	14	140
Cocktails				
Bloody Mary	5	14	5	116
Daiquiri	2	14	2	111
Manhattan	2	17	2	178
Martini	2.5	22	Trace	156
Old fashioned	4	26	Trace	180
Tom Collins	7.5	16	3	120

Adapted from Franz MJ: Alcohol and diabetes: Part II. Metabolism and guidelines, Diabetes Spectrum, 3:210-216, 1990.

*One alcohol equivalent is equal to the amount of alcohol in: 1½ ounces of distilled spirits, 4 ounces of dry wine, 2 ounces of dry sherry, 12 ounces of beer.

overconsumption. Some people appear more sensitive to sodium and at greater risk from high sodium intakes. For the population with diabetes, with an independent risk for hypertension, moderation in sodium intake is prudent.[78] The 1986 Recommendations advise a daily limit of 1000 mg/sodium per 1000 kcal.[2] For individuals with diagnosed hypertension, particularly associated with renal disease, sodium restriction is critical. In certain clinical conditions such as severe metabolic derangement, fluid imbalance, or postural hypotension, an increase in salt intake may be prescribed.

Vitamins and minerals

People with diabetes have the same requirements for vitamins and minerals as people who do not have diabetes. There is no evidence of a need for special supplementation that is unique to diabetes.[2] Vitamin and mineral supplementation is warranted when a low-calorie diet (less than 1200 calories) is prescribed or for individuals with unusual eating patterns or in special circumstances.

In summary, the ADA nutritional recommendations are general guidelines. They must be tailored to meet individual needs. The classification of diabetes is a primary factor to consider when applying these guidelines to individual diet plans.

CLASSIFICATION OF DIABETES AND NUTRITIONAL GUIDELINES

While principles of nutrition are the same for all individuals with diabetes, dietary approaches to normalizing blood glucose levels will differ by type of diabetes. Priorities vary according to insulin defect and metabolic goals. This chapter will present strategies for nutritional management of IDDM, NIDDM, and for pregnancy in gestational and overt diabetes.

Nutritional Management Of IDDM

IDDM represents an absolute dependence on exogenous insulin for survival. Diet and insulin prescriptions need to be integrated to achieve optimum energy metabolism and avoid hyperglycemia or hypoglycemia. Fortunately, modern insulin regimens and blood glucose monitoring allow increased flexibility in meal planning to accommodate individual lifestyles. IDDM is generally associated with youth as most people are diagnosed before age 30. People with IDDM, however, are of all ages and require dietary modifications appropriate for their chronologic age. Adjustments for metabolic changes resulting from the duration of diabetes may also be required.

Goals of nutritional management
Dietary treatment goals in IDDM are to:
- Achieve optimal blood glucose and lipid levels.
- Improve overall health through optimal nutrition.
- Promote normal growth and development in children and adolescents.
- Maintain reasonable body weight in adolescents and adults.[2]

Strategies for achieving these goals reflect the absolute insulin deficiency of IDDM, the need to integrate diet and exogenous insulin therapy in a life-style routine, and the young age of onset that describes this type of diabetes.

Nutritional strategies

Nutritional management of IDDM requires careful integration of diet, exercise, and insulin therapy in a treatment plan that promotes optimal metabolism but causes minimal intrusion in the individual's life-style. Specific strategies that will help achieve the nutritional goals for IDDM are to: (1) emphasize consistency in day to day nutrient intake, (2) determine a meal plan by diet history that is appropriate for the individual's life-style and integrates insulin therapy, and (3) modify the caloric and nutrient composition of the diet as needed to provide optimal nutrition, promote growth and development, and maintain desirable body weight.

Consistency in food intake   Flexible insulin regimens and SMBG now allow great latitude in meal planning for IDDM. The most sophisticated insulin regimen, however, still cannot mimic the exquisite secretory response of the pancreas and must rely on estimates of the amount of insulin required for metabolic balance. Therefore even with flexible regimens, day to day *consistency*—in meal times, in meal composition, and in caloric intake—is very important in the treatment of IDDM.

Consistency in eating patterns is needed to moderate the multiple factors that can influence glucose homeostasis. The greatest demand for insulin is during postprandial metabolism. In the postabsorptive state insulin requirements are minimal. When erratic eating patterns result in widely varying insulin demands, it is increasingly difficult to match insulin doses with metabolic needs. Changes in activity, emotional status, and other factors also effect insulin requirements; therefore consistency in the diet helps reduce the number of variables that can frustrate achieving glucose regulation.

Coordinating diet and insulin therapy   Meals, snacks, and the insulin regimen should be planned based on an assessment of the person's life-style. A child who is bused to and from school, a nurse on the evening shift, or a trial lawyer have very different schedules that direct when they inject their insulin and eat their meals. SMBG provides valuable information that patients can use to integrate diet, exercise, and insulin therapy into their daily routines and adjust for planned or unplanned changes in their usual activities. When developing individualized meal plans, certain fundamentals must be considered. First, the time and composition of a meal and the time, type, and amount of injected insulin must be coordinated. Second, availability of food varies and often dictates what and when people eat. Third, the ability and willingness of the individual to cooperate in the treatment regimen will have a direct effect on the therapeutic outcome.

Timing and composition of meals   Meal planning varies with the insulin regimen. When two injections of mixed short- and intermediate-acting insulins are prescribed, meals and snacks will need to correspond to four periods of insulin activity. On a daytime schedule using regular and NPH insulins, the pharmacokinetics of the regular and NPH in the morning injection cover breakfast and lunch, respectively, whereas the evening dose of regular insulin covers dinner. A bedtime snack is needed to compensate for the hypoglycemic potential of the evening NPH insulin. Additional snacks may be required to provide readily available glucose at insulin activity peaks of mid-morning and mid-afternoon. Intensive insulin therapy, by multidose insulin injections, continuous subcutaneous insulin infusion, or implanted pump provides low levels of insulin to mimic basal secretion and uses boluses of short-acting insulin before meals. Between-meal snacks usually are not required on these regimens.[82] The need for a bedtime snack varies by type of basal insulin and by individual metabolic differences. If a bedtime snack is indicated, or requested by personal preference, the need to bolus regular insulin also must be evaluated.

Snacks, to offset the caloric expenditure and hypoglycemic effect of exercise, are an important consideration in meal planning for IDDM. The frequency, intensity, time, and duration of exercise, individual weight, insulin regimen, and other food intake should be taken into consideration when planning exercise snacks. Guidelines for snacks are provided in Chapter 3, Exercise and Diabetes.

Availability of food   To facilitate adherence to the planned diet, practical consideration must be given to the availability of food.[58] Access to food can be restricted by job and school schedules, living conditions, travel, and other factors. The type of food available is limited when meals are prepared by others, eaten away from home, and by economic, social, religious, or ethnic constraints. The feasibility of making changes in food access or food type should be evaluated with the individual during the diet assessment. Diet planning and insulin therapy should be guided by realistic decisions on what modifications in food availability can, or will, be made.

Cooperation of patient in the treatment regimen   The willingness and ability of the individual to carry out the treatment plan must be considered. Diet and insulin therapies should be based upon the patient's goals, even when they appear in conflict with good diabetes management. The trial lawyer who may miss meals during court days, the teenager who is going to consume alcoholic beverages with peers, or the person with limited skills or limited desire to monitor self-care behaviors need diet and insulin regimens that will help them stay out of metabolic crises. Providing patients with modifications they can make in their diet plan based on SMBG values will enable them to adjust for expected and unexpected changes in their routine.[82,84] Use of SMBG in nutrition counseling is discussed later in this chapter.

Calories and nutrients to promote health   For children, caloric requirements increase from birth through the growth years, then stabilize and are more dependent on activity levels. Monitoring developmental growth and adjusting the diet plan to accommodate changing nutrient requirements are very important for the child with IDDM. Estimating the right number of calories is challenging since requirements vary dramatically with day to day activities, from season to season, and during growth spurts. Advocates for a nonstructured approach to the diet argue that an individual's appetite is more sensitive to caloric requirements than professional estimates.[26,64] However, some dietary guidelines, whether in a structured or unstructured teaching format, are needed to assure adequate nutrition and to assist in glucose control.

Excess weight gain can occur in IDDM patients of all ages but is most common in teenage women and in adults. Weight gain has been found to be an undesired side effect of improved metabolic control and has been most evident in patients changed to intensive insulin therapy.[38,82,99] This phenomenon has been attributed to improved utilization of glucose calories, increased experimentation with foods and meal patterns, and overtreatment of insulin reactions. Planning a weight-loss program for an individual with IDDM includes reducing food intake, increasing exercise, and decreasing the insulin dose. Information from SMBG can guide adjustments and help maintain stable diabetes control during the period of weight loss.

Eating disorders including bulimia and anorexia occur in diabetic individuals as they do in nondiabetic individuals. Some authors suggest that adolescents with diabetes are at increased risk because of the intense focus on diet required in diabetes.[94] Birk and Spencer[19] found the rate of anorexia and bulimia among 385 females with IDDM was within the range identified for the general population; however, they found approximately 5% used induced glycosuria as a purging method of weight control. The combination of IDDM and an eating disorder requires a team effort to provide psychologic, nutritional and metabolic counseling.

Nutritional Management of NIDDM

Nearly 90% of the diabetic population is composed of persons with type II, or non–insulin-dependent, diabetes (NIDDM). Since NIDDM generally manifests itself after age 40, nutritional issues are those of the adult individual. Yet, there is an increasing number of individuals who develop the disease in their 20s and 30s. Generally they are obese and have a family history of diabetes.

Goals for nutritional management
Dietary treatment goals in NIDDM are:
- To improve blood glucose levels (i.e., minimize glucose excursions and promote euglycemia).
- To improve overall health and improve, prevent or delay complications (i.e., control blood lipids, hypertension, proteinuria).
- To attain/maintain reasonable body weight.[2]

Since glucose intolerance and the incidence of diabetes increases with increasing body weight the primary treatment goal for at least 80% of individuals with NIDDM is weight loss. Indeed, losing weight will generally achieve all three goals.[77] For the remaining 10% to 20% of type II individuals who are already at a reasonable weight, promoting a healthy and active life-style with attention to an equally healthy diet is paramount.

Nutritional strategies
Nutrition strategies used to achieve these goals will vary with the individual. Life-style, eating habits, food preferences, medical condition, medications, and attitude toward health each affect the approach taken. Since NIDDM is characterized by insulin resistance, and normal, less than normal, or greater than normal levels of insulin secretion,

the level of glucose control can vary dramatically. Nearly 50% of persons with NIDDM may be on insulin or oral hypoglycemic agents that impact dietary strategies. As a rule the diet in NIDDM can be manipulated to improve blood glucose in the following ways:

1. Altering the composition of the diet (i.e., macronutrients).
2. Altering meal timing.
3. Altering the distribution of calories at meals and snacks.
4. Reducing calories to reduce body weight.

Composition of the diet   There remains no true consensus regarding the optimal nutrient composition of the diet for persons with NIDDM. Because of the heterogeneity of NIDDM it is probably unrealistic to expect that there should be. Since patients with NIDDM risk developing cardiovascular disease at a rate four to six times the general population, the dietary prescription must focus on reducing serum lipids levels. The ADA guidelines limiting fat to less than 30% of total calories is an excellent goal to strive to attain. Unfortunately, achieving this goal early in the dieting process is not always possible. People with NIDDM are older, averaging 55 years of age, and as a result bring with them years of dietary habits and food preferences. These generally are not abandoned overnight.

A gradual reduction in intake is usually most acceptable to the patient. Emphasis should be placed on concrete ways to alter fat intake (e.g., increase fish consumption, use skim milk dairy products, broil or bake foods as opposed to frying). Since NIDDM patients are almost always mature adults, it is important to include them in the goal setting process. The clinician needs to identify problems and guide the patient in committing to solutions.

Elevated triglycerides are particularly problematic in NIDDM and cannot be ignored. Data suggests that some NIDDM patients would be better off consuming less than 55% to 60% of calories as carbohydrate, thereby raising the percentage of calories from fat.[32,48] Diets as high as 40% to 45% fat (predominantly MUFA) have reduced triglycerides without lowering HDL cholesterol in NIDDM patients. This is a desirable effect, although long-term clinical studies have not been conducted. More studies need to examine the question of the efficacy of high-carbohydrate versus high monounsaturated–fat diets in NIDDM. At present, the clinician's best method to determine effectiveness is close follow-up. Periodic visits with laboratory evaluations of blood glucose and lipid values provides feedback as to the effectiveness of the diet plan chosen.

Most clinicians are taking a more liberal approach to the use of sucrose in the diet of the person with NIDDM. Since many of the foods recommended in the diet of a person with diabetes contain sugar from natural sources such as fruits, vegetables, and milk, the sugar intake may be as high as 10% of calories per day. Added sugar from desserts and table sweeteners are generally allowed to contribute 5% of carbohydrate calories.[77] For many older people, reducing or eliminating sugar may not be difficult. For others who have grown accustomed to a daily "sweet treat," sugar adds to their quality of life. Recent research into the glycemic response of various foods has led to the realization that an occasional sweet treat does not worsen blood glucose control and can therefore be included in the diet plan.[13,29,100]

The obese patient with NIDDM presents an interesting challenge when it comes to including sugar in the diet. Weight reduction diets cannot be nutritionally sound and include many sweets. Yet the restriction of sweets may lead to binging behavior. The concept of "good food, bad food" is generally a problem in obese people and becomes increasingly exaggerated in diabetes where sugar is usually considered bad. Human nature leads us to want what we cannot have. This is often the case in severely restricted weight reduction diets in which individuals are not taught how to deal with an occasional sweet or perceived "bad food." NIDDM patients should be taught not to use the description "I cheated" when describing an occasional desire and use of sweetened foods. This only adds to an already poor self-image from being obese.

Calorie and carbohydrate distribution   Because the pancreas of the person with NIDDM cannot secrete enough insulin after a meal to maintain normal glycemia, it has traditionally been considered best to distribute calories and carbohydrate evenly throughout the day. Three equal meals with one or two snacks has been considered ideal. The most common food intake pattern for an obese person is one of a small or nonexistent breakfast, a small lunch, and a large evening meal and snack in which the majority of the day's calories are consumed.[20] Since the majority of patients with NIDDM are obese, this pattern is not uncommon in this population. Some clinicians believe that this pattern of intake may be harmful in that it promotes obesity when excess calories consumed at night are stored as body fat, and that such a large carbohydrate and calorie consumption late in the day promotes hyperglycemia the next morning.

It remains to be seen whether the pattern in which food is consumed has an impact on blood glucose control or obesity in NIDDM. A recent study suggests that body weight may not be influenced by what time calories are consumed as long as calorie requirement is not exceeded.[16] When calories are held constant, mean blood glucose levels are similar in moderately well controlled NIDDM subjects regardless if they consume their daily calories as 3 equal meals or with 70% of calories consumed at the evening meal. If this is true then long-standing eating habits of the older NIDDM patients may not need to be altered to improve control. Once again, SMBG and close follow-up are required to evaluate the best way to distribute calories.

While snacks are often valuable in IDDM to prevent hypoglycemia between meals, this habit may not be of any value to the person with NIDDM. In type II diabetes, postprandial glucose responses are influenced by endogenous insulin production as well as peripheral glucose uptake. Snacking has been shown to delay or prevent blood glucose from returning to baseline values,[16] thus prolonging hyperglycemia throughout the day. Some individuals may prefer a small snack between meals to reduce hunger or reduce the fear of an insulin reaction. As individual responses may vary, blood glucose monitoring is necessary to evaluate whether snacks are necessary or how large they should be.

Meal timing   Because of a delayed and sluggish insulin response in NIDDM, generally 4 to 5 hours are required for enough insulin to be secreted to bring blood glucose down to baseline levels. As a result, it has been postulated that meals should be spaced 4 to 5 hours apart.[92] In theory this should allow blood glucose to fall to baseline before another glucose challenge from another meal or snack. This again is another theory that requires additional research.

Strict attention to consuming meals at specific times is not an issue for NIDDM patients who do not take insulin or oral agents. Consistency is required in those NIDDM individuals who take exogenous insulin just as in IDDM. As a rule, however, NIDDM patients have a better counter regulatory response and do not have problems with very severe hypoglycemic reactions. Planning ahead and not delaying or skipping meals is still important in NIDDM patients taking insulin, particularly in the elderly. It has been suggested that cognitive functioning decreases in the elderly. Hypoglycemia also alters cognitive functioning. Forgetting or delaying a meal may have serious implications in the elderly NIDDM patient.

Promoting reasonable body weight   Maintaining normal body weight is important to maintaining normoglycemia. As body weight increases, insulin resistance, glucose intolerance, and the propensity to develop diabetes increases. Since nearly 90% of patients with NIDDM are overweight, a hypocaloric diet to facilitate weight loss is the primary treatment goal for the majority of NIDDMs. Yet some 5% to 10% of NIDDM patients are normal weight at the time of diagnosis. For these individuals, making sure they are consuming an appropriate calorie level to *maintain* their normal body weight is important. Frequently improved glycemic control can result in weight gain as glucose calories are no longer lost in the urine.

Obesity is defined as an excess of body fat. Normal body fat content is approximately 15% to 17% in men and 22% to 25% in women.[70] Overfatness is defined as body fat in excess of 20% for men and 30% for women. Body fat content has a tendency to increase with advancing age. It is not clear if this is normal or merely reflects a decrease in muscle mass from inactivity and lack of use.

Development of the bioelectrical impedence technique for measuring body fatness has made it easier to determine actual percentage of body fat. This technique measures total body water and, in turn, lean body mass (LBM), by measuring resistance to a slight electrical current passed through the body. Since water is a good conductor of electricity, less resistance is present when more water is present—indicating more LBM. Use of this technique is increasing in frequency because it is painless, relatively accurate, and easy to perform.

Most health professionals, however, continue to rely on body mass index or relative body weight to determine degree of obesity. Body mass index (BMI) is an expression of weight where the effect of height is minimized (wt [kg] ÷ ht [m²]). It is considered more accurate than height-weight values. A BMI above 27 is generally indicative of obesity as it is equivalent to 20% above desirable weight. This term is not easily translated to the patient, therefore relative body weight is often used.

Relative body weight is the percentage of actual weight compared with ideal. Individuals above 20% of desirable body weight are considered obese. Controversy exists as to what is ideal body weight. Height and weight tables published by the Metropolitan Life Insurance Company are generally used as guides for desirable weight. Some clinicians are

Table 2-6 "Rule of Thumb" Method for Estimating Desirable Body Weight (DBW)

Height	Body frame	Adult men	Adult women
5 feet	Medium	106 lbs	100 lbs
Each inch above 5 feet	Medium	Add 6 lbs	Add 5 lbs
	Small	Subtract 10% of total	Subtract 10% of total
	Large	Add 10% of total	Add 10% of total

concerned over the fact that weights in the 1983 tables are higher than weights in the 1959 tables. The question often asked is "Are we accepting a heavier weight as normal when it is merely just reflecting a national trend toward obesity?" Many clinicians choose to use a general rule of thumb when estimating desirable body weight (Table 2-6).

Whenever body weight is being assessed, it is important to be realistic about what is a reasonable weight goal. This must be established with each individual patient based on age, degree of obesity, activity level, medical condition, and ability to restrict intake and alter life-style. Because most patients with NIDDM are older, realistic target weight goals are even more important.

Not only is the degree of obesity and body fatness significant in determining glucose intolerance, so is body fat distribution.[55] Individuals with body fat located at the waist and above generally have higher insulin, blood glucose, and serum lipid levels than individuals in whom body fat is located predominantly in the hips and thighs.[81,93] Such upper body obesity increases risk of cardiovascular disease, hypertension, and diabetes. Interestingly, upper body fat increases risk even at modest or slight levels of obesity (Fig. 2-4). Risk becomes greater as the degree of obesity increases.

Promoting weight loss An effective weight reduction diet for the obese patient with NIDDM should have several components. It should be safe, hypocaloric enough to promote a reasonable weight loss of 1/2 to 3 pounds/week, focus on developing healthy eating behaviors, enhance self-esteem, and promote increased physical activity. There are many weight loss approaches available that can in most instances be used in NIDDM patients. The most frequently used approach is the "exchange" plan in its many variations. This is an excellent approach since it promotes healthy eating choices and the consistency that is needed for individuals on hypoglycemic medication.

Experience suggests, however, that not all patients with NIDDM can be treated the same way when it comes to diet. Indeed, many individuals may have trouble with the exchange diet because of confusion about the concept of exchanges. The choices and flexibility that is the hallmark of this plan can be overwhelming to some individuals—they would prefer fewer choices and a less complicated approach such as individualized menus. Many older people in particular are less apt to experiment with new foods and prefer eating similar foods on a regular rotation.

Some individuals using exchange-type diets for weight loss like more flexibility in

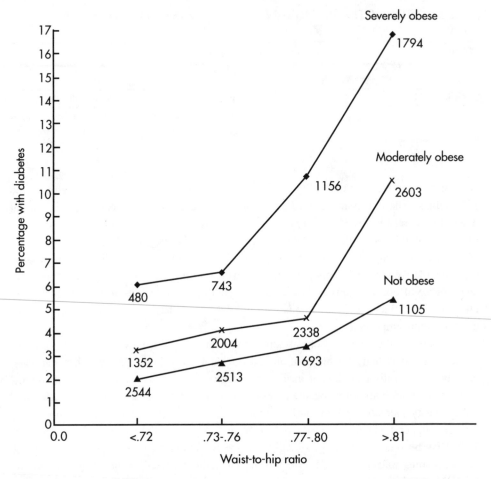

Fig. 2-4 The prevalence of diabetes according to relative weight and body fat distribution in 20,325 women. (From Hartz AJ and others: The association of girth measurement with disease in 32,856 women, Am J Epidemiol, 119:76, 1984.)

food choices between food groups. Since total calories and carbohydrate have the greatest impact on insulin requirements, some patients can be taught to cross-substitute between the milk group (12 g CHO, 90 kcal), the bread group (15 g CHO, 80 kcal), and the fruit group (15 g CHO, 60 kcal). This gives them more flexibility to alter the diet at a particular meal without compromising calorie intake.

Counting calories or counting grams of fat may be preferred by many NIDDM patients who are not on medication as these methods are simple to use. Patients can be taught to limit fat intake to 50 g/day or 25% to 30% of calories by using the exchange lists, nutrition labeling, and various other sources. This is often a good place to start with a newly diagnosed obese patient who may be easily overwhelmed by the many required diabetes self-care behaviors that include a diet.

Counting calories may be most effective when the patient is given guidelines for calorie distribution at meals, (e.g., breakfast, 300 kcal; lunch, 400; dinner, 500; and snacks, 300). A major drawback to this method of weight loss is the lack of control regarding sources of calories. There is no guarantee that food choices will be healthy. Using the 1990 Dietary Guidelines may be helpful.

The popularity of prepackaged and liquid diet regimens has had an impact on the approach to managing obesity in diabetes. These "no choices" approaches can be used in NIDDM patients under close medical and dietary supervision. Studies have demonstrated that very low–calorie diets (VLCDs) of less than 800 calories/day can be used successfully with obese diabetic patients.[11] These diets can produce rapid weight loss, dramatically improve blood glucose levels, and improve hypertension. Sustaining improved blood glucose responses with refeeding appears to depend largely on duration of diabetes and pancreatic insulin reserve.

Because of the drastic caloric restriction of these approaches, they should be limited to individuals who are at least 50 pounds overweight. Risks involved with use, such as cholecystitis, pancreatitis, and arrhythmias, are minimized by careful patient screening and close medical supervision.

The protein-sparing modified fast (PSMF) is a VLCD approach that has been used for years by many clinicians and involves real food in the form of lean meat, fish, and poultry. These high-protein foods are distributed as 2 to 3 meals per day in amounts to provide 1.2 to 1.5 g protein/kg ideal body weight. Fruits and vegetables may be incorporated to a level of 50 g carbohydrate/day. The result is similar to liquid regimens with the advantage of using real food. This allows the clinician and patient to focus on eating behaviors during the diet process. A major drawback to this approach is that supplements of vitamins and minerals are required and can sometimes be forgotten by even the most well-intending patient.

Careful monitoring of blood glucose is a must in patients who are taking insulin and on a calorie-restricted diet, regardless of the degree of restriction. Blood glucose levels generally decrease as soon as caloric restriction is initiated. If insulin doses are not tapered accordingly, the patient may develop hypoglycemia. To many individuals, including the elderly, this is a very unpleasant and fearful experience. As a result, they may often "feed" the insulin to prevent hypoglycemia. The patients' comfort level and trust can be enhanced if the insulin dose is reduced at the onset of a hypocaloric diet. Patients using VLCDs should have their insulin dose reduced by one-third to one-half on initiating the diet. Patients on oral hypoglycemic agents will need the dose reduced or discontinued. Failure to lose expected weight may be the result of frequent reactions that are overtreated with high-calorie foods.

One of the greatest concerns with any weight loss regimen (most recently the VLCDs) is the poor weight maintenance results. All successful weight loss regimens must focus on helping the patient develop permanent changes in eating and activity behaviors.

Cognitive restructuring of self-defeating thoughts is a concept receiving considerable attention in weight loss therapy. Obese patients with NIDDM can often have a poor self-image not only because of obesity but also because of the stigma of a chronic disease. Helping patients develop positive attitudes toward life in general can help weight loss efforts immensely.

Setting reasonable weight loss goals is one way to promote confidence and improve self-image in the obese persons with NIDDM. Generally, even small losses such as 10 to 20 pounds can substantially improve blood glucose levels. This improvement can be considered an important marker of success for the obese patient with NIDDM and can be used by the clinician to instill a sense of achievement in the patient. This is particularly true in the older individual in whom weight loss is frequently more difficult.

Weight goals should be kept reasonable in older patients who may have additional factors impacting their health. Clinicians differ as to their philosophy regarding weight goals in the elderly. Some believe that a few pounds over desirable weight may be better as it may act as a nutritional reserve in the event of illness, infection, or surgery. Current health status, degree of overweight, body fat distribution, and activity level should all be considered when determining the impact that individual body weight is having on the elderly person's health.

Nutritional Management of Pregnancy in Gestational and Overt Diabetes

Goals for nutritional management

Healthy babies and healthy mothers are the goals of nutritional management of diabetes during pregnancy. These goals are the same for pregnant women with previously diagnosed diabetes (IDDM and NIDDM) and women who develop gestational diabetes (GDM) during pregnancy. In nondiabetic individuals, glucose levels are lower during pregnancy than in the nonpregnant state.[88] The outcome of a healthy baby appears associated with achieving and maintaining these lower normal levels of blood glucose control during pregnancies complicated by diabetes. The risks for fetal abnormalities to occur during embryogenesis (gestational weeks 3 to 7) and for macrosomia to develop in the third trimester can be reduced with tight diabetes control.[6,88,69] The need for excellent blood glucose control during embryogenesis mandates that nutritional counseling for women with IDDM and NIDDM actually begins before conception.

Nutritional strategies

The nutritional recommendations for pregnancies complicated by diabetes are based upon guidelines from the National Research Council for healthy pregnancies. In the diabetes literature there are varying opinions on the number of calories that should be prescribed. Suggestions range from 24 to 37 kcal/kg of DBW in the first trimester to 24 to 40 kcal/kg DBW in the second and third trimesters.[6,59,88] Part of the variation in caloric requirements is related to the pregestational weight of the individual. Jovanovic-Peterson found that gestational women of normal weight (80% to 120% of IBW) remained ketone-free on a diet of 30 kcal/kg/day, whereas women less than 80% IBW required about 40 kcal/kg/day and women over 120% IBW could be managed on diets as low as 24 kcal/kg/day.[59] The Sweet Success California Diabetes and Pregnancy Program uses a formula of 30 kcal/kg/day in the first trimester raised to 36 kcal in the second and third trimesters for normal weight individuals and an initial 25 kcal/kg/day increased to 30 kcal/kg/day for obese individuals. Weight loss during pregnancy is not a goal of these lower caloric prescriptions. Rather, they are an attempt to avoid excessive weight gain due to overestimation of maternal requirements.

Composition and distribution   The amount of carbohydrate to be included in the diet is another issue for debate. The ADA recommendations for a carbohydrate intake of 55% to 60% are advocated by some authorities.[90] Others suggest that normoglycemia will be attained only if carbohydrate is limited to approximately 40% of total calories.[1,59] Individual tolerance of carbohydrate will need to be assessed. Starting with a carbohydrate intake of 45% to 50% is reasonable. Protein requirements during pregnancy increase by 10 g/day according to the RDAs.[44]

Strategies to achieve "tight glycemic control" while meeting maternal and fetal nutrient needs require careful meal planning by the registered dietitian and diligence on the part of the pregnant woman. The amount and type of carbohydrate in each meal must be carefully assessed. Whether the woman is taking exogenous insulin or relying on her endogenous supply, the need to minimize postprandial glycemic excursions is so critical that the glycemic effect of each meal must be considered. The distribution of carbohydrates among meals and snacks is also important. Recommendations vary. Some diabetes centers[88] ascribe to the three meal and bedtime snack regimen with a $2/7$, $2/7$, $2/7$, $1/7$ proportioning of carbohydrates, and others advocate a distribution of carbohydrate across six feedings eaten as three small meals with snacks in between and at bedtime.[6,42,76]

Morning insulin resistance, caused by growth hormone and cortisol, is greater during pregnancy, which means that carbohydrate tolerance at breakfast is especially limited. For this reason, restriction of quickly metabolized forms of carbohydrate such as fruit, fruit juices, and processed cereals in the breakfast meal is recommended by the Sweet Success Program. All fruits and starches are eliminated from the Jovanovic and Peterson dietary guidelines for breakfast.[59]

The tendency to ketosis, a common result of fetal demands on maternal fuel sources, requires routine monitoring of ketone as well as glucose levels to evaluate optimum energy metabolism. A positive test for ketones in the morning is a common result of the long period of time between the evening snack and breakfast. Adjustment of composition, size, and time of the evening snack may reduce morning ketonuria, but as adjustments are made, the effect on evening blood glucose values must be monitored. A 3 AM snack may give optimal therapy and, with the nocturia of pregnancy, may not be too inconvenient for the expectant mother.

It is important to recognize that pregnancy is marked by hormonal changes, which foster hypoglycemia in the first trimester and hyperglycemia in the latter trimester. Adjustments in the meal pattern from trimester to trimester may accommodate the changing hormonal effects. Patients can be instructed to select foods by fiber content or "glycemic index." SMBG will provide valuable feedback for all pregnant patients with diabetes and is essential for managing patients who are on insulin therapy.

Postpartum

The postpartum diet will reflect the status of diabetes and the mother's plans to breast feed. Breast feeding is feasible for women with pregestational and gestational diabetes. For women on insulin, the effect of breast feeding on blood glucose needs to be added to the usual list of factors influencing glycemia. From limited studies, it appears that blood glucose levels may vary widely during lactation, possibly in relation to the amount of milk produced and the frequency of feedings. The RDAs recommend an increase of 500 calories a day for lactation to include an additional 15 g/day of protein during the first 6 months of lactation and 12 g/day thereafter.[44] A caloric distribution of 50% to 60% carbohydrate, 12% to 20% protein, and 30% fat is appropriate. The calories should be distributed throughout the day. Adding between-meal snacks can help prevent hypoglycemia and may avert the need for increasing the insulin dose to cover larger meals.

Return to a normal weight is a postpartum goal for most women. For women with IDDM, the calories of the prepregnancy diet may need to be adjusted to allow for weight loss. Calorie restriction and exercise, coupled with careful monitoring of blood glucose, aid in the return to a desirable weight. For the woman with gestational diabetes, the tendency to be overweight and the potential for later development of NIDDM indicate that postpartum weight control counseling is very important. Nutritional counseling routinely should be provided to postpartum GDM women.

Recommendations for Children

In 1985 the American Academy of Pediatrics published a Summary Report, *Nutritional Management of Children & Adolescents with Insulin Dependent Diabetes Mellitus,* developed by a Diabetes Task Force of their Committee on Nutrition. Recommendations included distribution of calories in the meal plan as 50% to 60% carbohydrate, 15% to 20% protein, and 20% to 25% fat.[37] The report noted that investigations on use of dietary fiber, glycemic index, and lipid and protein reductions need to be confirmed in infants, children, and adolescents. No specific recommendation was given for dietary cholesterol intake in this report. The American Heart Association recommends reducing cholesterol intake to 200 mg/day for children. Rigorous restriction of dietary fat or cholesterol is not recommended for children under 2 years in whom metabolic processes are in developmental phases.[22]

INDIVIDUALIZATION OF DIET THERAPY

The Principles of Nutrition and the guidelines for nutritional management of IDDM, NIDDM, and GDM are generalizations. The true diet for diabetes is the nutrition regimen developed to meet physical, metabolic, and life-style requirements of an individual. The success of the nutrition intervention in diabetes depends on how well the diet fits the unique needs of the individual and how well the individual incorporates the diet plan into his or her life-style.

Assessment

Development of the nutrition regimen starts with an assessment of the patient (see accompanying box). Age, gender, and anthrophometric, biochemical, and physical measures di-

---

_____ COMPONENTS OF PATIENT ASSESSMENT _____

1. *Medical evaluation:* Identify those medical factors that have an impact on the dietary prescription. Review the problem list.
   Consider: Type of diabetes
   Weight, height history
   Growth curve
   Medications
   Insulin treatment
   Abnormal laboratory findings
   Significant physical findings
   Family history
2. *Nutritional assessment:* Identify the present nutritional status and factors that should be considered when developing a nutritional care plan. Evaluate the current dietary history and activity patterns.
   Consider: Average intake of: carbohydrate, protein, fat, and calories
   Saturated fat intake
   Nutritional density of intake
   Alcohol intake
   Food preferences/allergies
   Special needs, i.e., growth, stress
   Drug/diet interactions
3. *Educational assessment:* Identify preferred teaching methods and scope and level of proposed educational program.
   Consider: Motivational level
   Reading level
   Learning preferences
   Emotional status
4. *Evaluation of support systems available:* Identify significant problems the patient may encounter in implementing the dietary prescription.
   Consider: Facilities for food preparation
   Food budget
   Ethnic, cultural, social, religious background
   Life-style
   Support available from family and others

From Flood TM and others: Dietary management of diabetes. In Marble A and others: Joslin's diabetes mellitus, ed 12, Philadelphia, 1985, Lea & Febiger.

rect the basal caloric and nutrient composition of the diet. Information on the diabetes status suggests strategies in meal formats and times. Specific information on food intake, food preferences, and eating behaviors allows translation of the diet in foods and meal patterns that are familiar to the individual. A life-style profile identifies daily routines, socioeconomic conditions, cultural and religious beliefs, and other factors that influence how people eat. Collecting this data can be time consuming, but the information is so important that attention should be given to ways that it can be efficiently compiled. Questionnaires and records, completed by the diabetic individual or by a family member, can save time and may elicit more accurate information than verbal reporting.[66]

There are several common methods for obtaining information on food intake. Retrospective approaches include recall of all food consumed in a 24-hour period or the frequency in which a food is consumed in a specified time period (e.g., per day, week, or month). Prospective assessment, using food diaries kept for 3, 7, or more days, provides more accurate information on eating patterns and behaviors but is still subject to the bias of self-report or seasonal variation. Size of portion and method of preparation must be delineated to be able to determine caloric and macronutrient intake. Meal times and their relationship to medication, work, social and physical activity, and sleep patterns provide very useful information. This information can be obtained by inquiring about daily schedules for weekdays and weekends. Open-ended questions, such as, "When do you start your day? What is the first thing that you eat? What time is your first meal?" will provide valuable information that may not be elicited if the first question is "What do you usually eat for breakfast?" For patients who are on diabetes medication, a question asking when they take their medicine should be included. The value of learning that the patient is injecting the morning insulin dose at home, driving the 45 minute commute to work, and then eating breakfast is obvious.

Caloric Prescription

Diet planning starts with an estimation of the daily caloric requirement. An individual's caloric needs vary by body size, activity, and the demands for growth. For adults, the calorie level of the diet is estimated to be the number of calories that would maintain weight given the activity pattern of the individual. Several methods exist to determine caloric requirements.

Approaches that are fairly accurate calculate calories for basal or resting energy expenditure (REE), then add calories for physical activity. Harris-Benedict equations calculate REE using factors of gender, weight, height, and age:

Males: REE = $66.47 + (13.75 \times wt) + (5.03 \times ht) - (6.75 \times age)$

Females: REE = $655.1 + (9.56 \times wt) + (1.85 \times ht) - (4.68 \times age)$

Weight is measured in kilograms, height in centimeters, and age in years. Unfortunately REE has a tendency to overestimate requirements in the obese by as much as 12% when actual body weight is used.[43] In contrast, using ideal body weight underestimates requirements by as much as 38%. The RDAs use equations published by WHO that cal-

Table 2-7   Estimating Energy Requirements for Adults

Daily activity	Activity factor × REE	kcal/kg*	kcal/pound*
Sedentary	1.3	25-30	11-13
Moderate	1.6	31-38	14-17
Strenuous	2.0	39-47	18-21

Sedentary: majority of day seated or standing ≤2 hours walking or other light activity. Moderate: approximately 8 hours of day walking, gardening, house cleaning, exercising, carpentry, restaurant trades, electrical trades. Heavy: approximately 8 hours of day walking, digging, carrying load, manual labor, climbing, skiing, cycling.

*Calculation based on method of Pellet PL: Food energy requirements in humans, Am J Clin Nutr 51:717, 1990.

culate REE by weight, gender, and age in categories.[44] Both the Harris-Benedict equations and the WHO equations can be used in children. The Harris-Benedict equation for males should be used for both sexes in children under 10 years of age.[83]

Energy requirements for activity must be added to the REE or basal rate. Factors have been developed to calculate energy requirements based upon average daily activity. Table 2-7 gives factors for calculating calorie requirements for adults.

Energy requirements for children are more difficult to estimate. For children ages 1 to 8 an activity factor of 2.0 x REE estimates allowances consistent with intake.[83] After age 8 a steady decline in factors from 1.8 to 1.6 (adult level) at age 17 is suggested, with adolescent males having higher energy requirements than females. Another method for calculating calorie requirements of children is to allow 1000 calories for the first year and add 100 calories for each additional year up to puberty (age 12). Calorie requirements of adolescents (ages 12 to 15) are estimated at 1500 to 2000 calories plus 100 calories per year over age 12 for females and 2000 to 2500 calories plus 200 calories per year over 12 for males.[6] Independent of the method of calculation, the pediatric norms in height-weight grids should guide evaluation of caloric requirements of children.

Providing sufficient calories to promote growth has always been a primary concern when planning diets for diabetic children. Recently, being overweight has become a pediatric diabetes problem. This new condition in weight control is attributed to the technologies that allow tight blood glucose control and curtail loss of calories in the urine. Careful monitoring of actual calories consumed and of exercise patterns will provide valuable information for a weight management strategy and is a better approach than arbitrary reduction of a general estimate of caloric need. Often children eat high fat snacks that contribute more calories to the diet than planned.

To facilitate weight gain or weight loss, the calories estimated for maintaining weight are increased or decreased. A pound of body fat represents about 3500 calories; therefore adjustments of 500 calories a day should achieve a 1 pound a week change in weight. A greater reduction in calories would allow a faster rate of weight loss; however, minimum daily intakes of 1200 calories for women and 1500 for men are recommended. Diets with calorie levels below the recommended minimum may be nutritionally inadequate, require supplementation, and should be medically monitored.

Distribution of calories among the macronutrients (i.e., carbohydrate, protein, and fat) is guided by growth, metabolic status, and dietary habits. The ADA Nutritional Recommendations provide target goals.[2] When developing a diet prescription, the caloric and macronutrient values of current food intake should be calculated first, compared with the target values, then modified in consultation with the patient. Examples of calculations of a diet prescription for an adult male, a meal plan that meets the ADA Nutritional Recommendations, and a sample menu are provided in Appendix 2a.

TRANSLATING THE NUTRITION PRESCRIPTION INTO MEAL PATTERNS

The best-designed diet prescription is only as effective as the individual's ability and/or willingness to follow instructions. Adhering to a diet requires knowledge to make correct food choices and motivation to alter eating behaviors. Teaching materials and methods should be carefully selected for each person after an educational assessment to identify current knowledge, learning preferences, motivation to learn, reading level, visual acuity, and cultural eating patterns. A variety of meal planning approaches are available in a range of options from general guidelines for eating to complex programs providing detailed information on food, goal setting, and techniques for self-evaluation. More than one approach may be used with a single patient. For example, initial diet instruction may be limited to survival skills taught with general guidelines, followed by a more detailed meal-planning method introduced in subsequent counseling sessions to increase both precision and flexibility in diet therapy.

Teaching Materials

The Exchange Lists for Meal Planning

The Exchange Lists for Meal Planning, published by the American Diabetes Association and The American Dietetic Association, groups foods into six categories: starch/bread, meat, vegetable, fruit, milk, and fat. Each category lists measured foods of approximately the same nutritional value. One food portion on the list can be substituted or "exchanged" for another with minimum difference in calories or the amount of carbohydrate, protein, and fat it contains.[46]

The goal in developing the *Exchange Lists* was to construct an educational tool that would provide consistency in nutrient intake while allowing diversity in foods consumed. The *Exchange Lists* were initially published in 1950 and revised in 1976 and in 1986. The 1986 revision included added information on fiber and sodium and expanded the number of food items to include combination foods and foods for occasional consumption (high sugar or fat content). To use this teaching method, the dietary prescription of calories, carbohydrate, protein, and fat is calculated into servings from each of the lists. Selection of exchanges and distribution into meal patterns is guided by patient preference, life-style, nutrient composition, and glycemic effect. Individualization allows the same diet prescription to result in very different meal patterns. This flexibility creates confusion when patients perceive that all 1800 calorie diets for diabetes should be the same and interchangeable. Appendix 2a at the end of this chapter gives an example of planning a diet using the *Exchange Lists*.

As a teaching tool, the *Exchange Lists* give comprehensive information on basic nutrition, nutrient composition, and caloric density in user-friendly terms of common foods, household measures, and meal plans. The *Exchange Lists,* however, have limitations. Not all people can comprehend the concept of "exchanging" foods. Many people eat diets that are predominantly combination foods, often preprocessed by the manufacturer or in restaurants. Information on exchange values for home recipes and commercial foods is limited. Some people claim that the size of the current edition ($8\frac{1}{2} \times 10$ inches, 35 pages) makes it impractical to carry around as a reference guide. Others find the extensive information overwhelming. In response to these criticisms, variations of the *Exchange Lists* and companion materials have been published. The *Exchange Lists* are available in large print, in Spanish translation, and in a simplified pictorial version, *Eating Healthy Food.* In 1989, the *Exchange Lists* teaching method was expanded to include information on diets of various cultures with the introduction of "Ethnic and Regional Food Practices—a Series." Professional guides and client education pieces are included in this series. The concept of "exchanges" has been used in cookbooks written for persons with diabetes, modified in publications on diet in general, expanded in materials published by diabetes interest groups, and adopted by some food manufacturers in providing nutrient information on their products. See Appendix A for resource lists of major publishers of companion materials for the *Exchange Lists* teaching method.

Healthy Food Choices

Healthy Food Choices is a simplified meal planning tool developed in 1986 as part of the revision of the *Exchange Lists*. The pamphlet is designed to emphasize healthy eating and does not mention diabetes. Guidelines for making healthy food choices follow the Dietary Guidelines and emphasize eating more high-fiber foods and less fat, salt, and sugar. The *Exchange Lists* approach is used to categorize foods, but the terms "choice" and "group" replace "exchange" and "list." The caloric value of each group is given and general measures are provided for foods in each group (e.g., 1 fresh medium fruit, ½ cup fruit juice). The minimum number of daily choices from each group needed to provide a healthy diet are outlined and identified as a 1200-calorie diet. The format allows hanging as a poster or folding to be carried in a pocket or purse. Spaces are included for a health professional to enter individualized meal patterns and add information on favorite foods. *Healthy Food Choices* offers great flexibility as a teaching tool. It can be used as an introductory step in nutritional counseling for all classifications of diabetes, for NIDDM patients in whom weight loss is a primary goal, as the principal method of instruction for reinforcing individuals with established good eating practices, or for the person who is not capable of making major dietary changes. *Healthy Food Choices* does not provide the detailed information on food composition that may be required to achieve desired post-prandial blood glucose values for IDDM patients striving for optimum control or for management of GDM.

High Carbohydrate–High Fiber

A format similar to the *Exchange Lists* is used in the *High Carbohydrate–High Fiber* (HCF) exchange lists. Foods are divided into eight groups: milk, garden vegetables, fats, beans, proteins, cereals, starches, and fruits. Food portions in each group provide approximately the same calorie, carbohydrate, protein, and fat content. Emphasis is placed on the fiber content of foods. The high-fiber maintenance diet contains 25 grams of dietary fiber per 1000 calories. Developed by James W. Anderson, MD, in 1974, the HCF diet has been used to treat a variety of metabolic diseases, including diabetes, hyperlipidemia, obesity, and hypertension.

The Point System

The Point System, developed in 1944 by Virginia Stuckey, RD, is a structured meal planning approach that provides a simple method of counting daily intake of calories and/or selected other nutrients. For each nutrient, a point is defined as equal to a set amount of calories, or grams, or milligrams. Patients select foods equaling a certain number of nutrient points per day, or per meal. For example, 75 calories equals one point; therefore a 1500 calorie diet would equal 20 calorie points. The patient can be instructed to select foods to provide a total of 20 calorie points in a day or specifically 5 points at breakfast, 6 points for lunch, 7 points for dinner and 2 points as an evening snack. *The Point System* may be used to introduce calorie counting as an initial step and then may be expanded to counting of one or more nutrients, such as carbohydrate, protein, and fat. For a person with IDDM, a total number of calorie points could be defined for the day, then carbohydrate points assigned by meals. Guidelines for selecting a healthy diet must accompany instruction in *The Point System*. Food records are encouraged and provide the nutrition counselor a method for evaluating the nutritional adequacy of the patient's food choices.

Menu approaches

Several instructional methods have been developed that use menus to guide meal planning. Individualized menus often have been developed in conjunction with other teaching approaches, either as examples provided to the patient or as a return demonstration by the patient used to assess competencies. The sense of security found in a set of menus has led many hospitalized patients to collect them from their food trays to take home at discharge. Menus for daily meal planning can be purchased by subscription to services that provide sets, at various calorie levels, on a routine basis (generally monthly). The American Diabetes Association introduced a menu planner, *Month of Meals,* in 1989 and published a second edition in 1991.

Other meal-planning methods that have been developed, tested, and found to be effective in instructing patients with diabetes include TAG (total available glucose), *Kentucky Personal Guidelines,* and the *Food Choice Plan.* Materials developed for the general population such as the *four food groups* and *Dietary Guidelines* can be used effectively in diabetes nutritional counseling. A monograph, *Meal Planning Approaches in the Nutrition Management of the Person with Diabetes,* by Green and Holler, contains detailed information on a variety of meal-planning approaches including those discussed above and provides case studies to demonstrate patient characteristics and counseling situations in which each approach would be an appropriate choice. This monograph is published by The American Dietetic Association.

Expanding Nutritional Education

Persons following a diet for diabetes will most often eat a variety of foods in diverse settings. In addition to instructional materials used to teach the principles of diet, there are multiple forms of information that can help individuals follow their diets and enjoy favorite foods. There is a wealth of supplemental material that can be used to expand culinary options within the guidelines of the diet plan. Cookbooks, tips on dining out, suggestions for bagged lunches, and steps for converting recipes or nutritional label information into dietary measures (e.g., calories or exchanges) are available from many sources. Magazines such as Diabetes Forecast, Diabetes Self-Management and Diabetes in the News routinely offer menus and information on food products (The Resource list at the end of the text provides a resource directory).

Nutritional Counseling Strategies

Staged education

Nutrition education and counseling for diabetes is a continuous process. As people adjust to the diagnosis of diabetes and begin to master self-management skills, their needs for nutritional information will change and their interest in learning more about their diet usually will increase. The advice of educators and the experience of clinicians advocate a staged approach to diabetes nutrition counseling. Initial diet instruction should teach survival skills. The goal should be to provide knowledge and skills that enable the individual to select meals that will facilitate metabolic control. In-depth education in ways to improve the diet regimen with a wider variety of foods, with options for variations in daily schedules, and other modifications can be provided in follow-up sessions. *The Nutrition Guide for Professionals,* published by the American Diabetes Association and The American Dietetic Association, provides detailed objectives, methodologies, and outcomes for initial and in-depth and continuing nutrition education for IDDM and for NIDDM. Behavioral objectives for initial and in-depth nutrition education for IDDM, NIDDM, GDM, and for pregnancy in overt diabetes are outlined in *Goals for Diabetes Management,* published by the American Diabetes Association (See Resource List at the end of the text).

Behavior modification

The literature on diabetes contains an increasingly large number of articles written about patient compliance with treatment regimens. Health beliefs, social learning, motivation, family and societal influences, regimen complexity, and patient-provider relationships are among the many factors that have been studied as they relate to diabetes regimen adherence.[66] Recognition that changing eating behaviors is not easy, even for intelligent individuals, has encouraged use of a variety of behavioral techniques to promote dietary adherence. Behavior modification, goal setting, cognitive restructuring, and relapse prevention are techniques developed through theories of behavioral psychology. These techniques have been used in nutrition counseling for weight loss, hyperlipidemia, and diabetes. Decisions on which method to use should be made with the patient and guided by his or her past experiences with changing eating or other health behaviors. More detailed information on educational and behavioral theories that can be used in nutrition counseling is provided in other chapters of this text.

Self-monitoring of blood glucose

SMBG levels provides valuable feedback on the success of the diabetes treatment plan.[14] In nutrition counseling, test results can be used to evaluate the mix of foods in a meal or a snack, distribution of foods throughout the day, meal spacing, the effect of specific foods on an individual's blood glucose levels, and the relationship of meals with other therapeutic agents (i.e., medications and exercise). Use of SMBG records to evaluate therapy should be encouraged as a collaborative endeavor of the patient and the clinician. Too often, the person with diabetes (and some clinicians) view SMBG records as a "report card" of dietary compliance. The value of SMBG test records is their use to guide therapy.

When evaluating SMBG tests, patterns of blood glucose values should be determined before an adjustment is made. Common problems and optional regimen changes to consider are presented in Table 2-8. Changes in therapy generally are made after review of records from several days and are not based on a blood glucose value from a single test.[7]

SMBG can be used to evaluate the glycemic effect of a specific food or to compare two meal patterns, such as two breakfast menus. Premeal blood glucose values need to be similar if a comparison is to be made. To test the glycemic effect of particular foods in mixed meals, equivalent portions of all foods must be included in the meal on each occasion. Only one food should be changed at a time. To test the glycemic effect of a single food, such as a snack option, the portion size should be reasonable. In evaluating the adequacy of an evening snack, the morning fasting blood glucose value and ideally a 3 AM value should be considered.

PROBLEMS WITH METABOLIC CONTROL: DIET MODIFICATIONS
Sick-Day Management

During periods of illness and surgery, blood glucose levels become elevated and diabetes may get out of control. Counterregulatory hormones such as epinephrine, glucagon, nor-

Table 2-8   Options for Regimen Adjustments Based Upon Self-Monitoring Glucose Blood Tests

SMBG values	Regimen adjustments to consider
Hyperglycemia	
Fasting	Increase PM intermediate or long acting insulin dose, or time injection later*
	Reduce calorie intake to promote weight reduction and decrease insulin resistance and hepatic glucose secretion
	Decrease PM snack
Pre-lunch	Increase AM dose of short-acting insulin*
	Alter breakfast meal plan by:
	Decreasing size
	Adjusting composition†
	Divide into meal and AM snack
	Increase activity level in morning
Pre-dinner	Increase dose of AM intermediate-acting or prelunch short-acting insulin*
	Alter meal plan by:
	Decreasing or omitting afternoon snack
	Decreasing size of lunch
	Adjusting composition of lunch†
	Increase activity level in afternoon
Bedtime	Increase dose of PM short-acting insulin*
	Alter dinner meal plan by:
	Decreasing size
	Adjusting composition†
	Increase activity level after dinner
Hypoglycemia	
Fasting	Decrease PM intermediate- or long-acting insulin*
Pre-lunch	Decrease AM dose of short-acting insulin*
	Alter meal plan by:
	Increasing size of breakfast
	Adjusting composition of breakfast†
	Adding mid-morning snack
Pre-dinner	Decrease AM dose of intermediate-acting or prelunch short-acting insulin*
	Alter meal plan by:
	Increasing size of lunch
	Adjusting composition of lunch†
	Adding afternoon snack
	Adjust time of lunch
Bedtime	Decrease PM short-acting insulin dose*
	Alter meal plan by:
	Increasing size of dinner
	Adjusting composition of dinner†
	Increasing size of evening snack

Note: Oral hypoglycemia agents are not included in this table. The choice of an oral agent should be guided by the patient's eating pattern. SMBG patterns of hyper- or hypoglycemia can direct change to an oral agent with a different pharmacokinetic time frame.

*Options for insulin adjustments vary by regimens.

†Changes can be made in the amount or type of carbohydrate, or the amount of protein or fat, or fiber can be increased.

epinephrine, and cortisol increase in response to the stress of infection, illness, or injury. Hepatic glucose production increases dramatically and in turn raises insulin requirements. Thus the person with diabetes who normally takes insulin may need to increase the insulin dose while ill.[6] Likewise, the person not normally using insulin may need insulin coverage at least temporarily to control blood glucose well during illness.

Since food intake generally decreases during illness, it is not uncommon for individuals with diabetes to reduce or stop insulin under the false assumption that they do not need it because they are not eating as much as usual. All patients with diabetes should be taught to identify the signs and symptoms of hyperglycemia and be given personalized guidelines for managing diabetes during times of illness. This should increase their comfort level and skills needed to prevent serious problems with hyperglycemia during illness.

The goal of nutritional management during times of illness is to prevent dehydration and provide adequate nutrition to promote recovery. Carbohydrate intake is the most important concern during brief illness. In general, most diabetic patients should be taught to:

- Monitor blood glucose at least 4 times/day at the onset and throughout illness.
- Test urine for ketones when blood glucose is above 240 mg/dL.
- Continue to take their usual insulin or dose of oral hypoglycemic agent.
- Substitute easily digested liquids or semiliquid foods when solid foods are not tolerated. Replacing 15 g of carbohydrate from solids (starches, breads, or fruit) with 15 g of carbohydrate from liquids every 1 to 2 hours is usually sufficient (Table 2-9).
- 8 to 12 ounces of fluid should be sipped every hour. This may include a carbohydrate source as well as water, tea, broth, and diet soda.
- Call a physician if unable to eat normally for more than 24 hours or if diarrhea and vomiting persist for more than 6 hours.[7,67]

Treating Hypoglycemia

Hypoglycemia or low blood glucose is usually defined as a blood glucose concentration below 70 mg/dL. Hypoglycemia associated with diabetes is a man-made, or treatment-induced, phenomenon as it is produced from either exogenous insulin or oral hypoglycemic agents—thus the more common term *insulin reaction*. To produce an insulin reaction, circulating insulin levels must be elevated in relation to blood glucose levels. The primary causes are either too much insulin, too much exercise, or too little food. Occasionally insulin dosage may be increased inadvertently. During exercise, blood glucose is being used rapidly and hepatic glucose production is suppressed. Children and young adults are more susceptible to hypoglycemic reactions caused by variable and sporadic activity levels.

The most common cause of an insulin reaction is skipping or delaying meals or eating less than normal amounts of carbohydrate at a meal. In general, meals cannot be delayed more than 30 to 60 minutes without a drop in blood glucose when exogenous insulin is being administered. The tighter the blood glucose control, the greater the risk. A

Table 2-9   Food and Beverage Suggestions for Illness

Item	Measure	CHO/gm	Calories
Liquids			
Apple juice (unsweetened)	1/2 c	15	58
Beef broth	1 c	.1	16
Cola drink	1/2 c	14	53
Cranberry juice cocktail	1/2 c	19	74
Eggnog	1/2 c	17	171
Ginger ale	3/4 c	15	62
Grape juice	1/3 c	13	51
Instant breakfast + skim milk	1/2 c	17	101
Gatorade	1 c	15	50
Skim milk	1 c	12	90
Orange juice	1/2 c	13	56
Tomato juice	1 1/2 c	15	64
Semisolids			
Applesauce (unsweetened)	1/2 c	14	53
Cream of wheat	1/2 c	15	76
Cream soup	1 c	15	153
Custard	1/2 c	15	153
Frozen juice bar (DOLE)	1	16	70
Honey	1 T	16	64
Ice cream (vanilla)	1/2 c	16	135
Gelatin (regular)	1/2 c	16	80
Popsicle	1	10	40
Popsicle (sugar-free)	1	5	18
Pudding	1/2 c	30	180
Pudding (sugar-free)	1/2 c	16	103
Saltines	6	15	80
Graham crackers	3	16	80
Sherbet	1/4 c	15	68
Sugar	1 T	12	48
Yogurt (plain, low fat)	1 c	12	120
Yogurt (fruited, low fat)	1/2 c	20	112
Frozen yogurt	1/2 c	16	118
Frozen yogurt (sugar-free)	1/2 c	8	70

Source: Pennington J and Church H: Bowes and Church food values of portions commonly used, ed 15, Phildelphia, 1989, JB Lippincott Co.

snack should be consumed at the regular meal time if a meal is delayed more than 30 to 60 minutes.

Overweight NIDDM patients may experience hypoglycemia during weight reduction diets in which food intake is being reduced. If oral agent or insulin dosages are not reduced accordingly, frequent hypoglycemia may result. This is counterproductive to weight loss efforts since extra food must be eaten to treat a hypoglycemic reaction. Most insulin-requiring NIDDM patients benefit from a reduction in insulin dose at the onset of dieting. It provides the peace of mind they often need to suppress fears of hypoglycemic reactions and can motivate them to stay with their diet plan.

If hypoglycemia is suspected it should be identified by SMBG and treated quickly and appropriately. Most patients have learned to identify the "feeling" or symptoms of hypoglycemia specific to them. Identifying a reaction in small children, however, may be difficult because of their inability to describe or recognize symptoms. Family members can be taught to look for changes in behavior that are often the only clue to impending hypoglycemia. Severe hunger is one behavior. Good-natured children may suddenly become irritable and cranky. High-strung children may become quiet and lethargic. Whenever a reaction is suspected, a blood glucose test should be done quickly to confirm.

Most older individuals will rely on symptoms to forewarn a reaction. Yet, some individuals do not become symptomatic until blood glucose levels become dangerously low (i.e., neurologic changes occur.) Because of the unpleasantness of the experience, low blood glucose reactions are often overtreated with too much food to obtain quick relief. While the treatment goal is to raise blood glucose quickly, rebound hyperglycemia frequently follows a low blood glucose reaction.

Since food used to treat hypoglycemia should be in addition to regular daily intake, weight gain can result if reactions are too frequent or treated inappropriately. An astute clinician will look at SMBG records and frequency of reactions if weight gain is a problem for a person in normally good control.

Overtreating reactions can be avoided by teaching patients to use the 15/15 rule when blood glucose falls below 70 mg/dL:
- Eat 15 g of carbohydrate (Table 2-10).
- Wait 15 minutes then retest blood glucose—if still less than 70 mg/dL, repeat 15/15 rule—do this until blood glucose returns to normal range.
- If there is more than 1 hour to next meal, eat another 15 g of carbohydrate.[23]

Special "treat" foods such as ice cream, cake, and cookies should not be saved to be used only to treat reactions. A low blood glucose reaction can then be used to justify consuming sweets. These treats should be incorporated into the meal plan appropriately as they would be in any healthy diet plan.

Readily portable foods such as raisins, regular soft drinks, juice boxes, and low-fat candies are common foods used to treat reactions. Skim milk is preferred by some individuals but is not always accessible. Some health professionals choose to recommend pure glucose in the form of tablets, liquid, or gel. These products provide a rapid rise in glucose that is considered ideal. Studies suggest that it is the amount of available glucose in a food that determines its usefulness in treating a reaction. Carbohydrate sources that contain more glucose are preferred.

Patients should be taught to be prepared to treat a reaction at all times but that preventing a reaction is probably the best form of preparation. A regular eating schedule, plus anticipating extra exercise with extra food or reduced insulin dose are the best ways to prevent reactions. If hypoglycemia occurs too frequently (2 to 3 times/week), the meal plan and medication regimen need to be evaluated and adjusted if necessary.

Table 2-10   Glucose Sources for Treating Hypoglycemia

Source	Measure	CHO/gm
Glucose products		
Glucose tablets	3	15
Glutose	1-25 g tube	10
Insta glucose	1-31 g tube	30
Monoject gel	1-25 g packet	10
Dextro tabs	9 tablets	15
Foods/drinks		
Hard candy (Life Savers)	5	15
Jelly beans	6	15
Junior mints	7	15
Marshmallows	3 large	15
Raisins	2 T	14
Honey	1 T	17
Sugar	1 T	16
Gelatin (regular)	1/2 c	17
Juice (apple, orange)	1/2 c	14
Milk (skim)	1 c	12
Soft drinks (cola, lemon-lime)	1/2 c	13
Ginger ale	3/4 c	16
Gatorade	1 c	15

Source: Pennington J and Church H: Bowes and Church food values of portions commonly used, ed 15, Philadelphia, 1989, JB Lippincott Co.

A hypoglycemic reaction that leads to unconsciousness must be treated with glucagon or IV glucose. Individuals with IDDM and their families should be taught the use of a glucagon kit.

Nutrition Problems Related to Autonomic Neuropathy

A small number of people with diabetes may develop autonomic neuropathy that progresses to the point that nutritional health is compromised. Gastrointestinal motility can be either slowed or enhanced. Symptoms include heartburn, increased satiety and feeling of fullness, nausea, vomiting, anorexia, and constipation. Severe diarrhea may result in some. Because absorption of nutrients may be delayed or altered by changes in motility, blood glucose control becomes erratic. Blood glucose may peak or drop at unexpected times after eating (i.e., 3 to 4 hours) instead of the expected 2 hours. Careful SMBG and insulin adjustment is necessary to compensate.

Severe nausea, swallowing disorders, vomiting, and diarrhea can lead to fluid, electrolyte, and nutrition imbalances that must be treated appropriately. Nutrition intervention is limited to dividing food intake into frequent smaller meals of easily digested foods that are low in fat. Occasionally, pureed foods or tube feedings need to be used. Drugs such as metoclopromide and antidiarrheals are frequently prescribed.

THE TEAM APPROACH TO DIABETES NUTRITIONAL MANAGEMENT

Diabetes is a team disease. Therapy requires integration of expertise from a variety of medical disciplines. Ideally, a multidisciplinary health care team and the patient collaborate to develop a diabetes management plan that is tailored to his or her abilities, goals, and life-style. Although all members of the team have specific roles, the interrelated nature of diabetes therapy requires each health care member to be knowledgeable about all treatment modalities.

Role of the Patient

Patients must assume an active role in the design as well as in the implementation of their diabetes treatment regimen. Patient involvement has a special significance in planning diet therapy. Medications and monitoring are new skills patients need to learn from health professionals. By contrast, the health professionals must learn from patients about established dietary practices and changes they are willing or able to make in their food intake. The diet history provides the framework for nutrition therapy. When patients select the changes in their diet, they are more likely to assume responsibility for the diet plan and may be more motivated to adhere to the regimen.[54]

Role of the Dietitian

The registered dietitian provides the professional expertise to design the nutrition regimen, to translate it into a practical and flexible meal plan, and to counsel the patient in making dietary modifications. The importance of nutrition therapy to diabetes management has been demonstrated in studies showing dietary adherence is highly correlated with metabolic control.[27] Acquiring knowledge and skills to correctly follow a meal plan for diabetes requires time with a registered dietitian. Initial nutrition consultations are frequently scheduled to last an hour. Follow-up visits are planned according to needs of the individual and generally require from 15 to 30 minutes. Availability of registered dietitians varies, although many diabetes treatment centers include a registered dietitian on their staff. A growing number of dietitians are specializing in diabetes and are members of the Diabetes Care and Education Practice Group of the American Dietetic Association.

Role of the Health Care Team

Although other members of the health care team contribute their own expertise to management of the diabetic patient, they need to support the nutrition education process as well. Questions on diet relate to insulin therapy, exercise, illness, and other aspects of diabetes management. Questions on diet are asked when people think of them, which may be when they are being instructed on SMBG by the nurse or having their feet examined by the podiatrist. While technical questions can be referred to the dietitian as the authoritative member of the team, patients will benefit if their dietary education can be reinforced as often as possible by as many members of their health care team as possible.

REFERENCES

1. Abrams RS and Coustan DR: Gestational diabetes update, Clin Diabetes 8:17-24, 1990.
2. American Diabetes Association: Nutritional recommendations and principles for individuals with diabetes mellitus: 1986, Diabetes Care 10:126-132, 1987.
3. American Diabetes Association: Principles of nutrition and dietary recommendations for patients with diabetes mellitus: 1971, Diabetes Care 20:633-634, 1971.
4. American Diabetes Association: Principles of nutrition and dietary recommendations for individuals with diabetes mellitus: 1979, Diabetes Care 28:1027-1030, 1979.
5. American Diabetes Association: Glycemic effects of carbohydrates, Diabetes Care 7:607-608, 1984.
6. American Diabetes Association, Sperling MA, ed: Physicians guide to IDDM: Diagnosis and treatment, Alexandria, VA, 1988, American Diabetes Association.
7. American Diabetes Association/American Dietetic Association, Powers M, ed: Nutrition guide for professionals, Alexandria, VA and Chicago, 1988, American Diabetes Association/American Dietetic Association.
8. American Dietetic Association: Appropriate use of nutritive and non-nutritive sweeteners: technical support paper, J Am Diet Assoc 87:1690-1694, 1987.
9. American Dietetic Association: Position of the American Dietetic Association: health implications of dietary fiber—technical support paper, J Am Diet Assoc 88:217-221, 1988.
10. Anderson CE: Energy metabolism. In Schneider HA, Anderson CE, and Coursin DB, eds: Nutritional support of medical practices, ed 2, Philadelphia, 1983, Harper & Row Publishers.
11. Armatruda JM and others: The safety and efficacy of a controlled low-energy (very low calorie) diet in the treatment of NIDDM and obesity, Arch Intern Med 148:873-877, 1988.
12. Bantle JP: Clinical aspects of sucrose and fructose metabolism, Diabetes Care 12:56-61, 1989.
13. Bantle JP, Laine DC, and Thomas JW: Metabolic effects of dietary fructose and sucrose in type I and II diabetic subjects, JAMA 256:3241-3246, 1986.
14. Beebe CA: Self blood glucose monitoring: an adjunct to dietary and insulin management of the patient with diabetes, J Am Diet Assoc 87:63, 1987.
15. Beebe CA and others: Nutrition management for individuals with noninsulin-dependent diabetes mellitus in the 1990s: a review by the Diabetes Care and Education Dietetic Practice Group, J Am Diet Assoc 91:196-202, 1991.
16. Beebe CA and others: Effects of temporal distribution of calories on diurnal patterns of glucose levels and insulin secretion in NIDDM, Diabetes Care 13:748-755, 1990.
17. Bergman M, Gidez LI, and Eder HA: High-density lipoprotein subclasses in diabetes, Am Med J 81:488-492, 1986.
18. Bertorelli AM and Czarnowski-Hill JV: Review of present and future use of nonnutritive sweeteners, Diabetes Educ 16:415-420, 1990.
19. Birk R and Spencer ML: The prevalence of anorexia nervosa, bulimia, and induced glycosuria in IDDM females, Diabetes Educ 15:336-341, 1989.
20. Bray GA and others: Eating patterns of massively obese individuals, J Am Diet Assoc 70:94-97, 1980.
21. Brenner BM, Meyer TW, and Hostetter TH: dietary protein intake and the progressive nature of kidney disease, N Engl J Med, 307:652-659, 1982.
22. Brink SJ: Pediatric, adolescent and young adult nutrition issues in IDDM, Diabetes Care 11:192-200, 1988.
23. Brodows RG, Williams C, and Arakuda JM: Treatment of insulin reactions in diabetes, JAMA 252:3378-3381, 1984.
24. Caso EK: Calculation of diabetic diets: report of the committee on diabetic diet calculations, J Am Diet Assoc 26:575-583, 1950.
25. Castelli WP and others: HDL-cholesterol and other lipids in coronary heart disease: the cooperative lipoprotein phenotyping study, Circulation 55:767, 1977.

26. Chantelau E and others: Diet liberalization and metabolic control in Type I diabetic outpatients created by continuous subcutaneous insulin infusion, Diabetes Care 5:612-616, 1982.
27. Christensen NK and others: Quantitative assessment of dietary adherence in patients with insulin-dependent diabetes mellitus, Diabetes Care 6:245-250, 1983.
28. Ciavarella A and others: Reduced albuminuria after dietary protein restriction in IDDM patients with clinical nephropathy, Diabetes Care 10:407-413, 1987.
29. Colagiuri S, Miller JJ, and Edwards RA: Metabolic effects of adding sucrose and aspartame to the diet of subjects with NIDDM, Am J Clin Nutr 50:474-478, 1989.
30. Collings AJ: Metabolism of cyclamate and its conversion to cyclohexylamine, Diabetes Care 12:50-55, 1989.
31. Connor W and Connor S: The dietary prevention and treatment of coronary heart disease. In Connor W and Bristow JD, eds: Coronary heart disease: prevention, complications and treatment, Philadelphia, 1985, JB Lippincott.
32. Coulston AM and others: Persistence of hypertriglyceridemic effect of low-fat high-carbohydrate diets in NIDDM patients, Diabetes Care 12:94-101, 1989.
33. Coulston AM and others: Deleterious metabolic effects of high-carbohydrate, sucrose-containing diets in patient with non-insulin-dependent diabetes mellitus, Am Med J 82:213-220, 1987.
34. Crapo PA: Carbohydrate. In Powers MA, ed: Handbook of diabetes nutritional management, Rockville, MD, 1987, Aspen Publishers.
35. Crapo PA: Use of alternative sweeteners in diabetic diets, Diabetes Care 11:174-182, 1988.
36. Crapo PA, Reaven G, and Olefsky JM: Postprandial glucose and insulin responses to different complex carbohydrates, Diabetes 26:1723-1728, 1977.
37. Brink SJ, ed: Diabetes Task Force: nutritional management of children and adolescents with insulin-dependent diabetes mellitus, Elk Grove Village, IL, 1985, American Academy of Pediatrics.
38. DCCT Research Group: Weight gain associated with intensive therapy in the diabetes control and complications trial, Diabetes Care 11:567-573, 1988.
39. Dreon DM and others: Dietary fat: carbohydrate ratio and obesity in middle aged men, Am J Clin Nutr 47:995-1000, 1988.
40. Ducimetiere P and others: Relationship of plasma insulin levels to the incidence of myocardial infarction and coronary heart disease mortality in a middle-aged population, Diabetologia 19:205-210, 1980.
41. Evanoff GV and others: The effect of dietary protein restriction on the progression of diabetic nephropathy, Arch Intern Med 147:492-495, 1987.
42. Fagen C: Guidelines for nutritional management of diabetes, J Am Diet Assoc 90(suppl 9):A-147, 1990.
43. Feurer ID and others: Resting energy expenditure in morbid obesity, Ann Surg 197:17-21, 1983.
44. Food and Nutrition Board, National Academy of Sciences–National Research Council, Recommended Dietary Allowances, ed 10, 1989.
45. Franz MJ: Alcohol and diabetes. Part I: metabolism and guidelines, Diabetes Spectrum 3:136-144, 1990.
46. Franz MJ and others: Exchange lists: revised 1986, J Am Diet Assoc 87:28-34, 1987.
47. Fukargawa NK and Young VR: Protein and amino acid metabolism and requirements in older persons, Clin Geriatr Med 3:329-337, 1987.
48. Garg A and others: Comparison of a high-carbohydrate diet with a high-monounsaturated-fat diet in patients with noninsulin-dependent diabetes mellitus, N Engl J Med 319:829-834, 1988.
49. Ginsberg HN and others: Reduction of plasma cholesterol levels in normal men on an American Heart Association step 1 diet or a step 1 diet with added monounsaturated fat, N Engl J Med 322:574-579, 1990.
50. Glauber H and others: Adverse metabolic effect of omega-3 fatty acids in non-insulin dependent diabetes mellitus, Ann Intern Med 108:663-668, 1988.
51. Gordon T and others: High density lipoprotein as a protective factor against coronary heart disease: the Framingham Study, Am J Med 62:707-714, 1977.
52. Gore GP, Huff TA, and Stachuro ME: Pathophysiology. In Powers MS, ed: Handbook of diabetes nutritional management, Rockville, MD, 1987, Aspen Publishers.
53. Grundy SM: Comparison of monounsaturated fatty acids and carbohydrates for lowering plasma cholesterol, N Engl J Med 314:745-748, 1986.
54. Haire-Joshu D: Motivation and diabetes self-care: an educational challenge, Diabetes Spectrum 1:279-282, 1988.

55. Haffner SM and others: Do upper-body and centralized adiposity measure different aspects of regional body-fat distribution? Relationship to NIDDM, lipids and lipoproteins, Diabetes 36:43-51, 1987.

56. Heber D: Macronutrient nutrition for aging. In Morley JE, moderator: Nutrition in the elderly, Ann Intern Med 109:890-904, 1988.

57. Hendra TJ and others: Effects of fish oil supplements in NIDDM subjects, Diabetes Care 13:821-829, 1990.

58. Irvine AA and others: Validation of scale measuring environmental barriers to diabetes regimen adherence, Diabetes Care 13:705-711, 1990.

59. Jovanovic-Peterson L: Dietary manipulation as a primary treatment for gestational diabetic pregnancy, Diabetes Profess Winter:11-22, 1989-90.

60. Jenkins DJA and others: The glycemic response to carbohydrate foods, Lancet 2:388-391, 1984.

61. Jenkins DJA, Wolever TMS, and Jenkins AL: Starchy foods and glycemic index, Diabetes Care 11:149-159, 1988.

62. Jenkins DJA and others: Glycemic index of foods: a physiological basis for carbohydrate exchange, Am J Clin Nutr 34:362-366, 1981.

63. Kennedy AL and others: Relation of high-density lipoprotein cholesterol concentration to type of diabetes and its control, Br Med J 2:1191-1194, 1978.

64. Knowles H and others: The course of juvenile diabetes treated with unmeasured diets, Diabetes 14:239-273, 1965.

65. Kromhout D, Bosschieter EB, and Caulander C: The inverse relation between fish consumption and 20-year mortality from coronary heart disease, New Engl J Med 312:1205[]-1209, 1985.

66. Kurtz MS: Adherence to diabetes regimens: emperical status and clinical applications, Diabetes Educ 16:50-56, 1990.

67. Ley B and Goldman D: Sick-day management: a partnership in preparation for the expected, Clin Diabetes 8:25-30, 1990.

68. Lipid Research Clinics Program: The lipid research clinics coronary primary prevention trial results. II. The relationship of reduction in incidence of coronary heart disease to cholesterol lowering, JAMA 251:365-374, 1984.

69. Marshall RE: Infant of the diabetic mother: a neonatologist's view, Clin Diabetes 8:51-57, 1990.

70. McArdle WD, Katch FI, and Katch VL: Obesity and weight control: exercise physiology, energy, nutrition and human performance, Philadelphia, 1986, Lea & Febiger.

71. Mensick RD and others: Effects of monounsaturated fatty acids versus complex carbohydrates on serum lipoproteins and apoproteins in healthy men and women, Metabolism 38:172-178, 1989.

72. Mensink RP and Katan MB: Effect of monounsaturated fatty acids versus complex carbohydrates on high-density lipoproteins in healthy men and women, Lancet 1:122-125, 1987.

73. Miller SA and Frattali VP: Saccharin, Diabetes Care 12:75-80, 1989.

74. Munro HN and Crim MC:The proteins and amino acids. In Goodhart RS, ed: Modern nutrition in health and disease, Philadelphia, 1980, Lea & Febiger.

75. Nathan DM and others: Ice cream in the diet of insulin-dependent diabetic patients, JAMA 251:2825-2827, 1984.

76. Ney DM: Nutritional management of diabetes during pregnancy, Pract Diabetol 7:1-8, 1988.

77. National Institutes of Health: Consensus development conference on diet and exercise in NIDDM, Diabetes Care 10:639-644, 1987.

78. Nuttall FQ and Hollenbeck CB: Current issues in nutrition and metabolism, Part I, Diabetes Spectrum 2:123-128, 1989.

79. O'Dea K, Snow P, and Nestel P: Rate of starch hydrolysis in vitro as a predictor of metabolic responses to complex carbohydrate in vivo, Am J Clin Nutr 34:1991-1993, 1981.

80. Oldrizzi L and others: Progression of renal failure in patients with renal disease of diverse etiology on protein-restricted diets, Kidney Int 27:553-557, 1985.

81. Ostlund RE and others: The ratio of waist-to-hip circumference, plasma insulin level, and glucose intolerance as independent predictors of the HDL_2 cholesterol level in older adults, N Engl J Med 322:229-234, 1990.

82. Paige MS and Heins JM: Nutritional management of diabetic patients during intensive insulin therapy, Diabetes Educ 14:505-509, 1988.

83. Pellett PL: Food energy requirements in humans, Am J Clin Nutr 51:711-722, 1990.
84. Peters AL, Davidson MD, and Eisenberg K: Effect of isocaloric substitution of chocolate cake for potato in Type I diabetic patients, Diabetes Care 13:888-892, 1990.
85. Phillipson BE and others: Reduction of plasma lipids, lipoproteins, and apoproteins by dietary fish oils in patients with hypertriglyceridemia, N Engl J Med 312:1210-1216, 1985.
86. Pietri AO and others: The effect of continuous subcutaneous insulin infusion on very-low-density lipoprotein triglyceride metabolism in Type I diabetes mellitus, Diabetes 32:75-81, 1983.
87. Powers MA and Lane DC: Sweeteners. In Powers MA, ed: Handbook of diabetes nutritional management, Rockville, MD, 1987, Aspen Publishers.
88. Powers MA, Metzger BE, and Freinkel N: Pregnancy and diabetes. In Powers MS ed: Handbook of diabetes nutritional management, Rockville, MD, 1987, Aspen Publishers.
89. Rosenstock J and others: Reduction in cardiovascular risk factors with intensive diabetes treatment in insulin dependent diabetes mellitus, Diabetes Care 10:729-734, 1987.
90. Second International Workshop—Conference on Gestational Diabetes: Summary and recommendations, Diabetes 34:123-126, 1985.
91. Sims EAH and Danforth E: Expenditure and shortage of energy in man, J Clin Invest 79:1019-1025, 1987.
92. Skyler JS: Non–insulin-dependent diabetes mellitus: a clinical strategy, Diabetes Care 7(suppl 1):118-129, 1984.
93. Sparrow D and others: Relationship of fat distribution to glucose tolerance, Diabetes 35:411-415, 1986.
94. Stancin T, Link DL, and Reuter JM: Binge eating and purging in young women with IDDM, Diabetes Care 12:601-603, 1989.
95. Tinker LF: Dietary fiber: variables that affect its nutritional impact, Diabetes Spectrum 3:191-196, 1990.
96. Vinik AI and Jenkins DJA: Dietary fiber in management of diabetes, Diabetes Care 11:160-173, 1988.
97. Warshaw HS: Alternative sweeteners: past, present, pending and potential, Diabetes Spectrum 3:335-343, 1990.
98. Wheeler ML: Fiber and the diabetic diet. In Powers MA, ed: Handbook of diabetes nutritional management, Rockville, MD, 1987, Aspen Publishers.
99. Wing RR, Klein R, and Mars SE: Weight gain associated with improved glycemic control in population-based sample of subjects with type I diabetes, Diabetes Care 13:1106-1109, 1990.
100. Wise JE and others: Effect of sucrose-containing snacks on blood glucose control, Diabetes Care 12:423-426, 1989.
101. Witztum JL and others: Nonenzymatic glycosylation of low-density lipoprotein alters its biologic activity, Diabetes 31:283-291, 1982.
102. Zavaroni I and others: Risk factors for coronary artery disease in healthy persons with hyperinsulinenia and normal glucose tolerance, N Engl J Med 320:702-706, 1989.

Appendix 2a

PLANNING A DIET USING THE EXCHANGE LISTS

1. Identify desirable body weight using height-weight tables or Rule of Thumb (see Table 2-6).
2. Estimate daily calorie requirement (see Table 2-7). Adjust if weight loss or weight gain is desirable (± 500 calories = approximately $\pm$ 1 pound/week).
3. From diet history calculate current caloric intake using Exchange values.

Exchange list	Carbohydrate (g)	Protein (g)	Fat (g)	Calories
Starch/bread	15	3	trace	80
Meat				
Lean	—	7	3	55
Medium-fat	—	7	5	75
High-fat	—	7	8	100
Vegetable	5	2	—	25
Fruit	15	—	—	60
Milk				
Skim	12	8	trace	90
Low-fat	12	8	5	120
Whole	12	8	8	150
Fat	—	—	5	45

4. Compare usual intake with ADA Nutrient Recommendations and other therapeutic strategies for diabetes management. Consider:
   Calorie level.
   Calories from macronutrients.
   Distribution of food intake into meals and snacks to maximize efficiency of endogenous or exogenous insulin.
   Overall good nutrition.
   Diabetes medication.
5. Determine changes in usual intake, set goals with patient.
6. Using the nutrient values for each exchange list, calculate a meal plan to meet goals.

Example:

Sam Jones is a 45-year-old male, newly diagnosed with NIDDM.

Assessment:

Height:	5 feet 9 inches (172.5 cm)*
Weight:	162 pounds (73.6 kg)*
Frame:	medium
Activity:	sedentary—business requires out-of-town travel by car
Medication:	OTC for allergy
Health:	good—reports no other medical problems; father has NIDDM
Education:	college degree
Lifestyle:	married with two children; hobbies include fishing and reading

Step 1: Identify desirable body weight (see Table 2-6)

106 lbs plus 54 lbs = 160 lbs (73 kg)

Step 2: Estimate calories for weight maintenance (see Table 2-7, p. 59)

Harris-Benedict equation:

$$REE = 66.5 + (13.75 \times 73 \text{ kg}) + (5.03 \times 172.5 \text{ cm}) - (6.75 \times 45) = 1634.18$$

REE × Activity factor = Estimate of daily calorie requirement: 1634 × 1.3 = 2124 calories/day

Step 3: From diet history calculate current caloric intake using exchange values.

Diet history: Never followed a diet. Eats many meals away from home due to travel.

24 hour dietary recall

Breakfast:	Exchanges	Calories
1 egg, fried	1 meat, 1 fat	120
2 slices toast	2 bread	160
2 pats butter	2 fat	90
2% low-fat milk, 8 oz.	1 lowfat milk	120
Lunch: (Fast food chain)		
Hamburger, quarter pounder	3 high-fat meat	300
	2 bread	160
French fries, large	2 bread + 2 fat	250
Soft drink, 10 oz.	no exchange	120
Dinner:		
Roast beef—2 large slices (4 oz)	4 meat	300
Mashed potatoes with gravy	1 bread + 1 fat	125
Roll with butter	1 bread + 1 fat	125
Green beans	1 vegetable	25
Salad with dressing	free food + 2 fat	90
Ice tea with 2 t. sugar	no exchange	32
Snack:		
Ice Cream, 1 c.	2 bread + 2 fat	250
	Total	2267

*Conversion table: inches × 2.5 = centimeters; pounds ÷ 2.2 = kilograms.

Step 4: Compare usual intake with ADA Nutrient Recommendation and therapeutic strategies for diabetes management:

Calorie level: current intake is close to estimate, weight OK, needs to increase activity

Calories from macronutrients: high intake of fat, protein, and simple carbohydrate

Distribution of food among meals: appears adequate for diet therapy

Overall good nutrition: diet is low in fruits, vegetables, and fiber

Diabetes medication: none prescribed at this time

Step 5: Determine changes in usual intake and discuss with patient.

Goal: Reduce fat intake to 30% of calories, modify protein intake, increase fiber intake and consumption of fruits and vegetables. Increase activity.

Discuss options with patient: High-fiber breakfast cereals, whole grain bread and lean meat selections are acceptable. Fruits and vegetables OK. Will initiate walking program.

Step 6: Using nutrient values for each exchange list, calculate a meal plan to meet goals.

Worksheet for Calculating a Meal Plan

Food Group	Breakfast	Snack	Lunch	Snack	Dinner	Snack	Total servings/day	CHO (g)	Protein (g)	Fat (g)	Calories	Fiber (g)
Starch/Bread	3		3		2	1	9	135 ^{15}	27 ^{3}	9 ^{1}	720 ^{80}	18 ^{2}
Meats/Substitutes			2		3		5		35 ^{7}	25 ^{5}	375 ^{75}	
Vegetables					2		2	10 ^{5}	4 ^{2}		50 ^{25}	4 ^{2}
Fruits	3		3		2	2	10	150 ^{15}			600 ^{60}	20 ^{2}
Milk	1						1	12 ^{12}	8 ^{8}	1	90 ^{90}	
Fats	1		2		3	1	7			35 ^{5}	315 ^{45}	
Total								307	74	70	2150	42
Calories								$^{\times 4} = $ 1228	$^{\times 4} = $ 296	$^{\times 9} = $ 630		
Percent calories								57	14	29		

SAMPLE MENU PLAN
———————— **(MAINTENANCE DIET FOR 160-POUND MALE)** ————————

Breakfast

1 cup of bran flakes
1 cup milk, skim/low fat
½ banana
1 slice whole wheat toast
1 tsp. margarine

Lunch

2 oz. lean beef roast
2 slices whole wheat bread
Lettuce and tomato for sandwich
1 tsp. mayonnaise
1 nectarine
2 small chocolate chip cookies
1 cup apple juice

Dinner

3 oz. chicken breast
1 baked potato
1 slice whole wheat bread
1 cup broccoli
1 cup lettuce salad
2 tsp. margarine
1 tbsp. Italian salad dressing
1 cup canned pears (juice pack)

Snack

3 cups popcorn (air popped)
1 tsp. margarine
1 large apple

CHAPTER **3** _____

Exercise and Diabetes

MARION J. FRANZ

INTRODUCTION

Over the past 10 years interest in the role that exercise plays in diabetes management has increased. Just as the general public's interest and participation in exercise have increased, the interest and participation in exercise of persons with diabetes have increased as well. As a result, professionals are reexamining the role of exercise in diabetes management—both its benefits and risks. In addition, with more research available, health care providers have been better able to prepare guidelines to assist persons with diabetes to exercise safely. However, the response to exercise is still highly variable and requires a participant who is willing and able to monitor the individualized effects of exercise on metabolic parameters.

This chapter begins by reviewing the metabolic and hormonal adaptations of exercise in nondiabetic persons and the alterations that occur in persons with diabetes mellitus. Research related to strategies recommended to help persons with diabetes exercise safely is reviewed next. Special situations, such as exercise recommendations during pregnancy, for the elderly, for persons with long-term complications of diabetes, and for the athlete with diabetes, will also be discussed.

The purpose of this chapter is to (1) identify three sources of fuel substrate used by exercising muscle; (2) list hormones involved with exercise and discuss their role in maintaining glucose balance; (3) discuss the metabolic and hormonal responses to exercise in persons with diabetes; (4) explain five factors related to the effects of exercise in persons with insulin-dependent diabetes mellitus (IDDM); (5) compare five strategies that can be used to assist persons with IDDM exercise safely; (6) assess five strategies that can be used by athletes with diabetes to exercise safely; (7) discuss the benefits and risks of exercise for persons with non–insulin-dependent diabetes mellitus (NIDDM); (8) summarize five strategies that can be used to assist persons with NIDDM exercise safely; (9) describe precautions women with diabetes should take if exercising during pregnancy; (10) describe precautions for elderly persons with diabetes and persons with complica-

80

tions of diabetes during exercise; and (11) identify the components of an exercise program.

In persons with IDDM, metabolic control is best achieved by a regular or consistent life-style that includes regular meals and snacks covered by the appropriate amount of insulin on a day-to-day basis. Adding exercise to this equation often increases the difficulty of maintaining metabolic control since exercise, especially acute exercise bouts, can drastically alter the delicate balance of glucose. However, this does not mean that persons with IDDM should be discouraged from exercising. Instead, assistance from health care providers may be necessary for them to be able to exercise safely and thus receive the same benefits and enjoyment from exercise as persons without diabetes receive.

In contrast, in persons with NIDDM, exercise has been shown to be a useful adjunct to diet for improved metabolic and weight control and to lessen the risk for cardiovascular disease. The beneficial effects of exercise on blood glucose levels are, however, of a short duration and appear to result primarily from the overlapping acute effects.[76] This emphasizes the importance of regular exercise. For exercise to be of benefit, it must be performed regularly (a minimum of three to four times a week) and on a long-term basis. If exercise is to be performed correctly and safely, persons with NIDDM will also require assistance from professionals.

FUEL METABOLISM DURING AND AFTER EXERCISE

During exercise it is necessary to ensure the delivery of oxygen and metabolic fuels to working muscles as well as the removal of metabolic end-products. Increased oxygen delivery and carbon dioxide removal are accomplished by increased respiration, increased cardiac output, redistribution of blood flow, and increased capillary perfusion of working muscles. Changes in the use of metabolic fuels is a more complex process.

For example, blood glucose during long-duration exercise in nondiabetic persons is maintained at a fairly stable level despite what can be a twentyfold increase in whole body oxygen, five- to sixfold increase in cardiac output, and an even greater increase in blood flow and oxygen consumption in the working muscles.[65]

Muscle Metabolism During Exercise

In the resting state, skeletal muscle accounts for 35% to 40% of total oxygen consumption. During exercise, consumption of oxygen and metabolic fuels in muscle increases dramatically to provide adenosine triphosphate (ATP), the energy necessary for muscle contractions. At the start of exercise the muscle cell uses fuel stored locally in the form of glycogen and triglycerides (see Fig. 3-1), these substances being readily available as sources of fuel for the glycolytic pathway and the citric acid cycle.

The rapid breakdown of muscle glycogen stores is stimulated by activation of the sympathetic nervous system and is enhanced by adrenaline (epinephrine)[66] and by a high preexercise glycogen contribution.[69] It may be inhibited by high concentrations of free fatty acids (FFA).[20] The regulation of muscle triglyceride use during exercise has not

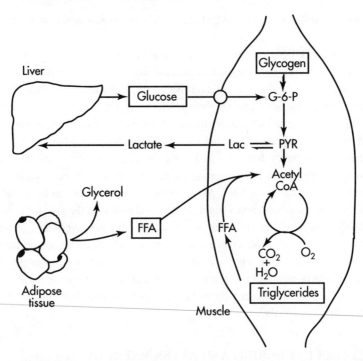

Fig. 3-1 Muscle cell fuel sources. A schematic diagram of the muscle cell and its intracellular and extracellular fuel sources. During exercise the use of both carbohydrate and lipid fuels increases and nearly all steps in the pathway of glucose metabolism are enhanced. Some of the glucose not oxidized by muscle is released into the circulation as lactate which, in turn, may be used for glucose synthesis by the liver (Cori cycle). Glycerol derived from the hydrolysis of adipose tissue triglyceride may also be used by the liver for gluconeogenesis. (Reprinted with permission from Richter EA, Ruderman NB, and Schneider SH: Diabetes and exercise, Am J Med 70:202, 1981.)

been studied thoroughly. Because intracellular fuel sources are limited, muscle cells soon depend on fuel sources from circulating blood as well as from tissue stores.

Following an overnight fast, the major fuel of resting muscle is FFA released from adipose tissue.[1] During exercise, use of carbohydrate as fuel increases, and the increase is greater as the intensity of exercise increases.[87] As shown in Fig. 3-1, glycogen breakdown and glucose uptake into the muscle cell are increased, as is the flux of glucose through the glycolytic pathway, the conversion of pyruvate to acetyl coenzyme A (CoA) and the oxidation of acetyl CoA in the citric acid cycle. Some of the glucose not oxidized by muscle is released into the circulation as lactate, which may be used for glucose synthesis by the liver (Cori cycle). During exercise the use of lipid fuels also increases, and glycerol derived from the hydrolysis of adipose tissue triglycerides may also be used by the liver for gluconeogenesis.[60,67]

The mechanism that accounts for the increase in glucose uptake in contracting muscle is thought to involve both an increase in membrane permeability for glucose[64] and an increase in the activity of the enzymes involved in glucose disposal.[46] The transport of glucose into the muscle cell is almost exclusively by facilitated diffusion, brought about by a process involving membrane-associated glucose-transporter units that facilitate hexose transport through the membrane.[92] The rate of glucose transport increases in response to both insulin and muscle contractions.[91]

It was thought that muscle contractions would only increase this glucose transport and uptake with the availability of some small, but necessary amount of insulin. However, research in isolated perfused rat muscle has shown that muscles contracting in the absence of insulin can increase transport and uptake of glucose into muscle cells, although this effect is short-lived.[60] Despite this, in persons with diabetes, insulin-deficient ketotic states impair peripheral glucose use. This has been ascribed to the exaggerated counterregulatory hormone response that acts to further augment hepatic glucose production.[94] Additionally, a rise in the concentration of FFA and ketone bodies seen during ketosis decreases glucose uptake.[62] These responses, rather than impairment of membrane permeability for glucose per se, produce a progressive hyperglycemia and can lead to ketoacidosis in ketoacidosis-prone diabetic patients.[10]

The pattern of muscle fuel use (see Fig. 3-2) is triphasic, in which muscle glycogen,

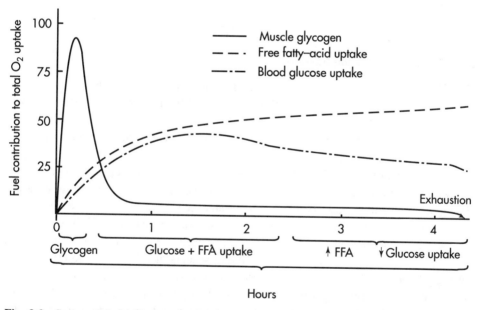

Fig. 3-2 Stages of fuel utilization by muscle in prolonged exercise. The relative contribution of muscle glycogen and blood glucose and free fatty acids to oxidative energy during various time periods of exercise. (Reprinted with permission from Felig P and Koivisto VA: Metabolic response to exercise. Implications for diabetes. In Lowenthal DT, Bhradwaja K, and Oaks WW, ed: Therapeutics through exercise, New York, 1979, Grune & Stratton, Inc.)

blood glucose, and FFA successively predominate as the major fuel substrate. During the first 5 to 10 minutes of exercise, muscle glycogen is the major fuel consumed.[45] As exercise continues and blood flow to muscle increases, blood-borne substrates become increasingly important sources of energy. If exercise continues for 10 to 40 minutes, glucose uptake by muscle rises to 7 to 20 times the basal level and accounts for 30% to 40% of total oxygen consumed by muscle.[86] This is comparable to the need for blood-borne FFA, which provides an additional 40% of oxidizable fuel. The remainder continues to be from nonblood-borne fuels (muscle glycogen and intramuscular lipids). Beyond 40 minutes of exercise, glucose use increases until it peaks at 90 to 180 minutes and then declines slightly.[1] FAA use continues to increase during 1 to 4 hours of exercise as the uptake of FFA by muscles rises to approximately 70%. Thus, after 4 hours of continuous mild exercise, FFA contribute twice the fuel as does glucose.[30]

Blood Glucose Use During Exercise

Blood glucose concentrations change little during mild to moderate exercise, but may increase 1.1 to 1.7 mM (20 to 30 mg/dL) with more intense exercise. However, if exercise continues 90 minutes or more, blood glucose levels may decrease 0.5 to 2.2 mM (10 to 40 mg). Hypoglycemia (blood glucose <2.2 mM [40 mg/dL]) is rare, however, in nondiabetic persons.[30]

Liver Metabolism During Exercise

To maintain euglycemia and to prevent hypoglycemia during exercise, the increase in glucose use at the cellular level must be counterbalanced by an increase in hepatic glucose output (see Fig. 3-1). The increase in glucose production at the beginning of exercise mainly results from glycogenolysis, but as exercise continues, gluconeogenesis plays an increasingly important role.[1]

At rest, approximately 75% of the hepatic glucose output comes from glycogenolysis, with the remaining 25% to 30% from gluconeogenesis. During short-term exercise, liver glucose output increases two to five times and keeps pace with the use of glucose by muscle tissue. This is primarily as a result of additional glycogenolysis.[86] The liver usually contains no more than 50 to 100 grams of glycogen, and if exercise is prolonged and intense, it will be completely expended. (During 4 hours of exercise, 50 to 60 grams of liver glycogen can be mobilized—a 75% or more depletion of total liver glycogen stores.) When this occurs, glucose can be derived only from gluconeogenesis. Therefore gluconeogenesis becomes more important during prolonged exercise and may account for 40% to 50% of hepatic glucose output. The principal gluconeogenic precursor during exercise is lactate released by the contracting, and also by the resting, muscles in heavy exercise.[2] However, alanine and glycerol may also be used, especially during the later stages of prolonged exercise.[29]

Table 3-1 Sources of Fuel for Exercise

Exercise duration	Source of fuel	Substrate
First 5 to 10 minutes	Intramuscular	Glycogen (triglycerides)
10 to 40 minutes	Circulating substrates	Glucose and FFA
40 minutes and longer	Tissue stores	
	Liver	Glucose from glycogenolysis and gluconeogenesis
	Adipose tissue	Triglycerides FFA

Reprinted with permission from Franz MJ: Exercise and diabetes mellitus. In Powers MA ed: Handbook of diabetes nutritional management, Rockville, Md, 1987, Aspen Publishers, Inc.

Fuel Sources for Exercise

An orderly sequence of fuel use takes place during prolonged exercise. At first, intramuscular fuels are the primary source. As exercise continues, the blood-borne fuels of glucose and eventually FFA become increasingly important. As exercise progresses, circulating substrates are also limited, requiring mobilization of substrates from tissue stores, that is, glycogen from the liver and fat in the form of triglycerides stored in adipose tissue. (See Table 3-1 for a summary of sources of fuel for exercise.) This switch from local to circulating fuels and from carbohydrates to lipid is important for endurance capacity, since extramuscular fat stores are the most abundant energy source. Ketone bodies can be used, but they do not normally make a substantial contribution to the overall energy supply.[40]

In a nonobese man, fat accounts for 80% to 85% of body fuel stores (approximately 140,000 kcal in a 70 kg man).[30] Metabolizing this fat requires a substantial amount of oxygen, which means exercise intensity must be reduced and some carbohydrate made available. To the endurance athlete an important function of fat metabolism is glycogen sparing. With training the body develops the ability to sustain long periods of muscle contractions by using fat for 50% to 85% of energy needs. Glycogen stores are thereby conserved.

However, the oxidation of fat-derived fuels cannot fully replace the use of glucose, even during prolonged exercise. When the supply of carbohydrate is limited the oxidation of fat is incomplete, resulting in the production of ketone bodies. These ketone bodies can later be reused in the fatty acid oxidation cycle of skeletal musculature, but may also be excreted in the urine, resulting in a net energy loss.

The major problem with glucose as the primary fuel source is its limited storage capacity. In contrast to stored fat, stored carbohydrate accounts for approximately 1500 kcal—300 to 400 grams of muscle glycogen (approximately 15 g/kg muscle), 50 to 100 grams of liver glycogen, and 20 grams of glucose in extracellular water.[88] Muscle glycogen can only be used to meet the energy needs of the muscle in which it is contained.

Liver glycogen, however, can be used gradually during periods of starvation or rapidly mobilized in response to exercise or hypoglycemia.

Physical training enhances the body's ability to store and use carbohydrate; however, even trained athletes store only approximately 2000 kcal in the body as blood glucose and liver and muscle glycogen. If carbohydrates were the only fuel used during exercise, sports activities lasting more than 2 hours would be impossible because overwhelming fatigue and exhaustion occur when muscle glycogen becomes depleted. Why glycogen depletion coincides with fatigue is not clear since large amounts of circulating substrate in the form of FFA are still available.[30]

Carbohydrate is the main fuel for short-duration, high intensity exercise. Its glucose structure contains more oxygen than other nutrients. This allows for rapid oxidation and release of energy. Glucose is the only substrate that can be used in anaerobic glycolysis and is the main substrate serving the energy needs of the brain and nervous system.

Protein combustion during exercise is generally believed to be insignificant, provided the exercise is not excessively heavy or prolonged. Protein accounts for 15% to 20% of body fuel stores (30,000 to 40,000 kcal). Its usefulness as a fuel is limited because its consumption would necessitate the breakdown of muscle or other tissue.[30]

Hormonal Response to Exercise

In the resting state, glucose production is modulated by the balance between insulin and the counterregulatory hormones. Increases in plasma insulin and glucose inhibit hepatic glucose production, whereas increases in glucagon, glucocorticoids, and catecholamines and decreases in insulin and glucose promote it. These factors also influence hepatic glucose output during exercise.[36]

The plasma concentration of insulin decreases during exercise of an intensity above approximately 50% $Vo_{2\ max}$, 66% of which is due to alpha-adrenergic inhibition of insulin secretion, and 33% of which is due to an enhanced insulin removal rate.[94,37] This, in combination with the increase in counterregulatory hormones, induces an impressive increase of glucose output from the liver and may also contribute to the increase in adipose tissue lipolysis, as well as act as a restraint on glucose use by nonexercising muscle.

The precise role of various neuroendocrine responses to exercise in the regulation of carbohydrate metabolism is unclear. A number of hormones probably play a role and it is their interaction with each other and with the autonomic nervous system that regulates glucose homeostasis.

The counterregulatory hormones—glucagon, growth hormone, cortisol, norepinephrine, and epinephrine—play an important role in glucose homeostasis during exercise. Norepinephrine, reflecting sympathetic nervous system activation, is of major importance in stimulating glycogenolysis in both liver and muscle and in stimulating lipolysis in adipose tissue.[27] Epinephrine increases in response to high-intensity exercise or declining blood glucose and also stimulates hepatic glycogenolysis and lipolysis.[37]

Growth hormone and cortisol are less important in response to short-term exercise,

Table 3-2   Hormonal Response to Exercise

Hormone	Effect	Result
Insulin	Decreased	Increases glucose output from the liver
		Stimulates glucose utilization by exercising muscle cells
		Increases adipose tissue lipolysis
		Restrains glucose utilization by nonexercising muscle cells
Counterregulatory hormones		
Epinephrine	Increased	Stimulates rapid breakdown of muscle glycogen stores at the start of exercise
		In response to high-intensity exercise of declining blood glucose—stimulates hepatic glycogenolysis and adipose tissue lipolysis
Norepinephrine	Increased	Stimulates glycogenolysis in both liver and muscle
		Stimulates lipolysis in adipose tissue
Growth hormone and cortisol	Increased	Less important in short-term exercise—increases lipolysis and decreases glucose uptake in peripheral tissues
		Over longer periods of exercise—increases gluconeogenesis
Glucagon	Increased	Stimulates glucose production by the liver

but they increase lipolysis, decrease insulin-stimulated glucose uptake in peripheral tissues, and increase hepatic gluconeogenesis over longer periods of exercise.[37]

Studies with dogs[93] and rats[68] have suggested that glucagon plays a role in increasing hepatic glucose production during exercise. However, in humans, some evidence suggests that glucagon *does not play* an important role in increasing hepatic glucose production.[14] These studies report that a glucagon deficiency does not significantly impair the early glycogenolytic response to exercise. Plasma concentrations of glucagon increased late during prolonged exercise at a time when plasma glucose concentrations began to decrease.[67] Their potential effect is to play a significant role in stimulating gluconeogenesis at this point in exercise.[14] The more traditional view of the role of glucagon during exercise is that it is the primary hormone for the stimulation and maintenance of increased hepatic glucose production, increasing both glycogenolysis and gluconeogenesis to prevent hypoglycemia as a result of increased muscle glucose uptake.[36] It has been demonstrated that glucagon is responsible for 75% of the increase in hepatic glucose production during exercise.[88] (See Table 3-2 for a summary of hormonal responses to exercise.)

Postexercise Response

After exercise of an intensity that depletes muscle glycogen stores, replenishment becomes a high metabolic priority. This happens by an increase, lasting several hours, in insulin sensitivity of the exercised muscles and by a noninsulin-dependent increase in muscle glucose uptake. Whole-body insulin sensitivity has been found to be increased for at least 48 hours following 1 hour of bicycling at a moderate intensity.[54] This increase in insulin sensitivity after exercise may contribute to hypoglycemia in persons with IDDM.

Upon cessation of exercise, blood flow is redistributed from previously exercising muscles, and blood flow to the splanchnic bed increases. The overall effect is to initiate repletion of glycogen stores in muscle as well as in the liver. Glucose uptake by muscle remains 3 to 4 times the basal level for at least 40 minutes after exercise. Repletion of liver glycogen is facilitated by a rapid decline in splanchnic glucose output, which reaches basal levels by 40 minutes.[30] At the same time, uptake of gluconeogenic substrates increases. Thus liver glycogen can be repleted even in the absence of glucose ingestion.

The hormonal response to the cessation of exercise is characterized by a rapid increase in insulin levels within 2 to 10 minutes.[85] In contrast, glucagon concentration remains at the same high level during recovery[31] and may contribute to the increase in hepatic uptake of gluconeogenic precursors.

ALTERATIONS IN FUEL METABOLISM IN PERSONS WITH IDDM DURING AND AFTER EXERCISE

During exercise, the working muscles use their own store of glycogen and triglycerides as well as glucose released by the liver and FFAs derived from adipose tissue lipolysis. Changes in the use of these metabolic fuels can occur in persons with diabetes, especially persons with IDDM.

Muscle Glycogen Use

Direct measurements of muscle glycogen content in acutely insulin-deprived persons with diabetes indicate that the rate of glycogen use is the same as in nondiabetic persons. However, resynthesis is an insulin-dependent process. Thus, in the absence of insulin therapy, muscle glycogen repletion is minimal in persons with diabetes, whereas with insulin the rate of repletion is the same.[88]

Blood Glucose Levels During Exercise

Before the advent of insulin, accumulated evidence showed that in insulin-deficient persons with diabetes, exercise resulted in a more pronounced hyperglycemia, hyperketonemia, and glycosuria; in fact, strenuous exertion occasionally led to coma.[88] After the introduction of insulin, it soon became apparent that in persons treated with insulin, blood glucose levels fell during exercise and that regular insulin reduced the exogenous insulin requirement.

The metabolic and hormonal response to exercise varies depending on the degree of metabolic control at the start of exercise, more specifically the availability of insulin. In nonketotic persons with diabetes with mild-to-moderate hyperglycemia (>15 mm

[270 mg/dL]), moderately heavy exercise 24 hours after insulin withdrawal causes blood glucose to fall. In contrast, in persons with more severe hyperglycemia and mild keto-nemia (blood ketones 2-3 mM), exercise causes a significant rise in blood glucose concentration.[10] This may reflect either an overproduction of glucose from the liver or under-use by the working muscles, or both. Furthermore, since lipolysis is also enhanced during insulin deficiency, FFA and ketone body concentrations rise in the blood, resulting in an inhibition of glucose uptake by muscle, which counterbalances the effect of exercise in the glucose transport process.[32,62]

Liver Metabolism During Exercise

The rise of hepatic glucose output in response to exercise is similar in persons with and without diabetes.[89] However, in persons with diabetes, the use of gluconeogenic precursors during short-term exercise rises 2 to 3 times the basal level; in persons without diabetes, it remains the same. Thus gluconeogenesis was estimated to account for 30% of the liver glucose output in persons with diabetes compared with no more than 11% for those without diabetes. As a result, *the influence of brief (40 minutes) exercise on hepatic glucose metabolism in persons with diabetes is comparable to that of prolonged (4 hours) exercise in nondiabetic subjects.*[88]

Free Fatty Acid Levels

Plasma concentrations of FFA increase at low insulin levels, such as what occurs during exercise or with uncontrolled diabetes, and the use of FFA in muscles increases during these two conditions. In general, the importance of FFA as a fuel relative to carbohydrate increases with the duration of exercise and decreases as exercise intensity increases.[40] During prolonged exercise of low intensity (40% of maximal aerobic capacity [$Vo_{2\ max}$]), FFA oxidation accounts for approximately 60% of muscle oxygen consumption.[1] The uptake of FFA is not insulin-dependent but is proportional to the concentration of FFA in plasma. Thus, in poorly controlled diabetes with elevated levels of FFA, the uptake and oxidation of FFA during exercise are increased relative to that of glucose.[40]

In nonketotic diabetic persons with mild hyperglycemia, as well as in nondiabetics, an initial decline in FFA concentration is followed by a modest gradual rise as exercise continues.[10] In contrast, persons with diabetes with marked hyperglycemia and ketosis already show an elevated FFA level at rest, and the rise during exercise is more marked.[89] As a result of this greater availability of FFA, uptake of FFA by working muscle is increased. In mildly ketotic persons with diabetes, a sevenfold increase in FFA uptake by muscles was shown, as compared with a three to fourfold increment in nondiabetics.[89]

Ketone Body Use

The short-chain fatty acids, 3-hydroxybutyric acid, and acetoacetic acid are present in plasma in low amounts normally, and during exercise ketone bodies make no net contribution to the fuel supply of muscles.[64] However, mildly ketotic persons with diabetes use ketone bodies during exercise. In severely insulin-deficient persons with diabetes with marked hyperketonemia, strenuous exercise causes a further rise in blood ketone body levels.[10,89]

The mechanism for this rapid development of ketosis is not altogether clear. Recent studies suggest that a defect in peripheral clearance of ketones rather than a marked increase in ketogenesis during exercise in insulin-deprived individuals is the major factor.[33]

Hormonal Changes with Exercise in Persons with IDDM

Plasma insulin levels may be much higher in persons with diabetes as compared with those without diabetes. In such a setting hepatic glucose production is inhibited and glucose clearance is enhanced by peripheral glucose uptake and stimulated glucose oxidation by the exercising muscle. As a result, plasma glucose falls. Its major effect is inhibition of glucose production, and both glycogenolysis and gluconeogenesis are inhibited by the high insulin levels. Although counterregulatory hormone response may be excessive, the hepatic glucose production cannot match the rate of peripheral glucose use, and blood glucose falls.

Whether this decrease in plasma glucose is large enough to produce signs of neuroglucopenia depends on factors such as initial plasma glucose levels, intensity and duration of exercise, actual plasma insulin concentrations, and relation of exercise to the last meal. Furthermore, the setpoint of the glucoregulatory system may be higher in persons with diabetes, and as a result they may experience symptoms of neuroglucopenia when their plasma glucose concentration is normal or even in the hyperglycemic range.[23] However, some persons with diabetes have poor counterregulatory defense mechanisms, possibly due to autonomic neuropathy, and these persons are especially prone to develop frank hypoglycemia.[21] This fall in blood glucose with mild-to-moderate exercise may be beneficial to some persons with diabetes but, with more prolonged exercise, hypoglycemia may result. This is a problem particularly in persons who are also glucagon deficient.

Persons who exercise when in moderately poor control of their diabetes induce an abnormally increased secretion of the glucoregulatory hormones. Insulin deficiency plus a high concentration of counterregulatory hormones enhances gluconeogenesis at levels 2 to 3 times those seen in nondiabetic persons, resulting in an exaggerated increase in hepatic glucose production and circulating plasma glucose concentrations.[88]

Postexercise Hypoglycemia

Campaigne and associates[18] investigated the effects of different diets and insulin adjustments in nine persons with IDDM. When hypoglycemia occurred, it was noted 5 hours after exercise 5 out of 8 times. MacDonald[51] selected 300 young people with IDDM for study. Postexercise, late-onset hypoglycemia (PEL) occurred in 48 of the subjects during the 2-year study period. The incidence of hypoglycemia varied from 3 to 31 hours after exercise but was most common 6 to 15 hours after exercise. Hypoglycemia during exercise, or 1 to 2 hours after exercise, was relatively uncommon. Furthermore, persons who experienced hypoglycemia did not appear to be in "tighter" control than those who did not. Exercise was usually vigorous or prolonged and often occurred after a period of relative inactivity.

Causes for PEL include: (1) muscle and/or liver glycogen depletion from unusually intense or long exercise, (2) increased insulin sensitivity in those making a transition from the untrained to a trained state, (3) ongoing glucose use following exercise, (4) defective counterregulatory response, (5) inappropriate adjustments in insulin or food before or after exercise, (6) lack of blood glucose monitoring postexercise, which might have allowed for preventive intervention (e.g., increased caloric intake or subsequent decreased insulin), or (7) a combination of all of the above.

EXERCISE AND IDDM

Considering the complexity of fuel flux during exercise and the important regulatory role played by insulin and the counterregulatory hormones, it is not surprising that persons with diabetes, especially IDDM, can run into management problems when exercising. Because of the increased risks of exercise, experts still debate whether exercise should be recommended for all persons with IDDM.

Benefits of Exercise

Persons with diabetes experience the same benefits that persons without diabetes gain from a regular exercise program, namely, improved fitness and psychologic state, change in body composition, weight control, and improved physical work capacity. For persons with diabetes, exercise has additional benefits; for example, increased insulin sensitivity results in a potential reduction in insulin dosage,[88] as well as in a reduction of risk factors for atherosclerosis.[44]

Acute Effects of Exercise

Insulin taken by injection clearly does not duplicate the normal secretion of insulin from the pancreas, which can vary acutely depending on food intake and the performance of physical activity. Sporadic exercise can exert acute or short-term effects on fuel metabolism in persons with IDDM as a result of variable states of insulin excess and insulin deficiency. When insulin deficiency and ketosis are present, exercise can cause an increase in plasma glucose and accelerated ketone body formation. In contrast, with a relative excess of insulin in the circulation, blood glucose levels decrease during and after exercise, and exercise-induced hypoglycemia occurs.

Training Effects of Exercise

With training, clinical observations suggest that the risk of hypoglycemia with exercise is reduced. Several factors may contribute to this decreased risk: (1) the meal plan is adjusted so that snacks are planned to coincide with usual exercise times; (2) insulin dosages are reduced because of the decreased need for insulin with exercise; (3) higher levels of counterregulatory hormones exist in trained persons[53]; or (4) a combination of the above. Futhermore, postexercise hypoglycemia is also reduced with training.[51]

A limited number of studies have been done on the effect of exercise training on long-term metabolic control in IDDM. Most studies focus on the acute effects of exercise and suggest that physical training can increase insulin sensitivity and glucose storage as well as improve lipoprotein concentrations. Long-term effects of exercise, such as improved blood glucose control as measured by glycosylated hemoglobin, have not been demonstrated.

The lack of a long-term beneficial effect of exercise in persons with IDDM, as measured by glycosylated hemoglobin, is somewhat unexpected because of the acute glucose-lowering effect that can occur with each exercise session. It was hoped that this acute response would have a summation effect on overall control. Zinman and others[97] reported that although 45 minutes of supervised exercise was undertaken 3 times a week for 12 weeks in 13 persons with IDDM, fasting blood glucose and HbA_{1c} values remained unchanged with training. This lack of improvement was attributed to the increased intake of approximately 300 kcal on exercising days.

Wallberg-Henriksson and others[90] reported a similar lack of unchanged glucose control related to exercise. They studied 9 men with IDDM who participated in a training program consisting of 1 hour of exercise 2 to 3 times a week for 16 weeks. Despite increased peripheral insulin sensitivity, decreased total cholesterol, and increased high-density lipoprotein cholesterol, there was no improvement in glycosylated hemoglobin, glycosuria, or 24-hour urinary glucose excretion. Subjects also consumed a snack of approximately 400 kcal after exercise. They concluded that, although other benefits from exercise were noted, *in the absence of efforts to alter food intake and insulin administration, physical training by itself does not improve blood glucose control in persons with IDDM.*

The long-term effect of physical activity among persons with IDDM on other risks from diabetes is not known. LaPorte and others[49] studied the relationship of physical activity and diabetes complications in 696 persons with IDDM. They reported that the long-term effect of physical activity does not appear to accelerate development of severe eye disease, coronary heart disease, or death. On the contrary, it may be beneficial. Because persons with IDDM have at least a sevenfold increased risk of these complications, any factor associated positively with prevention has important implications.

More recent, unpublished data reported by LaPorte[48] has linked reduced levels of physical activity to the risk of early mortality. On the basis of epidemiologic data collected on historical physical activity in 600 persons with IDDM, he reported that any increase in physical activity appears to be associated with a decreased occurrence of nephropathy and macrovascular disease as well as a reduced risk of death. Furthermore, it appears that only a small increase in activity (such as engagement in team sports in high school, resulting in more physical activity as adults than those who were not team-sports participants) was associated with a reduced risk of complications.

FACTORS RELATED TO THE EFFECTS OF EXERCISE IN PERSONS WITH IDDM

The metabolic response to exercise is highly variable even in the same individual because of the many variables related to exercise as well as to metabolic homeostasis. Exercise variables include exercise intensity, type and duration, timing of exercise in relation to meals, the time of day exercise is performed, and time of exercise in relation to insulin injections.

Metabolic Control

A major determinant of the response to exercise is related to insulin availability. Aside from the effects of this on metabolic control at the start of exercise, which have already been discussed, diabetes also influences the size of the body fuel reserves, primarily the carbohydrate store. The amount of carbohydrate stored is related to the degree of glycemic control. Insulin availability determines the extent of glycogen storage and depletion in both liver and muscles; therefore a person experiencing frequent bouts of hypoglycemia or hyperglycemia may have inadequate hepatic and muscle glycogen stores available for exercise. The degree of glycogen depletion is intimately related to the extent of insulin deprivation.[10,88] These persons can be more susceptible to fluctuations in blood glucose levels, especially hypoglycemia, and they should be advised to avoid prolonged exercise until diabetes control is improved.

Food Intake

Stratton and others[82] studied adolescents with IDDM who entered a structured 8-week exercise program held after their usual afternoon snack. Food intake was not increased on exercise days. Although glycosylated hemoglobin values did not improve, glycosylated serum albumin, which is a more sensitive index of glycemic changes over a shorter period of time, showed a significant decline. Blood glucose concentrations before exercise were also significantly lower in the last 3 weeks of the program as compared with the first 3 weeks. Stratton and colleagues attributed this improvement to better control of food intake.

Timing of Exercise

Free-insulin levels in persons with IDDM tend to be lower before breakfast than before subsequent meals or bedtime. As a result, less hypoglycemia in response to exercise before breakfast, as opposed to late afternoon exercise, might be expected. Ruegemer and others[71] studied persons with IDDM at rest and when exercising before breakfast and at 1600 hours. Plasma glucose increased from 6.7 ± 0.4 to 9.1 ± 0.4 mM (121 ± 7 to 164 ± 7 mg/dL) during morning exercise as compared with no change in plasma glucose during afternoon exercise. However, there was a 0.3 to 1.0 mM (5 to 18 mg/dL) decrease with afternoon exercise in *half* of the individuals. They concluded that the risk of exercise-induced hypoglycemia is lowest before breakfast. The hyperglycemia induced by prebreakfast exercise is mild and short-lived and thus would likely have a minimal impact on overall glucose control.

Type of Exercise

Recommendations for exercise programs for persons with diabetes usually emphasize aerobic programs. The effects of strength training on metabolic control and fitness capacity has not been well studied. Resistance training is usually not emphasized because of the acute response associated with high-intensity–type training (e.g., hyperglycemia[56] and increased blood pressure). However, Durak and others[25] reported that a supervised strength-training program 3 days a week for 10 weeks for men with IDDM was associated with no morbidity, increased strength, reduced blood glucose and glycosylated hemoglobin with no change in insulin dose, and lower cholesterol levels.

Amount of Insulin Injected

Schiffrin and Parikh[75] studied persons with near-normal glycosylated hemoglobins who exercised moderately 1½ hours after breakfast (2 hours after insulin injections). They reported that a 30% to 50% reduction of premeal insulin dose appeared to accommodate 45 minutes of exercise without hypoglycemia. When adjustments in insulin are not feasible, they suggested that 15 grams of glucose before each 45 minutes of unplanned exercise and 15 to 30 grams of glucose after physical activity would be appropriate to prevent hypoglycemia.

Duration and Intensity of Exercise

Brief, intense exercise tends to induce mild hyperglycemia, whereas prolonged exercise can result in hypoglycemia, both in persons with diabetes and in those persons without diabetes, in whom circulating insulin levels can change.

Mitchell and others[56] found that periods of intense exercise (80% $Vo_{2 max}$) in nondiabetic subjects produce sustained postexercise hyperglycemia, 20% above basal, with a 100% increase in plasma insulin. In persons with IDDM incapable of generating that rise in insulin by increased secretion, postexercise hyperglycemia was greater and sustained longer. Thus, in the recovery period after intense exercise, glycemia may be raised rather than improved. In persons with IDDM exercising to exhaustion at 80% $Vo_{2 max}$, when preexercise plasma glucose was normal (4.8 $\pm$ 0.2 mM [86 $\pm$ 4 mg/dL]), hyperglycemia rose to 7.0 ± 1.5 mM (127 ± 7 mg/dL) and was sustained for 2 hours postexhaustion. When plasma glucose was 8.3 ± 0.5 mM (149 + 9 mg/dL), it rose progressively throughout the 2 hours to 12.7 ± 1.5 mM (229 ± 28 mg/dL). The type of sport that most closely resembles exercise of the intensity used in this study would involve sprints or repeated short bouts of exercise, such as in hockey or basketball.

Injection Sites

In persons with diabetes, plasma insulin concentrations do not decrease during exercise and may even increase substantially if exercise is undertaken within 1 hour or so after an insulin injection. This is caused by increased absorption of insulin from the subcutaneous tissue, particularly if regular insulin is used and the injection site is in an exercising part of the body. However, when 40 minutes have elapsed after injection of regular insulin and before exercise has begun, more than half the administered insulin has been mobilized. In addition, intermediate insulins are also unaffected when exercise is begun 2½ hours after injection.[11] Since in reality exercise rarely occurs immediately after an insulin injection, it appears to be unnecessary to recommend rotating insulin sites to parts of the body that are not involved in physical activity to prevent exercise-induced hypoglycemia. However, exercising at peak action times of any insulin can still lead to hypoglycemia.

Physical Fitness

Inactivity has long been shown to be a cause of glucose intolerance and insulin resistance. Arslanian and others[7] studied adolescents with IDDM and adolescents without diabetes and reported that insulin-mediated glucose disposal was positively related to the state of physical fitness as assessed by $Vo_{2\ max}$ and negatively related to diabetes control as assessed by HbA_1. However, for similar degrees of physical fitness, adolescents with diabetes had lower total body insulin-mediated glucose metabolism than did controls. They concluded that adolescents with IDDM are insulin-resistant as compared with nondiabetics, and this resistance is attributable to the state of diabetes control. However, the level of physical fitness explains a major part of the interindividual variations in insulin action in adolescents both with and without IDDM.

Meinders and others[53] also studied trained athletes with diabetes performing activities of long duration, and compared them to well-trained nondiabetics during a 3-hour marathon-training run. Insulin was withheld the morning of the run, but a normal breakfast was eaten 2½ hours before the start of the run. All subjects ate a banana after 90 minutes and a 3-gram dextrose tablet after 150 minutes of running. Blood glucose dropped from 17 mM to 5 mM (306 to 90 mg/dL) after 150 minutes of running. However, the runners with diabetes had higher peripheral serum concentrations of counterregulatory hormones as compared with those of controls, which presumably helped to prevent hypoglycemia. This may help explain why well-trained persons with diabetes are less prone to hypoglycemia than athletes with diabetes who are not well trained.

PRECAUTIONS WITH EXERCISE FOR PERSONS WITH IDDM

It is important that persons with diabetes who want to exercise be encouraged to participate in either recreational or competitive activities. However, physical exercise is not without risks to individuals with IDDM. Hypoglycemia, hyperglycemia, ketosis, cardiovascular ischemia and arrhythmia, exacerbation of proliferative retinopathy, and lower-extremity injury are potential complications of exercise.[44]

Participants should undergo a thorough medical evaluation before undertaking unusual or particularly vigorous exercise programs. This is especially important for persons who are over age 35 and/or those who have had diabetes for more than 10 years.[5] Individuals should be screened carefully for the presence of cardiovascular disease, proliferative retinopathy, and nephropathy, all of which present risks for exercise. Some types of exercise should be avoided if specific risks are present. With exercise, blood pressure may rise higher in persons with IDDM than in nondiabetic individuals, placing the patient with retinopathy at risk. Furthermore, those with proliferative retinopathy should not participate in heavy lifting or straining and should avoid head-low positions or excessive jarring of the head, all of which may precipitate a vitreous hemorrhage. Those with peripheral neuropathy should be particularly careful to avoid cuts, blisters, and pounding exercises of the lower extremities, and those with autonomic neuropathy should be careful to maintain appropriate fluid and electrolyte balance during exercise in a warm climate.[5] Exercise has also been shown to result in proteinuria in persons with diabetes[57]; this is probably a transient hemodynamic response and it is unknown if exercise has any deleterious effect on the progression of renal disease.[44]

STRATEGIES TO ASSIST PERSONS WITH IDDM EXERCISE SAFELY

Although each individual responds differently to exercise, general guidelines are important so persons can begin to exercise safely. As individuals gain experience with exercise, they can adapt specific issues to meet their needs. Ideally, exercise should be performed at about the same time each day, but for practical reasons, this is often not possible. Therefore the goal is to assist persons to exercise safely at times of the day that are convenient for them. Persons who are trained will also find they have fewer problems when exercising.

A good general "rule of thumb" regarding exercise concerns blood glucose levels, food intake, and insulin adjustment. If blood glucose is <5.5 Mm (100 mg/dL) before exercise, eat a pre-exercise snack. If blood glucose is 5.5 to 8.3 Mm (100 to 150 mg/dL), go ahead and exercise and, if necessary, eat a snack afterwards. If blood glucose is >14 Mm (250 mg/dL), check urine for ketones. If ketones are positive, improve control by adjusting insulin. Do not exercise until ketones are negative.[34]

Self-monitoring of blood glucose levels is essential. Blood glucose monitoring before, during (if exercise is of long duration), and after exercise is essential if persons are to determine their response to exercise. Monitoring records are the most effective tool for

Table 3-3   Preexercise and Postexercise Snacks

Food	Amount	Carbohydrate content (gm)	Exchanges
Bagel or English muffin	½	14	1 starch/bread
Graham cracker squares	3	15	1 starch/bread
Snack crackers	4-5	15	1 starch/bread
Muffin	1	17	1 starch/bread, 1 fat
Pretzels	6 3-ring	14	1 starch/bread
Soup (not cream)	1 cup	15	1 starch/bread
Yogurt (plain or sweetened with NutraSweet®)	1 cup	16	1 milk
Apple	1 medium	22	1½ fruit
Banana	1 small	22	1½ fruit
Dried fruit	¼ cup	10	1 fruit
Orange	1 medium	18	1 fruit
Raisins	2 Tbsp	15	1 fruit
Fruit juice	½ cup	15	1 fruit

Source: Adapted with permission from Franz MJ and Norstrom J: Diabetes actively staying healthy. Your game plan for diabetes and exercise, Wayzata, MN, 1990, Diabetes Center, Inc.

determining a particular pattern of response to exercise. Patterns can then be used to adapt food or insulin to the time and amount of exercise planned. Carefully finding out how exercise affects blood glucose levels will decrease the risk of hypoglycemia.

Food intake may need to be increased to accommodate activity or exercise. The individual's meal plan should take into consideration the person's exercise pattern. If exercise is done regularly, the snacks should be a part of the usual meal plan. In general, persons with IDDM tend to overeat before exercise. Well-trained individuals who regularly exercise at about the same time each day need less additional food than persons who exercise only occasionally. (See Table 3-3 for suggestions of pre- and/or postexercise snacks.)

Guidelines for increasing food intake for exercise need to be based on blood glucose levels before and after exercise, the duration of the exercise, the proximity of unscheduled exercise to scheduled meals, the times of day, and the regularity of exercise sessions. It may be best to delay consumption of extra food until after exercise, when testing of blood glucose can help determine how many (if any) calories are needed. In general, 10 to 15 g of carbohydrate—one fruit or starch/bread exchange—should be eaten before 1 hour of moderate exercise, such as tennis, swimming, jogging, cycling, or gardening. For more strenuous activity of a 1 to 2-hour duration, such as football, hockey, racquetball, basketball, strenuous cycling or swimming, 30 to 50 g of carbohydrate—half a meat sandwich with one milk or fruit exchange—may be needed. Mild exercise, such as walking a half mile, will probably not require any extra food.[35] (See Table 3-4 for general guidelines on increasing food intake for exercise that is not done regularly.)

Table 3-4   Suggested General Guidelines for Making Food Adjustments for Exercise for Persons with IDDM

Type of exercise and examples	If blood glucose is	Increase food intake by	Suggestions of food to use
Exercise of short duration and of low to moderate intensity (walking a half mile or leisurely bicycling for less than 30 minutes)	Less than 100 mg/dL 100 mg/dL or above	10 to 15 gm of carbohydrate per hour Not necessary to increase food	1 fruit or 1 starch/bread exchange
Exercise of moderate intensity (one hour of tennis, swimming, jogging, leisurely bicycling, golfing, etc)	Less than 100 mg/dL	25 to 50 gm of carbohydrate before exercise, then 10 to 15 gm per hour of exercise	½ meat sandwich with a milk or fruit exchange
	100 to 180 mg/dL 180 to 300 mg/dL 300 mg/dL or above	10 to 15 gm of carbohydrate Not necessary to increase food Do not begin exercise until blood glucose is under better control	1 fruit or 1 starch/bread exchange
Strenuous activity or exercise (about one to two hours of football, hockey, racquetball, or basketball games; strenuous bicycling or swimming; shoveling heavy snow)	Less than 100 mg/dL	50 gm of carbohydrate, monitor blood glucose carefully	1 meat sandwich (2 slices of bread) with a milk and fruit exchange
	100 to 180 mg/dL	25 to 50 gm of carbohydrate, depending on intensity and duration	½ meat sandwich with a milk or fruit exchange
	180 to 300 mg/dL 300 mg/dL or above	10 to 15 gm of carbohydrate Do not begin exercise until blood glucose is under better control	1 fruit or 1 starch/bread exchange

Reprinted with permission from Franz MJ and Norstrom J. Diabetes actively staying healthy. Your game plan for diabetes and exercise, Wayzata, MN, 1990, Diabetes Center, Inc.

Persons with IDDM should be careful not to overeat with exercise. Many persons use exercise as an opportunity to liberalize their usual food intake with foods they might normally avoid, such as desserts, candy bars, or regular soft drinks.

Strenuous exercise over an extended period may require a decrease in insulin dosage. A conservative recommendation is to begin decreasing the insulin acting during the time of the activity (morning or afternoon) by 10% of the total insulin dose per day. If the person is active during the entire day, both the short-acting and intermediate-acting insulin can be decreased by 10%, for a total of 20%.[34]

Because blood glucose continues to decrease after exercise, it is important to continue testing blood glucose after exercise is completed. Blood glucose levels can continue to decrease for up to 30 hours after exercise, especially after vigorous or prolonged exercise or exercise that is not done regularly. The most frequently reported time for hypoglycemia is 4 to 10 hours after exercise. Hypoglycemia during exercise, or even 2 hours after exercise, is not as common as hypoglycemia later. Replacing stored liver and muscle carbohydrate used during exercise can take from 24 to 48 hours. Blood glucose testing is essential for the person to determine whether to eat extra food and/or decrease insulin dosage after exercise.

Timing is also a factor in making decisions about exercise. Depending on the time of day that exercise is done and the blood glucose level before exercise, various changes in blood glucose can occur. For example, exercising late in the afternoon may cause a greater drop in blood glucose values than exercising before or after breakfast. When possible, exercise should be scheduled so it will improve postprandial hyperglycemia. Ideally, exercise should occur 1 to 3 hours after a meal, when blood glucose is >5.5 mM (100 mg/dL). An excellent time to exercise may be before or after breakfast because blood glucose levels are often elevated during this time.

Peak times of injected insulin and the excessive lowering of blood glucose levels that exercise may produce at these times must be considered. Exercising when insulin is at peak effect can result in a precipitous fall in blood glucose, and additional carbohydrate may be needed to prevent hypoglycemia.

Fluid intake is important. Persons with IDDM often become so preoccupied with replacing carbohydrate that they forget that the most important nutrient needed during exercise is water. Individuals whose diabetes is not well controlled are particularly prone to dehydration when exercising, especially on warm days. Cool water, sports drinks, or diluted fruit juices are good choices. A half cup of fruit juice (15 grams of carbohydrate) diluted with a half cup of water, for a total of 1 cup per hour, or as often as needed, is an excellent way to take in both carbohydrate and fluid when exercising. For every pound of weight lost during exercise, 2 cups of fluid are needed for replacement.

Persons should have adequate metabolic control. When an insulin deficiency results in poor metabolic control (BG >13.8 to 16.6 mM [250 to 300 mg/dL]), especially with ketonuria, the production of glucose and the breakdown of fat to ketones exceed the ability of the muscles to use them. This is of particular concern when diabetes control has been suboptimal over several days or more.

Injection sites are not a major concern, unless the injection is given in a part of the body that will be exercising immediately. If it has been more than 40 minutes between the injection of regular insulin and the start of exercise, more than half of the injected insulin will be mobilized from the injection site. Likewise, absorption of intermediate-acting insulin remains unaffected when exercise is begun 1½ hours after an injection. If exercise if performed immediately after an insulin injection, the injection should be given in an area that is not involved in the exercise, such as the abdomen.

All individuals should carry adequate identification and a source of readily available carbohydrate. (See box on the opposite page for a summary of strategies to assist persons with IDDM exercise safely.)

STRATEGIES FOR ATHLETES WITH IDDM

Athletes with IDDM find that if they begin training gradually and extend it over a period of time, their bodies adapt physically as well as metabolically. As a result, there can be gradual adjustments (usually decreases) in insulin, and food intake can be adapted. When training for more than 60 minutes at a time, insulin dosage may need to be reduced even further.

An exercising body uses carbohydrate as its main fuel source. In athletes who do not have diabetes, blood glucose reaches a point at which noticeable fatigue sets in after about 90 to 180 minutes of exercise. At that point they also will perform better with a carbohydrate replacement. This can delay the onset of fatigue by slowing depletion of muscle glycogen stores. For athletes with IDDM, a carbohydrate replacement may be needed after approximately 60 minutes of exercise to prevent hypoglycemia, especially if blood glucose was in the normal range before exercise.

Drinks containing 5% to 10% carbohydrate are absorbed best. Concentrated drinks that exceed 10% carbohydrate can cause gastrointestinal upset such as cramps, nausea, diarrhea, or bloating.[19] Fruit juices and most regular soft drinks contain about 12% carbohydrate, so they need to be diluted. The advantage of sports drinks or glucose polymer drinks is that they average 6% to 7% carbohydrate. In events lasting less than 60 minutes, plain cold water is usually the beverage of choice. In events lasting longer than 60 minutes, athletes with diabetes should try to consume 10 to 15 g of carbohydrate every hour.[34] The athlete should not wait for symptoms of hypoglycemia to develop. Loss of consciousness is not only embarrassing but may go unnoticed or be misunderstood in the excitement of an athletic event.

Hypoglycemia can be prevented if some of the carbohydrate is eaten during rather than before exercise. This may result in increased use of blood glucose with a proportionate slowing of muscle glycogen use.[19] For events of long duration, such as cross-country skiing, marathons, and so on, the limited stores of liver and muscle glycogen, even after supercompensation, are not sufficient to complete the event. Carbohydrate ingestion is essential for the successful completion of the event. After exercise, a bigger snack, such as a sandwich with milk or fruit, may be needed to prevent postexercise hypoglycemia.[34]

STRATEGIES TO ASSIST PERSONS WITH IDDM
TO EXERCISE SAFELY

1. Adequate metabolic control should be established before an exercise program is initiated.
2. Self-monitoring of blood glucose levels is essential.
3. Food intake may need to be increased to accommodate exercise. In general, 10 to 15 g of carbohydrate should be eaten before or after 1 hour of moderate activity.
4. Strenuous exercise over an extended period may require a decrease in insulin dosage.
5. Testing of blood glucose after exercise is completed is important to prevent postexercise hypoglycemia.
6. Timing of exercise can also be a factor in making decisions about exercise.
7. Peak times of injected insulin and the possible decrease in blood glucose levels at that time must be considered.
8. Fluid intake is important.
9. Injection sites are not a major concern unless the injection is given in a part of the body that will be exercising immediately.
10. All persons should carry adequate identification and a source of readily available carbohydrate.

Along with ingestion of additional carbohydrate in events of long duration, athletes with IDDM may also have to omit their usual short-acting insulin dose and start with an elevated blood glucose concentration that gradually falls to a normal range during the first 60 to 90 minutes of exercise. As long as insulin deficiency is not severe enough to result in ketosis before exercise, metabolic fuel regulation during exercise is fairly normal. The counterregulatory hormones, including glucagon, catecholamines, growth hormone, and cortisol, increase more in persons with diabetes than in those without diabetes. This counterregulatory response may be a key factor in preventing hypoglycemia from occurring.[44]

Furthermore, to prevent hypoglycemia, especially PEL hypoglycemia, athletes with IDDM may need to take longer and make a more gradual progression to a higher level of training than is generally prescribed. This may allow the athlete to tolerate more intense and longer duration activities than usual. This higher level of fitness may offer some protection from PEL hypoglycemia, or at least may lower the individual's sensitivity to unusual increases in intensity or duration of exercise. A more gradual progression from the untrained to the trained state may also offer some protection for athletes in the training progression who may be more likely to experience PEL hypoglycemia.[51] (See box on p. 102 for a summary of strategies that can be used to assist athletes with diabetes to exercise safely.)

STRATEGIES TO ASSIST ATHLETES WITH IDDM
─────────────── TO EXERCISE SAFELY ───────────────

1. Begin training gradually and over an extended period.
2. To prevent hypoglycemia during exercise of long duration, carbohydrate may be needed after approximately 60 minutes of exercise. Drinks containing 5% to 10% carbohydrate are absorbed better than are more concentrated carbohydrate drinks.
3. Adjustments in insulin doses may aiso be needed for events of long duration.
4. Athletes with IDDM may need to take longer and make a more gradual progression to a higher level of training than is generally prescribed. The higher level of fitness may allow the athlete to tolerate more intense and longer duration activities than usual and may offer protection from PEL hypoglycemia as well.

EXERCISE AND NIDDM

Hyperglycemia in IDDM is primarily the result of an absolute insulin deficiency, whereas in NIDDM hyperglycemia is the result of insulin resistance and impaired insulin secretion. Many persons with NIDDM are hyperinsulinemic and many are obese. Therefore any form of therapy that reverses or lessens insulin resistance and assists in weight loss has potential benefit. Furthermore, the prevention of NIDDM in genetically predisposed persons and the prevention of cardiovascular disease are also desirable goals. Increased activity levels or exercise has the potential to assist in any or all of the above.

Most studies [42,63,78,84] suggest that exercise is most effective in persons with impaired glucose tolerance or mild-to-moderate diabetes (i.e., fasting glucose levels <11.1 mM [200 mg/dL]). Hyperinsulinemic patients also respond best to exercise, which is consistent with the observation that exercise acts by reversing insulin resistance.

Benefits of Exercise

Exercise and Insulin Resistance

Regularly performed vigorous exercise can result in significant improvement in glucose tolerance within a relatively short time (less than 7 days) in some persons with NIDDM.[55,78] The improvement in glucose tolerance appears to be caused by a decrease in insulin resistance—that is, to a greater susceptibility to the action of insulin. This can occur even without changes in body weight, body fat content, or $Vo_{2\ max}$. Regular exercise has been shown to result in decreased insulin levels in nondiabetic, obese persons and in persons with impaired glucose tolerance (IGT).[12]

Improvements in glycemic control and glucose tolerance associated with exercise in persons with NIDDM occur *without* a decrease in elevated insulin levels, consistent with improved insulin sensitivity in trained persons.[13,74] It has been shown that in persons with NIDDM training improves glucose tolerance, but the effect is short-lived.[17]

In studies on obese, insulin-resistant men and in persons with NIDDM, Devlin and others[24] have shown that a single bout of glycogen-depleting exercise can significantly increase insulin sensitivity and increase the rate of glucose disposal.

In studies by Schneider and others[76] 6 weeks of training, 3 times a week at 60% $Vo_{2\ max}$ for 30 minutes, diminished fasting glucose levels and improved glucose tolerance for 12 hours but not for 72 hours after the last exercise session. Glycosylated hemoglobin levels were also slightly reduced by training. Similar results have been obtained in several other recent studies.[22,63,84]

Exercise and Weight Loss

Exercise can be an effective adjunct to weight loss and weight control regimes. Wing and others[96] have shown that a combination of diet and exercise improves weight loss in persons with NIDDM and allows for greater reduction in hypoglycemic medication. Exercise may affect weight loss in several different ways. First, exercise increases calorie expenditure during the exercise bout. Second, it may offset the effect of calorie restriction on energy expenditure. Another possibility is that moderate levels of exercise may decrease appetite. Exercise may also promote dietary adherence and may improve mood and self-esteem, leading to more control over dietary intake. Although the mechanism is still unclear, exercise seems to be effective in promoting long-term weight loss and has consistently been one of the strongest predictors of long-term weight control.[95]

Prevention of NIDDM

Physical training may be of significant value in preventing or delaying the development of overt NIDDM in genetically predisposed persons. Exercise may be a means of delaying the onset of insulin resistance cardiovascular disease, and NIDDM in persons at high risk,[70] including those with a positive family history of NIDDM or hypertriglyceridemia, women who have had gestational diabetes, and persons with android-type obesity.[6]

Although obesity and genetics have been identified as possibly the most powerful contributing factors to the epidemic explosion of NIDDM in certain populations, changes in life style have also been implicated. Populations at high risk include the Pima Indians and other North American Indians, Tamil-speaking Eastern Indians in South Africa, and some Pacific Island populations.[28] Life style changes are characterized by a decrease in physical activity and high consumption of calories that have given way to obesity. Although obesity is generally regarded as the risk factor, decreased physical activity independent of obesity has also been identified as a risk factor for NIDDM.

Taylor and others[83] found that in Melanesian and Indian men in the Fiji Islands the occurrence of NIDDM was twice as high in sedentary as in physically active men, an effect that could not be ascribed to differences in body weight.

Prevention of Cardiovascular Disease

Diabetes is a major risk factor for macrovascular disease (see Chapter 6). Cerebrovascular, coronary, and peripheral artery disease are more common in diabetes and occur at an earlier age.[70] In addition, diabetes eliminates the relative protection from coronary problems possessed by premenopausal women. Coronary heart disease is approximately doubled for persons with IGT. Hyperinsulinemia and insulin resistance have been implicated as risk factors for atherosclerosis. Glucose intolerance may also contribute to atherosclerotic risk by the nonenzymatic glycosylation of lipoproteins, both low-density lipoprotein (LDL) and high-density lipoprotein (HDL).[77]

Epidemiologic studies suggest that endurance-type exercise diminishes the mortality and morbidity from macrovascular disease in nondiabetic populations.[50,59] In persons with diabetes, it is not known whether physical training is associated with decreased cardiovascular disease, but the cardiovascular risk factors can be reduced, making physical training especially beneficial for persons with diabetes. By enhancing body sensitivity to insulin, plasma insulin levels are reduced. If hyperinsulinemia is indeed a risk factor for macrovascular disease, as has been postulated, lower insulin levels may help prevent macrovascular complications.

Most studies of persons with NIDDM undergoing physical training report a significant decrease in plasma triglyceride levels and very low–density lipoproteins (VLDL). Plasma cholesterol and HDL-cholesterol levels appear to not change significantly. In a clinical study by Schneider and Kanj[77] of 108 patients followed in a diabetes exercise program, an average fall in plasma triglyceride levels of 15% from the basal level was found over three months with no change in cholesterol and HDL-cholesterol levels. The time course of changes in plasma triglyceride levels suggests that, as with glucose, many of the benefits of exercise training are caused by the summed effects of individual bouts of exercise. In Schneider's studies, a significant decrease in plasma triglyceride was consistently noted 12 hours after a typical exercise training bout, but 72 hours later the improvement was no longer measurable.

The fact that exercise training has not been consistently found to result in elevated HDL-cholesterol in persons with NIDDM may be because the exercise required to elevate plasma HDL levels in persons with NIDDM is of a longer duration and greater intensity than is usually recommended, or current studies may not have been conducted long enough to realize this benefit.[77]

Lowering Blood Pressure

Exercise and diet therapy have been shown to be effective in reducing blood pressure of hypertensive persons with NIDDM resulting in a mean reduction of 10 to 15 mm Hg of diastolic blood pressure.[77] The mechanism by which exercise reduces blood pressure is poorly understood at the present time.

Psychologic Benefits

As previously noted, exercise training and improved cardiorespiratory fitness are associated with decreased anxiety, improved mood and self-esteem, an increased sense of well-being, and an enhanced quality of life.[6] These and other benefits suggest the need for careful incorporation of exercise into the therapeutic regimen of persons with NIDDM.

Acute Effects of Exercise

The effect of a single exercise session in persons with NIDDM is to lower blood glucose concentrations. The acute decrease in plasma glucose levels leading to improvements in glucose metabolism may persist for hours to days, possibly related to an increase in insulin sensitivity in muscles and other tissues that persists for several hours following the exercise. This is related to both the need for replenishment of decreased muscle and liver glycogen stores and to increased glucose metabolism in muscle. Minuk and others[55] determined that 45 minutes of moderately intense exercise (60% $Vo_{2\ max}$) resulted in a significant decrease in plasma glucose concentration during glucose turnover determinations in persons who were being treated with diet and oral hypoglycemic agents. The reduction in plasma glucose level was about 1.9 mM (35 mg/dL) and persisted during the recovery study period of 60 minutes.

Devlin and others[24] studied the effects of exercise until muscle fatigue, at 1900 hours, compared with no exercise in persons with NIDDM, and reported that on the mornings following exercise, endogenous glucose production rates were 20% lower than on days with no exercise the evening before. Because increased endogenous glucose production that occurs overnight is believed to be a primary cause of fasting hyperglycemia in NIDDM, a single bout of evening exercise can have clinical significance 12 to 16 hours later.

Blake and others[15] compared blood pressure changes during mild-to-moderate exercise in persons with NIDDM and nondiabetic persons. Both groups were sedentary and usually normotensive. A greater exercise-induced systolic blood pressure (mean maximum 208 ± 6 versus 177 ± 3 mm Hg) occurred in the NIDDM group. Neither pulse rate nor diastolic pressure differed between the groups before or during exercise. Return to basal pulse and blood pressure was also similar. They suggest that in investigations of exercise as a therapeutic modality in diabetes, intraexercise blood pressure should be considered in assessing the safety of this form of treatment.

Training Effects of Exercise

Several factors may contribute to the lack of improvement in glucose tolerance after endurance exercise training. In the studies with NIDDM patients in whom there was little improvement in glucose tolerance, the exercise stimulus in terms of intensity and duration of exercise training was relatively low. Furthermore, glucose tolerance was also measured 4 to 7 days after the last bout of exercise. More recently Holloszy[42] determined that 12 months of vigorous exercise training resulted in normalization of oral glucose tolerance and reduced insulin resistance in a group of patients with NIDDM and a group with IGT. The data are consistent with the concept that *improved glycemic control is the result of the summed effects of the individual bouts and not the state of aerobic fitness per se.* Improved aerobic fitness may potentiate and prolong the metabolic effects of an acute exercise bout. Thus physical training may play an indirect role in enhancing glucose tolerance.

Bogardus and others[16] elucidated the mechanism for improved insulin sensitivity with exercise. The major effect of training, compared with diet alone, was to increase the peripheral use of glucose during hyperinsulinemia. The improved glucose disposal was primarily caused by an increase in the nonoxidative pathways of glucose metabolism, presumed to represent predominantly glycogen synthesis. This is important because the body's capacity to increase carbohydrate storage in response to insulin is greater than its capacity to increase carbohydrate oxidation rates.[43,72]

Physical endurance training results in not only an increased capacity for aerobic exercise but an improved cardiovascular system as well. From studies in persons with NIDDM it appears their response to physical training is qualitatively similar to that in nondiabetic persons.[90,73]

PRECAUTIONS WITH EXERCISE FOR PERSONS WITH NIDDM

Persons with NIDDM should be examined thoroughly for diabetic complications before starting an exercise program. Those who are about to start an exercise program should have a preexercise evaluation specifically designed to uncover previously undiagnosed hypertension, neuropathy, retinopathy, nephropathy, and, particularly, silent ischemic heart disease.[4] Further evaluation is essential for diabetic persons with a history of angina or for those who develop marked fatigue or dyspnea with exercise.[58] An evaluation of peripheral sensitivity and circulation should be done, and individuals with peripheral neuropathy or decreased circulation should avoid forms of exercise that involve trauma to the feet.

Myocardial ischemia can be present during exercise without chest pain in a substantial number of persons with diabetes. Therefore it may be prudent to consider whether cardiovascular autonomic neuropathy is present when advising individuals about exercise goals in order to avoid too great a stress during routine exercise. Because of this higher prevalence of silent ischemic heart disease, an exercise stress electrocardiogram is recommended in all subjects over 35 years of age.[4] This test is also helpful for identifying persons who have an exaggerated hypertensive response to exercise and/or who develop postexercise orthostatic hypertension.[6]

Persons with NIDDM have been shown to have unexpectedly low $Vo_{2\ max}$ both before and after 6 weeks of training.[78] Whether this is secondary to metabolic abnormalities or is independent of and precedes them remains to be established. This may also be caused by subtle autonomic dysfunction in persons with NIDDM.

Schneider and others[78] also report that standard tables of maximal heart rates based on nondiabetic populations correlate poorly with maximal heart rate in individuals with NIDDM. They report a maximal heart rate 15% to 20% lower than in age-matched controls in the absence of clinically evident neuropathy or coronary heart disease. Autonomic neuropathy or beta-blocker drugs may further impair maximal heart rate and aerobic exercise performance. Exercise programs should be initiated at the lower target pulse and gradually increased to the desired pulse rate over 2 to 3 weeks.

People taking oral medications or insulin should self-monitor their glycemic response to exercise. Those treated with sulfonylureas are at some increased risk of developing hypoglycemia during or following exercise, although this is less of a problem than that which occurs with insulin treatment. Individuals using insulin or oral medications have higher than normal insulin concentrations during exercise that may inhibit hepatic glucose production sufficiently and result in hypoglycemia. They must follow the same precautions as persons with IDDM, however, because they are still producing endogenous insulin, their blood glucose levels are not as unstable as those of the person who produces no endogenous insulin.

Special precautions should be taken if individuals use drugs that can produce hypoglycemia, such as alcohol. The recognition of hypoglycemia may also be retarded or obscured by beta-adrenergic receptor-blocking drugs such as propranolol and nadolol, that may prevent glycogenolytic responses that normally correct hypoglycemia.[47]

Blood glucose regulation during exercise in persons with NIDDM controlled by diet alone is not significantly different from that in persons without diabetes. During mild to moderate exercise, elevated blood glucose concentrations fall toward normal but do not reach hypoglycemic levels. There is no need for supplementary food before, during, or after exercise, except when exercise is exceptionally vigorous and of long duration. In this case, extra food may be beneficial just as it is in persons who do not have diabetes.

STRATEGIES FOR SAFE EXERCISE FOR PERSONS WITH NIDDM

Because many individuals with NIDDM may have been sedentary for many years, they are frequently deconditioned and unable to exercise continuously for any period of time. It is important that these individuals be encouraged to start with a mild exercise program, such as walking or riding a stationary bicycle, and be urged to rest if they feel out of breath. A program of gradually increasing exercise sessions, beginning with sessions of 5 to 10 minutes, is most successful and safest for this group. It is important to encourage any increase in activity and to help the individual continue exercising during the sometimes lengthy period before improvement is actually evident.

Available evidence suggests that to improve insulin sensitivity and glycemic control individuals should exercise at least three days per week or every other day. When no exercise is performed for 24 hours, glucose tolerance declines significantly. *Exercise should therefore be performed more than three times a week to achieve continuous improvement in glucose control.* Muscle-strengthening exercises may also lead to improved glucose disposal and lipid levels.

If weight reduction is a major goal, exercise 5 to 6 days per week is probably necessary. The goal is to burn 250 to 300 kcal per exercise session. Rhythmic aerobic exercises recommended for weight loss include brisk walking, jogging, swimming, bicycling, and aerobic dance. It is important that exercise be low impact in nature, thus avoiding injury to bones and joints.

The most efficient way to burn fat with exercise is to exercise at a level that results in no shortness of breath and to exercise continuously for a minimum of 20 to 30 minutes. Exercise of low intensity and long duration (for more than 20 to 30 minutes) uses stored

---

STRATEGIES TO ASSIST PERSONS WITH NIDDM
—————————— TO EXERCISE SAFELY ——————————

1. Start with mild and gradually increasing exercise sessions, such as walking or riding a stationary bicycle.
2. To improve insulin sensitivity and glycemic control, exercise should be done at least 3 days/week or every other day.
3. For weight control, persons should exercise 5 to 6 days/week.
4. Exercise should not result in shortness of breath and should be done continuously for a minimum of 20 to 30 minutes.
5. Exercise should be at 65% to 80% maximal heart rate. Intensity of exercise should be limited so that blood pressure does not exceed 180 mm Hg.
6. Aerobic exercise that is of low impact should be performed.
7. Muscle-strengthening exercises may also lead to improved glucose disposal.

---

fat as its major energy source. Exercise of short duration (for less than 2 to 3 minutes) and high intensity uses glycogen as the major energy source.

Exercise at 50% to 70% $Vo_{2\ max}$ is usually prescribed if complications of diabetes permit and the blood pressure response is not excessive.[6] (According to Pollock and others,[61] 50% to 70% of $Vo_{2\ max}$ would be approximately equal to 65% to 80% of maximum heart rate.) However, exercise at $<50\%$ $Vo_{2\ max}$, (i.e., walking) may also be beneficial if carried out for prolonged periods of time.[59,70] Intensity should be limited so blood pressure does not exceed 180 mm Hg. (See the box above for a summary of strategies to assist persons with NIDDM to exercise safely.)

EXERCISE IN SPECIAL CIRCUMSTANCES

Pregnancy, Diabetes, and Exercise

Pregnant women with IDDM have traditionally been denied the option of exercising during pregnancy primarily because of fear of affecting the fetus. However, women who are doing regular exercise before becoming pregnant can usually continue their exercise program during pregnancy, with appropriate timing of exercise to balance insulin action and food intake. It has been suggested that exercise may be another tool to facilitate the maintenance of optional blood glucose levels during pregnancy.[8] However, Hollingsworth and Moore,[41] in a study of 42 pregnant women with IDDM and 28 nondiabetic controls who participated in a postprandial walking exercise program, reported no significant improvement in glycemic control in women with IDDM. Exercise patients were instructed to walk 20 minutes (1 mile) after each meal. Exercise was associated with lower fasting cholesterol and triglyceride values in both groups and with significantly lower fasting plasma triglyceride levels in the diabetic exercise group. There were no adverse effects of postprandial walking exercise in mothers or infants.

It would seem prudent to advise women who wish to exercise during pregnancy to exercise at a lower intensity than nonpregnant diabetic women. Target heart rates for exercise prescription are not available for pregnancy; however, heart rates at 50% of target rate are believed to be of adequate intensity.[8] Guidelines published by the American College of Obstetricians and Gynecologists[4] also caution about exercise with ballistic movements (jerky, bouncy movements) and deep flexion or extension of joints because of connective tissue laxity during pregnancy.

Exercise appears to be effective in normalizing glucose tolerance only in patients who still have an adequate capacity to secrete insulin and in whom insulin resistance is the major cause for abnormal glucose tolerance. Thus it is perhaps reasonable to suggest that exercise in pregnancy might be more beneficial for pregnant women with NIDDM (but "insulin requiring" during pregnancy) and for women with gestational diabetes mellitus (GDM).[41]

Since most women with GDM are diagnosed at approximately 28 weeks, they probably have not undergone any supervised training program. Although exercise should not be too vigorous to cause maternal or fetal complications (such as increased core temperature, excessive fatigue, fetal heart rate arrhythmias, and so on) it should be of adequate intensity to cause some change in blood glucose levels independent of other metabolic factors, such as calorie intake and time of day of exercise.[26]

For women with GDM, mild aerobic exercise does not seem to have an adverse effect on the pregnant woman or her fetus. An exercise program done three to four times weekly could be used to attain improved glucose control and reduce the need for exogenous insulin. Because it is often difficult to maintain blood glucose levels in the desired range after breakfast, a mild exercise program, such as a brisk walk, may be especially beneficial at this time.

Exercise for the Older Person with Diabetes

In his review, Schwartz[79] states that guidelines for exercise training for the older patient with diabetes are difficult because no published data pertain directly or specifically to this issue. Extrapolation from information on the effects of exercise on the elderly in general, as well as the effects of exercise on persons with diabetes, must be used. Because most elderly persons with diabetes have NIDDM, the data from this group become of particular interest.

Maximal aerobic capacity ($V_{O_2 \, max}$) declines with age in all persons, but evidence suggests that the slope of the decline can be significantly reduced with exercise training.[39] This can be of substantial importance in the elderly because symptoms of fatigue, weakness, and breathlessness as related to percent $V_{O_2 \, max}$ limit task performances. In training studies of elderly persons (over 65 years of age) researchers have usually demonstrated significant training effects with improvements of $V_{O_2 \, max}$ of up to 30%.[9]

Improvements in risk factors for atherosclerosis are potentially even more important than the increase in $V_{O_2 \, max}$ after training for the elderly person with diabetes, who is already at increased risk for atherosclerosis because of diabetes.[81]

Lean body mass declines with age, and a reduction in adipose tissue and an accompanying increase in lean body mass occur after exercise training. Of equal importance may be the change in the distribution of adiposity. Abdominal obesity is associated with an increased risk for cardiovascular disease. A decrease in the waist/hip ratio and a greater than 20% decline in central fat areas after an intensive exercise training program in elderly persons has been reported.[80]

Because of the potential risks of exercise in persons with diabetes, especially an elderly person, a thorough evaluation by a physician should be performed before an exercise training program is begun. Diabetes treatment, complications, and glucose control should be evaluated. An exercise stress test (with blood pressure and 12-lead electrocardiogram monitoring) should be done to uncover any unknown coronary artery disease. The stress test can also be used to obtain a maximal heart rate measure that can then be used as the basis of a specific exercise prescription. It is recommended that exercise begin at 50% to 60% of target heart rate, with a gradual increase in exercise every 2 to 4 weeks, as tolerated, to 70% to 80% of target heart rate. Appropriate stretching, warm-up, and cool-down periods should accompany all exercise.[79]

Long-Term Complications of Diabetes and Exercise

Disuse syndrome results from disruption of the normal balance between rest and physical activity, thereby decreasing the optimal functioning capacity of an individual. Disuse syndrome can develop within as few as 3 days of immobilization and glucose intolerance in nondiabetic persons begins within 72 hours of absolute bedrest. Disuse combined with diabetes generally yields more disability than would be predicted by diabetes alone, increasing the cost of medical care and home health programs.

Exercise can assist in preventing or reversing disuse syndrome and can be provided for persons with diabetes, even those with severe complications. Unfortunately disuse syndrome is easier to prevent than to correct. Graham and Lasko-McCarthey[38] have recently reviewed the role of exercise for persons with diabetic complications.

Peripheral Vascular Disease/Claudication

Assessment of the arterial circulation of a diabetic patient with periperal vascular disease (PVD) should be conducted before engaging in a physical activity program. Interval training (e.g., 2-minute walk, 1-minute rest, 2-minute walk), swimming, stationary cycling, walking on a slow treadmill at 1 mile/hr, and chair exercises are all options for diabetic persons with PVD. Chair exercises or upper body exercises can be performed by those unable to use the lower extremities because of PVD and claudication. Exercise that provokes intense pain should be discontinued immediately.

Retinopathy

Before diabetic persons with proliferative retinopathy begin an exercise program, submaximal testing should be conducted under the guidance of trained personnel to establish a training heart rate according to blood pressure response.

Aerobic exercise for patients with retinopathy includes stationary cycling, low-intensity rowing on a rowing machine, swimming, and walking. A guide wire or guide person may be needed for assistance with walking or jogging if vision is lost or badly impaired. Resistive exercise using standard weight-lifting equipment is not recommended. Exercise is contraindicated if the person has recently undergone retinal photocoagulation or eye surgery.

Nephropathy

The elevated risk factors for cardiovascular disease in patients with neuropathy indicate a role for exercise. However, goals need to be established on the basis of the patient's limitations, since exercise capacity is usually exceptionally low.

Low hemoglobin and hematocrit values and abnormal cardiac function are characteristic for this population and contribute to a low physical work capacity. Exercise must be done at mild-to-moderate levels. Renal osteodystrophy begins very early when renal function begins to decline. Thus, weight-bearing exercises, done with dynamic physical activity, may result in improvements in bone volume.

Hemodialysis patients may benefit from aerobic-type activities such as brisk walking, cycling, and swimming; however, anemia, cardiovascular dysfunction, and low physical working capacity underscore the importance of a gradual, progressive training program. No exercise training should begin until the patient is stabilized on a program of medication, dialysis, and diet. Exercises that involve fluid changes, that damage weakened bones, or cause sustained elevations in blood pressure should be avoided.

Sensorimotor Neuropathy

Although exercise cannot reverse symptoms of sensorimotor neuropathy, it can prevent the loss of physical fitness associated with disuse syndrome. Adaptive shortening of connective tissue can be caused by disuse and immobilization. Daily range-of-motion exercises for the major joints, such as the ankle, knee, hip, shoulder, wrist, and trunk area, are essential for preventing or minimizing contractures. Loss of sensation to the extremities can create a greater susceptibility to overstretching in muscles and connective tissue. Stretching exercises should be performed gently through the pain-free range of motion at all times.

The frequent incidence of blisters, stress fractures, red and hot spots, and muscle strains requires inspection of the feet after every workout session and frequent observations of the feet as part of the daily hygiene routine.

Autonomic Neuropathy

Exercise tolerance with autonomic neuropathy may be severely limited because of impairment of the sympathetic and parasympathetic nervous systems that normally augment cardiac output and redirect peripheral blood flow to the working muscles. Commonly the person becomes easily fatigued with little exertion.

Cardiac denervation syndrome (sudden death, silent myocardial infarction) has been attributed to the neuropathic diabetic syndrome in which the heart becomes unresponsive to nerve impulses. In autonomic neuropathy, the counterregulatory response may also be impaired, putting the individual at increased risk with exercise. Clinically this state is recognized by a fixed heart rate of 80 to 90 beats/minute while the patient rests or exercises.

Activities to be avoided are those that cause rapid changes in body position or that elicit and require rapid and significant changes in heart rate or blood pressure. As exercise tachycardia is often blunted, high-intensity exercise should be avoided.

EXERCISE PRESCRIPTION

The goal of exercise training is to achieve optimal cardiovascular, muscular, and metabolic adaptations to aerobic stimulus. Cardiovascular fitness to prevent or minimize the long-term complications related to diabetes is of obvious importance for persons with diabetes. Flexibility in persons with diabetes can be impaired if muscle collagen becomes glycosylated. Warm-up and cool-down components, which increase flexibility, therefore take on added significance. Muscle strength may deteriorate as a result of neuropathy; muscle-strengthening exercise can improve muscle strength. Furthermore, increased muscle mass resulting from strength training may also result in a reduction of plasma insulin concentrations, but despite the lower insulin concentrations, glucose tolerance improves and peripheral glucose disposal increases as well.

Each exercise session should begin with a warm-up and end with a cool-down period. A warm-up period of at least 5 minutes is adequate for circulatory adjustment to exercise and to minimize potential arrhythmias, 5 to 7 minutes of stretching and cardiovascular warm-up are added to this initial period. This is followed by aerobic activity. Aerobic activities require large amounts of oxygen and usually involve movement of many large muscles. An exercise prescription clearly specifies type, intensity, duration, and frequency of the activity in days per week.

Heart rate (pulse rate) and perceived exertion (PE) are two methods used to determine the intensity of exercise. PE involves having individuals rate how hard (strong) they "perceive" they are exercising and how tired they are. The original scale, developed by psychologist Gunnar Borg, allows persons to rate their activity on a scale from 6 to 20. In 1986, the American College of Sports Medicine released a revised scale from 0 ("nothing at all") to 10 ("very, very strong").[3] See Table 3-5 for the scale and the written description for rating the degree of perceived exertion. Table 3-6 lists target heart rates for exercise related to the desired exercise intensity.

Muscle-strengthening exercises are usually performed after the aerobic portion of exercise and take on added importance for persons with diabetes. The exercise session should end with a cool-down period of 10 to 12 minutes, consisting of cardiovascular cool down, specific muscle strengthening exercises, and exercises for flexibility and relaxation. Fig. 3-3 details a typical exercise session.

Adherence to a regular exercise program, like most other lifestyle changes, is difficult to maintain.[52] Approximately 50 of enrolled persons drop out within the first few months.

Table 3-5 American College of Sports Medicine Revised Scale for Rating Perceived Exertion

Rating	Description
0	Nothing at all
0.5	Very, very weak
1.0	Very weak
2	Weak
3	Moderate
4	Somewhat strong
5	Strong
6	
7	Very strong
8	
9	
10	Very, very strong
	Maximal

Reprinted with permission from Borg GAV: Psychophysical bases of perceived exertion, Med Sci Sports Exer 14:380, 1982.

Table 3-6 Target Heart Rates During Exercise: Ten-Second Heartbeats

Intensity	Age											
	15	20	25	30	35	40	45	50	55	60	65	70
60%	20	20	19	19	18	18	17	17	16	16	15	15
75%	25	25	24	23	23	22	22	21	20	20	19	19
85%	29	28	27	27	26	25	25	24	23	22	22	21

Reprinted with permission from Franz MJ: Diabetes and exercise: guidelines for safe and enjoyable activity, Wayzata, MN, 1985, Diabetes Center, Inc.

Suggestions to improve adherence include:
1. making the exercise program an enjoyable social experience.
2. providing enthusiastic leadership.
3. giving personalized feedback and praise.
4. promoting spouse and family support.
5. setting flexible goal.
6. preparing attendance contracts.
7. using distraction techniques (music).

It may also be helpful to provide persons with a set of strategies to cope with the problem of relapse at the beginning of the program, thus minimizing the likelihood of a complete relapse.

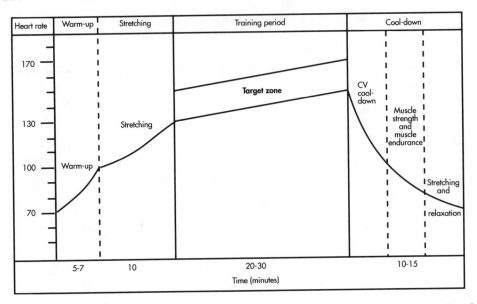

Fig. 3-3   Training pattern for an exercise session. (Reprinted with permission from Franz MJ and Norstrom J: Diabetes actively staying healthy. Your game plan for diabetes and exercise, Wayzata, MN, 1990, Diabetes Center Inc.)

SUMMARY

Persons with diabetes experience the same benefits from exercise that persons without diabetes gain from a regular exercise program, namely, improved fitness and psychologic state, change in body composition, weight control, and improved physical work capacity. For persons with diabetes, exercise has additional benefits; for example, increased insulin sensitivity and improved glucose tolerance, potential reduction in insulin dosage, reversal of resistance to insulin, reduction of risk factors for atherosclerosis, and a potential lowering of blood pressure.

The goals of an exercise program are (1) to allow individuals with diabetes to experience the same benefits and enjoyment that people without diabetes gain from a regular exercise program, (2) to maintain or improve cardiovascular fitness, (3) to improve flexibility and muscle strength, (4) to allow persons with IDDM to safely participate in and enjoy physical and/or sporting activities, and (5) to assist in blood glucose and weight control and overall diabetes management in people with NIDDM.

Above all, exercise should be fun. It should be presented as part of a reasonable health care plan. Regular exercisers stick with it because they enjoy it. It may take time to develop this attitude toward exercise, but eventually the rewards are worth it.

REFERENCES

1. Ahlborg G, and others: Substrate turnover during prolonged exercise, J Clin Invest 53:1080-1090, 1974.
2. Ahlborg G and Felig P: Lactate and glucose exchange across the forearm, legs, and splanchnic bed during and after prolonged leg exercise, J Clin Invest 69:45-54, 1982.

3. American College of Sports Medicine. Guidelines for Exercise Testing and Prescription, Philadelphia, 1986, Lea & Febiger, p 23.

4. American College of Obstetricians and Gynecologists. Exercise During Pregnancy and the Postnatal Period (AGOG Home Exercise Program), Washington, DC, 1985, AGOG.

5. American Diabetes Association Position Statement. Diabetes mellitus and exercise, Diabetes Care 13:804-805, 1990.

6. American Diabetes Association Technical Review. Exercise and NIDDM, Diabetes Care 13:785-789, 1990.

7. Arslanian S and others: Impact of physical fitness and glycemic control on in vivo insulin action in adolescents with IDDM, Diabetes Care 13:9-15, 1990.

8. Artal R, Wiswell R, and Romen Y: Hormonal response to exercise in diabetic and nondiabetic pregnant patients, Diabetes 34 (suppl 2):78-80, 1985.

9. Barenhop DT and others: Physiologic adjustments to higher-or lower-intensity exercise in elders, Med Sci Sports Exerc 15:496-502, 1983.

10. Berger M, and others: Metabolic and hormonal effects of muscular exercise in juvenile type diabetics, Diabetologia 13:355-365, 1977.

11. Berger M and others: Absorption kinetics and biological effects of subcutaneously injected insulin preparations, Diabetes Care 5:77-91, 1982.

12. Bjorntorp P and others: Effects of physical training on glucose tolerance, plasma insulin and lipids and body composition in men after myocardial infarction, Acta Med Scand 192:439-443, 1972.

13. Bjorntorp P, daJounge K, and Sjostrom L: The effect of physical training on insulin production in obesity, Metabolism 19:631-637, 1970.

14. Bjorkman 0 and others: Influence of hypoglucagonemia on splanchnic glucose output during leg exercise in man, Clin Physiol 1:43-57, 1981.

15. Blake GA, Levin SR, and Koyal SN: Exercise-induced hypertension in normotensive patients with NIDDM, Diabetes Care 13:799-801, 1990.

16. Bogardus C and others: Effects of physical training and diet therapy on carbohydrate metabolism in patients with glucose intolerance and non–insulin-dependent diabetes mellitus, Diabetes 33:311-318, 1984.

17. Burstein R and others: Acute reversal of the enhanced insulin action in trained athletes: associate with insulin receptor changes, Diabetes 34:756-760, 1985.

18. Campaigne BN, Wallberg-Henrikssen H, and Gunnarsson R: 12-hour glycemic response following acute physical exercise in type I diabetes in relation to insulin dose and caloric intake, Diabetes Care 10:716-721, 1987.

19. Costill DL: Carbohydrate nutrition before, during and after exercise, Fed Proc 44:364-368, 1985.

20. Costill DL and others: Effects of elevated plasma FFA and insulin on muscle glycogen usage during exercise, J Appl Physiol 43:695-699, 1977.

21. Cryer PE: Hypoglycemic glucose counterregulation in patients with insulin-dependent diabetes mellitus, J Lab Clin Med, 99:451-456, 1982.

22. DeFronzo RA, Ferrannini E, and Koivisto V: New concepts in the pathogenesis and treatment of NIDDM, Am J Med 74:52-81, 1983.

23. DeFronzo RA, Hendler R, and Christensen NJ: Stimulation of counterregulatory hormonal responses in diabetic man by a fall in glucose concentration, Diabetes 29:125-131, 1980.

24. Devlin JT and others: Enhanced peripheral and splanchnic insulin sensitivity in NIDDM after single bout of exercise, Diabetes 36:434-439, 1987.

25. Durak E, Jovanovic-Peterson L, and Peterson CM: Randomized crossover study of effect of resistance training on glycemic control, muscular strength, and cholesterol in type I diabetic men, Diabetes Care 13:1039-1043, 1990.

26. Durak EP, Jovanovic-Peterson L, and Peterson CM: Physical and glycemic response of women with gestational diabetes to a moderately intense exercise program, Diabetes Educator 16:309-312, 1990.

27. Edwards AV: The sensitivity of the hepatic glycogenolytic mechanism to stimulation of the splanchnic nerves, J Physiol (Lond) 220:315, 1977.

28. Ekoe J-M: Overview of diabetes mellitus and exercise. Med Sci Sports Exerc 21:353-355, 1989.

29. Felig P: The glucose-alanine cycle, Metabolism 22:179-207, 1973.

30. Felig P and Wahren J: Fuel homeostasis in exercise, N Engl J Med 293:1078-1084, 1975.

31. Felig P and others: Plasma glucagon levels in exercising man, N Engl J Med 287:184-185, 1972.

32. Ferrannini E and others: Effect of fatty acids on glucose production and utilization in man, J Clin Invest 72:1737-1747, 1983.

33. Fery F, deMaertelaer V, and Balasse EO: Mechanism of hyperketonaemic effect of prolonged exercise in insulin-deprived Type I (insulin-dependent) diabetic patients, Diabetologia 30:298-304, 1987.
34. Franz MJ and Norstrom J: Diabetes Actively Staying Healthy. Your Game Plan for Diabetes and Exercise. Wayzata, MN, 1990, Diabetes Center, Inc.
35. Franz MJ: Diabetes and Exercise: Guidelines for Safe and Enjoyable Activity. Wayzata, MN, 1988, Diabetes Center, Inc.
36. Franz MJ: Exercise and diabetes mellitus. In Powers MA, ed: Handbook of Diabetes Nutritional Management. Rockville, Md, 1987, Aspen Publishers.
37. Galbo H: Hormonal and metabolic adaptations to exercise, Stuttgart, New York 1983, Georg Thieme Verlag.
38. Graham C and Lasko-McCarthey P: Exercise options for persons with diabetic complications, The Diabetes Educator 16:212-219, 1990.
39. Hagberg JM: Effect of training on the decline of Vo_{2max} with aging, Fed Proc 46:1830-1833, 1987.
40. Hagenfeldt L: Metabolism of free fatty acids and ketone bodies during exercise in normal and diabetic man, Diabetes 28 (suppl 1):66-70, 1979.
41. Hollingsworth DR and Moore TR: Postprandial walking exercise in pregnant insulin-dependent (type I) diabetic women: Reduction of plasma lipid levels but absence of a significant effect on glycemic control, Am J Obstet Gynecol 157:1359-1363, 1987.
42. Holloszy JO and others: Effects of exercise on glucose tolerance and insulin resistance, Acta Med Scand Suppl 711:55-65, 1986.
43. Holloszy JO and Coyle EF: Adaptation of skeletal muscle to endurance exercise and their metabolic consequences, J Appl Physiol 56:831-838, 1984.
44. Horton ES: Exercise and diabetes mellitus, Med Clin North Am 72:1301-1321, 1988.
45. Hultman E: Studies on muscle metabolism of glycogen and active phosphate in man with special reference to exercise and diet, Scand J Clin Lab Invest 19:1-63, 1967.
46. Issekutz B: Clearance rate of metabolizable and nonmetabolizable sugar in insulin-infused dogs and in exercising dogs, Diabetes 29:348-354, 1980.
47. Koivisto VA: Diabetes in the elderly: What role for exercise? Geriatrics 36:74-83, 1981.
48. LaPorte RE: American Diabetes Association Exercise Council, Unpublished data, June 1990.
49. LaPorte RE and others: Pittsburg insulin-dependent diabetes mellitus morbidity and mortality study: Physical activity and diabetic complictions, Pediatrics 78:1027-1033, 1986.
50. Leon AS and others: Leisure-time physical activity levels and risk of coronary heart disease and death: the multiple risk factor intervention trial, JAMA 258:2388-2395, 1987.
51. MacDonald MJ: Postexercise late-onset hypoglycemia in insulin-dependent diabetic patients, Diabetes Care 10:584-588, 1987.
52. Martin JE and Dubbert PM: Adherence to exercise. Exerc Sport Sci Rev 13:137-167, 1985.
53. Meinders AE, Willekens FLA, and Heere LP: Metabolic and hormonal changes in IDDM during long-distance run, Diabetes Care 11:1-7, 1988.
54. Mikines KJ and others: Insulin sensitivity and responsiviness after acute exercise in man, Clin Physiol 5 (suppl 4): A67, 1985.
55. Minuk HL and others: Glucoregulatory and metabolic response to exercise in obese noninsulin-dependent diabetes, Am J Physiol 240:E458-E464, 1981.
56. Mitchell TH and others: Hyperglycemia after intense exercise in IDDM subjects during continuous subcutaneous insulin infusion, Diabetes Care 11:311-317, 1988.
57. Morgensen CE and Vittinghus E: Urinary albumin excretion during exercise in juvenile diabetes, Scand J Clin Lab Invest 35:295-300, 1975.
58. Nesto RW and others: Angina and exertional myocardial ischemia in diabetic and nondiabetic patients: Assessment by exercise thallium scintigraphy, Ann Intern Med 108:170-175, 1988.
59. Paffenbarger RS and others: Physical activity, all-cause mortality and longevity of college alumni, N Engl J Med 314:605-613, 1986.
60. Plough T, Galbo H, and Richter EA: Increased muscle glucose uptake during contractions: no need for insulin, Am J Physiol 247:E726-E731, 1984.
61. Pollock ML, Wilmore JH, and Fox SM: Exercise in Health and Disease Evaluation and Prescription for Prevention and Rehabilitation, Philadelphia, 1984, WB Saunders.
62. Randall PJ, Newsholme EA, and Garland PB: Regulation of glucose uptake by muscle. 8. Effects of fatty

acids and ketone bodies and pyruvate acid of alloxan-diabetes and starvation on the uptake and metabolic fate of glucose in rat heart and diaphragm muscle, Biochem J 93:652-655, 1964.

63. Reitman JS and others: Improvement of glucose homeostasis after exercise in NIDDM, Diabetes Care 7:434-441, 1984.
64. Rennie MJ, Paik DM, and Salaiman WR: Uptake and release of hormones and metabolites by tissues of exercising leg in man. Am J Physiol 231:967-973, 1976.
65. Richter EA and Galbo H: Diabetes, insulin and exercise. Sports Medicine 3:275-288, 1986.
66. Richter EA and others: Muscle glycogenolysis during exercise: dual control by epinephrine and contractions, Am J Physiol 242:E25-E32, 1982.
67. Richter EA, Ruderman NB, and Schneider S: Diabetes and exercise, Am J Med 70:201-209, 1981.
68. Richter EA and others: Significance of glucagon for insulin secretion and hepatic glycogenolysis during exercise in rats, Horm Met Res 13:323-326, 1981.
69. Richter EA and Galbo H: Rate of glycogen breakdown and lactate release in contracting isolated skeletal muscle is dependent on glycogen concentration, Clin Physiol 5 (suppl 4):82,1985.
70. Ruderman NB and Haudenschild C: Diabetes as an atherogenic factor, Prog Cardiovasc Dis 16:373-412, 1984.
71. Ruegemer JJ and others: Differences between prebreakfast and late afternoon glycemic responses to exercise in IDDM patients, Diabetes Care 13:104-110, 1990 .
72. Saltin B: Physiologic adaptation to physical conditioning: old problems revisited, Acta Med Scand (Suppl) 711:11-24, 1986.
73. Saltin B and others: Physical training and glucose tolerance in middle-aged men with chemical diabetes. Diabetes 28(Suppl 1):30-32, 1979.
74. Sato Y, Igudi A, and Sakamoto N: Biochemical determination of training effects using insulin clamp technique, Horm Metab Res 16:483-486, 1984.
75. Schiffrin A and Parikh S: Accommodating planned exercise in type I diabetic patients on intensive treatment, Diabetes Care 8:337-342, 1985.
76. Schneider SH and others: Studies on the mechanism of improved glucose control during regular exercise in type 2 (noninsulin-dependent) diabetes, Diabetologia 26:355-360, 1984.
77. Schneider SH and Kanj H: Clinical aspects of exercise and diabetes mellitus, Curr Concepts Nutr 15:145-182, 1986.
78. Schneider SH and others: Abnormal glucoregulation during exercising in type II (noninsulin-dependent) diabetes. Metabolism 36:1161-1167, 1986.
79. Schwartz RS: Exercise training in treatment of diabetes mellitus in elderly patients, Diabetes Care 13 (suppl 2):77-85, 1990.
80. Schwartz RS, and others: Intensive exercise training in the elderly decreases body fat and control fat distribution, Clin Res 37:149A, 1989, (Abst.).
81. Seals DR and others: Effects of endurance training on glucose tolerance and plasma lipid levels in older men and women, JAMA 252:645-649, 1984.
82. Stratton R and others: Improved glycemic control after supervised 8-wk exercise program in insulin-dependent diabetic adolescents. Diabetes Care 10:589-593, 1987.
83. Taylor R and others: Physical activity and prevalence of diabetes in Melanesian and Indian men in Fiji. Diabetolgoia 27:578-582, 1984.
84. Trovati M and others: Influence of physical training on blood glucose control, glucose tolerance, insulin secretion and insulin action in NIDDM, Diabetes Care 7:416-420, 1984.
85. Wahren J: Glucose turnover during exercise in healthy man and in patients with diabetes, Diabetes 28 (suppl 1):82-88, 1979.
86. Wahren J and others: Glucose metabolism during leg exercise in man, J Clin Invest 50:2715-2725, 1971.
87. Wahren J and others: Glucose and amino acid metabolism during recovery after exercise, J Appl Physiol 34:838-845, 1973.
88. Wahren J, Felig P, and Hagenfeldt L: Physical exercise and fuel homeostasis in diabetes mellitus, Diabetologia 14:213-222, 1978.
89. Wahren J, Hagenfeldt L, and Felig P: Splanchic and leg exchange of glucose, amino acids, and free fatty acids during exercise in diabetes mellitus, J Clin Invest 55:1303-1314, 1975.
90. Wallberg-Henriksson H, and others: Increased peripheral sensitivity and muscle mitochondrial enzymes but unchanged blood glucose control in type I diabetics after physical training, Diabetes 31:1044-1050, 1982.

91. Wallberg-Henriksson H, and others: Glucose transport into rat skeletal: interaction between exercise and insulin, J Appl Physiol 65:909-913, 1988.
92. Wardzala LJ, Cushman SW, Salans LB: Mechanisms of insulin action on glucose transport in the isolated rat adipose cell, J Biol Chem 253:8002-8005, 1978.
93. Wasserman DH, Lickley HL, and Vranic M: Interactions between glucagon and hypoglycemia exercise in dogs, J Clin Invest 74:1404-1413, 1984.
94. Wasserman DH and Vranic M: Interaction between insulin and counterregulatory hormones in control of substrate utlllzatlon ln health and diabetes during exercise, Diabetes Metab Rev 1:359-384, 1986.
95. Wing RR: Behavioral strategies for weight reduction in obese type II diabetes patients, Diabetes Care 12:139-144, 1989.
96. Wing RR and others: Behavior change, weight loss, and physiological lmprovements in type II diabetic patients, J Consult Clin Psychol 53: 111-122, 1985.
97. Zinman B, Zuniga-Guajardo S, and Kelly D: Comparison of the acute and long-term effects of exercise on glucose control in type I diabetes, Diabetes Care 7:515-519, 1984.

CHAPTER 4

Pharmacologic Therapies in the Management of Diabetes Mellitus

JOHN R. WHITE, JR. AND R. KEITH CAMPBELL

Effective pharmacologic management of diabetes mellitus is a relatively recent development. Before the 1920s a diagnosis of insulin-dependent diabetes mellitus (IDDM) carried with it the grave prognosis of a rapid downhill course. The first effective treatment was realized, and research into the prevention and treatment of diabetes burgeoned with Banting's and Best's discovery in 1922[7] of insulin and its hypoglycemic properties. In the early 1920s a patient requiring insulin therapy was subjected to multiple daily injections of a crude animal insulin extract with reusable and often dull needles. Today a patient may use a myriad of various highly purified animal or human insulins with a choice of time action profile injected with microfine needles and disposable syringes or delivered via internal or external insulin pump. The first oral agent, Synthalin, was synthesized in the 1920s by Frank and others.[11] Synthalin has long since been replaced by the less toxic sulfonylurea agents. Currently in the United States there are two generations of sulfonylurea agents in use. Outside the United States two biquanide compounds (buformin and metformin) are being used as well. Significant advances have been made, but unfortunately there is still no cure for diabetes. Insulin and the sulfonylurea agents can decrease morbidity and mortality when used appropriately but are far from the wanted panacea.

This chapter will review the pharmacology, clinical dosing, and monitoring of insulin and the oral hypoglycemic agents available to the clinician in the United States. Specific chapter objectives will (1) discuss the normal physiologic effects of insulin; (2) list the clinical indications for exogenous insulin use; (3) differentiate sources and the adverse effect profiles for various insulin sources; (4) counsel a patient as to the appropriate procedure for insulin storage, dose preparation, and administration; (5) discuss the pros and cons of the various insulin regimens; (6) list the various compilations of insulin, and state the treatments of the complications; (7) discuss the

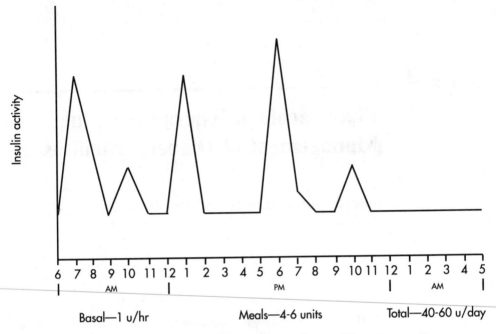

Fig. 4-1 Normal physiologic insulin secretion.

physiologic effects of the sulfonylureas; (8) choose an oral hypoglycemic agent and regimen for a given patient; (9) list the complications associated with sulfonylureas; and (10) discuss the potential drug interaction types associated with oral hypoglycemic agents.

INSULIN
Structure and Production

Preproinsulin is produced in the β-cells of the islets of Langerhans in the pancreas. It is a large molecular weight (mw ≈ 12,000) protein with a half-life of approximately one minute. Pre-proinsulin is cleaved to form proinsulin (mw ≈ 9000). Proinsulin is in turn cleaved to form equimolar amounts of insulin and C-peptide.[32] Insulin is a proteinaceous molecule composed of 51 amino acids arranged in two polypeptide chains (A and B) that are connected via disulfide bonds. The plasma half-lives of insulin and C- peptide are ≈4 and ≈30 minutes, respectively.[35,36,38]

Approximately 200 units of insulin are stored in the normal human pancreas, while virtually none is found in the pancreas of the patient with IDDM after approximately 7 years of disease.[14] The normal human pancreas has a basal insulin secretory rate of 1 to 2 units per hour, with postprandial rates increasing to 4 to 6 units per hour (Fig. 4-1). Normal daily total amounts of secreted insulin range from 40 to 60 units. Clearance of insulin takes place in the periphery, the liver, and the kidneys. Patients who suffer diabetic nephropathy may require downward adjustments in their insulin regimens caused by decreases in renal insulin metabolism that parallel renal failure.

C-peptide measurement is useful in both the clinical and the research setting. The measurement of C-peptide may be utilized in the differential of hypoglycemia when factitious insulin administration is a possibility. It is also useful as an indicator of residual β-cell function in patients receiving exogenous insulin and in the evaluation of pancreatectomy status.

Physiologic Effects of Insulin

Insulin exerts an effect on carbohydrate, fat, and protein metabolism. Therefore, disruption of insulin secretion or disposition or action such as encountered with diabetes mellitus results in abnormal carbohydrate, fat, and protein disposition and utilization. These metabolic abnormalities are closely linked to the acute and chronic complications encountered in the patient with diabetes.[19]

The effects of insulin on carbohydrate metabolism include: (1) enhanced rate of glycogen synthesis and storage in the liver, skeletal muscle, and other tissue and (2) increased facilitated transport of glucose from the systemic circulation into skeletal muscle, adipose tissue, and some smooth muscle organs. Insulin is not required for glucose transport in the central nervous system, intestinal mucosa, ocular lens, and renal tubular epithelium. Therefore, when hyperglycemia is present, these tissues are subjected to high intracellular glucose concentrations. Lack of insulin or insulin activity results in hyperglycemia caused by impaired glucose transport and glycogen storage. A relative intracellular hypoglycemia in insulin-dependent tissue triggers the liberation of hepatic glucose (glycogenolysis), thus escalating the systemic hyperglycemia.[17,19,39]

Insulin affects protein synthesis and storage in a variety of ways: (1) insulin suppresses the formation of glucose from amino acids (gluconeogenesis); (2) insulin depresses the rate of protein catabolism; (3) the presence of insulin favors the transport of amino acids into cells; and (4) insulin affects mRNA to, in turn, increase the rate of protein production. Lack of insulin results in an increase in protein catabolism coupled with a decreased ability to form new proteins from constituent amino acids. Hyperglycemia is again escalated, but in this case, it is secondary to increased rates of gluconeogenesis.[17,19,39]

Insulin also effects fat metabolism. Lipase enzymes are inhibited by insulin. Lipase is responsible for the breakdown of triglycerides into free fatty acids. Insulin also promotes the transport of glucose into fat cells. A fraction of this glucose is utilized to synthesize free fatty acids, while another fraction eventually is converted to glycerol. Glycerol is essential in the formation of triglycerides from free fatty acids. Therefore, insulin is lipogenenic and promotes fat storage. Lack of insulin results in depletion of fat stores and high concentrations of circulating free fatty acids.[17,19,39]

Table 4-1   Amino-Acid Sequences of Various Insulins

Source	A chain	B chain
	Position 8/10	Position 30
Human	Threonine/isoleucine	Threonine
Beef	Alaninine/valine	Alanine
Pork	Threonine/isoleucine	Alanine

Indications for the Clinical Use of Exogenous Insulin

Insulin is indicated for use in the following situations:
1. All persons with IDDM require exogenous insulin.
2. Women with gestational diabetes, if diet alone does not adequately control blood glucose levels (see Chapter 9).
3. Persons with non–insulin-dependent diabetes (NIDDM) who are not controlled by diet or oral hypoglycemic agents.
4. Persons with NIDDM who are experiencing stress such as infection or surgery, or require corticosteroid therapy.
5. Treatment of diabetic ketoacidosis (see Chapter 8).
6. Treatment of hyperosmolar nonketotic syndrome.
7. Individuals who are receiving parenteral nutrition or who require high caloric supplementation to meet increased intermittent energy needs may require exogenous insulin.[3,4]

Sources of Insulin

The three species sources of insulin that are currently clinically utilized are beef, pork, and human. The six product types include beef, pork, beef/pork combination, biosynthetic recombinant human derived from bacteria, biosynthetic recombinant human derived from yeast (available in Europe), and semisynthetic human insulin derived from pork. Structurally, pork and beef insulin differ from human insulin by one and three amino acids, respectively (see Table 4-1).[39,40]

Human insulin is currently produced by two different methods in the United States. Human insulin of recombinant DNA origin (Eli Lilly and Company) is produced by *Escherichia coli* into which plasmids bearing the sequencing information for human proinsulin have been inserted. The bacteria are then placed into an appropriate medium under conditions conducive to multiplication and proinsulin production. The proinsulin is harvested, enzymatically cleaved, and the I resultant insulin purified.[13]

Semisynthetic human insulin (Novo-Nordisk) is produced by enzymatic transpeptidation of pork insulin at position 30 of the B chain with the substitution of threanine for alanine.[30]

Clinically, human insulins differ from animal source insulins with respect to antigenicity and solubility. Human insulins are less antigenic than pork insulins; in turn, pork insulins are less antigenic than beef insulins. Theoretically, decreased antigenicity parallels a decreased incidence of lipoatrophy, local and systemic allergic reactions, and antibody production. While it is clear that persons treated with human insulin produce lower titers of insulin antibodies, the clinical significance is uncertain. Insulin antibodies, when present in high titers, may cause insulin resistance. Some clinicians believe that insulin antibodies may bind and subsequently release insulin, resulting in erratic time action profiles. Human insulin is more soluble than animal source insulins, and thus displays a slightly different pharmacokinetic pattern. [24,27,34] A higher rate of subcutaneous absorption and a shorter duration of action have been observed with human insulin as compared with animal source insulins. Thus, the individual with diabetes switching from one species source to another must be closely monitored and subsequently have doses adjusted appropriately. Insulin requirements may decline as antibody titers wane in persons switched from animal source insulin to human insulin because of immunologically mediated insulin resistance.

There is a great deal of discussion as to which insulin source is the most efficacious. Insulins from all sources are apparently equally effective in normalizing blood glucose levels. Human insulin, however, has the most acceptable side effect profile of all the insulins. Lower titers of antibodies and resolution of lipoatrophy may be seen in the individual who is switched from animal source to human insulin. At this time there is no evidence that supports an across-the-board switch to human insulin; thus, persons who are maintained without problems on animal source insulin should probably remain on those insulins. Human insulin is indicated in the following situations.

1. Persons who use insulin temporarily (i.e., individual with IDDM undergoing surgery).
2. Persons who have a history of drug allergies.
3. Persons with an active allergic response to animal source insulin (including lipoatrophy and insulin resistance).
4. Persons with religious or ethical aversion to animal source products.
5. Newly diagnosed persons with IDDM.
6. Pregnant women with diabetes or those planning pregnancy.

It should be noted that human insulin was produced in part as a response to the US Diabetes Advisory Board's findings in 1978. An insulin shortage in the 1990s was predicted by this group, based on figures of expected population growth and anticipated decreases in red meat consumption in the Western world.[1] With the continued population expansion, decreases in red meat consumption, advances in biotechnology, and side-effect profile of human insulin, it is reasonable to predict that animal source insulins will eventually be completely phased out.

Preparations

Insulins are available in short-, intermediate-, and long-acting preparations (Table 4-2). The time action profile of each of these categories is obviously different (Fig. 4-2). Ad-

Table 4-2   Insulins Available in the United States

Product	Manufacturer	Strength
Short-acting		
Beef		
Iletin II regular	Lilly	U-100
Semilente	Novo-Nordisk	U-100
Pork		
Iletin II regular	Lilly	U-100,-500
Regular	Novo-Nordisk	U-100
Purified pork regular	Novo-Nordisk	U-100
Velosulin	Novo-Nordisk	U-100
Beef/pork		
Iletin I regular	Lilly	U-40,-100
Iletin I semilente	Lilly	U-40,-100
Human		
Humulin regular	Lilly	U-100
Humulin BR	Lilly	U-100
Novolin R	Novo-Nordisk	U-100
Velosulin human R	Novo-Nordisk	U-100
Intermediate-acting		
Beef		
Iletin II lente	Lilly	U-100
Iletin II NPH	Lilly	U-100
Lente	Novo-Nordisk	U-100
NPH	Novo-Nordisk	U-100
Pork		
Iletin II lente	Lilly	U-100
Iletin II NPH	Lilly	U-100
Purified pork lente	Novo-Nordisk	U-100
Purified pork NPH	Novo-Nordisk	U-100
Insulatard NPH	Novo-Nordisk	U-100
Beef/pork		
Iletin I NPH	Lilly	U-40,-100
Iletin I lente	Lilly	U-40,-100

ditionally, the time action profile of the various preparations in each category will vary slightly. Last, the time action profile of each particular insulin preparation varies with different injection sites, changes in ambient temperature, among individuals, and with source. These three categories are used for ease of classification, and should not imply that insulins within a given category are interchangeable without proper monitoring and

Table 4-2 Insulins Available in the United States—cont'd.

Product	Manufacturer	Strength
Human		
Humulin L (lente)	Lilly	U-100
Humulin N (NPH)	Lilly	U-100
Novulin L (lente)	Novo-Nordisk	U-100
Novulin N (NPH)	Novo-Nordisk	U-100
Insulatard NPH human	Novo-Nordisk	U-100
Long-acting		
Beef		
Iletin II PZI	Lilly	U-100
Ultralente	Novo-Nordisk	U-100
Pork		
Iletin II PZI	Lilly	U-100
Beef/pork		
Iletin I PZI	Lilly	U-40,-100
Iletin I ultralente	Lilly	U-40,-100
Human		
Humulin U (ultralente)	Lilly	U-100
Fixed combinations (all are U-100 insulins)		
		NPH-REG
Pork		
Mixtard	Novo-Nordisk	70/30
Human		
Humulin 70/30	Lilly	70/30
Novolin 70/30	Novo-Nordisk	70/30
Mixtard human 70/30	Novo-Nordisk	70/30

dosage adjustment. Clinicians are cautioned against relying too heavily on chart descriptions of time action profiles of insulin and should base dosage adjustments on the person's self-monitoring of blood glucose (SMBG).

The short-acting insulins include regular, buffered regular, and Semilente. When administered subcutaneously, the onset of action of these insulins is $\approx$ ½ to 1 hour, peak activity is $\approx$ 2 to 4 hours, and duration is $\approx$ 6 to 8 hours (Fig. 4-2). Regular and buffered regular are formulations containing solubilized crystalline insulin. These formulations are solutions; their appearance should thus be clear. *Regular insulin is the **only** insulin that may be administered intravenously, since all other insulin formulations are suspensions.*

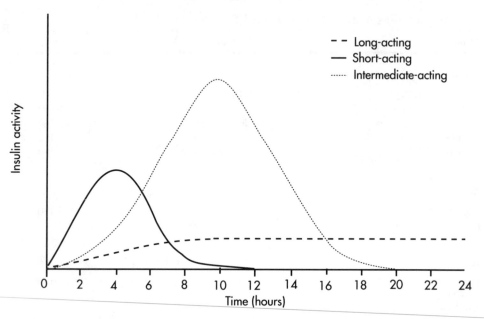

Fig. 4-2 Insulin time action profiles: short- versus intermediate- versus long-acting.

Buffered regular is the insulin of choice for continuous subcutaneous insulin infusion devices (CSII). Semilente is a suspension containing an amorphous precipitate of insulin and zinc. Semilente insulin has a slightly delayed onset and peak and a longer duration than Regular insulin.[16,17]

The intermediate-acting insulins include Lente, and Neutral Protamine Hagedorn (NPH), also known as isophane. The intermediate-acting insulins have an onset of ≈ 1 to 4 hours, a peak effect at ≈ 6 to 8 hours, and a duration of ≈ 10 to 16 hours (Fig. 4-2). Some clinicians consider human Ultralente to be an intermediate-acting preparation because its time action profile falls between the "classic" intermediate-acting preparations and long-acting preparations. This difference in time action profile is secondary to the greater solubility and enhanced absorption of human insulin.[16,17]

NPH insulin was introduced in 1946 by researchers at Nordisk laboratories in Denmark.[26] NPH insulin contains a combination of zinc-insulin crystals and protamine sulfate in a ratio such that the solid phase is composed of insulin, zinc, and protamine. Protamine is a protein derived from fish sperm. This foreign protein, which causes an allergic response in a small fraction of patients, helped prompt researchers to develop Lente insulins.[20] Lente insulin is a 70→30 combination of Ultralente and Semilente. Lente insulin is a useful intermediate-acting formulation, particularly in those patients sensitive to protamine. Both NPH and Lente display time action profiles that favor their use in two daily injection regimens.

Long-acting insulins include Protamine Zinc Insulin (PZI) and Ultralente. These insulins have an onset of between 6 and 14 hours and a duration that may range from 18 to

36 hours (Fig. 4-2). The long-acting insulins are not usually associated with a peak effect but instead provide a sustained, relatively consistent insulin release.

Strength and Purity

Insulin is available in the United States in three strengths: (1) U-40, (2) U-100, and (3) U-500 (by special order from Eli Lilly and Company). The strength correlates to the number of units of insulin per milliliter of product. In the past, a U-80 insulin was available, but it was decertified in 1980 by the Food and Drug Administration. Currently, the vast majority of insulin-requiring patients utilize U-100, with less than 2% using U-40 products. Some persons who require small doses of insulin prefer U-40 strength; however, with the release of 50-unit and 30-unit U-100 syringes, the justification for U-40 insulins is further weakened. There is a general agreement shared by the FDA, the American Diabetes Association, and the American Pharmaceutical Association that U-40 insulin should be phased out. The elimination of U-40 products would decrease dosage errors associated with use of the wrong insulin strength or the wrong syringe type (U-40 syringes and U-100 syringes are calibrated differently).[9]

Persons traveling abroad should be cautioned that in many countries only U-40 insulin is available, and sometimes specific insulin types are limited. In this situation, it is advised that the individual carry sufficient quantities of insulin and syringes for the entire trip, continue to wear a Med-Alert bracelet, and carry prescriptions for both extra insulin and syringes.

Persons resistant to insulin who require greater than 100 units of insulin per injection may be treated with U-500 insulin. U-500 insulin is a legend medication, and therefore requires a prescription. Also, U-500 is not routinely stocked in pharmacies and must be specially ordered from the manufacturer, Eli Lilly and Co.

Insulin purity is measured in terms of parts per million (ppm) of proinsulin. Contamination by proinsulin is considered representative of noninsulin contaminants; since precise measurement of proinsulin is possible, it is utilized as the standard of purity.[31]

Insulin was purified by means of crystallization prior to the 1960s. Currently insulin products undergo extensive purification by chromatographic processes that yield highly purified products. Standard insulins today contain less than 10 ppm proinsulin, while most insulin products contain $\leq$ 1 ppm and are associated with a reduced incidence of allergic responses. Many allergic responses associated with insulin today are probably caused by differences in species or exogenous components such as protamine. However, some persons experience lipotrophy while using standard insulin ($<$ 10 ppm proinsulin) that resolves with the use of highly purified products such as human insulin or purified pork ($\leq$ 1 ppm proinsulin).[31]

Stability and Storage

Insulin must be refrigerated by the manufacturer, the distributor, and the dispenser. Insulins are stable at room temperature (68° to 75° F) for several months. Higher temperatures will cause an accelerated degradation of the insulin product and may induce flocculation. Persons living in areas subjected to high temperatures should be warned against leaving their insulin in automobiles or in any location where extreme temperatures may occur. Freezing insulin will alter the physical suspension characteristics of modified insulins and is not recommended. Refrigeration at $\approx 40°$ F is the best method for insulin storage, although persons may keep bottles of insulin they are using at room temperature for up to 1 month.[17] Individuals who refrigerate their insulin should be instructed to roll the insulin syringe between their palms after the appropriate dose has been withdrawn, to warm the insulin, making the injection more comfortable.

Flocculation and frosting of various intermediate-acting insulins has been reported with recombinant human insulin, semisynthetic human insulin, and purified pork insulin. When flocculation occurs, the insulin loses its homogeneous characteristics and appears as large clumped particles. Frosting is characterized by a frosted or crystalized appearance on the inner wall of the vial. Flocculation and frosting usually occur in vials that are less than half full and that have been in use for 3 to 6 weeks. Factors that may contribute to flocculation and frosting include excessive agitation of the insulin vial, temperature extremes, and zinc/insulin ratios. Persons should be instructed to examine insulin products prior to use and not use insulin products with a flocculated or frosted appearance. The expiration date, stamped on each bottle, should be examined carefully prior to use. A slight loss in potency may occur if the bottle has been used for more than 30 days, and if it has been stored at room temperature. Unexplained fluctuations in blood glucose may be related to reduced insulin potency.[2]

Mixing Insulins

Many intensive insulin regimens are based on multiple daily injections of various types of insulin. Mixing of two insulin types in one syringe or vial is a simple procedure that sometimes circumvents the need for an excessive number of injections. This technique is not without risk, because any combination may result in physical or chemical changes in the components, which may in turn alter the predicted physiologic response. The questions concerning the appropriateness of insulin mixtures have been difficult to answer because of problems associated with measuring free insulin and its effects. The recent introduction of improved assay techniques, coupled with a number of well-designed clinical studies, have answered some previously unresolved questions.

The Lente insulins (Semilente, Lente, Ultralente) may be mixed in any ratio, with the clinical response of each of the constituents preserved. Mixtures of Lente insulins remain stable for as long as 18 months.[10]

Regular insulins may be mixed with NPH in any ratio while retaining the time action profiles of the components. This is probably the combination of choice when a mixture of short-acting and intermediate-acting insulins is required. Currently in the United States, premixed insulins are available in a ratio of 70% NPH and 30% regular. Mixtures in the ratios of 90→10, 80→20, 60→40, 50→50 NPH→regular in addition to the 70→30 are available in Europe.[10]

When regular insulins are mixed with Lente insulins, a binding phenomenon occurs between the excess zinc in the Lente and the free insulin from the regular insulin, causing a blunting of the regular insulin's effect. [8,16,32] The binding begins within 15 minutes after injection and continues for as long as 24 hours. The amount of attenuated regular insulin is dependent on the ratio of regular to Lente. The greater the Lente concentration, the greater the amount of binding. If this type of mixture is to be used, it is recommended that mixtures be allowed to stand for 24 hours prior to injection to assure consistency between the regular→Lente interaction from injection to injection. In the past, it has been recommended that as an alternative to the 24-hour waiting period, this type of mixture be injected immediately. This immediate injection method is not currently recommended because when human insulins are used, the interaction begins immediately,[33] and with all source insulins, the interaction may continue once the mixture is in the subcutaneous reservoir, resulting in inconsistent time action profiles. This interaction also occurs when Ultralente is mixed with regular. One solution to the problem is to have the patient inject the two types separately. This solution obviates binding interactions, but does not always meet with acceptance by the individual.

The combination of regular and Protamine Zinc Insulin yields a mixture that is unpredictable in nature. Mixtures of 1→1 regular→PZI results in a formula which has a time action profile similar to PZI alone. Ratios of 2→1 yield mixtures with the characteristics of NPH insulin. Mixtures of > 2→1, Regular→PZI have time action profiles similar to Regular:NPH combinations.[33]

*Buffered insulins such as NPH, PZI, Human BR, and all Novo-Nordisk insulins should **never** be mixed with Lente insulins*. Precipitation of zinc from the suspension by phosphorus will result in an increase in Regular insulin in the mixture. This shift may cause hypoglycemia in the patient. Buffered Regular insulin, formulated specifically for insulin pumps, should never be mixed with other insulins. See box on p. 130 for guidelines for mixing insulin.

INSULIN REGIMENS
Initiation of Treatment

Initial insulinization of the person with diabetes should be aimed at eliminating hyperglycemic symptoms and re-establishment of metabolic and fluid balance without causing hypoglycemia. In the past, most persons were hospitalized during initial treatment. Today, many individuals begin insulin therapy on an outpatient basis unless their presentation is with diabetic ketoacidosis (DKA). Education at this point is extremely important because these individuals are establishing habits that affect their long-term outcome. Unfortunately, approximately 10% to 20% of newly diagnosed persons do not receive even rudimentary education about insulin dose preparation or injection, but are simply handed a prescription. It is probably best to begin a newly diagnosed person on a twice-daily regimen and to immediately teach self-monitoring of blood glucose. Some clinicians prefer to stabilize the individual by initiating therapy with twice-daily injections of NPH, switching later to a split mixed regimen.

GUIDELINES FOR MIXING INSULIN

According to the American Diabetes Association,[2] the following guidelines for mixing insulin should be followed:

Individuals with diabetes who are well controlled on a particular mixed-insulin regimen should maintain their standard procedure for preparing their insulin doses.

No other medication or diluent should be mixed with any insulin product unless approved by the physician.

Use of commercially available premixed insulins is preferred to extemporaneously mixing by the individual with diabetes if the insulin ration is appropriate to the individual's insulin requirements.

Currently available NPH and regular insulin formulations may interact when mixed.

Lente insulins do not interact with each other.

Mixing of regular and Lente insulin is not recommended except for patients already adequately controlled on such a mixture. This is caused by the binding of lente insulins with regular insulin, delaying onset of action.

Phosphate buffered insulins should not be mixed with Lente insulins.

There is no rationale for mixing animal with human insulin.

Insulin formulation may change; therefore the manufacturer should be consulted in cases in which recommendation appear to conflict with the American Diabetes Association guidelines.

Initial diabetes education should include cursory information about the disease, complications, and the importance of treatment and monitoring. Education should also include teaching of insulin injection technique, preparation of insulin doses, information about storage of insulin, and recognition and treatment of hypoglycemia. Individuals who have access to comprehensive diabetes education programs offered by health care organizations should be strongly encouraged to enroll in such programs.

Insulin should be initiated at a dose of 0.5 units/kg/day. Based on this recommendation a person weighing 70 kg would begin therapy with a total daily dose of 35 units of insulin. A person receiving this amount of insulin in two divided doses is less likely to become hypoglycemic than the individual who receives the entire amount as a single injection. Two thirds of the total daily dose should be given in the morning, and one third of the dose should be taken around the evening meal. The ratio of AM→PM doses may be adjusted, based on blood glucose monitoring. It should be anticipated that this dose will eventually need to be titrated upward toward the 1 unit/kg/day range especially for persons with NIDDM. Persons (20% to 30%) often experience a "honeymoon" or remission phase within weeks after their diagnosis that is characterized by a temporary recovery of β-cell function.[5] During this time insulin requirements may decline to the point at which no exogenous insulin is needed. Most clinicians prefer to continue insulin at very small doses rather than discontinue insulin altogether. Total discontinuance of insulin may give the individual a false impression of cure and may also result in immunologic problems associated with intermittent insulin administration. Individuals who do not monitor blood glucose levels and have insulin doses adjusted accordingly during the honeymoon period run a high risk of the hypoglycemia.

Administration of Insulin

Insulin may be administered with traditional syringes, jet injectors, pumps, or modified syringes (pen injectors). The vast majority of persons administer insulin via subcutaneous injection with disposable plastic syringes with small-gauge lubricated needles. Dosage preparation and administration should be explained to the individual; he or she should then be asked to explain the procedure to the health care provider. This will assure that the individual understands what is being taught and will allow the clinician to detect problems. See box below for insulin administration guidelines to stress with patients.

INSULIN ADMINISTRATION GUIDELINES

Wash hands.

Insulin vials should be checked for flocculation or frosting and expiration date.

Intermediate-acting and long-acting insulins should be resuspended by gently rolling the vial between the palms—DO NOT SHAKE.

Clean the tops of the insulin vials with an alcohol swab.

After the alcohol has dried, an amount of air equal to the dose of insulin required should be drawn up and injected into the vial. When mixing insulins, put sufficient amount of air into both bottles.

Insert the syringe into the vial, invert the vial, and pull back the plunger untll the appropriate amount has been withdrawn. Withdraw-appropriate amount of intermediate insulin. When mixing insulins, the clear short-acting insulin should be drawn into the syringe first.

If bubbles appear, tap the side of the syringe and inject the bubbles back into the vial, then withdraw the needed amount of insulin.

Carefully recap syringe.

Cleanse injection site with alcohol and allow alcohol to dry.

Pinch a fold of skin at the injection site with one hand (pinching lifts fat off of muscle and circumvents intramuscular or intravenous injection that may cause hypoglycemia). Hold the syringe like a pencil in the other hand. Insert the needle with the beveled edge pointed up at a 45° to 90° angle (the angle will depend on the level of subcutaneous fat—the greater the fat, the more perpendicular the injection may be).

Smoothly and continuously press plunger in as far as it will go; routine aspiration is not necessary.

Withdraw needle and gently apply pressure with cotton swab.

Record dose, time, and injection site.

Discard syringe in an appropriate manner.

Syringe Reuse

Because the sterility of the syringe cannot be guaranteed, manufacturers of disposable syringes recommend that they be used only once. However, some individuals prefer to reuse syringes several times. If reuse is planned, the needle must be recapped after each use, demonstrating a technique that supports the syringe in the hand and replaces the cap with a straight motion of the thumb and forefinger. The individual should be instructed to discard the syringe if the needle becomes dull, bent, or has contact with any surface other than the skin. Syringe reuse is not recommended for persons exhibiting poor personal hygiene, acute concurrent illness, open wounds, or decreased resistance to infection for any reason.[2]

Selection of Sites

Insulin absorption is affected by a number of factors.
1. Injection site—the predictability and completeness and rate of absorption is >abdomen >deltoid >thigh >hip.
2. Ambient temperature—the greater the temperature, the greater the rate of absorption.
3. Exercise or massage—may increase absorption.

The above-mentioned factors must all be considered when designing a patient regimen. In the past, most clinicians agreed that injection sites should be routinely rotated from one area to another as rotation of sites is important to the prevention of lipohypertrophy or lipoatrophy. However, since an injection in the abdominal area may elicit a different time action profile than an injection in the hip, dosage response observations may be difficult to interpret. Therefore, some clinicians now recommend that individuals with IDDM inject in a given area (i.e., abdominal area) and systematically rotate sites within the area before moving to a different area (for example, the individual would systematically use abdominal sites before moving on to using sites identified in the deltoid). Persons who exercise should avoid injecting into subcutaneous tissue adjacent to the muscles to be used. Rapid absorption can lead to hypoglycemia.

In the newly diagnosed individual, one method of teaching injection technique is for the instructor to self-inject using sterile water. This graphically demonstrates to the individual that the technique is virtually painless, and with the use of sterile water the patient can practice a few injections, thus lowering his or her apprehension in a less than pleasant situation.

Regimens and Dosage Adjustments

Normal insulin secretion is depicted in Fig. 4-1 and is best described as a continuous basal release with superimposed bolus doses triggered by food intake or blood glucose concentration changes. Insulin replacement regimens should seek to mimic this secretory pattern. The most effective method of achieving this goal will probably be via a closed

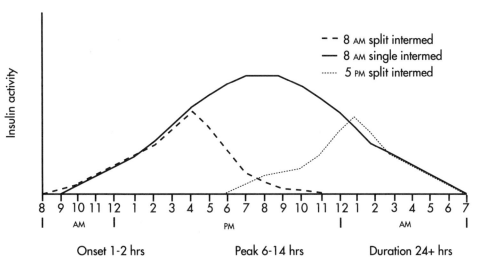

Fig. 4-3   Insulin time action profile: intermediate-split versus single.

loop pump system that constantly monitors blood glucose levels and adjusts insulin infusion rates accordingly. Unfortunately, at this time a closed loop system of this nature is much too large and expensive to be considered pragmatic. The regimen that most closely resembles physiologic secretion and is used to any great degree is the external insulin pump in combination with frequent (usually at least 4 times per day) blood glucose monitoring.

One-injection regimens

Unfortunately, one of the most frequently encountered insulin regimens is the once-daily intermediate-acting insulin regimen. Many clinicians learned this method during their initial training and continue to make use of it today even in light of new evidence that strongly suggests that it is suboptimal. Persons with diabetes who have not been educated about the long-term implications usually resist changing to more complex but much more efficacious regimens. In order to understand the shortcomings of such a regimen, one simply needs to examine the time action profile for intermediate-acting insulins (Figs. 4-2 and 4-3). The individual taking an injection in the early morning upon arising has no insulin coverage until around the midday meal and no coverage the following morning before the next injection. Since the entire insulin dosage is given as one dose, a large peak effect that may cause severe hypoglycemia will occur 8 to 12 hours after the dose. In persons with IDDM, a single injection per day of an intermediate-acting insulin is predictably almost always insufficient. In individuals with an active insulin reserve, the single-injection regimen may at times prove beneficial.

Two-injection regimens

Two injections per day is probably the minimum number to adequately cover the patient with IDDM. The total daily insulin dose (0.5 to 1.0 units/kg) is typically divided

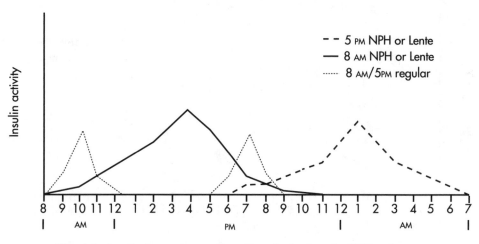

Fig. 4-4   Insulin time action profile: split and mixed regular/NPH or Lente.

into a morning dose of two thirds to one half of the total daily dose, and an evening dose of the remaining one third to one half of the total daily dose. The two injections may consist of intermediate-acting insulin alone (see Fig. 4-3) but are much more effective if given as a mixture of intermediate- and short-acting insulins (Fig. 4-4). Mixtures of intermediate- and short-acting insulins are usually given initially in a ratio of 2→1, respectively. This ratio and the total daily dose must be adjusted based on blood glucose monitoring. If Lente is used in place of NPH, the ratio may need to be adjusted to increase the activity of the fast-acting insulin. Doses should be adjusted based on information obtained under stable exercise and diet conditions, in the absence of other stressors. Preprandial blood glucose determinations are more consistent than postprandial blood glucose determinations and are probably the routine test of choice. Refer to Table 4-3 for dosage adjustment guidelines.

Currently premixed formulations of NPH and regular insulin are available in the United States in a ratio of 70→30 NPH→regular. While this mixture is an improvement over twice-daily injections of NPH alone, it does not offer the needed flexibility to adjust doses on an as-needed basis. This mixture may be appropriate for the individual who cannot or will not utilize the split and mix approach. In the future, there may be a variety of mixed ratios available in the U.S. In Europe, ratios of 50→50, 60→40, 70→30, 80→20, and 90→10 NPH→regular are available.

Three-injection regimens

In some individuals on the mixed dose two-injection regimen, the intermediate-acting insulin administered with the evening meal is not sufficient to control the individual's blood glucose throughout the following night. The resulting fasting hyperglycemia can be countered by further splitting the regimen into an evening meal short-acting insulin dose and a bedtime intermediate-acting dose. When early morning hyperglycemia is encountered, the Somogyi effect should first be ruled out before regimen changes are made.

Table 4-3   Split and Mixed Regimen Dose Adjustment

	Test time				
	Fasting	**Prelunch**	**Predinner**	**Prebedtime**	**Early morning**
Insulin dose	Evening NPH If elevated check early AM BG	Morning regular	Morning NPH	Evening regular	Evening NPH
Meal or snack	Late-night snack	Breakfast	Lunch Snack	Dinner	Dinner Late snack

Insulin doses and meals or snacks that may affect blood glucose levels at the above mentioned times are listed.

This table assumes the patient is on a normal 8 to 5 schedule, with regular meals and snacks.

If fasting blood glucose levels are elevated, consider Somogyi effect and dawn phenomenon (see Chapter 8), evaluate with early AM levels. The clinician should usually attempt to correct one unacceptable level at a time. Goals should be approached slowly. Increase or decrease insulin dose 1 to 2 units for every 40 to 50 mg/dL desired change in blood glucose level.

When this regimen is used, persons with diabetes usually take two thirds of their total daily insulin in their morning dose, one sixth with their evening meal, and one sixth at bedtime.

Multidose regimens

Basically there are two multidose regimens that may be used. The first is a regimen of four daily doses of rapid-acting insulin given before each meal and at bedtime. Initially the daily dose is divided into four equal doses. Doses are then adjusted from this baseline. One of the problems with this regimen is that the evening dose regular insulin (especially human regular) may not provide sufficient coverage throughout the night, particularly if the dose is taken early. If larger doses are given, the individual may experience early morning (2 to 3 AM) hypoglycemia during the peak effect of the short-acting insulin. An alternative is to give injections of short-acting insulin before each meal with a single morning injection of long-acting insulin such as PZI or Ultralente. The long-acting insulin dose should initially comprise two fifths of the total daily dose, and will provide a basal amount of insulin. Most clinicians recommend using Ultralente with this regimen, while very few will recommend PZI. Each short-acting insulin dose in this regimen comprises approximately one fifth of the total daily dase. Inasmuch as individuals with diabetes can adjust doses of regular insulin to compensate for various meals, this regimen offers good glycemia control and flexibility of lifestyle. It does, however, require multiple injections and frequent blood glucose monitoring that some individuals find burdensome. Please refer to Fig. 4-5 for a graphic description of this regimen.

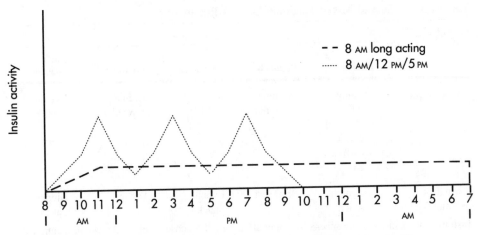

Fig. 4-5   Insulin time action profile: split regular with long-acting insulin.

Continuous subcutaneous insulin infusion

Continuous subcutaneous insulin infusion (CSII) devices, both internal (experimental) and external, can be programmed to release a basal amount of insulin and bolus doses on an as-needed basis. Most available pumps can be programmed with about the same amount of difficulty as a programmable wristwatch and contain alarms for malfunctions (such as low batteries) and dosage ceilings to prevent accidental overdose. Subcutaneous access may be achieved by a small needlelike catheter or a flexible plastic catheter (inserted with a needle). The catheters may be used for 2 to 3 days before they are replaced. Only regular insulin should be used in a pump, preferably human buffered regular. Pumps offer tight control and great flexibility of life-style for those health care providers and patients motivated enough to learn about the functioning and maintenance of CSII.

Goals

The short-term goals for insulin therapy can be divided into four categories: blood glucose levels, glycosylated hemoglobin levels, urine test results, and symptoms. Symptoms of hyperglycemia such as polydipsia, polyphagia, and polyuria should completely resolve with near normalization of blood glucose levels. This resolution of hyperglycemic symptoms should be attained without the induction of hypoglycemia. Three degrees of acceptability have been delineated for blood glucose levels measured at various times for the different types of regimens. Simplistically, the more intensive the regimen, the closer to normal ranges the blood glucose levels and glycosylated hemoglobin levels should be. The three levels of treatment and/or expected short-term outcomes are minimal, average, and intensive. An example of minimal treatment would be the use of a single injection of intermediate-acting insulin in an individual with IDDM. Given this common situation, one could expect that the person's glycated hemoglobin would measure between 11% and 13%, urine glucose loss would be common, and blood glucose measurements would often be in the 300 mg/dL range. The individual would at times be symptomatic, and if still growing may do so at a slower rate than an age-, weight-, and genetically matched counterpart. Under normal circumstances (i.e., without infection, surgery, etc.), this individual would not develop diabetic ketoacidosis.

With average treatment (possibly two injections of intermediate-acting insulin) the same person would have average preprandial blood glucose levels in the range of 160 to 200 mg/dL with glycated hemoglobin levels of 8% to 10%. The individual would not usually be symptomatic, would experience self-treatable hypoglycemia every week or so, and would grow at a normal rate. If treated in an intensive manner, this same person would be seen with a blood glucose diary that reveals preprandial glucose concentrations in the range of 80 to 120 mg/dL, and with a hemoglobin A_{1c} in the range of 6% to 8%. The patient would note a sense of increased energy and well being, but would probably have an increased incidence of hypoglycemic episodes.

Setting goals for the individual with diabetes is much more meaningful for all involved if the person is educated about various levels of treatment, the consequences, and the costs (in money, time, and commitment) and has an input into their formulation. Overall, the goal should be to maintain all measurable parameters as close to the euglycemic values as possible while maintaining the individual's quality of life and not running too great a risk of hypoglycemia.

Dose Adjustments

When evaluating an individual's blood glucose levels, several questions must be answered.

1. Are these concentrations taken from the individual's normal situation? (For instance, is infection, a large meal or snack, or a missed insulin dose a factor?)
2. Was the insulin dose, time administered, and time of glucose concentration measurement recorded accurately?
3. Is the person's SMBG technique acceptable?
4. Are the presented values believable? Do they generally correspond to glycated hemoglobin concentration?

Persons with diabetes should routinely monitor blood glucose levels at least 4 times per day when therapy is being adjusted, at fasting in the morning, prelunch, predinner, and prebedtime. They should also check their early morning (2 to 3 AM) blood glucose levels upon initiation of treatment, with adjustments of evening insulin doses, and to intermittently rule out early morning hypoglycemia. Postprandial glucose levels are more difficult to interpret, but may be beneficial on occasion, particularly in persons undergoing intensive therapy.

In a two-injection split and mixed regimen, the individual's SMBG diary should be evaluated and the adjustment of insulin doses should then be made based on observed trends. When possible, persons with diabetes may also be taught to adjust their own insulin doses as needed. Goals should be approached carefully, and in most cases only one dose should be altered at a time. A patient-specific algorithm should be established. An insulin dose change of two units may affect two different persons in dramatically different degrees. A change of one to two units of insulin will usually cause a difference of 40 to 50 mg/dL of glucose.

Complications of Insulin Therapy

Complications associated with insulin therapy can be divided into two categories—immunologically mediated and nonimmunologically mediated. The nonimmunologically mediated complications include hypoglycemia, insulin edema, and lipohypertrophy that are effects directly attributable to the pharmacologic effects of insulin. Immunologically mediated side effects of insulin include local dermatologic reactions, systemic immunologic response, and antibody-induced insulin resistance and lipotrophy. With the introduction of better purification methods and the use of human insulin, the incidence of immunologically mediated problems would be expected to decrease.

Hypoglycemia

The most significant and common adverse effect of insulin therapy is hypoglycemia. Almost all persons with diabetes who undergo exogenous insulin therapy will at some time in their therapeutic course experience hypoglycemia. Approximately 1 of 10 people with diabetes will experience at least one episode of hypoglycemia on a yearly basis severe enough to require the assistance of another person for recovery. As many as 59% of insulin-treated patients who were evaluated had nocturnal hypoglycemia, many of whom were asymptomatic. [15] About 3% of the deaths in patients with IDDM are attributed to hypoglycemic reactions.

Signs and symptoms of hypoglycemia include mental confusion, nervousness, sweaty palms, dizziness, blurred vision, anxiety, hunger, and tingling and numbness around the mouth. Nocturnal hypoglycemia sometimes presents with nightmares, a feeling of "hangover" in the morning upon awakening, morning headache, night sweats, or restless sleep. Signs and symptoms of hypoglycemia may be very predictable in a given individual (based on history) or may be quite erratic. A person is usually considered to be hypoglycemic when his or her blood glucose drops below 60 mg/dL. Symptoms are sometimes not noted until the concentration falls below 40 mg/dL, with coma and seizures resulting from levels of less than 20 mg/dl. Hypoglycemia may result in permanent brain damage or may induce cardiac arrhythmias or even myocardial infarction. Central nervous system impairment secondary to hypoglycemia can result in injury or accident. The hyperglycemic response to hypoglycemia (Somogyi effect) may be a cause of prebreakfast hyperglycemia and ketonuria. Fear of development of hypoglycemia may deter the person from achieving good glycemia control.

Normally, glucose counterregulatory hormones work to maintain glucose homeostasis in the plasma. Counterregulatory hormones include glucagon, epinephrine, growth hormone, and cortisol. Under normal conditions, the secretion of these hormones prevents the development of hypoglycemia. Glucagon and epinephrine are the dominant hormones in the counterregulatory system, having rapid onsets of action and being activated as soon as blood glucose levels begin to decline. The effects of growth hormone and cortisol are not noticed until approximately 2 hours after the hypoglycemic event.

In addition to the potential hypoglycemic problems caused by injections of exogenous insulin, the person with diabetes may also have impaired counterregulatory responses to insulin-induced hypoglycemia. Deficits in counterregulatory response are common in the IDDM population and have been well documented.[18] Reduction or loss of glucagon response is usually present in patients who have had diabetes for 5 years or more. Attenuation of the sympathetic response also frequently occurs in persons who have been treated with insulin for a number of years. The individual who has a blunted counterregulatory response will have "hypoglycemic unawareness" and may undergo periods of prolonged hypoglycemia. Persons who are treated with intensive management regimens have a higher incidence of hypoglycemia. See box below for possible causes of hypoglycemia.

Hypoglycemia may be treated in the conscious person by the administration of 10 to 15 g of oral carbohydrate (see Chapter 2). Examples of food sources providing 10 g of carbohydrate include ½ cup of orange juice or 6 to 8 Life Saver candies. Resolution of symptoms usually occurs in 15 to 20 minutes. If the patient remains hypoglycemic after 15 minutes, he or she should be instructed to ingest another 15 g of oral carbohydrate, and, if a mealtime is 2 hours or more away, the person should also consume a small complex carbohydrate/protein snack.

The unconscious person with diabetes may be treated with either intravenous 25 g glucose or 1 mg glucagon subcutaneously, intramuscularly, or intravenously. Since glucose administration requires intravenous access, glucagon is the drug of choice for the unconscious hypoglycemic patient in the home setting. All individuals utilizing exogenous insulin who have a teachable significant other or a home caretaker should have a glucagon kit. Unfortunately, only one of 90 persons who receive insulin therapy own a glucagon kit. The procedure for preparing and administering glucagon is simple and can

---

POSSIBLE CAUSES OF HYPOGLYCEMIA

1. Excessive or incorrect insulin dose.
2. Altered sensitivity to insulin (e.g., an individual switched to less antigenic insulin with resulting decrease in antibodies).
3. Insulin clearance decreased (e.g., renal-failure patients may require dose reductions as renal failure progresses).
4. Glucose intake decreased.
5. Hepatic glucose production decreased.
6. Injection inadvertently given IM or IV.
7. Drug interactions.
8. Increased physical exertion.
9. Ethanol ingestion.

be taught in minutes. The individual receiving the medication must always be placed in a position to prevent aspiration, since glucagon may induce emesis. Because of the relatively short duration of action of glucagon, the individual should be fed immediately upon awakening.

Lipodystrophies

Lipodystrophies can be divided into two categories, lipoatrophy and lipohypertrophy. Lipohypertrophy or hypertrophic lipodystrophy is nonimmunologically mediated and will be discussed first.

Lipohypertrophy is characterized by a fatty, tumorlike growth at or around the injection site. In advanced cases, the skin around the hypertrophied area becomes anesthetized. These spongy growths are thought to be caused by the lipogenous properties of insulin when it has been repeatedly injected into a single area. No evidence uncovered thus far implicates an immunologic cause for this problem. Apparently, persons who focus their injections in a single area eventually develop lipohypertrophy, and then magnify the problem by continuing to inject into this area because of the loss of pain sensation. The treatment of lipohypertrophy consists of systematically rotating injection sites. Switching to human insulin should have no effect on this condition.

Lipoatrophy, or a loss of fatty tissue at-or distant from the site of insulin injection, is a problem that is probably of immunologic origin. Persons treated with unchromatographed insulins have a much higher incidence of this problem than patients treated with highly purified pork insulins or human insulins. A high percentage of individuals who have insulin allergy also experience lipoatrophy. Locally injected steroids sometimes will result in the resolution of lipotrophy. Histologic studies also indicate that an active immunologic process is taking place with lipoatrophy.

Lipoatrophy is more common in females than males and is most often reported in young females. The treatment of choice is human insulin injected at the borders of the lipoatrophic area. Use of the least antigenic insulin will theoretically attenuate the immunologic response and allow the lipogenous properties of insulin to be elicited. Resolution sometimes begins after two weeks of therapy but usually requires 4 to 6 months of therapy for complete resolution. After complete resolution, the individual should be instructed to continue to inject into the area every 2 to 3 weeks to avoid recurrence. A small percentage of persons will not respond to human insulin therapy. Unfortunately, these individuals do not show favorable outcomes when treated with local steroids.

Antibodies, allergy, and resistance

Insulin allergy may reveal itself as a small, local subdermal nodule or may, on rare occasions, present as a full-blown anaphylactic reaction. Allergies to alcohol (or any skin preparation), protamine, and zinc may sometimes be mistaken for insulin allergy. The most common type of allergic response is a local cutaneous reaction to insulin at the injection site that is evident 4 to 8 hours after the injection, is erythematous and indurated, and resolves in a few days. Other forms of dermatologic reactions to insulin include late-phase and Arthus reactions. On rare occasions, a person with diabetes may present with an anaphylactic reaction to insulin. This type of reaction is mediated by IgE antibodies and is treated with epinephrine, antihistamines, and corticosteroids. Desensitization is almost always required in these patients, even if switched to human insulin.

Persons who require greater than 200 units of insulin per day for more than several days in the absence of ketoacidosis, infection, or coma are said to be insulin resistant. Insulin resistance is caused by insulin-binding antibodies (IgG) but may also be observed secondary to obesity, glucocorticoid administration, Cushing's syndrome, acromegaly, and several other rare causes. Immunologically mediated insulin resistance is typically observed in persons who have been treated intermittently with insulin or who have had other allergic problems. The treatment of choice of immunologically mediated insulin resistance is treatment with either human insulin or purified pork insulin. Immunologically mediated insulin resistance usually resolves soon after the person has been begun treatment with a less antigenic insulin. Persons who require large doses of insulin may be treated with a special U-500 insulin available by special order from Eli Lilly and Company. In some cases the individual may be treated with a short course of corticosteroids (40 to 80 mg of prednisone or equivalent daily for one to 3 weeks), with improvement being observed in about 75% of reported cases. Non-immunologically mediated insulin resistance such as is observed with obesity does not respond to alterations in insulin types but may be managed by caloric restriction.

Drug interactions

Many compounds may alter the effects of insulin. Unexpected alterations in glucose levels, either positive or negative, may adversely affect diabetes care. Nonselective beta blockers may cause prolonged hypoglycemia, while at the same time masking some of the signs and symptoms of hypoglycemia. Ethanol ingestion, particularly large quantities taken without food, may accentuate the effects of insulin resulting in profound hypoglycemia. Corticosteroids and diuretics are among the list of agents that may increase blood glucose levels. Complete medication histories should be taken on all persons with histories being screened for potential reactions (Table 4-4).

ORAL HYPOGLYCEMIC AGENTS

There are two types of oral hypoglycemic agents—biguanides and sulfonylureas. In the United States, sulfonylurea agents are the only oral hypoglycemic medications available. Phenformin, a biguanide, was removed from the U.S. market in 1977 because of its association with lactic acidosis. Sulfonylureas can be divided into two categories—first generation and second generation. The second-generation agents were introduced later (1984) than the first-generation agents and display about 100 times the potency of the first-generation agents. However, there is no evidence to suggest that the second-generation agents are more effective than the first-generation agents. All of the agents differ by dose, dosing interval, route of metabolism and excretion, and activity of metabolites.

Table 4-4   Potential Pharmacokinetic and Pharmacodynamic Interactions Altering Blood Glucose Levels

Intrinsic hyperglycemic effect	Beta blockers
	Caffeine (with large doses)
	Corticosteroids
	Diazoxide
	Diuretics (thiazide>loop>K^+ sparing)
	Epinephrine-like compounds (decongestants)
	Glucagon
	Niacin
	Oral contraceptives
	Pentamidine (beta cell toxic—see also hypoglycemia)
	Phenytoin
	Sugar-containing syrups
Intrinsic hypoglycemic effect	Beta blockers noncardioselective > cardioselective
	Chloroquine
	Disopyramide
	Ethanol
	MAO inhibitors
	Pentamidine
Displacement of sulfonylureas from binding sites (hypoglycemia)	Clofibrate
	Phenylbutazone
	Salicylates (large doses)
	Sulfonamides
Decreased hepatic metabolism of sulfonylureas	Chloramphenicol
	Dicumerol
	Phenylbutazone
Increased hepatic metabolism of sulfonylureas	Ethanol (chronic use)
	Thyroid
Decreased renal excretion of sulfonylureas	Allopurinol
	Probenecid
	Phenylbutazone
	Salicylates
	Sulfonamides
Decreased insulin absorption	Nicotine

Physiologic Effects

The exact mechanism of action of each of the sulfonylurea agents is still controversial. Initially, sulfonylureas stimulate insulin release. This increased secretion lasts for only a few months during continued use. Glipizide may have an extended effect on insulin secretion, but it is doubtful that this is clinically significant. Fasting hyperglycemia in the individual with NIDDM is primarily a result of overproduction of glucose by the liver. Sulfonylurea agents have been shown to normalize hepatic glucose production. Lastly, sulfonylureas partially normalize both receptor and postreceptor defects. Persons with NIDDM have lower than normal insulin receptor populations on insulin-sensitive tissue. In addition to this insulin resistance, those with NIDDM probably also have defective insulin receptor (or postreceptor) activity. Sulfonylureas increase the numbers of insulin receptors and also decrease the insulin resistance by apparently altering postreceptor function. Since sulfonylurea agents work in concert with existing beta cells and insulin, they are of no use in the individual with IDDM or those who have been pancreatectomized.

Indications

Sulfonylurea agents are indicated in the person with NIDDM who has not responded to a reasonable course of exercise and diet therapy. Older persons, obese persons, and those with lower plasma glucose levels should be subjected to longer trials of diet and exercise than the individual who is close to ideal body weight or one with very high plasma glucose levels. Those with NIDDM who have fasting plasma glucose levels of greater than 250 mg/dL should have their glucose levels brought under control with a few weeks of insulin therapy. Once plasma glucose levels are controlled, the individual may be switched to an oral agent.

Contraindications

Individuals who meet the following criteria should not be treated with oral agents but, instead, should use insulin.
- Women with gestational diabetes.
- Persons with IDDM.
- Pregnant or lactating women.
- Ketosis-prone individuals.
- Persons in whom rapid glucose control is desired.
- Persons with severe infections or surgery (sliding scale—insulin is the treatment of choice).
- Use oral agents with extreme caution in individuals with a history of allergic response to sulfa or sulfonylurea compounds.

Predictors of Outcome

There are several factors that have been shown to be predictive of a positive or negative response to sulfonylureas. These include age, weight, duration of disease, prior treatment with insulin, and fasting blood glucose levels.[21,28,29] Persons are more likely to respond to sulfonylurea therapy if their diagnosis of NIDDM is recent (within 5 years). Age of the individual being treated is sometimes predictive of response, with persons greater than 40 years of age responding better than younger patients. Body weights of between 110% and 160% of ideal body weight and fasting blood glucose levels of less than 200 mg/dL are predictive of a positive outcome. Individuals who have in the past required insulin and were stabilized with doses of less than 40 units per day tend to respond more favorably than those who require greater than 40 units per day. Physically active persons who follow a meal plan respond more favorably than sedentary persons who do not adhere to a meal plan.

Of all individuals treated with sulfonylureas, approximately 60% to 75% will respond favorably. When persons are chosen according to the above criteria, the rate of successful treatments rises to 85%.[29] Primary treatment failures are those individuals not responding to a one month trial of oral sulfonylurea given at maximum doses. Of the persons who respond favorably in the initial months of treatment, 5% to 10% per year will experience secondary treatment failures. After 10 years of treatment with oral sulfonylureas, 50% of the initial positive responders will become secondary treatment failures. Secondary treatment failure may be a result of the natural progression of diabetes or may be induced by other treatable causes, such as drug interactions, infection, weight gain, or surgery. For the person with secondary treatment failure without an explainable underlying cause, a different oral agent may be substituted, or a small dose of evening intermediate-acting insulin may be added. Persons who do not respond initially or who experience secondary treatment failure when being treated with tolazamide, tolbutamide, or acetohexamide, may respond to glyburide, glipizide, or chlorpropamide. Substitution will probably not affect persons already being treated with maximum doses of glyburide, glipizide, or chlorpropamide.

Specific Agents

There is no evidence that suggests that one sulfonylurea is the most efficacious, and indeed all of the agents seem to be equally effective when given in equipotent doses. The differences in the agents arise from the various pharmacokinetic and side effect profiles. Care must be taken when choosing a sulfonylurea for a particular person (Table 4-5).

Acetohexamide (Dymelor) should be dosed two times daily with total daily doses ranging from 250 to 1500 mg. It is metabolized to a metabolite, hydroxyhexamide, the activity of which is equal to or greater than the parent compound.[12,21] This active metabolite is excreted via the kidney; therefore, dosage adjustment is necessary with renal failure.

Chlorpropamide (Diabinese) has the longest duration of action (24 to 72 hours) of all the sulfonylureas and is dosed once daily.[21] Daily dosage range is from 100 to 500 mg. Average elimination half lives of chlorpropamide are $\approx$33 hours; therefore, time required to reach steady state is 7 to 10 days. Chlorpropamide is both metabolized to slightly active metabolites and excreted unchanged by the kidneys. Dosage adjustment is required in the elderly and in patients with renal failure. When compared with other sulfonylureas, chlorpropamide is associated with the highest incidence of severe hypoglycemic reactions (4% to 6% of patients treated). Approximately 50% of all reported cases of sulfonylurea-induced hypoglycemia can be attributed to chlorpropamide. Chlorpropamide is also noted for its disulfiram-like effect in 33% of patients treated.[25] Last, chlorpropamide has also

Table 4-5   Sulfonylurea Comparison

Drug	Total daily dose	Number of doses per day	Considerations
Acetahexamide (Dymelor)	250-1500 mg	1-2	Renally excreted metabolite may have greater activity than parent compound; adjust dose for renal failure
Chlorpropamide (Diabenese)	100-500 mg	1	Highest incidence of side effects; longest duration; adjust dose in presence of renal failure
Glipizide (Glucotrol)	2.5-40 mg	1-2	Metabolized to inactive metabolites that are excreted renally
Glyburide (Diabeta, Micronase)	1.25-20 mg	1-2	Metabolized to less active forms; 50% excreted renally, 50% via feces
Tolbutamide (Orinase)	500-3000 mg	2-3	Shortest acting; metabolites inactive
Tolazamide (Tolinase)	100-1000 mg	1-2	Converted to inactive metabolites

been associated with syndrome of inappropriate antidiuretic hormone secretion (SIADH) that can result in severe hyponatremia.

Glipizide (Glucotrol), a second-generation sulfonylurea, is normally given in daily doses of from 2.5 to 40 mg. Persons receiving less than 15 mg per day may take their medication as a single dose, while patients taking greater than 15 mg per day should take two divided doses. Glipizide is completely metabolized by the liver to inactive metabolites that are renally excreted. Twelve percent of the dose is excreted via the feces.[6]

Glyburide (Diabeta, Micronase) is also a second-generation sulfonylurea. Its normal daily dosage range is from 1.25 to 20 mg. Because it has an effective duration of action of up to 24 hours, glyburide may be dosed on a once-daily basis. If doses of greater than 10 mg per day are required, the dose should be divided. Glyburide is metabolized by the liver to 3 metabolites, 1 retaining about 15% activity; the metabolites are excreted by both the renal and biliary routes in a ratio of 1:1. Accumulation of the partially active metabolite may cause hypoglycemia in the renal failure patient. [11,34]

Tolazamide (Tolinase) is administered 1 to 2 times daily with a total daily dose of 100 to 1000 mg. It is metabolized to three metabolites with varying degrees of activity that are renally excreted.[18] Tolazamide has a slower absorption rate than the other sulfonylureas and therefore displays a delayed onset of action.

Tolbutamide (Orinase) is the least potent and shortest acting of all the sulfonylureas. It must be administered 2 to 3 times daily with a total daily dose of between 500 to 3000 mg.[12,21] Tolbutamide is metabolized to less active forms that are excreted renally. Tolbutamide may be a reasonable choice for the person in whom prolonged hypoglycemia is likely.

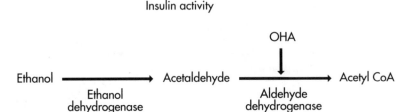

Fig. 4-6   Oral hypoglycemic agent-induced disulfiram-like reaction.

Side Effects

Overall, sulfonylureas are very well tolerated, with only 2% of patients experiencing side effects sufficient to warrant discontinuance of the medication.[21] The most common side effects associated with the sulfonylurea agents include hypoglycemia, a diuretic effect (sometimes leading to hyponatremia), gastrointestinal disturbances, and a disulfiram-like effect. Less common adverse effects include rashes, pruritis, and, rarely, hematologic reactions (hemolytic anemia and bone marrow aplasia).

The disulfiram-like activity of chlorpropamide has been well documented and occurs in approximately one third of individuals who ingest ethanol while being treated with chlorpropamide. This reaction occurs in fewer than 5% of patients taking tolbutamide and at an even lower frequency in those being treated with the second-generation agents.

The complete mechanism for this reaction is still the subject of research, but most agree that chlorpropamide inhibits acetaldehyde dehydrogenase, with a resultant build up of acetaldehyde (Fig. 4-6). The reaction is elicited about 15 minutes after the ingestion of ethanol and is associated with a flushed and tingling sensation in the neck that may extend to the arms. Occasionally the flush will be accompanied by headache, nausea, and breathlessness. The reaction, that is not dose dependent, rarely progresses to vomiting and hypotension; and tolerance does not usually develop.[23]

Hypoglycemia is the most common, severe reaction associated with sulfonylurea administration. In one study it was estimated that 20% of treated persons experienced a minimum of one severe episode of hypoglycemia during a 6-month evaluation period.[22] Chlorpropamide, the sulfonylurea with the longest history of use and the longest duration of action, is responsible for 50% of recorded cases of hypoglycemia.[25] Risk factors for the development of hypoglycemia include advanced age (greater than 60 years), poor nutrition, alcohol use, multidrug regimens, hepatic dysfunction, and renal dysfunction. Sulfonylurea-induced hypoglycemia can be severe and prolonged, requiring treatment with intravenous glucose.[18]

Chlorpropamide and tolbutamide have been associated with an increased release and increased activity of antidiuretic hormone. Chlorpropamide has been linked to SIADH and may cause hyponatremia severe enough to elicit weakness, headache, nausea, vomiting, confusion, and even coma. Risk factors for the development of SIADH include age (greater than 60 years), gender (female > male), and diuretic use. Tolazamide, acetohexamide, glyburide, and glipizide all exert a mild diuretic effect.

Drug Interactions

Several varieties of drug interactions are possible with the sulfonylurea agents. Pharmacodynamic interactions are possible with any medication that may increase or decrease blood glucose levels. Pharmacokinetic interactions can occur with agents that cause displacement of sulfonylureas from plasma protein-binding sites (which is less problematic with second-generation agents), compounds that alter hepatic enzyme activity (either ↑ or ↓), or medications that alter renal elimination (Table 4-4).

Combination Therapy

Multiple studies have evaluated the use of combination therapy with insulin and sulfonylureas. Insulin requirements may be reduced in the person who receives both insulin and sulfonylureas. In the majority of sulfonylurea treatment failures, cost-effective treatment that achieves better glycemic control is possible with the use of insulin alone when appropriate doses of insulin are administered. Combination therapy is probably indicated only in persons who fail optimal regimens of oral agents and insulin given independently.

REFERENCES

1. A Study of Insulin Supply and Demand. A Report of the National Diabetes Advisory Board, publication No. 78-1588. Washington, DC, 1978, US Dept of Health, Education, and Welfare.
2. American Diabetes Association: Clinical Practice Recommendations, Diabetes Care (suppl 1) 13:28-31, 1990.
3. American Diabetes Association: Physicians guide to insulin-dependent (type I) diabetes, Alexandria, VA, 1988, ADA.
4. American Diabetes Association: Physicians guide to insulin-dependent (type II) diabetes, Alexandria, VA, 1988, ADA.
5. Agner T, and others: Remission in IDDM: prospective study of basal C-peptide and insulin dose in 268 consecutive patients, Diabetes Care 10:164 1987.
6. Balant L, and others: Behaviour of glibenclamide on repeated administration to diabetic patients, Eur J Clin Pharmacol 11:19-25, 1977.
7. Banting FG, and others: Pancreatic extracts in the treatment of diabetes mellitus: a preliminary report, Can Med Assoc J 12:141-146, 1922.
8. Binder C, and others: Insulin pharmacokinetics, Diabetes Care 7:188-199, 1984.
9. Campbell RK: Why you've got to become involved in diabetes patient care. US Pharm Guide Diabetes Manage Nov. suppl:36-47, 1988.
10. Campbell RK: Mixing Insulins in 1990. Submitted to The Diabetes Educator March, 1990.
11. Fabre J, and others: Hypoglycemic activity of the main metabolite of glibenclamide: influence of renal insufficiency, Kidney Int 13:435, 1978 (abst).
12. Ferner RE and Chaplin S: The relationship between the pharmacokinetics and the pharmacodynamic effects of oral hypoglycaemic drugs, Clin Pharmacokinet 12:379-401, 1987.
13. Frank BH, and others: The production of human proinsulin and its transformation to human insulin and C-peptide. In Rich DH and Gross R, eds: Peptides: synthesis-structure-function. Proceedings of the Seventh American Peptide Symposium, Rockford, Illinois, 1981, Pierce Chemical Co.
14. Fredichs H and Creutzfeldt W: Hypoglycemia: insulin secreting tumors, Clin Endocrinol Metab 5:747, 1976.

15. Gale E and Tattersall R: Unrecognized hypoglycemia in insulin-treated diabetes, Lancet 1:1049-1052, 1979.
16. Galloway JA, and others: Mixtures of intermediate-acting insulin (NPH and Lente) with regular insulin:an update. In Skyler JS, ed, Insulin Update: 1982, Proceedings of a Symposium, December 7-9, 1981, Key Biscayne, Fla, Princeton NJ, 1982, Excerpta Medica.
17. Galloway JA, Potvin JH, and Shuman CR, eds: Diabetes mellitus, ed 9, Indianapolis, IN, 1988, Eli Lilly and Company.
18. Gerich JE: Oral hypoglycemic agents, N Engl J Med 321:1231-1245, 1989.
19. Guyton AC: Textbook of medical physiology, Philadelphia, 1986, WB Saunders Co.
20. Hallas-Moller K: The Lente insulins, Diabetes 5:7-14, 1956.
21. Jackson JE and Bressler R: Clinical pharmacology of sulfonylurea hypoglycaemic agents, Drugs 22:211-245; 295-320, 1981.
22. Jennings AM, Wilson RM, and Ward JD: Symptomatic hypoglycemia in NIDDM patients treated with oral hypoglycemic agents, Diabetes Care 12:203-208, 1989.
23. Johnston C and others: Chlorpropamide-alcohol flush: the case in favor, Diabetologia 26:1, 1984.
24. Kemmer FW and others: Absorption kinetics of semisynthetic human insulin and biosynthetic (recombinant DNA) human insulin, Diabetes Care 5(suppl 2):23, 1982.
25. Koda-Kimble MA and Rotblatt MD: Diabetes mellitus. In Young LYY and Koda-Kimble MA, eds: Applied therapeutics, the clinical use of drugs, ed 4, Vancouver, WA, 1988, Applied Therapeutics Inc.
26. Krayenbuhl C and Rosenberg T: Crystalline protamine insulin, Rep Steno Mem Hosp 1:60-73, 1946.
27. Krosnick A: Newer insulins, insulin allergies and the clinical uses of insulins. In Bergman M, ed: Principles of diabetes management, New Hyde Park, NY, 1986, Medical Examination Publishing Co.
28. Leahy JL, and others: Chronic hyperglycemia is associated with impaired glucose influence on insulin secretion: a study of normal rats using chronic in vivo glucose infusions, J Clin Invest, 77:908-915, 1986.
29. Lebovitz H: Clinical utility of oral hypoglycemic agents in the management of patients with noninsulin-dependent diabetes mellitus, Am J Med 75 (suppl 5B):94-99, 1983.
30. Markussen J, and others: Human insulin (Novo): chemistry and characteristics, Diabetes Care 6(suppl 1):4-8, 1983.
31. Notes from the Meeting of the Medical Advisory Board of the Food and Drug Administration Concerning Standards for Insulin Purity, Washington, DC, December, 1979.
32. Nolte MS, and others: Reduced solubility of short-acting soluble insulins when mixed with longer-acting insulins, Diabetes 32:1177-1181, 1983.
33. Olsson PO, Arnqvist H, and Von Schenck H: Miscibility of human semisynthetic regular and Lente insulin and human biosynthetic regular and NPH insulin, Diabetes Care 10:473-477, 1987.
34. Pearson JG, and others: Pharmacokinetic disposition of 14C-Glyburide in patients with varying renal function, Clin Pharmacol Ther 39:318-324, 1986.
35. Permutt MA and Kipnis DM: Insulin biosynthesis. I. On the mechanism of glucose stimulation, J Biol Chem 247:1194, 1972.
36. Polonsky K and Rubenstein A: C-peptide as a measure of the secretion and hepatic extraction of insulin: pitfalls and limitations, Diabetes 33:486, 1984.
37. Pramming S, and others: Absorption of soluble and isophane semisynthetic human and porcine insulin in insulin-dependent diabetic subjects, Acta Endocrinol 105:215, 1984.
38. Robbins D, Tager H, and Rubenstein A: Biologic and clinical importance of proinsulin, N Engl J Med 310:1165, 1984.
39. Schade DS, Santigo JV, and Skyler J: Intensive insulin therapy, Princeton, NJ, 1983, Excerpta Medica.
40. Steil CF: Drug therapy for diabetes mellitus. US Pharm Guide Diabetes Manage Nov. Suppl:36-47, 1988.

CHAPTER 5

Microvascular Complications of Diabetes

WILLIAM H. HERMAN AND DOUGLAS A. GREENE

The prevalence of diabetes and the occurrence of microvascular complications associated with diabetes have far-reaching impacts for the individual with diabetes in terms of morbidity and mortality. Extensive research in this area has been critical to identifying complication course and avenues for preventive care and education, diagnosis, and treatment. The purpose of this chapter is to: (1) identify microvascular complications associated with diabetes and the current state of research with regard to the occurrence and treatment of these complications; (2) describe clinical manifestations associated with these complications; (3) discuss treatment options, including preventive as well as acute measures; and (4) identify education principles critical to preventive self-care.

DIABETIC RETINOPATHY

Diabetic eye disease is the leading cause of new cases of legal blindness in American adults. Sight-threatening retinopathy may exist even when a patient has good vision. Better understanding of the risk factors for retinopathy and recent advances in treatment have provided the rationale for developing an approach to prevent visual loss. This approach requires that diabetic patients at risk for visual loss be systematically examined, referred, and treated.[53]

Clinical Manifestations

The clinical manifestations of diabetic retinopathy are outlined in the box on p. 150. The earliest clinical sign of diabetic retinopathy seen with the ophthalmoscope is the retinal microaneurysm, a small out-pouching of a retinal capillary that appears as a small red dot in

_____ **CLINICAL MANIFESTATIONS OF DIABETIC RETINOPATHY** _____

Nonproliferative diabetic retinopathy

Microaneurysms
Blot hemorrhages
Hard exudates
Occasional soft exudates

Preproliferative diabetic retinopathy

Multiple large blot hemorrhages
Multiple soft exudates
Venous beading and venous duplications
Multiple intraretinal microvascular abnormalities

Proliferative diabetic retinopathy

New vessels on the disc (NVD)
New vessels elsewhere (NVE)
Fibrous tissue proliferation
Preretinal or vitreous hemorrhage

the retina. Retinal microaneurysms are usually not a threat to vision. Retinal blot hemorrhages and hard exudates may also occur early in the course of diabetic retinopathy. Both may occur in other types of retinal disease, especially hypertension, and neither is specific for diabetes. Retinal blot hemorrhages, which are larger than microaneurysms, are round with blurred edges. They represent hemorrhagic infarcts secondary to retinal ischemia and result from extravasation of blood from retinal capillaries into the retina. Retinal hard exudates or waxy exudates are variable in size, usually yellow in color, and may be scattered, aggregated, or ringlike (circinate) in their distribution. Hard exudates are thought to arise from leakage of lipoprotein material from retinal capillaries into the outer retinal layer.

In more advanced retinopathy, closure of retinal capillaries and arterioles may occur. These changes cause ischemic swelling of the nerve fiber layer of the retina. These appear as white or grayish white areas with ill-defined borders and are termed soft exudates or cotton wool spots. Other manifestations of advanced nonproliferative diabetic retinopathy include intraretinal microvascular abnormalities (IRMA), venous beading, and venous duplications.

Proliferative diabetic retinopathy is a more advanced form of retinopathy characterized by proliferation of new vessels and fibrous tissue. Contraction of fibrous tissue may be associated with hemorrhage or retinal detachment as a result of traction. Proliferative retinopathy is thought to be associated with retinal hypoxia. The appearance of cotton wool spots and other manifestations of retinal ischemia should thus be considered warning signs of impending proliferative diabetic retinopathy.[63-65]

Pathogenesis

The primary effect of diabetes on the retina appears to be on its capillaries. Functional changes in the retinal circulation precede structural changes. These include alterations in retinal blood flow and breakdown in the blood retinal barrier. The mechanisms responsible for the structural changes associated with diabetic retinopathy are not well understood. Pericyte dropout has been suggested as a cause of microaneurysm formation. Alterations in aldose reductase activity in vascular endothial cells, nonenzymatic glycosylation of retinal proteins, defects in vascular autoregulation, and hemodynamic factors including increased red blood cell and platelet aggregation, have been suggested as possible pathophysiologic mechanisms leading to retinal ischemia.

Diagnostic Criteria

Nonproliferative diabetic retinopathy may be diagnosed when retinal microaneurysms, hard exudates, blot hemorrhages, soft exudates, or intraretinal microvascular abnormalities are present.

Preproliferative retinopathy is a more advanced form of nonproliferative diabetic retinopathy. Preproliferative retinopathy may be diagnosed when multiple soft exudates, venous caliber abnormalities, and intraretinal microvascular abnormalities are present. Eyes with preproliferative changes have an increased risk of progressing to proliferative retinopathy.[53]

Proliferative retinopathy may be diagnosed when new vessels develop on the surface layer of the retina. Prospective studies have defined characteristics associated with proliferative diabetic retinopathy that increase the risk of severe visual loss. These characteristics, termed high-risk characteristics, are: (1) the development of new vessels and preretinal or vitreous hemorrhage, and (2) the development of new vessels on or within one disc diameter of the optic disc equaling or exceeding one-fourth to one-third disc area in extent, even in the absence of preretinal or vitreous hemorrhage.[32]

Any of the pathologic processes associated with diabetic retinopathy may affect the macula, the parafoveal region of the retina responsible for sharp central vision. This condition is referred to as diabetic maculopathy. The diabetic maculopathies have been classified into two groups: the intraretinal maculopathies and vitreoretinal maculopathies. The intraretinal maculopathies may occur in the presence of nonproliferative or proliferative retinopathy. They are associated with leakage or occlusion of the retinal capillaries and arterioles in the macula and appear clinically as macular edema, hard exudate deposition, and macular ischemia. The vitreoretinal maculopathies occur in the presence of proliferative retinopathy. They arise when fibrovascular proliferation and contraction cause macular distortion or detachment. Diabetic maculopathy is designated as being "clinically significant" if any of the following characteristics apply: (1) thickening of the retina at or within 500 microns of the center of the macula, (2) hard exudates at or within 500 microns of the center of the macula, if associated with thickening of adjacent retina, or (3) a zone or zones of retinal thickening one disc area or larger, any part of which is within one disc diameter of the center of the macula.[37]

Occurrence

In insulin-dependent diabetes mellitus (IDDM), the prevalence of nonproliferative diabetic retinopathy varies from 17% in persons with diabetes for less than 5 years to 98% in those with diabetes for 15 or more years.[63] The prevalence of proliferative retinopathy varies from 1% in persons with IDDM for less than 10 years to 67% in those with IDDM for 35 or more years.[63] The prevalence of macular edema varies from 0% in those with IDDM for less than 5 years to 29% in those with IDDM for 20 to 64 or more years.[65] In IDDM, both retinopathy and macular edema are associated with longer duration of diabetes, higher glycosylated hemoglobin levels, higher blood pressure, presence of proteinuria, and male gender.[63,65]

In non–insulin-dependent diabetes (NIDDM), the prevalence of nonproliferative diabetic retinopathy varies from 29% in those with diabetes for less than 5 years to 78% in those with diabetes for 15 or more years.[64] The prevalence of proliferative diabetic retinopathy varies from 2% in those with NIDDM for less than 5 years to 16% in those with diabetes for 15 or more years.[64] The prevalence of macular edema varies from 3% in those who have had NIDDM for less than 5 years to 28% in those with diabetes for 20 or more years.[64] Nonproliferative and proliferative diabetic retinopathy and diabetic macular edema are more common in insulin-treated than in non–insulin-treated subjects with NIDDM.[64,65] In NIDDM, retinopathy is associated with longer duration of diabetes, younger age at diagnosis, higher glycosylated hemglobin levels, higher systolic blood pressure, and presence of proteinuria.[64] In NIDDM, presence of macular edema is associated with longer duration of diabetes, higher glycosylated hemoglobin levels, higher systolic blood pressure, and presence of proteinuria.[65]

It is estimated that in IDDM, 1.4% of subjects have moderate visual impairment (best corrected visual acuity in the better eye of 20/80 to 20/160) and 3.6% are legally blind (visual acuity in the better eye of 20/200 or worse).[66] In IDDM, visual impairment and legal blindness are associated with older age, longer duration of diabetes, presence of proliferative retinopathy, and presence of senile cataracts.[66] In NIDDM, approximately 3% of subjects have moderate visual impairment and 1.6% are legally blind.[66] In NIDDM, visual impairment and legal blindness are associated with older age, longer duration of diabetes, presence of senile cataracts, presence of macular edema, and proliferative diabetic retinopathy.[66] When assigning causes of legal blindness, diabetic retinopathy is the sole or contributing cause in about 86% of subjects with IDDM and in about 33% of subjects with NIDDM.[66] In subjects with NIDDM, macular edema, cataracts, glaucoma, and macular degeneration are more important contributors to legal blindness.[66]

Progression of Retinopathy

In a population-based study of the incidence and progression of diabetic retinopathy, 59% of subjects with IDDM who were initially free of retinopathy developed it in 4 years, and 11% of those initially free of proliferative retinopathy developed it in 4 years.[70] Overall, worsening of retinopathy occurred in 41% of the population in 4 years and improvement occurred in 7%.[70] Among insulin-using subjects with NIDDM, 47% of those who did not have any retinopathy developed it in 4 years, and 7% of those initially free from proliferative retinopathy developed it.[71] Worsening of retinopathy occurred in 34% over 4 years.[71] Among non–insulin-using subjects, 34% of those who did not have any retinopathy developed it in 4 years, whereas 2% of those initially free from proliferative retinopathy developed it in 4 years, and 25% had worsening of retinopathy over 4 years.[71] The 4-year incidence of macular edema in subjects with IDDM was 8.2%, in subjects with insulin-treated NIDDM was 8.4%, and in non–insulin-treated subjects was 29%.[72]

Prospective follow-up studies have demonstrated that the risk of progression of retinopathy is higher in those with the highest glycosylated hemoglobin levels compared to those with the lowest glycosylated hemoglobin levels.[60,70,71,72,99] The association between progression of retinopathy and glycosylated hemoglobin persists after controlling for duration of diabetes, age, sex, and baseline retinopathy status. Other studies have shown associations between proliferative diabetic retinopathy, difficulty in managing diabetes, and less effort expended in managing diabetes. Hypertension is associated with progression of background retinopathy in both IDDM and NIDDM.[60,75,99] Pregnancy has been prospectively determined to be a progression of diabetic retinopathy[69] as has nephropathy.[25,73] In IDDM, proliferative retinopathy has also been associated with the HLA-DR phenotypes 4/0, 3/0, or X/X. These results support a multifactorial model for the development of proliferative diabetic retinopathy, which includes both metabolic and genetic risk factors.

Management and Treatment

The results of the Diabetes Control and Complications Trial will clarify whether near normoglycemia can prevent the development of diabetic retinopathy or slow its progression. To date, there are no prospective studies that demonstrate that the incidence of retinopathy may be reduced by controlling blood glucose or blood pressure levels. In the absence of prospective data, it is prudent for health care providers to work with their patients to achieve good blood glucose and blood pressure control. Such efforts should be intensified in patients with evidence of diabetic nephropathy. Although diabetic retinopathy cannot be prevented, therapies exist that can prevent visual loss and restore vision in diabetic patients with proliferative diabetic retinopathy, vitreous hemorrhage, and diabetic macular edema.

The Diabetic Retinopathy Study Research Group demonstrated that panretinal laser photocoagulation reduces the 5-year incidence of severe visual loss (visual acuity, 5/200 or worse) by more than 50%, and from 49% to 22% in people with proliferative diabetic retinopathy and high risk characteristics (see earlier).[32] Side effects of treatment are relatively mild. Panretinal photocoagulation may lead to some long-term loss of peripheral and night vision, and about 10% of treated patients have minor reductions in visual acuity. This reduction in visual acuity is especially prominent in eyes with pre-existing macular edema and is more common in intensively treated eyes than in less intensively treated eyes.

Vitrectomy is performed in people with advanced proliferative diabetic retinopathy. The role of vitrectomy in the treatment of diabetic retinopathy has been defined by the Diabetic Retinopathy Vitrectomy Study.[34] When eyes with advanced, active, proliferative diabetic retinopathy and visual acuity of 10/200 or better were randomly assigned to either early vitrectomy or conventional management, the percentage of eyes with a visual acuity of 10/20 or better was 44% in the early vitrectomy group and 28% in the conventional management group. The proportion with very poor visual outcome was similar in the two groups. The advantage of early vitrectomy tended to increase with increasing severity of new vessels.

In persons with IDDM and vitreous hemorrhage with severe visual loss, there is a clear-cut advantage to early vitrectomy, as reflected in the percentage of eyes recovering visual acuity of 10/20 or better (36% in the early group versus 12% in the deferred group).[33] In persons with NIDDM, spontaneous clearing of vitreous hemorrhage occurs more frequently than in patients with IDDM (29% versus 16%), and there is no advantage to early vitrectomy (16% recovery of visual acuity of 10/20 or better in the early group versus 18% in the deferred group).[33]

The Early Treatment Diabetic Retinopathy Study Research Group demonstrated that focal photocoagulation of clinically significant diabetic macular edema (see above) substantially reduces the risk of visual loss even if visual acuity is not reduced.[37] At 3 years, 12% of those with eyes with clinically significant diabetic macular edema assigned to immediate focal photocoagulation had lost greater than or equal to three lines of visual acuity, and 24% of those in whom photocoagulation was deferred had lost greater than or equal to three lines. Focal treatment increases the chance of visual improvement, decreases the frequency of persistent macular edema, and causes only minor visual field losses.

Guidelines For Preventive Care

As a rule, diabetic retinopathy is asymptomatic in its most treatable stages. Patient education is therefore critical to preventive care. Patients should be reminded to report ocular symptoms, since essentially any symptom may be associated with diabetic retinopathy. Blurred vision while reading may indicate changes in hydration of the lens associated with changes in blood glucose control, but it may also indicate macular edema. The presence of floaters may indicate hemorrhage, and flashing lights may indicate retinal detachment. Persons should also be informed of the relationship between glycemic control, hypertension, and diabetic retinopathy and the importance of continuing treatment of hypertension. Most importantly, individuals should understand the natural history of diabetic retinopathy, the importance of regular eye examinations, and the benefits of timely therapy in reducing the risk of visual loss.[55]

Despite compelling evidence that treatment may prevent visual loss or restore vision in people with diabetic eye disease, many people with diabetes do not receive adequate eye care. In one large population-based survey, it was discovered that approximately one-fourth of subjects with IDDM and one-third of those with NIDDM had never had an ophthalmologic examination.[127] Risk factors for not having had an ophthalmologic examination included being older at time of diagnosis of diabetes, having a shorter duration of diabetes, having better visual acuity, having fewer years of education, receiving diabetes care from a family or general practitioner, and living in a nonmetropolitan county.[27] Barriers to care perceived by persons with diabetes in need of ophthalmic care include failure to be told of the benefits of care or needs for care, denial, dislike of the examination, cost, and distance.[68]

Because significant retinopathy may be present without symptoms, the responsibility to screen the patient with diabetes for retinopathy is significant. Shortly after the initial publication of the results of the Diabetic Retinopathy Study, there was a lack of awareness of the study results among primary care physicians and a failure to incorporate the findings of the study into clinical practice.[117] More recently, there has been controversy as to how best to diagnose diabetic retinopathy. Studies have examined the ability of ophthalmic opticians,[14] optometrists,[74] medical residents, internists, diabetologists, ophthalmologists,[118] nonmydriatric fundus photography,[67] and stereoscopic fundus photography[96] to diagnose diabetic retinopathy. Although difficult to compare, these studies suggest that either a thorough clinical examination performed by a well-trained examiner through dilated pupils or nonstereoscopic retinal photography through a pharmacologically undilated pupil provides a reasonable measure of the severity of retinopathy as assessed by stereoscopic fundus photography. In both cases, follow-up or referral for definitive diagnosis of patients with positive screens is necessary.

Consensus Guidelines (including principles for patient education) now exist for ophthalmic care for persons with diabetes.[55] Patient education is critical to the promotion of eye care (see box on p. 156). All patients with IDDM of more than 5 years' duration and all those with NIDDM should have a baseline eye examination. After the initial eye examination, persons with diabetes should receive complete eye examinations at least once a year. The examination should include a history of visual symptoms, measurement of visual acuity, measurement of intraocular pressure, dilation of the pupils, and thorough retinal examination including stereoscopic examination of the macula. Because stereoscopic examination of the macula requires dilation of the pupils and binocular indirect ophthalmoscopy or other specialized techniques, referral to an ophthalmologist or optometrist skilled in the diagnosis and classification of diabetic retinopathy is preferred.

Persons with nonproliferative retinopathy entering puberty and women with diabetes who are planning pregnancy should be examined by a practitioner who is experienced in the diagnosis and classification of diabetic retinopathy, because of the tendency of retinopathy to progress more rapidly under these conditions. A woman with known diabetes who becomes pregnant should be examined for diabetic retinopathy in the first trimester

---

———————————— **EYE CARE: EDUCATION PRINCIPLES** ————————————

Inform persons with diabetes that sight-threatening eye disease is a common complication of diabetes and may be present even with good vision.

Remind them to report all ocular symptoms, since any symptoms may be diabetic in origin.

Blurred vision while reading may indicate macular edema.

Floaters may indicate hemorrhage.

Flashing lights may indicate retinal detachment.

Inform patients that early detection and appropriate treatment of diabetic eye disease greatly reduces the risk of visual loss.

Explain the possible relationship between glycemic control and the subsequent development of ocular complications.

Tell persons with diabetes about the association between hypertension and diabetic retinopathy.

Stress the importance of the diagnosis and continuing treatment of hypertension.

Help persons with diabetes understand the natural course and treatment of diabetic retinopathy.

Stress the importance of yearly eye examinations.

Tell persons with diabetic retinopathy about the availability and benefits of early and timely laser photocoagulation therapy in reducing the risk of visual loss.

Inform individuals about their higher risks of cataract formation, open-angle glaucoma, and neovascular glaucoma.

Tell individuals with any visual impairment (including blindness) about the availability of visual, vocational, and psychosocial rehabilitation programs.

Adapted from Herman WH, ed: The prevention and treatment of complications of diabetes mellitus: a guide for primary care practitioners, 1991, Atlanta, Dept of Health and Human Services, Public Health Services, Centers for Disease Control, Center for Chronic Disease Prevention and Health Promotion.

and, at the discretion of the examiner, every 3 months until parturition. All individuals with preproliferative retinopathy, proliferative retinopathy without high risk characteristics, and macular edema should be under the care of ophthalmologists and will require more frequent follow-up.

Persons with significant retinal disease or those who have lost vision from retinopathy should continue to receive regular eye care. Proper refraction, low vision evaluation, optical aids, and other techniques and devices are available to enable a person to use even severely limited vision. Referral to optometrists or ophthalmologists specializing in low vision may be appropriate. Support groups for the visually impaired and organizations providing vocational rehabilitation are available in most areas (see Appendix A).

DIABETIC NEPHROPATHY

Diabetic nephropathy is a clinical syndrome characterized by albuminuria, hypertension, and progressive renal insufficiency. In the United States, diabetic nephropathy is the lead-

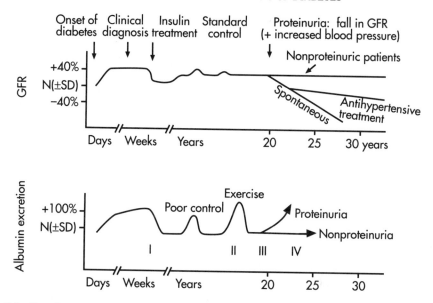

Fig. 5-1 Development of kidney function changes in juvenile diabetes mellitus: GFR and albumin excretion. (Adapted from Morgenson CE, Christensen CK, and Vittinghus E: The stages of diabetic renal disease with emphasis on the stage of incipient diabetic nephropathy, Diabetes 32(suppl 2):64-78, 1983.)

ing cause of new cases of end-stage renal disease that requires dialysis or transplantation for survival. The number of new cases of diabetic end-stage renal disease has increased at an epidemic rate from approximately 2200 in 1980 to nearly 9000 in 1986. At present, the pathogenic mechanisms responsible for the development of diabetic nephropathy are poorly understood, and strategies for the prevention of diabetic nephropathy are limited. Better understanding of the risk factors for nephropathy and the elucidation of treatments to slow the progression of nephropathy have provided the rationale for developing an approach to delay the onset of end-stage renal disease. This approach requires that patients with early diabetic nephropathy be identified, counseled, and treated.[55]

Clinical Manifestations

In IDDM, the natural history of diabetic nephropathy has been well characterized (see Fig. 5-1).[89]

Stage I is the hyperfiltration-hyperfunction stage, found early after the diagnosis of IDDM. Glomerular size and kidney size are both increased. The glomerular filtration rate is high at this stage but returns toward normal with treatment. Slightly elevated urinary albumin excretion rates (microalbuminuria) may be present, but urinary albumin excretion is normalized by insulin treatment.

Stage II is an asymptomatic stage during which renal lesions may be observed without clinical signs or symptoms. This stage is found as early as 2 years after the onset of IDDM. Glomerular basement membrane thickening and mesangial expansion are observed. The GFR remains high. Microalbuminuria may occur during poor metabolic control and exercise.

Stage III is the stage of high risk for diabetic nephropathy, also referred to as the stage of incipient nephropathy. It occurs 10 to 15 years after the diagnosis of IDDM in persons destined to develop overt diabetic nephropathy. GFR remains high, the blood pressure begins to rise, and urinary albumin excretion increases. Intervention at this stage is very important to slow the progress of disease.

Stage IV is the stage of overt diabetic nephropathy. It develops 15 to 25 years after onset of diabetes in about 40% of people with IDDM. Hypertension almost invariably occurs. Clinical signs are now apparent. GFR steadily decreases. Levels of albuminuria greater than 300 mg per 24 hours are observed. Even at this stage, intensified treatment can reduce the rate of decline in GFR and delay progression to stage V.

Stage V is end-stage renal disease (ESRD). Renal function is insufficient to sustain life, and to survive the patient must begin dialysis treatment or receive a renal transplant.

In IDDM, the course of diabetic nephropathy is quite consistent. About 80% of patients who progress to stage III (incipient nephropathy) progress to stage IV (overt nephropathy) over 10 years and essentially all of those progress to stage V (ESRD) within 5 to 10 years.[92]

In NIDDM, some major differences have been described in the natural history of diabetic nephropathy. A population-based study of older subjects with diabetes, older subjects with occult fasting hyperglycemia, and age- and sex-matched controls did not find evidence of hyperfiltration or hyperfunction early in the course of diabetes (stage I).[28] A light microscopy study of glomerular morphology found no evidence of increased glomerular volume early in the course of NIDDM (stage I).[114] In addition, albuminuria appears to be a less specific marker for diabetic nephropathy in older persons with NIDDM. Elderly nondiabetic subjects have a wide range of urinary albumin excretion rates.[28] Only about 22% of patients with NIDDM and microalbuminuria (stage III) progress to overt nephropathy (stage IV) within 10 years[91,92] and only 1 in 8 subjects with NIDDM and overt nephropathy (stage IV) have progressive renal insufficiency.[41] It appears that in NIDDM, the 20-year cumulative incidence of diabetic nephropathy is 25% to 50%.[9,80,128] However, the incidence of ESRD in NIDDM is significantly less than that observed in IDDM. In 1 study, the 10-year risk of ESRD was 5.8% for subjects with IDDM and 0.5% for subjects with NIDDM.[26] When ESRD is observed in persons with NIDDM, it generally develops at an older age but after a shorter duration of known diabetes than that seen in IDDM. These differences in the clinical course of nephropathy in IDDM and NIDDM may be partially explained by the frequently asymptomatic nature of NIDDM, which may result in its remaining undiagnosed for many years, and the selective mortality of subjects with NIDDM and diabetic nephropathy.[58] Nevertheless, it is possible that real differences exist in the clinical course of nephropathy in IDDM and NIDDM.

Pathogenesis

The pathogenesis of diabetic nephropathy has not been defined. Both metabolic and genetic factors appear to be involved. One hypothesis has proposed that intrarenal hypertension is important in the initiation and progression of diabetic nephropathy.[57] Hyperfunction is stimulated by some of the features of the diabetic state such as extracellular fluid volume expansion (caused by hyperglycemia), renal hypertrophy, and increased levels of growth hormone and glucagon. Increases in the glomerular plasma flow rate and the glomerular transcapillary pressure gradient are responsible for hyperfiltration. Hyperfiltration leads to albuminuria and mesangial protein deposition. The latter effect promotes mesangial expansion and ultimately leads to glomerulosclerosis. The loss of functioning nephrons leads to further compensatory hyperfiltration in surviving glomeruli, contributing to their eventual destruction. Other metabolic theories for the pathogenesis of diabetic nephropathy have focused on the altered polyol pathway metabolism and nonezymatic glycosylation of glomerular proteins.[57]

None of these hypotheses can account for the observation that diabetic nephropathy develops in less than half of all patients with diabetes. As a result, studies have also focused on heredity as a possible risk factor for diabetic kidney disease. Some investigators have noted family clustering of nephropathy in IDDM, independent of duration of diabetes, glycemic control, and blood pressure.[115] Most studies have not, however, found associations between HLA type and the presence of nephropathy in IDDM.[10,105] A number of recent studies have found an association between family history of essential hypertension and nephropathy in IDDM.[78,83] In addition, increased rates of erythrocyte sodium-lithium countertransport, a marker for essential hypertension in Caucasian populations, have been found in patients with IDDM and increased glomerular filtration rates,[17] microalbuminuria,[62] and diabetic nephropathy.[78,83,84]

Despite these recent advances in current understanding of the pathogenesis of diabetic nephropathy in IDDM, the exact pathogenic factors responsible for the condition remain unknown. Little work has been done in NIDDM.[93]

Occurrence

In IDDM, overt diabetic nephropathy is unusual before 10 years' duration of diabetes but occurs in 30% to 50% of those with IDDM for 20 or more years. In IDDM, the cumulative incidence of overt nephropathy plateaus after about 25 years and the risk of ever developing nephropathy is low in patients with IDDM who have not developed nephropathy after 25 years' duration of diabetes.[7]

Three recent studies of nephropathy in NIDDM have found a cumulative incidence similar to that observed in IDDM. In a population-based study in Rochester, Minnesota, the 20-year cumulative incidence of persistent proteinuria in NIDDM was 25%.[9] In a clinic-based series from Michigan, the 20-year cumulative incidence of nephropathy in NIDDM was 34%.[128] Among the Pima Indians, the 20-year cumulative incidence of diabetic nephropathy was 50%.[80] Data in NIDDM suggest that the cumulative incidence of nephropathy may not plateau after 25 years' duration and that the risk of diabetic nephropathy may increase with increasing duration of diabetes to approximately 75% after 35 years.[128]

Population-based cross-sectional studies have found that in IDDM approximately 6% of patients with durations of diabetes less than 10 years have evidence of nephropathy compared with 34% of those with durations more than 15 years. In contrast, in NIDDM, about 12% of those with durations less than 10 years and 19% of those with durations more than 15 years have evidence of diabetic nephropathy.[69] Clinic-based studies of patients with IDDM and NIDDM[41,76,88,89] have reported similar findings. The apparent discrepancy between the high cumulative incidence of nephropathy in NIDDM and the low cross-sectional prevalence is probably related to selective mortality among subjects with NIDDM and nephropathy. A number of groups have now reported an association between microalbuminuria and mortality in NIDDM.[61,90] In these studies, patients with NIDDM and microalbuminuria have been found to have a twofold increased mortality as compared with subjects with NIDDM who did not have microalbuminuria. In all studies, cardiovascular disease appears to be the major cause of death. A study performed among the Pima Indians demonstrated that subjects with NIDDM and proteinuria had a death rate 3.5 times higher than those without proteinuria after controlling for age, sex, and diabetes duration.[97,98] Mortality rates from uremia and cardiovascular disease were significantly higher in Pima Indians with diabetes with proteinuria than in those without.[97,98]

Data from the Medicare End-Stage Renal Disease System in the United States have shown that the number of incident cases of diabetic ESRD have increased steadily each year from 2202 in 1980 to 8994 in 1986.[35] Using the estimated diabetic population as the denominator, the age-adjusted incidence per 100,000 people with diabetes increased from 38 in 1980 to 138 in 1986.[35] Compared with white females, the age-adjusted incidence ratios were 1.3 for white males, 2.2 for black females, and 2.1 for black males.[35] Rates of diabetic ESRD are even higher among native Americans and Hispanics. Two studies have compared the incidence of end-stage renal disease in IDDM and NIDDM. In these studies, the incidence of ESRD as a result of diabetic nephropathy was approximately 12-fold greater among patients with IDDM compared with those with NIDDM.[26,109] Most of the excess incidence of diabetic ESRD among blacks occurs among patients with NIDDM.[26] Blacks with NIDDM are approximately four times more likely to develop ESRD than are whites with NIDDM.[26] Blacks with IDDM are approximately 1.6 times more likely to develop ESRD than are whites with IDDM.[26]

Diagnosis

In monitoring persons with diabetes, the health care provider should maintain data so that trends in urinary protein or albumin secretion, serum creatinine, and blood pressure can be readily assessed.

A clinical diagnosis of diabetic nephropathy can be made when an individual who has had diabetes for more than 5 years and has evidence of diabetic retinopathy develops clinically apparent albuminuria or proteinuria. Because albuminuria and proteinuria may be caused by the presence of other complicating renal diseases, a person who does not meet these criteria or has evidence of other kidney disease may require a kidney biopsy. In general, however, a clinical diagnosis of diabetic nephropathy can be made without performing a kidney biopsy.[55]

Because early persistent subclinical increases in urinary albumin excretion can identify persons at risk for developing diabetic nephropathy and cardiovascular disease, and because early intervention may slow or prevent the progression of diabetic nephropathy, there has been emphasis on the use of sensitive quantitative measures of urinary albumin excretion (microalbuminuria). Traditional urine dipstick methods are insensitive and only semiquantitative and, therefore, cannot be used to detect mild to moderate increases in urinary albumin excretion or to detect changes in urinary albumin excretion.[54]

Urinalysis should be performed at the diagnosis of diabetes. If infection is present, the urine should be cultured and the patient treated appropriately. When infection is not present, urinary albumin excretion (UAE) should be measured quantitatively. If UAE is normal, UAE and renal function (serum creatinine and/or glomerular filtration rate) should be measured yearly. If UAE is abnormal, it should be measured quantitatively on at least 3 occasions over 6 months. Clinical laboratories offer an array of sensitive quantitative techniques for measuring UAE, including radioimmunoassay, enzyme-linked immunosorbent assay (ELISA), and turbidimetry or nephelometory-immunoassay. New semiquantitative techniques are also being developed.[54]

UAE can be measured in a variety of different urine samples including first-morning urine samples, random urine samples, and from urine samples collected over timed periods. The results can be expressed as rates, in terms of albumin/creatinine ratios, or as concentrations. All techniques have advantages and disadvantages, and the choice of technique and the selection of sample depend largely on local experience. Efforts must be made to ensure that different methods give comparable results and that the value chosen to define increased urinary albumin excretion should not misclassify healthy diabetic and nondiabetic subjects.[54] Table 5-1 summarizes criteria for the stages of diabetic nephropathy as defined by urinary protein and albumin concentrations, urinary protein and albumin excretion rates, and urinary protein to creatinine and albumin to creatinine ratios.

Management/Treatment

At present, strategies for preventing diabetic nephropathy must be viewed as limited in their effectiveness because the exact pathogenic factors responsible for this condition are unknown. It is hoped that in the next few years, the results of the Diabetes Control and Complications Trial will determine whether or not improved glycemic control can prevent or delay the development of diabetic nephropathy. It is, however, clear that in patients with albuminuria, blood pressure control is of critical importance in slowing the progression of disease. Other strategies that may slow the progression of renal disease include limiting dietary protein consumption, promptly treating urinary tract infections, and avoiding potentially nephrotoxic drugs and radiographic dyes.[4]

Table 5-1   Criteria for the Diagnosis of Diabetic Nephropathy

	Urinary albumin (u albumin)			
	Concentration µg/ml	Rate µg/min	mg/24°	Ratio u albumin/ u creatinine
Normal	<20	<20	<30	<0.02
Microalbuminuria	20-200	20-200	30-300	0.02-0.2
Diabetic nephropathy	>200	>200	>300	>0.2
	Urinary protein (u protein)			
	Concentration µg/ml	Rate µg/min	mg/24°	Ratio u protein/ u creatinine
Normal	<30	<30	<50	<0.03
Microproteinuria	30-300	30-300	50-500	0.03-0.3
Diabetic nephropathy	>300	300	>500	>0.3

Education

All persons with diabetes should be informed about the potential renal complications of diabetes and the possible relationship between poor glycemic control and the development of diabetic kidney disease. Patients with diabetic kidney disease should know about the association between hypertension and accelerated kidney disease and should understand the critical importance of treating hypertension. They should be aware of the need for regular blood pressure monitoring and should be encouraged to measure their own blood pressures at home. In addition, they should know their target blood pressure levels. Patients with diabetic kidney disease should be informed about the role of excessive dietary protein in the progression of diabetic kidney disease and should be counseled to consume no more than the recommended daily allowance for protein. All persons with diabetes should know the symptoms and signs of urinary tract infections and pyelonephritis and should be instructed to contact their health care provider if such symptoms occur. Patients with diabetic kidney disease should also know which drugs are potentially nephrotoxic and should be made aware of the risks of radiographic dye studies. Persons with diabetic kidney disease should also know the natural history of the condition and understand the therapeutic options for ESRD.

Blood Pressure

In patients with evidence of incipient nephropathy or overt diabetic nephropathy, blood pressure should be carefully monitored and hypertension should be aggressively treated.[20,21,87,103] Blood pressure greater than 140/90 mm Hg should be treated, and treatment should be considered in patients with significant increments in blood pressure (20/10 mm Hg) on careful follow-up.

Although some theoretic evidence and limited clinical data suggest that angiotension-converting enzyme (ACE) inhibitors (Mason N) and calcium channel blockers[30] may be preferred in the treatment of hypertension in patients with diabetic nephropathy, any drug that effectively lowers blood pressure without undue side effects or further impairment in renal function may be used. Before any antihypertension medication is prescribed, the dosage schedule, potential side effects, and cost should be discussed with the patient.

Dietary Measures

Since recent studies in small numbers of subjects with IDDM and NIDDM have suggested that dietary protein restriction may reduce the rate of rise of urinary albumin excretion and slow the rate of decline of renal function,[39,130] patients with incipient nephropathy or overt diabetic nephropathy should be encouraged to adhere to the recommended dietary allowance (RDA) for protein[3,108] (see Chapter 2). For children aged 7 to 14 this is 1.0 g of protein per kilogram of body weight per day, and for males age 15 to 18 this is 0.9 g of protein per kilogram of body weight per day. Females age 15 to 18 require 0.8 g of protein per kilogram of body weight per day. Pregnant women require approximately 10 g more protein per day, and lactating women require approximately 15 g more protein per day. For adults over age 19, the recommended daily allowance for protein is 0.8 g per kilogram of body weight per day. Adherence to these guidelines can be assessed by dietary history or by measurement of 24-hour urinary urea nitrogen. The grams of protein ingested per day can be estimated from the urinary urea nitrogen by the formula: protein intake (g/day) equals 24-hour urinary urea nitrogen (g/24 hours) times 6.25 and then divided by 0.80.

Metabolic Control

Because a number of small clinical trials in subjects with IDDM and microalbuminuria have suggested that improved glycemic control may slow the rate of progression of renal disease,[27,44,77] efforts to improve glycemic control should be considered in patients with microalbuminuria. The potential benefits of therapy must be weighted against the increased risks of hypoglycemia. Improved glycemic control does not appear to affect the course of overt diabetic nephropathy.

Risk Reduction

Because of the associations among diabetic nephropathy, retinopathy, and cardiovascular disease, complete eye examinations should be performed at least yearly for subjects with nephropathy, and risk factors for coronary heart disease, including hypertension, hyperlipidemia, and cigarette smoking, should be assessed and treated as needed.

Urinary tract infection should be promptly treated in patients with diabetes, and a urine culture should be repeated after treatment to ensure that the infection has resolved. In addition, potentially nephrotoxic drugs and radiographic dyes should be avoided when possible in patients with diabetes and especially in those with diabetic nephropathy. Persons with diabetes with pre-existing renal insufficiency are at increased risk for exacerbation of renal failure following radiocontrast studies. Clinical series have demonstrated that 10% to 70% of diabetic persons with serum creatinine levels greater than or equal to 1.5 mg/dL will develop deterioration in renal failure following radiocontrast studies. Up to 95% of subjects with diabetes with serum creatine levels greater than 5 mg/dL may develop acute renal failure.[51,102,125]

Persons with Renal Disease

The management of diabetes in persons with renal disease requires special attention.[5] As renal insufficiency develops, many persons with diabetes require a reduction in their dose of insulin or sulfonylurea. Since approximately one-third of insulin is metabolized and cleared by the renal parenchyma and the half-life of all sulfonylureas is prolonged with renal disease, it is generally prudent to reduce the insulin dose and/or use a sulfonylurea that has a short half-life and is converted by the liver into inactive metabolites (Glipizide) as renal insufficiency supervenes. It is also important to recognize that uremia may be associated with anorexia, weight loss, and bowel dysmotility. Decreased calorie intake, erratic nutrient absorption, and decreased gluconeogenesis may also contribute to the risk of severe hypoglycemia.

Subjects with impending renal failure (serum creatine greater than 2 mg/dL and/or glomerular filtration rate less than 40 ml/min) should be referred for renal consultation. Patients with diabetes who have developed ESRD will require dialysis or kidney transplantation to prolong their lives. Because diabetic complications—especially retinopathy and neuropathy—progress more rapidly with the onset of renal failure, dialysis is instituted earlier for people with diabetes than for those without diabetes. In general, treatment is initiated when the serum creatinine reaches about 6 mg/dL. Kidney transplantation is preferable to dialysis when a living relative of the patient is available as a donor. The patient's chances of survival are otherwise about equal given peritoneal dialysis, hemodialysis, or cadaveric renal transplant. The ultimate choice of treatment will require the input of the patient, the patient's family, and a health care team.

Compared with nondiabetic patients with ESRD, diabetic patients with ESRD have a significantly shorter 5-year survival rate (28% versus 40%).[52] In general, survival decreases with increasing age at onset of ESRD. The difference in survival between nondiabetic and diabetic patients is greatest among older persons.[52] The higher mortality observed among diabetic patients with ESRD and the increasing age-specific mortality among diabetic ESRD patients are probably the result of a higher prevalence of comorbid conditions including cerebral vascular disease, atherosclerotic heart disease, and peripheral vascular disease.[23]

DIABETIC NEUROPATHY

Diabetic neuropathy can be defined as peripheral nerve dysfunction that occurs in people with established diabetes, is of a type known to be more prevalent among people with diabetes than among people without diabetes, and cannot be attributed to any other disease process. Diabetes is probably the most common cause of neuropathy in the United States, and diabetic neuropathy is a major cause of suffering, disability, and lower extremity amputation. In the past, lack of consistency in the classification of diabetic neuropathy retarded efforts to define its occurrence, causes, prevention, and treatment. In recent years, there has been an emerging consensus as to the classification of diabetic neuropathy, and there have been improvements in current understanding of its biochemical and vascular bases.

Classification

Diabetic neuropathy can be best understood as a group of clinical syndromes. The clinical syndromes of diabetic neuropathy each have characteristic presentations, symptoms and signs, and courses. Although each syndrome is distinct, the syndromes may coexist in the same patient, making classification difficult. The classification of diabetic neuropathy is based upon its presumed underlying pathophysiology.[36] Diabetic neuropathy may be classified as being either diffuse or focal (see box below).

Distal symmetric sensorimotor polyneuropathy is a form of diffuse neuropathy. It is the most common type of neuropathy associated with diabetes. It is primarily a sensory neuropathy but may be associated with distal motor abnormalities and with autonomic dysfunction. Sensory deficits appear first in the toes and feet and progress proximally. Involvement of the fingers and hands is a relatively late finding. In advanced disease, distal portions of the truncal nerves may become involved, and sensory deficits may occur in a vertical band on the anterior chest. The symptoms and signs of distal symmetric sensorimotor polyneuropathy vary depending on the classes of nerve fibers involved. Three over-

---

————————— **SYNDROMES OF DIABETIC NEUROPATHY** —————————

Diffuse neuropathy

Distal symmetric sensorimotor polyneuropathy
Acute painful neuropathy
Small fiber neuropathy
Large fiber neuropathy
Autonomic neuropathy
Sudomotor dysfunction
Abnormal pupillary function
Cardiovascular autonomic neuropathy
Gastrointestinal autonomic neuropathy
Genitourinary autonomic neuropathy
Hypoglycemia unawareness

Focal neuropathy

Cranial neuropathy
Radiculopathy
Plexopathy
Mononeuropathy multiplex
Mononeuropathy

lapping clinical syndromes have been described: (1) an acute painful neuropathy without evidence of significant neurologic deficits, (2) a small fiber neuropathy characterized by diminished pain and temperature sensation, and (3) a large fiber neuropathy characterized by loss of light touch, vibration, and position sensation.[120]

Diabetic autonomic neuropathy is a second form of diffuse neuropathy. It may involve virtually any sympathetic or parasympathetic autonomic function. Manifestations of diabetic autonomic neuropathy may include abnormal sweating, abnormal pupillary function, cardiovascular autonomic neuropathy, gastrointestinal autonomic neuropathy, genitourinary autonomic neuropathy, and hypoglycemia unawareness.[40]

Focal diabetic neuropathy is associated with deficits in the distribution of a single nerve (mononeuropathy), multiple peripheral nerves (mononeuropathy multiplex), the brachial or lumbosacral plexuses (plexopathy), or the nerve roots (radiculopathy). Individual cranial nerves may also be involved (cranial nerve palsies).[8]

Occurrence

The epidemiology of diabetic neuropathy has not been well defined because of a lack of standardization of diagnostic methods and a lack of consensus in diagnostic criteria.[86] In IDDM, the prevalence of diabetic distal symmetric sensorimotor polyneuropathy appears to parallel the duration and severity of hyperglycemia. This is not the case in NIDDM, in which patients may present with symptoms or signs of peripheral neuropathy and only later be found to have NIDDM. This is probably explained by the frequently asymptomatic nature of NIDDM, which may result in its remaining undiagnosed for many years. In 1 population-based study of NIDDM, the cumulative incidence of distal symmetric sensorimotor polyneuropathy was 4% after 5 years and 15% after 20 years.[101] Clinic-based series have reported a 40% prevalence of distal symmetric sensorimotor polyneuropathy after 20 years of diabetes.[106] Population-based studies of diabetic autonomic neuropathy and diabetic focal neuropathy are not available. Clinic-based series have found that the prevalence of cardiovascular autonomic neuropathy occurs in up to 20% of persons with diabetes and sexual dysfunction in up to 50% of men and 30% of women with diabetes. The focal neuropathies appear to be uncommon, but they are often misdiagnosed. Their prevalence may be higher than is generally recognized.

Pathogenesis

Distal symmetric sensorimotor polyneuropathy

Pathologic studies of diabetic distal symmetric sensorimotor polyneuropathy suggest that longer myelinated axons are preferentially involved. The diffuse nature and progressive course of distal symmetric sensorimotor polyneuropathy suggest a metabolic basis. A number of hypotheses have been proposed to explain the pathogenesis of the condition. Two leading hypotheses are the sorbitol-myo-inositol-sodium-potassium ATPase hypothesis and the nonenzymatic glycation hypothesis.[49,50]

The sorbitol-myo-inositol-sodium-potassium ATPase hypothesis has linked acute hyperglycemia, metabolic abnormalities in peripheral nerve, nerve conduction slowing, and neuroanatomic defects in peripheral nerves.

Another metabolic process that has been proposed to explain the pathogenesis of diabetic neuropathy is nonenzymatic glycation. Nonenzymatic glycation occurs in various tissue proteins as a result of increased ambient glucose concentrations. Nonenzymatic glycation of peripheral nerve protein has been described, although its role in clinical diabetic neuropathy has not been critically examined.[49,50]

Autonomic neuropathy

Autopsy studies of people with diabetic autonomic neuropathy have demonstrated axonal degeneration and fiber loss in the sympathetic and parasympathetic systems. The intrinsic nerves of the gastrointestinal and genitourinary systems are also affected. The diffuse nature and chronic progressive course of autonomic neuropathy suggest a metabolic basis, and, as in the case in distal symmetric sensorimotor polyneuropathy, alterations in sorbitol-myo-inositol-sodium-potassium ATPase and nonenzymatic glycation of nerve proteins have been hypothesized as pathogenetic mechanisms.[49,50] Complement-fixing antisympathetic ganglia antibodies and antivagus nerve antibodies have recently been described in subjects with IDDM and cardiovascular autonomic neuropathy, and it has been postulated that autoimmunity may also play a role in the pathogenesis of diabetic autonomic neuropathy.[107]

Focal neuropathy

The pathogenesis of the focal diabetic neuropathies has not been extensively studied but appears to be vascular. The natural history of the focal neuropathies, with sudden onset, gradual resolution, and confinement to a single nerve root, nerve, or plexus is consistent with a vascular etiology. Serial sections of the cranial nerves of two patients with diabetes who died after developing isolated third-nerve palsies revealed local thickening and occlusion of arterioles. Focal acute demyelinating lesions were also present. A second autopsy report of a patient with diabetes, who died shortly after developing femoral neuropathy, revealed multiple microinfarcts of the nerve, vessel wall thickening, and occlusion of the vasa nervora. Thus it appears that vascular pathology in diabetic nerve and ischemic injury are critical in the pathogenesis of focal neuropathy.[49,50]

Clinical Manifestations, Diagnosis, and Treatment of Distal Symmetric Sensorimotor Polyneuropathy

Clinical manifestations

The symptoms and signs of distal symmetric sensorimotor polyneuropathy vary depending on the classes of nerve fibers involved.

Acute painful neuropathy is an uncommon and extremely unpleasant complication of diabetes. It may occur early in the course of diabetes with institution of insulin or sulfonylurea therapy. It is often associated with precipitous weight loss. Most commonly, persons experience distal paresthesias (spontaneously occurring uncomfortable sensations), dysesthesias (uncomfortable sensations on contact), and pain. At times, the pain is described as superficial and burning, shooting or stabbing, or aching or tearing. Often the pain is worse at night, producing insomnia. Because damage is limited to the small myelinated fibers, objective signs of neuropathy may be minimal. Sensory loss may not be striking, vibration sensation may be intact, motor weakness may be absent, and conduction velocity may not be dramatically impaired. The presence of painful symptoms in the absence of striking neurologic deficits appears somewhat paradoxic. Pain may, however, reflect increased fiber regeneration. In general, pain subsides in months and is preceded by weight gain. Relapses are uncommon.[120]

Small-fiber neuropathy may appear after only a few years of diabetes. Pain may occur and may be described as burning, shooting, or aching. Paresthesias may occur. Alternatively, patients with small-fiber neuropathy may present with subjective symptoms of numbness or feelings of "cold feet." The extent of peripheral nervous system damage is generally not severe. Objectively, patients have diminished pinprick and temperature sensation. Soft touch, vibration, and position sensation are generally spared. Motor weakness is usually not marked. If motor weakness occurs, it involves the most distal intrinsic muscles of the feet and hands as a rather late feature. Mild autonomic dysfunction may occur. If autonomic dysfunction occurs, it may be associated with abnormal sweating and dry skin on the feet. Patients with advanced small-fiber neuropathy may occasionally present with undetected trauma of the extremities such as burns or abrasions of the feet or with cigarette burns of the fingers. Neuropathic ulcers may occasionally occur at sites of trauma.[120]

Large-fiber neuropathy occurs insidiously or, at times, quite rapidly in the setting of small-fiber neuropathy. Subjective symptoms of paresthesias and pain are usually absent. Involvement of large fibers leads to impairment of touch, pressure, discriminative sense, vibration, and position sense. The ankle reflexes are depressed or lost. In more severe instances, there is sensory ataxia and a positive Romberg's test. This condition is referred to as a "pseudotabetic" form of diabetic neuropathy. Large-fiber neuropathy is often associated with distal motor and autonomic abnormalities that manifest themselves as deformed feet with dry, thickened, and cracked skin. Since pain is generally not associated with large-fiber neuropathy, patients with large-fiber neuropathy are least likely to have complaints referable to their feet. Large-fiber neuropathy is, however, most strongly associated with the development of neuropathic foot ulcers and neuropathic arthropathy (Charcot joint), and patients with large-fiber neuropathy are at greatest risk for amputation[120] (see Chapter 7).

Diagnosis

To detect distal symmetric sensorimotor polyneuropathy, the clinician should conduct an interview at each visit to determine whether the patient is experiencing pain, paresthesias, numbness, or weakness. Because patients with large-fiber neuropathy may have no symptoms, the clinician should also remove the patient's shoes and socks and inspect the feet for deformities, dry skin, and ulcers. At least once a year, the clinician should perform a physical examination to assess sensation, muscle strength, and deep-tendon reflexes. Temperature sensation may be assessed by touching a cool piece of metal (such as a tuning fork) to the patient's foot and by asking the patient to describe the object's temperature. Pinprick sensation may be assessed by holding a clean straight pin lightly between the thumb and forefinger and touching it to the patient's foot. The patient is asked to say when a sensation is felt and whether it is sharp or dull. Vibration sensation may be assessed with a 128 HZ tuning fork applied to the distal first metatarsal head or the malleoli of the ankles. The patient is asked to report when the vibration ceases. Position sensation is assessed by having the patient describe the toe's position as it is alternately flexed and extended.[55]

The diagnosis of diabetic distal symmetric sensorimotor polyneuropathy requires that the patient have diabetes mellitus and have symptoms or signs of peripheral nerve dysfunction that are not attributable to any other cause. Since there are no features that are unique to diabetic distal symmetric sensorimotor polyneuropathy, other causes of peripheral neuropathy must be excluded by careful history and physical examination and by appropriate diagnostic tests (see box on p. 170).[49,50] Occasionally, nerve conduction studies with needle electromyography may help in the diagnosis.

Treatment

Current therapy for diabetic distal symmetric sensorimotor polyneuropathy is palliative and is directed at reducing pain. Troubling pain generally improves spontaneously within a number of months, although some patients have persistent disabling pain. Although a number of studies have shown that improved glycemic control is associated with improvement in nerve conduction velocity,[27,116] it is not clear that improved glycemic control reduces pain. Nevertheless, pending the results of definitive studies, it appears prudent to strive to achieve good glycemic control in patients with painful diabetic neuropathy while attempting to minimize undue side effects from hypoglycemia. Transcutaneous electrical nerve stimulation (TENS) is rarely effective in the treatment of painful neuropathy but deserves consideration because of its lack of systemic side effects. Various pharmacologic agents have been recommended for the treatment of painful neuropathy, including simple analgesics, antidepressants alone or with phenothiazines, mexiletine, capsaicin, and anticonvulsants.

Among simple analgesics, both ibuprofen (600 mg orally, 4 times daily) and sulindac (200 mg orally, twice daily) have been shown to be more effective than placebo in the treatment of painful diabetic neuropathy.[22] Numerous clinical trials have demonstrated the efficacy of tricyclic antidepressants in the treatment of painful diabetic neuropathy.[38,47,81,84,129] These medications appear to relieve the pain of diabetic neuropathy independent of any effect on mood.[84] Onset of analgesia is variable, but may take days to several weeks. For this reason, a low dosage of medication should be started and the dosage increased in small steps until the patient's symptoms are relieved or the patient reaches the highest tolerable dose. Side effects common to all of the tricyclic antidepressants include drowsiness, dry mouth, orthostatic hypotension, constipation, and urinary retention. Studies have shown that the combination of a tricyclic antidepressant and a phenothiazine (nortriptyline and fluphenazine) are effective in the treatment of painful

DIFFERENTIAL DIAGNOSIS OF DISTAL SYMMETRIC
SENSORIMOTOR POLYNEUROPATHY

Metabolic

Diabetes mellitus
Uremia
Hypothyroidism
Folic acid/cyanocobalamin deficiency
Acute intermittent porphyria

Toxic

Medications
Alcohol
Heavy metals (lead, mercury, arsenic)
Industrial hydrocarbons

Infectious or inflammatory

Sarcoidosis
Leprosy
Periarteritis nodosa
Other connective tissue diseases (e.g., systemic lupus erythematosus)

Other

Amyloidosis
Dysproteinemias
Leukemias and lymphomas
Psychophysiologic disorders (e.g., severe depression, hysteria)
Hereditary neuropathies

neuropathy[47] and that the addition of fluphenazine or clonazepam to a tricyclic antidepressant may provide relief of pain when a tricyclic antidepressant alone has not relieved pain.[129] More recently, mexiletine, an oral antiarrhythmic agent that is structurally similar to lidocaine, has been shown to be effective in the treatment of 1 diabetic neuropathy at a dose of 10 mg per kilogram of body weight per day.[29] Mexiletine is contraindicated in the presence of preexisting atrioventricular heart block (if no pacemaker is present) and is associated with reversible gastrointestinal and central nervous system side effects. Recently, there have been anecdotal reports of the successful treatment of painful diabetic neuropathy with topical capsaicin applied to the affected areas four times daily,[110] but there are concerns regarding possible neurotoxicity associated with its use.[82] Although anticonvulsant medications are used widely in the treatment of chronic pain,[119] and although they have been found to be effective in uncontrolled studies of the treatment of diabetic neuropathy, they have not proved to be effective in controlled clinical trials.[18,113] Small, short-term trials of aldose reductase inhibitors and myo-inositol supplementation have yielded conflicting results.[12,46,100,112] Vitamins are not effective in the treatment of painful diabetic distal symmetric sensorimotor polyneuropathy.

Clinical Manifestations, Diagnosis, and Treatment of Diabetic Autonomic Neuropathy

The symptoms and signs of diabetic autonomic neuropathy are protean, and the manifestations of diabetic autonomic neuropathy range from the annoying to the disabling and life-threatening.[49,50]

Sudomotor dysfunction

Autonomic sudomotor dysfunction may produce absence of sweating in a stocking-glove distribution and increased sweating in the face or trunk. Gustatory sweating—abnormal sweating associated with eating—is uncommon but may be quite bothersome to the patient. Distal anhydrosis is often associated with distal symmetric sensorimotor polyneuropathy and is of clinical significance because it causes dry skin and diminished skin lubrication and may contribute to the development of plantar ulcers. Abnormal sweating may also contribute to decreased thermoregulation and may predispose to heat stroke or hyperthermia.[49,50] Unless the history is carefully elicited and the feet are examined, patients rarely report abnormal sweating. Diagnosis is important so that affected patients can be counseled to prevent foot lesions, heat stroke, and hyperthermia. Patients with dry, thickened skin should be instructed in foot care and the use of lubricating oils or creams. Patients with thermoregulatory dysfunction should be counseled to avoid intense heat and humidity.[49,50]

Abnormal pupillary function

The pupillary iris is innervated by both parasympathetic and sympathetic fibers. Parasympathetic fibers cause pupillary constriction, and sympathetic fibers cause pupillary dilatation. Diabetic autonomic neuropathy of the eye is associated with abnormalities of both parasympathetic and sympathetic tone, but sympathetic tone is more severely affected. As a result, diabetic patients with autonomic dysfunction tend to have small pupils that dilate slowly in the dark. These changes may be apparent if the practitioner attempts to perform an undilated ophthalmoscopic examination in a darkened room and finds that the pupil dilates slowly. Patients themselves may note poor dark adaptation and should be counseled to allow themselves more time when entering poorly illuminated areas and to use lights when walking at night. Otherwise no specific therapy is required.[49,50]

Cardiovascular autonomic neuropathy

Cardiovascular autonomic neuropathy is associated with abnormalities of heart rate control and vascular dynamics. Parasympathetic tone slows the heart rate and sympathetic tone speeds the heart rate and increases the force of cardiac contraction. Sympathetic tone also stimulates the vascular tree and increases blood pressure. There are three syndromes of cardiovascular autonomic neuropathy: (1) cardiac denervation syndrome, (2) postural hypotension, and (3) abnormal exercise-induced cardiovascular performance.[49,50]

Cardiac denervation produces a fixed heart rate that does not change with stress, exercise, or sleep. Both parasympathetic and sympathetic tone are affected in cardiac denervation syndrome. Initially, parasympathetic tone decreases, resulting in a relative increase in sympathetic tone and an increase in the heart rate. Early in the course of cardiac denervation syndrome, patients have a fixed resting heart rate of 100 to 120 beats/min. Progressive loss of sympathetic tone results in a gradual slowing of the heart rate. Finally, when both parasympathetic and sympathetic tone are impaired, cardiac denervation syndrome exists and patients have a fixed heart rate of 80 to 90 beats/min.

Cardiac denervation can be diagnosed by checking the pulse during slow deep breathing (6 breaths per minute) or before and after exercise. Persons with cardiac denervation syndrome lack normal sinus rhythm and have no heart rate variation during deep breathing and have no pulse change before or after exercise. Persons with cardiac denervation syndrome are also at increased risk for cardiac arrhythmias, sudden death, and painless myocardial ischemia.

Normally, blood pressure is maintained when a person stands by the "postural reflex," in which baroreceptors initiate a sympathetic reflex that increases heart rate and peripheral vascular resistance in association with an increase in the plasma norepinephrine level. Postural hypotension is defined as a fall of systolic blood pressure of more than 30 mm Hg or a fall of diastolic blood pressure of more than 10 mm Hg on changing from lying to standing position. Postural hypotension may or may not be associated with symptoms.

Symptoms of postural hypotension include postural faintness, weakness, visual impairment, or syncope in the absence of hypoglycemia or arrhythmia. Measurement of the supine and standing blood pressure and pulse is critical in the evaluation of diabetic patients with postural symptoms. Postural hypotension as a result of cardiovascular autonomic neuropathy is a diagnosis of exclusion and requires a careful history and physical examination and appropriate laboratory testing to rule out other potential causes (see box below). Volume depletion can be differentiated from cardiovascular autonomic neuropathy by evaluating the heart rate response and/or the plasma norepinephrine response to standing. In volume depletion, the heart rate and catecholamine levels increase in response to standing. In cardiovascular autonomic neuropathy, the heart rate and catecholamine levels are unchanged in response to standing.

The treatment of diabetic postural hypotension includes avoiding volume depletion by improving glycemic control to control glucosuria and by ensuring the intake of adequate dietary salt. Salt intake can be assessed by measuring 24-hour urinary sodium excretion. Mechanical measures such as waist-high elastic stockings, plasma volume expansion with salt supplementation and/or fludrocortisone,[15] and pharmacologic treatment with sympathetic agonists such as phenylephrine, ephedrine and Neosynephrine nasal spray may occasionally be necessary. Beta blockers,[11] clonidine,[1] metoclopramide,[79] and somatostatin analog[56] have also been reported to be useful in the treatment of diabetic postural hypotension but have not been evaluated in large controlled clinical trials.

The cardiovascular response to exercise may be abnormal in patients with diabetes with cardiovascular autonomic neuropathy. Such patients may fail to increase their cardiac output or vascular tone with exercise and may develop hypotension in response to exercise. Persons with abnormal exercise-induced cardiac performance should be counseled not to attempt aerobic exercise.[49,50]

Gastrointestinal autonomic neuropathy

There are many gastrointestinal manifestations of diabetic autonomic neuropathy. Parasympathetic nervous system activity stimulates esophageal and gastric peristalsis. Dopaminergic intervention inhibits gastric peristalsis and sympathetic nervous system activity inhibits gastric emptying. Abnormalities in any of these pathways may result in abnormal gastrointestinal function.[49,50]

Upper gastrointestinal motility disorders may involve the esophagus, stomach, and proximal small intestine. Patients may complain of symptoms of dysphagia, heartburn, reflux, anorexia, bloating, early satiety, upper abdominal pain, nausea, and vomiting. Associated signs may include weight loss, gastric splash, and erratic glycemic control. The usual pattern of erratic glycemic control in insulin-treated patients with gastroparesis is one of postprandial hypoglycemia and late hyperglycemia reflecting normal insulin action but delayed nutrient absorption. Persons with gastroparesis are also at risk for developing bezoars that may be associated with early satiety, gastric outlet obstruction, and vomiting.

Diabetic gastroparesis is a diagnosis of exclusion (see box on p. 174). Upper gastrointestinal (GI) endoscopy or a barium upper GI series may be necessary to rule out obstruction. An abnormal barium upper GI series, which measures liquid-phase gastric emptying, almost always implies the existence of abnormal solid-phase emptying. Conversely, a normal liquid-phase emptying study does not exclude abnormal solid-phase emptying. A nuclear medicine solid-phase gastric emptying study, which uses a radiolabeled solid food (egg or chicken liver), is the most sensitive and specific way to diagnose delayed gastric emptying.

Treatment of gastroparesis includes improvement of glycemic control and correction of other metabolic abnormalities such as ketosis and hypokalemia. It also includes dietary modification with small, low-fat, low-fiber, and/or liquid meals.[45] Pharmacologic treatment with metoclopramide,[85] domperidone, cisapride, and erythromycin has also been shown to be effective in the treatment of diabetic gastroparesis.[19,45,60,85,124]

Constipation

Constipation is probably the most common gastrointestinal symptom associated with diabetes and has been reported by up to 60% of patients with long-standing diabetes. The pathogenesis of constipation is poorly understood. Measurement of distal colonic myoelectrical and motor activity have shown absent gastrocolic responses to feeding.[49,50] Other possible contributing factors must be excluded (see box on p. 174). Three stool specimens should be tested for occult blood, and patients should have careful digital examinations. Women should have pelvic examinations with careful bimanual examinations. If occult blood is detected, a complete blood count, iron, total iron-binding capac-

DIFFERENTIAL DIAGNOSIS OF AUTONOMIC NEUROPATHY

Orthostatic hypotension

Hypovolemia
Medications (diuretics, antihypertensives, tricyclic antidepressants)
Panhypopituitarism
Pheochromocytoma
Shy-Drager syndrome
Idiopathic orthostatic hypotension

Gastroparesis

Medications
Acute metabolic disturbances
Gastric or intestinal obstruction

Constipation

Medications
Dehydration
Intestinal obstruction

Diarrhea

Medications
Dietary sorbitol or lactose
Bacterial overgrowth
Pseudomembranous colitis
Enteric pathogens
Primary intestinal diseases
Pancreatic exocrine insufficiency

Impotence

Medications
Hormonal abnormalities
Vascular disease
Psychogenic disease

Hypoglycemia unawareness

Medications
Liver disease
Renal disease
Adrenocortical insufficiency
Lack of knowledge about hypoglycemia

ity (TIBC), and proctosigmoidscopy and barium enema or colonoscopy should be performed. Treatment of diabetic constipation includes improvement of glycemic control with correction of glycosuria, adequate hydration, high-fiber diet, psyllium, and stool softeners.

Diarrhea

Diabetic diarrhea is an uncommon but troubling complication of diabetes. Diabetic diarrhea may be preceded by abdominal cramps. It is severe and watery and may occasionally be associated with steatorrhea. It is generally not associated with weight loss, is often worse at night, and may fluctuate from season to season. It is intermittent, and during remissions the individual may experience constipation. It characteristically lasts from a few hours to several weeks. It may be associated with fecal incontinence (see below). Its pathogenesis appears to be multifactorial, as autonomic neuropathy, microangiopathy, and functional mucosal abnormalities may all contribute.[49,50] History, physical examination, and laboratory testing should rule out diarrhea resulting from other causes (see box on p. 174). The history should focus on ingestion of lactose, nonabsorbable artificial sweeteners such as sorbitol and mannitol, and antacids, all of which may be associated with diarrhea. When appropriate, history and laboratory studies should be obtained to rule out bacterial overgrowth pseudomembranous colitis enteric pathogens, primary intestinal disorders such as inflammatory bowel disease and celiac disease, and pancreatic exocrine insufficiency.

The diagnosis of diabetic diarrhea is established only by excluding other causes of diarrhea and by confirming the presence of autonomic neuropathy. The intermittent nature of diabetic diarrhea makes it difficult to assess the effectiveness of treatment. As a result, much of the treatment for diabetic diarrhea is empiric. Since afferent denervation may contribute to the problem, a bowel program that includes regular efforts to move the bowels should be tried. Fiber and psyllium may be used to increase stool bulk and consistency; codeine, loperamide, or diphenoxylate hydrochloride and atropine sulfate may be used to slow gastrointestinal motility. Use of broad-spectrum antibiotics with anaerobic coverage such as tetracycline or metronidazole hydrochloride have been reported to be beneficial.[48] If there is no improvement, then bile salt binders such as cholestyramine and colestipol may be tried since patients with gallbladder atony have inappropriate spillage of bile salts into the gut between meals, and that may result in diarrhea.[24] Clonidine, an alpha-2 adrenergic blocker, has also been reported to increase intraluminal fluid absorption and to decrease diarrhea.[42] Finally, somatostatin analog has been used successfully in some cases.

Fecal incontinence is a devastating complication of diabetes. Patients with fecal incontinence will often become homebound and avoid social contact. Fecal incontinence is associated with a reduced threshold of conscious rectal sensation, low basal internal anal sphincter pressure, and reduced voluntary external anal sphincter squeeze pressure.[31] Patients do not generally volunteer a history of fecal incontinence, so the clinician must actively elicit a history of problems controlling the bowels. In patients with diarrhea and fecal incontinence, diarrhea should be assessed because treatment of diabetic diarrhea may reduce the severity of fecal incontinence. In addition, anorectal function may be evaluated by anorectal manometry, which quantitiates maximal basal sphincter pressure and the rectal anal inhibitory reflex. Continence for solids and liquids may be assessed by simulating the stress of stools with a solid sphere or rectally infused saline. Patients with intact rectal sensation and good motivation may benefit from biofeedback training.[31]

Genitourinary autonomic neuropathy

Genitourinary autonomic neuropathy can affect bladder function and sexual function. Afferent autonomic fibers transmit sensation of bladder fullness. Efferent parasympathetic fibers promote bladder contraction during urination. Efferent sympathetic fibers maintain sphincter tone. Parasympathetic function mediates erections and vaginal lubrication. The sympathetic nervous system mediates both orgasm and ejaculation.[49,50]

Diabetic bladder dysfunction generally occurs in association with distal symmetric sensorimotor polyneuropathy and, in males, with impotence. Symptoms of diabetic bladder dysfunction develop insidiously and progress slowly. Initially, there may be lengthened intervals between voiding and increased urinary volume. Later the urinary stream may become weak and prolonged. Evaluation for diabetic bladder dysfunction should be performed in any patient with diabetes with recurrent urinary tract infections, recurrent pyelonephritis, incontinence, or a palpable bladder. Evaluation should include assessment of renal function, urine culture, and measurement of a postvoiding residual. A postvoiding residual of greater than 150 ml is diagnostic of abnormal bladder function. It may be detected by postvoiding catheterization or a postvoiding sonogram. Postvoiding catheterization is invasive and may produce bacteriuria. Postvoiding sonograms can accurately and noninvasively evaluate the residual urine retained within the bladder.

The aim of treatment of diabetic bladder dysfunction is to improve bladder emptying and to reduce the risk of urinary tract infection. The patient with a grossly overdistended bladder should undergo an initial period of catheter drainage to improve bladder contractility. Care should be taken to avoid the introduction of infection, and, if infection exists, it should be treated. Thereafter, the person should be instructed to void by the clock rather than waiting for a conscious sensation of bladder distention. Pressure applied to the bladder (Credes maneuver) will often facilitate emptying. Cholinergic agents (Bethanechol) and intermittent self-catheterization may also be used to facilitate bladder emptying. Recurrent urinary tract infections may be treated with chronic suppressive antibiotic therapy.[49,50]

Sexual dysfunction in males

Sexual dysfunction is common in diabetic men and women. In men, sexual dysfunction most often involves changes in libido, erectile ability, and ejaculation. Change in libido may result from chronic illness in patients with multiple diabetic complications. Impotence, defined as impairment or loss of penile erection sufficient for vaginal intercourse, may occur as a result of genitourinary autonomic neuropathy but is a diagnosis of exclusion (see box on p. 174). The history should focus on use of ethanol and medications associated with impotence such as antihypertensive and antidepressant medications. A history of pelvic surgery, especially prostate surgery, should be elicited.

Penile blood flow should be assessed by auscultating for bruits over the abdominal aorta and measuring the penile blood pressure with a Doppler probe. To rule out androgen deficiency, libido, virilization, and testicular size and consistency should be assessed. Prolactin, LH, and testosterone levels should be measured. In impotence associated with diabetic autonomic neuropathy, there is usually a gradual progression from partial to complete erectile failure over about 2 years. Impotence is not partner specific and it is characterized by the absence of erections even during sleep. Impotence associated with diabetic autonomic neuropathy is often associated with diminished or absent testicular pain sensation to pressure, loss of perineal sensation (anal wink reflex and bulbocarvernosus reflex), and neurogenic bladder dysfunction.

Therapy for impotence may include use of a suction apparatus, yohimbine, prostheses, and injections. Suction devices apply vacuum to the penis, which draws blood into the penis and results in tumescence.[2] Yohimbine is an alpha-2 adrenergic blocker that increases vascular blood flow within the corpus of the penis and results in tumescence and rigidity. It is, however, associated with hypertension, and use of this medication requires close monitoring of blood pressure.[94,95]

There are several types of penile prostheses currently available. These include semirigid, malleable, inflatable, and self-contained devices. Each has advantages and disadvantages but each requires a surgical procedure of insertion. Injections of papaverine plus phentolamine into the corpus of the penis can also be used to produce tumescence. This method has, however, been associated with priapism.[122] Ejaculatory failure caused by autonomic neuropathy is important if fertility is desired. Retrograde ejaculation is an unusual complication that results from damage to the efferent sympathetic nerves that normally coordinate the simultaneous closure of the internal vesicle sphincter and relaxation of the external vesicle sphincter during ejaculation. Retrograde ejaculation may be diagnosed by the presence of oligospermia or azospermia and the finding of sperm in the postcoitally voided urine. If retrograde ejaculation is incomplete or of recent onset, the patient should be instructed to have intercourse with his bladder distended. Sometimes ejaculation can be restored with use of an antihistamine or desipramine.[6,13]

Sexual dysfunction in females

Sexual dysfunction in women has not been investigated as extensively as that in men. Diabetic women have been identified as having three basic sexual difficulties, including arousal, painful intercourse, and a nonorgasmic response. While it would seem unlikely that diabetes might affect orgasm in women, there is the possibility of related problems associated with lack of vasocongestion and clitoral engorgement. However, methodologies for assessing vaginal and clitoral circulation have not been developed substantially for the study of women with diabetes.[49,50]

Diabetic women have an increased likelihood of some dyspareunia from vaginal infections. Monilial infections are also common in these women. Therapy for female sexual dysfunction may include the use of over-the-counter lubricants or estrogen creams. Estrogen creams have the advantage of providing lubrication and thickening the vaginal mucosa, which may decrease dyspareunia.[49,50]

Hypoglycemia unawareness

The metabolic response to hypoglycemia is mediated largely by the autonomic nervous system. The acute counterregulatory response to hypoglycemia consists of an increase in the secretion of glucagon, epinephrine, growth hormone, and corticol and an increase in glucose production by the liver (see Chapter 8). Patients with defective hypoglycemia counterregulation may present with hypoglycemia unawareness. Patients with hypoglycemia unawareness do not have typical adrenergic warning signs such as anxiety, nervousness, sweating, and palpitation. Instead, when hypoglycemic, they develop symptoms of neuroglycopenia, including irritability, mental dullness, lethargy, confusion, amnesia, loss of consciousness, and/or seizures. Patients with hypoglycemia unawareness are at increased risk of severe life-threatening hypoglycemia, and patients with past histories of severe hypoglycemia are at increased risk for future occurrences.

Little is known about glucose counterregulation in NIDDM. In IDDM, the normal glucagon response to hypoglycemia deteriorates within approximately 5 years of the diagnosis of diabetes. The epinephrine response to hypoglycemia also declines with increasing duration of IDDM and in some patients is diminished or lost after 15 to 30 years. Absent glucagon and epinephrine responses to hypoglycemia greatly diminish glucose counterregulation and increase the risk for severe hypoglycemia.[49,50]

Hypoglycemia unawareness as a result of autonomic neuropathy is a diagnosis of exclusion (see box on p. 174). All persons who use oral hypoglycemic agents or insulin should understand the symptoms, signs, causes, and treatment of hypoglycemia (see Chapters 2 and 8). They should wear identification that identifies them as having diabetes and carry sugar or some other source of simple carbohydrate that can be used to promptly treat hypoglycemia. Patients with hypoglycemia unawareness should monitor their blood glucose levels at frequent intervals so that unexpected episodes of hypoglycemia can be recognized early and more severe hypoglycemia forestalled. Persons with hypoglycemia unawareness should have glucagon available, and family members and friends should know how and when to administer it. Adjustment of the goals of glycemic control should be considered for patients with hypoglycemia unawareness who have histories of severe hypoglycemia, and for those who do not understand the educational details of avoiding or treating hypoglycemia, or whose lifestyles make them vulnerable to life-threatening episodes of hypoglycemia.[55]

Clinical Manifestations and Diagnosis of Focal Neuropathies

A number of focal and multifocal neuropathies occur in association with diabetes mellitus.[104] The onset is typically acute and often heralded by pain. Most occur in middle-aged or older patients with NIDDM but seem to be correlated to the duration of control of diabetes. The neurophysiologic hallmark of focal neuropathy is the finding of abnormal nerve conduction in a distribution corresponding to the distribution of a single nerve, multiple peripheral nerves, the brachial or lumbosacral plexuses, or nerve roots. Focal neuropathies are often superimposed upon diffuse symmetric sensorimotor polyneuropathy. Needle electromyography is a sensitive indicator of axonal degeneration and is very useful to document the presence of superimposed focal neuropathies. It can also be used to examine muscles inaccessible or poorly accessible to nerve conduction studies, including paraspinal, abdominal, and proximal extremities muscles. The subjective interpretation of the results of needle electromyography also allows differentiation of acute, subacute, and chronic peripheral disorders.[49,50]

Cranial neuropathies

Third-nerve palsy, often termed "diabetic opthalmoplegia," is the most common cranial mononeuropathy. Headache, eye pain, or prickling dysesthesias on the upper lid may proceed a palsy by 1 or several days. Onset is usually abrupt. Ptosis is marked, the eye is deviated laterally by approximately 10 degrees, and the patient is unable to move the eye medially, up, or down. The pupil, however, is usually spared.

Progressive diminution of pain and return of oculomotor motor function is the rule, even in elderly patients. In general, findings persist for several weeks and then begin to improve gradually. Full resolution often takes 3 to 5 months. Differential diagnosis of isolated third-nerve palsy includes lesions of the midbrain, posterior circle of Willis, the cavernous sinus, the base of the brain, and the posterior orbit. Aneurysms and tumors must be considered (see box on p. 180). High-resolution CT scanning or MRI are usually sufficient to rule out other potential causes.[8]

Radiculopathy

Diabetic radiculopathy presents with dermatomal pain and loss of cutaneous sensation. Although usually singular and unilateral, the syndrome may involve multiple dermatomol levels and may be bilateral in some cases. It may be associated with significant weight loss. Most often the pain is localized to the chest (truncal neuropathy) but may also affect the abdominal wall. Truncal neuropathy generally has an abrupt onset over days or weeks. Pain or dysethesia are heralding features. It is unusual to have sudden worsening with cough, sneezing, straining, or physical activity, but pain is almost universally worse at night. Since the clinical picture is that of pain, the issue of cardiopulmonary disease and visceral malignancy are usually raised. The condition also resembles herpes zoster infection in the prevesicular phase. On examination, there may be hypesthesia to pinprick in the segments of greatest pain. The differential diagnosis of radiculopathy includes compressive lesions such as disc disease and cardiopulmonary and gastrointestinal disease, including pneumonia, pleurisy, myocardial infarction, cholecystitis, peptic ulcer disease, or appendicitis (see box on p. 180). Not uncommonly, multiple diagnostic procedures and even exploratory surgeries are performed before the correct diagnosis is made. Prognosis for recovery is generally good. Spontaneous resolution of both symptoms and signs is the rule, usually within 6 to 24 months.[8,49,50]

——————— **DIFFERENTIAL DIAGNOSIS OF FOCAL NEUROPATHY** ———————

Cranial neuropathy

Increased intracranial pressure
Intracranial mass
Carotid aneurysm

Radiculopathy

Cardiopulmonary disease
Visceral malignancy
Acute abdomen
Degenerative spinal disc disease
Pagets disease

Plexopathy

Degenerative spinal disc disease
Pagets disease of the spine
Intrinsic spinal cord mass lesion
Cauda equina lesions
Coagulopathies

Mononeuropathy multiplex and mononeuropathy

Vasculidities
Amyloidosis
Hypothyroidism
Acromegaly
Coagulopathies

Plexopathy

In diabetes, the most commonly encountered plexopathy is that involving the lumbosacral plexus. The condition is relatively uncommon and of sudden onset. Patients are generally in older age groups. The condition, also termed *femoral neuropathy,* often involves motor and sensory deficits at the level of the sacral plexus as well as the femoral nerve. The relative excess of motor involvement differentiates diabetic femoral neuropathy from that seen in other conditions. The pain may develop insidiously or episodically and may be worse at night. Pain and sensory impairment occur in the anterior thigh and medial calf. This is associated with disabling weakness of thigh flexion and knee extension. The plantar response may be extensor, and areflexia is present. In general, pain is not present on straight leg raising, thus distinguishing diabetic femoral neuropathy from sciatica. Nevertheless, because of the similarities between diabetic femoral neuropathy and other conditions, diabetic femoral neuropathy remains a diagnosis of exclusion. Differential diagnosis includes space-occupying lesions, trauma, retroperitoneal hemorrhage, and nondiabetic vasculopathies (see box on p. 180). Nearly complete recovery is the rule, though not universal, and the syndrome may persist for several years or recur.[49,50]

Mononeuropathy and mononeuropathy multiplex

Isolated peripheral neuropathies are more common in diabetes. It appears that diffuse diabetic neuropathy predisposes to focal nerve damage. This hypothesis is supported by the finding that 40% of unselected patients with clinically overt diffuse diabetic neuropathy have electrophysiologic or clinical evidence of superimposed focal nerve damage at common entrapment or compression sites. There is also evidence that the risk of developing carpal tunnel syndrome is more than doubled in diabetic patients. Nerves not commonly exposed to compression or entrapment occasionally demonstrate focal impairment in patients with diabetes. This may simply reflect coincidental occurrence of diabetes and mononeuropathy.[49,50]

The most common mononeuropathies associated with diabetes include those of the median nerve at the wrist (carpal tunnel syndrome associated with the pain and weakness in the hand), the ulnar nerve at the elbow (associated with weakness and loss of sensation over the palmar aspect of the fourth and fifth fingers), the radial nerve in the upper arm (associated with weakness of the upper arm, wrist drop, and loss of sensation on the back of the hand), the lateral cutaneous nerve of the thigh in the inguinal region (associated with pain in the thigh), and the peroneal nerve at the fibular head (associated with foot drop). Diagnosis of mononeuropathy or mononeuropathy multiplex should be confirmed by electrodiagnostic studies. Other nondiabetic causes should be excluded including hypothyroidism, vasculitis, and coagulopathy (see box on p. 180).[49,50]

Treatment of focal neuropathies

Diabetic cranial neuropathies, radiculopathies, and plexopathies generally resolve spontaneously. Reassurance often makes the pain more tolerable. If diabetic ophthalmoplegia causes diplopia, patching of the affected eye may help. Simple analgesics, antidepressants, and anticonvulsant medications can be used on a short-term basis for pain management. Physiotherapy is important to preserve range of motion and to prevent contractures for patients with femoral neuropathy. Compression and entrapment palsies in diabetic patients respond to standard conservative or surgical management. Treatment of other mononeuropathies is essentially supportive. For example, patients with peroneal neuropathy should be fitted with ankle braces. Because diffuse diabetic neuropathy predisposes to focal nerve damage, protection against additional mechanical trauma is important.[49,50] For example, patients with carpal tunnel syndrome should wear neutral wrist splints, and patients with ulnar neuropathy should avoid applying pressure to their elbows and/or wear elbow pads.

General principles of preventive education

Were it not for a set of secondary complicating disorders, diabetic distal symmetric sensorimotor polyneuropathy would often be nothing more than an incidental finding on

---

——————————— NEUROPATHY: EDUCATION PRINCIPLES ———————————

Inform persons with diabetes about the possible relationship between poor glycemic control and the subsequent development of diabetic neuropathy.

Explain possible risk factors (such as smoking, alcohol) and concomitant neural insults that may hasten the development or progression of diabetic neuropathy.

Stress that sensory or motor neuropathy may be asymptomatic.

Explain that routine evaluation is necessary even for patients who have no symptoms of neuropathy.

Explain that diabetic neuropathy can contribute to the development of other complications.

Inform patients who have lost sensation in their feet about the importance of caring for their feet and wearing proper shoes.

Stress the importance of proper exercise.

Discuss the signs and symptoms of autonomic neuropathy.

Explain the benefits of treatment to patients with autonomic neuropathy.

Adapted from Herman WH, ed: The prevention and treatment of complications of diabetes mellitus: a guide for primary care practitioners, 1991, Atlanta, Dept of Health and Human Services, Public Health Services, Centers for Disease Control, Center for Chronic Disease Prevention and Health Promotions.

clinical examination. There are, however, a number of extremely serious consequences of sensory and/or motor denervation, many of which can be prevented through good self care. For this reason, prophylaxis must be a major goal of diabetes patient education,[49,50] the principles of which are noted in the box above.

Foot ulcers are a major complication of diabetic distal symmetric sensorimotor polyneuropathy (see Chapter 7). Diabetic foot ulcers arise as a result of traumatic damage to the skin and soft tissues of the feet. Insensitivity to pain is critical in the development of diabetic foot ulcers. Diminished proprioception and muscle strength, decreased sweating, and vascular factors also contribute.[49,50] In patients with distal symmetric sensorimotor polyneuropathy, neurogenic atrophy of the intrinsic muscles of the feet results in chronic flexion of the metatarsal-phalangeal joints, thereby drawing the toes into a cocked-up position. Autonomic dysfunction and distal anhydrosis result in decreased foot lubrication. Weight bearing is thus shifted to the metatarsal heads, and, in the absence of pain, thick callouses form over the bony prominences. With repeated trauma, the dry skin over these abnormal pressure points breaks down, and the resulting ulcers may go unnoticed even when secondary infection develops.[49,50]

A second complication associated with distal symmetric sensorimotor polyneuropathy is neuroarthropathy, also called Charcot's joint. Neuroarthropathy occurs in any condition in which sensation is impaired but motor function is left relatively intact. Diabetic neuroarthropathy primarily involves the ankle, metatarsal, or metatarsal-phalangeal joints. Patients with neuroarthropathy often present with painless swelling and redness of the foot in the absence of fever or leukocytosis. Large-fiber neuropathy is almost universally present. Pedal pulses are generally intact and often quite strong. Unhealed fractures are often evident radiographically. In later stages, patients may present with gross architectural distortion of the foot, and in the most advanced stages there are multiple fractures accompanied by extensive bone demineralization and reabsorption. The pathogenetic mechanism is presumed to be multiple recurrent traumatic insults of the joint that are not noticed by the patient because of insensitivity to pain (see Chapter 7).[49,50]

Patient education

Persons with insensitive feet may not be aware of foot problems. Therefore, at each visit, the health care provider should inquire for symptoms of peripheral neuropathy, and the shoes and socks must be removed at every visit—at least four times a year—and the feet inspected for dryness, calluses, deformities, ulcers, and evidence of neuroarthropathy. At least once a year, the health care provider should assess the patient's ability to sense temperature, pinprick, pressure, touch, and vibration and should test muscle strength and deep-tendon reflexes.[55]

Persons with diabetes with evidence of distal symmetric sensorimotor polyneuropathy must learn foot hygiene and how to protect the feet. Patients who spend a lot of time on their feet or who do a great deal of walking and those who jog for exercise may need to change their activity. Patients with deformed feet almost always require specially molded, extra-depth shoes. Deformed feet will not fit into ordinary shoes, although the patient, because of loss of sensation, may think they fit. The wearing of ordinary shoes on deformed feet may result in abrasions, ulcerations, and infection, which can lead to gangrene and amputation.[55]

When patients present with foot ulcers, the ulcers should be vigorously debrided to establish the depth. Radiographs should be used to exclude the possibility of embedded foreign objects or osteomyelitis. If osteomyelitis is suspected, follow-up radiographs and appropriate scans should be used to help establish the diagnosis. Where there is significant infection, parenteral antibiotics should be used. Since anaerobes frequently occur in the foot ulcers of diabetic patients, aerobic and anaerobic bacterial cultures should be obtained to help select appropriate antibiotics.[55]

Patients with foot ulcers should not put weight on the affected foot. Those who do not feel pain will likely continue to walk, and the resulting pressure on the foot will prevent healing. Total bedrest or the use of crutches may be required. Total-contact casts have been shown to help patients with foot ulcers ambulate while ulcers heal. The casts redistribute pressure so that the area of the ulcer bears much less weight than it would otherwise.[55]

Prophylactic measures to prevent neuroarthropathy include avoiding prolonged weight bearing, avoiding strenuous weight-bearing exercise or athletic activities, ambulating only over well-lighted, smooth terrain, and wearing cushioned shoes. Therapy is directed at removal of continued trauma by removing the involved extremity from weight bearing, either by decreasing ambulation or providing other means of weight bearing. The use of a bivalved ankle/foot orthosis and the use of a cane, crutches, or wheelchair is often necessary.[49,50]

All diabetic patients should be informed about the possible relationship between poor glycemic control and diabetic neuropathy and the role of diabetic neuropathy in the development of other complications, including foot ulcers and amputation. Patients should also be informed of the importance of routine clinical evaluations for diabetic neuropathy, even when they have no symptoms. Individuals with distal symmetric sensorimotor polyneuropathy should understand that other factors such as consumption of ethanol and exposure to chemical toxins may hasten the progression of neuropathy. Persons with insensitive feet should also understand the importance of caring for their feet, wearing proper shoes, and getting appropriate exercise. They should also be aware of the possible signs and symptoms of autonomic neuropathy and understand the availability and benefits of treatment for autonomic neuropathy.[55]

PERIODONTAL DISEASE

Periodontal diseases progresses more rapidly in persons with uncontrolled diabetes, but occurs with equivalent incidence in persons with controlled diabetes or without diabetes.[126] Periodontal diseases fall into two major classifications: (1) gingivitis, an inflammation of the gum tissues, caused by aerobic gram-positive bacteria, and (2) periodontitis, inflammatory parts found in gingivitis, which reaches the bone and causes further bone destruction. Saadoun[111] found, following an extensive review of the literature, that periodontal diseases are more severe in those with uncontrolled diabetes than in those persons without diabetes. However, persons with well-controlled diabetes have the same incidence of periodontal disease as does the general population. In addition, persons with diabetes who have periodontitis fare worse than those persons without diabetes. The reason for this seems to be related to the same microangiopathic process and changes that occur in the retina, kidney, and muscle vessels found in the tissues. In addition, several studies report that persons who have retinopathy exhibit more severe periodontal lesions than those who do not.[126]

All persons with diabetes should be counseled as to possible periodontal problems, with prevention a major focus of counseling. Careful review of oral care guidelines, reinforcement of proper daily oral hygiene practices, and frequent follow-up is important to patient education.[55] The person with diabetes should be instructed to inform his or her dentist of the diabetes and to provide the dentist with the diabetes health care provider's name and telephone number. The importance of scheduling dental appointments that do not interfere with the patient's insulin and meal schedule (the best time for an appointment may be a few hours after breakfast) and maintenance of good control of blood glucose levels should be encouraged. In addition, persons with diabetes should be instructed on proper oral care guidelines, including (1) brushing their teeth with a soft toothbrush and a fluoridated toothpaste at least twice a day, especially before going to sleep, and using dental floss as recommended; (2) rinsing their toothbrush thoroughly and replacing it at least every 3 months; (3) emphasizing the importance of seeking regular preventive dental care at least every 6 months (or according to the dentist's recommended schedule); and (4) seeing a dentist if they have bad breath, an unpleasant taste in the mouth, bleeding gums, sore gums or teeth, or red or swollen gums. Once periodontal disease is diagnosed, active therapy involves removal of bacteria via simple cleaning or, in later stages, more extensive procedures, including surgical intervention.

The prevalence of microvascular complications in diabetes makes the role of preventive education critical. The health care provider needs to carefully and regularly assess patient status with regard to the occurrence of complications and take care to provide frequent and regular patient and family education with regard to preventive or ongoing care. In order to ensure such systematic and quality care, all members of the health care team need to carefully work with the person with diabetes and his or her family to ensure principles of education and preventive guidelines of care are followed. The emphasis on education, leading to routine preventive follow-up care, is critical to assist the person with diabetes in achieving his or her optimal level of well-being.

REFERENCES

1. Abram DR: Decreased alpha-2 adrenergic receptors on platelet membranes from diabetic patients with autonomic neuropathy and orthostatic hypotension, J Clin Endocrin Metab 63:906-912, 1986.
2. Al-Juburi AZ and O'Donnell PD: Synergist erection system: clinical experience, Urology 35:304-306, 1990.
3. American Diabetes Association: Nutritional recommendations and principles for individuals with diabetes mellitus: 1986, Diabetes Care 10:126-132, 1987.
4. American Diabetes Association: Consensus statement—diabetic neuropathy, Diabetes Care 13(suppl 1):47-52, 1990.
5. Amico JA and Klein I: Diabetic management in patients with renal failure, Diabetes Care 4:430-434, 1991.
6. Andaloro VA, Jr and Dube A: Treatment of retrograde ejaculation with brompheniramine, Urology 5:520-522, 1975.
7. Andersen AR and others: Diabetic nephropathy in type I (insulin-dependent) diabetes: an epidemiologic study, Diabetologia 25:496-501, 1983.
8. Asbury AK: Focal and multifocal neuropathies of diabetes. In Dyck PJ and others, eds: Diabetic neuropathy, Philadelphia, 1987, WB Saunders Co.
9. Ballard DJ and others: Epidemiology of persistent proteinuria in type II diabetes mellitus: population-based study in Rochester, Minnesota, Diabetes 37:405-412, 1988.
10. Barbosa J: Is diabetic microangiopathy genetically heterogeneous? HLA and diabetic nephropathy, Hormone Metab Res 11:77-80, 1981.
11. Boesen F and others: Treatment of diabetic orthostatic hypotension with pindolol, Acta Neurol Scan 66:386-91, 1982.
12. Boulton AJ, Levin S, and Comstock J: A multicentre trial of the aldose-reductase inhibitor, tolrestat, in patients with symptomatic diabetic neuropathy, Diabetologia 33:431-437, 1990.
13. Brooks ME, Berezin M, and Braf Z: Treatment of retrograde ejaculation with imipramine, Urology 15:353-355, 1980.
14. Burns-Cox CJ and Hart JC: Screening of diabetics for retinopathy by ophthalmic opticians, Br Med J 290:1052-1054, 1985.
15. Campbell IW, Ewing DJ, and Clarke BF: A-alpha-fluorohydrocortisone in the treatment of postural hypotension in diabetic autonomic neuropathy, Diabetes 24:381-384, 1975.
16. Campbell RK and Baker DE: New drug update: capsaicin, Diabetes Educ 16:313-316, 1990.
17. Carr S and others: Increase in glomerular filtration rate in patients with insulin-dependent diabetes and elevated erythrocyte sodium-lithium countertransport, N Engl J Med 322:500-505, 1990.
18. Chakrabarti AK and Samantaray SK: Diabetic peripheral neuropathy: nerve conduction studies before, during, and after carbamazepine therapy, Aust NZ Med 6:565-568, 1976.
19. Champion MC: Management of idiopathic, diabetic, and miscellaneous gastroparesis with cisapride, Scand J Gastrointerol 165(suppl):44-52, 1989.
20. Christensen CK and Mogensen CE: Effect of antihypertensive treatment on progression of disease in incipient diabetic nephropathy, Hypertension 7:109-114, 1985.

21. Christensen CK and Mogensen CE: Antihypertensive treatment: long-term reversal of progression of albuminuria in incipient diabetic nephropathy. A longitudinal study of renal function, J Diab Complic 1:45-52, 1987.

22. Cohen KL and Harris S: Efficacy and safety of nonsteroidal anti-inflammatory drugs in the therapy of diabetic neuropathy, Arch Int Med 147:1442-1444, 1987.

23. Collins AJ and others: Changing risk factors demographics in end-stage renal disease patients entering hemodialysis and the impact on long-term mortality, Am J Kidney Dis 25:422-432, 1990.

24. Condon JR and others: Cholestyramine and diabetic and post-vagotomy diarrhoea, Br Med J 4:423, 1973.

25. Constable IJ and others: Assessing the risk of diabetic retinopathy, Am J Ophthalmol 97:53-61, 1984.

26. Cowie CC and others: Disparities in incidence of diabetic end-stage renal disease according to race and type of diabetes, New Engl J Med 321:1074-1079, 1989.

27. Dahl-Jorgensen K and others: Effect of near normoglycemia for two years on progression of early diabetic retinopathy, nephropathy, and neuropathy: the Oslo study, Br Med J 293:1195-1199, 1986.

28. Damsgaard EM and Mogensen CE: Microalbuminuria in elderly hyperglycaemic patients and controls, Diabetic Med 3:430-435, 1986.

29. Dejgard A, Petersen P, and Kastrup J: Mexiletine for treatment of chronic painful diabetic neuropathy, Lancet 1:9-11, 1988.

30. Demarie BK and Bakris GL: Effects of different calcium antagonists on proteinuria associated with diabetes mellitus, Ann Int Med 113:987-988, 1990.

31. DePonti F, Fealey RD, and Malagelada JR: Gastrointestinal syndromes due to diabetes mellitus. In Dyck PJ and others, eds: Diabetic neuropathy Philadelphia, 1987, WB Saunders Co.

32. Diabetic Retinopathy Study Research Group: Photocoagulation treatment of proliferative diabetic retinopathy: clinical application of Diabetic Retinopathy Study (DRS) findings, DRS Report Number 8, Ophthalmology 88:583-600, 1981.

33. Diabetic Retinopathy Vitrectomy Study Research Group: Early vitrectomy for severe vitreous hemorrhage in diabetic retinopathy: two-year results of a randomized trial, Diabetic Retinopathy Vitrectomy Study Report 2, Arch Ophthalmol 103:1644-1652, 1985.

34. Diabetic Retinopathy Vitrectomy Study Research Group: Early vitrectomy for severe proliferative diabetic retinopathy in eyes with useful vision, Diabetic Retinopathy Vitrectomy Study Report 3, Ophthalmology 95:1307-1320, 1988.

35. Division of Diabetes Translation: Diabetes surveillance, 1980-1987, Atlanta, 1990, US Department of Health and Human Services, Public Health Service, Centers for Disease Control.

36. Dyck PJ and others: Diabetic neuropathy, Philadelphia, 1987, WB Saunders Co.

37. Early Treatment Diabetic Retinopathy Study Research Group: Photocoagulation for diabetic macular edema: Early Treatment Diabetic Retinopathy Study Report Number 1, Arch Ophthalmol 103:1796-1806, 1985.

38. Egbunike IG and Chaffee BJ: Antidepressants in the management of chronic pain syndromes, Pharmacotherapy 10:262-270, 1990.

39. Evanoff G and others: Prolonged dietary protein restriction in diabetic nephropathy, Arch Intern Med 149:1129-1133, 1989.

40. Ewing DJ and Clarke BF: Diabetic autonomic neuropathy: A clinical viewpoint. In Dyck PJ and others, eds: Diabetic neuropathy, Philadelphia, 1987, WB Saunders Co.

41. Fabre J and others: The kidney in maturity onset diabetes mellitus: a clinical study of 510 patients, Kidney Int 21:730-738, 1982.

42. Fedorak RN, Filed M, and Chang BB: Treatment of diabetic diarrhea with clonidine, Ann Intern Med 102:197-199, 1985.

43. Feldman M and Schiller LR: Disorders of gastrointestinal motility associated with diabetes mellitus, Ann Intern Med 98:378-384, 1983.

44. Feldt-Rasmussen B, Mathiesen ER, and Deckert T: Effect on the progression of diabetic renal disease during two years of strict metabolic control in insulin-dependent diabetes, Lancet 2:1300-1304, 1986.

45. Gentry P and Miller PF: Nutritional considerations in a patient with gastroparesis, Diabetes Educ 15:374-376, 1989.

46. Gills JS and others: Effect of the aldose reductase inhibitor, ponalrestat, on diabetic neuropathy, Diabetes Metab 16:296-302, 1990.

47. Gomez-Perez FJ and others: Nortriptyline and fluphenazine in the symptomatic treatment of diabetic neuropathy. A double-blind cross-over study, Pain 23:395-400, 1985.

48. Green PA, Berge KG, and Sprague RG: Control of diabetic diarrhea with antibiotic therapy, Diabetes 17:385-387, 1968.

49. Greene DA, and others: Diabetic neuropathy. In Rifkin H and Porte D, Jr, eds: Ellenberg and Rifkin's diabetes mellitus, theory and practice, ed 4, New York, 1990, Elsevier Publishing Co.

50. Greene DA and others: Diabetic neuropathy. In Rifkin H and Porte D, Jr, eds: Ellenberg and Rifkin's diabetes mellitus, theory and practice, ed 4, New York, 1990, Elsevier Publishing Co.

51. Harkonen S and Kjellstrand CM: Exacerbation of diabetic renal failure following intravenous pyelography, Am J Med 63:936-946, 1977.

52. Held PJ, and others: Five-year survival for end-stage renal disease patients in the United States, Europe, and Japan, 1982-87, Am J Kidney Dis XV:451-457, 1990.

53. Herman WH and others: An approach to the prevention of blindness in diabetes, Diabetes Care 6:608-613, 1983.

54. Herman WH and others: Consensus statement. Proceedings from the International Symposium on Preventing the Kidney Disease of Diabetes Mellitus: public health perspectives, Am J Kidney Dis 13:2-6, 1989.

55. Herman WH, editor: The prevention and treatment of complications of diabetes mellitus: a guide for primary care practitioners, Atlanta, 1991, Department of Health and Human Services, Public Health Service, Centers for Disease Control, Center for Chronic Disease Prevention and Health Promotion.

56. Hoeldtke RD, Boden G, and O'Dorisio TM: Treatment of postural hypotension with a somatostatin analogue (SMS 201-995), Am J Med 81(suppl 6B):83-87, 1986.

57. Hostetter TH, Rennke HG, and Brenner BM: The case for intrarenal hypertension in the initiation and progression of diabetic and other glomerulopathies, Am J Med 72:375-380, 1982.

58. Humphrey LL and others: Chronic renal failure in non–insulin-dependent diabetes mellitus: a population based study in Rochester, Minnesota, Ann Intern Med 111:788-796, 1989.

59. Janka HU and others: Risk factors for progression of background retinopathy in long-standing IDDM, Diabetes 38:460-464, 1989.

60. Janssens J and others: Improvement of gastric emptying in diabetic gastroparesis by erythromycin: preliminary studies, N Engl J Med 332:1028-1031, 1990.

61. Jarrett RJ and others: Microalbuminuria predicts mortality in non-insulin-dependent diabetes, Diabetes Med 1:17-19, 1984.

62. Jones SL and others: Sodium-lithium countertransport in microalbuminuric insulin-dependent diabetic patients, Hypertension 15:570-575, 1990.

63. Klein R and others: The Wisconsin Epidemiologic Study of Diabetic Retinopathy. II. Prevalence and risk of diabetic retinopathy when age at diagnosis is less than 30 years, Arch Ophthalmol 102:520-526, 1984.

64. Klein R and others: The Wisconsin Epidemiologic Study of Diabetic Retinopathy. III. Prevalence and risk of diabetic retinopathy when age at diagnosis is 30 or more years, Arch Ophthalmol 102:527-532, 1984.

65. Klein R and others: The Wisconsin Epidemiologic Study of Diabetic Retinopathy. IV. Diabetic macular edema, Ophthalmology 91:1464-1474, 1984.

66. Klein R and others: Visual impairment in diabetes, Ophthalmology 91:1-9, 1984.

67. Klein R and others: Diabetic retinopathy as detected using ophthalmoscopy, a nonmydriatic camera and a standard fundus camera, Ophthalmology 92:485-491, 1985.

68. Klein R, Moss SE, and Klein BEK: New management concepts for timely diagnosis of diabetic retinopathy treatable by photocoagulation, Diabetes Care 10:633-638, 1987.

69. Klein R and others: Proteinuria in diabetes, Arch Intern Med 148:181-186, 1988.

70. Klein R and others: The Wisconsin Epidemiologic Study of Diabetic Retinopathy. IX. Four-year incidence and progression of diabetic retinopathy when age at diagnosis is less than 30 years, Arch Ophthalmol 107:237-234, 1989.

71. Klein R and others: The Wisconsin Epidemiologic Study of Diabetic Retinopathy. X. Four-year incidence and progression of diabetic retinopathy when ae at diagnosis is 30 years or more, Arch Ophthalmol 107:244-249, 1989.

72. Klein R and others: The Wisconsin Epidemiologic Study of Diabetic Retinopathy. XI. The incidence of macular edema, Ophthalmology 96:1501-1510, 1989.

73. Klein BEK, Moss SE, and Klein R: Effect of pregnancy on progression of diabetic retinopathy, Diabetes Care 13:34-40, 1990.

74. Kleinstein RN and others: Detection of diabetic retinopathy by optometrists, J Am Optom Assoc 58:879-882, 1987.

75. Knowler WC, Bennett PH, and Ballintine EJ: Increased incidence of retinopathy in diabetics with elevated blood pressure, N Engl J Med 302:645-650, 1980.

76. Knowles HC: Magnitude of the renal failure problem in diabetic patients, Kidney Int 1:(suppl)2-7, 1974.

77. The Kroc Collaborative Study Group: Blood glucose control and the evolution of diabetic retinopathy and albuminuria. A preliminary multicenter trial, N Engl J Med 311:365-372, 1984.

78. Krolewski AS and others: Predisposition to hypertension and susceptibility to renal disease in insulin-dependent diabetes mellitus, New Engl J Med 318:140-145, 1988.

79. Kuchel O and others: Treatment of severe orthostatic hypotension by metoclopramide, Ann Intern Med 93:841-843, 1980.

80. Kunzelman CL and others: Incidence of proteinuria in type 2 diabetes mellitus in Pima Indians, Kidney Int 35:681-687, 1989.

81. Kvinesdal B and others: Imipramine in treatment of painful diabetic neuropathy, JAMA 251:1727-1730, 1984.

82. Levy DM, Abraham RR, and Tomlinson DR: Topical capsaicin in the treatment of painful diabetic neuropathy, N Engl J Med, 324:776-777, 1991.

83. Mangili R and others: Increased sodium-lithium countertransport activity in red cells of patients with insulin-dependent diabetes and nephropathy, N Engl J Med 318:146-150, 1988.

84. Max MD and others: Amitriptyline relieves diabetic neuropathy pain in patients with normal and depressed mood, Neurology 37:589-596, 1987.

85. McCallum RW and others: A multicenter placebo-controlled clinical trial of oral metaclopramide in diabetic gastroparesis, Diabetes Care 6:463-467, 1983.

86. Melton LJ, III and Dyck PJ: Epidemiology. In Dyck PJ and others, eds: Diabetic neuropathy, Philadelphia, 1987, WB Saunders Co.

87. Mogenesen CE: Long-term antihypertensive treatment inhibiting progression of diabetic nephropathy, Br Med J 285:685-688, 1982.

88. Mogensen CE: Complete screening of urinary albumin concentration in an unselected diabetic outpatient clinic population, Diabet Nephropathy 2:11-18, 1983.

89. Mogensen CE, Christensen CK, and Vittinghus E: The stages in diabetic renal disease: with emphasis on the stage of incipient diabetic nephropathy. Diabetes 32(suppl):64-78, 1983.

90. Mogensen CE: Microalbuminuria predicts clinical proteinuria and early mortality in maturity-onset diabetes, N Engl J Med 310:356-360, 1984.

91. Mogensen CE and Christensen CK: Predicting diabetic nephropathy in insulin-dependent patients, N Engl J Med 311:89-93, 1984.

92. Mogensen CE: Microalbuminuria as a predictor of clinical diabetic nephropathy, Kidney Int 31:673-689, 1987.

93. Mogensen CE, Schmitz A, and Christensen CK: Comparative renal pathophysiology relevant to IDDM and NIDDM patients, Diabetes Metab Rev 4:453-483, 1988.

94. Morales A, Surridge DH, Marshall PG: Yohimbine for treatment of impotence in diabetes, N Engl J Med 305:1221, 1981.

95. Morales A and others: Is yohimbine effective in the treatment of organic impotence? Results of a controlled trial, J Urol 137:1168-1172, 1987.

96. Moss SE and others: Comparison between ophthalmoscopy and fudus photography in determining severity of diabetic retinopathy, Ophthalmology 1985; 92:62-67, 1985.

97. Nelson RG and others: Incidence of end-stage renal disease in type 2 (non–insulin-dependent) diabetes mellitus in Pima Indians, Diabetologia 31:730-736, 1988.

98. Nelson RG and others: Effect of proteinuria on mortality in NIDDM, Diabetes 37:1499-1504, 1988.

99. Nelson RG and others: Proliferative retinopathy in NIDDM: incidence and risk factors in Pima Indians, Diabetes 38:435-440, 1989.

100. O'Hare JP and others: Aldose reductase inhibitor in diabetic neuropathy: clinical and neurophysiological studies of one year's treatment with sorbinil, Diabetic Med 5:537-542, 1988.

101. Palumbo PJ, Elveback LR, and Whisnant JP: Neurologic complications of diabetes mellitus: transient ischemic attack, stroke, and peripheral neuropathy, Adv Neurol 19:593-601, 1978.

102. Parfrey PS and others: Contrast material induced renal failure in patients with diabetes mellitus, renal insufficiency, or both, N Engl J Med 320:143-149, 1989.

103. Parving HH and others: Early aggressive antihypertension treatment reduces rate of decline in kidney function in diabetic nephropathy, Lancet 1:1175-1179, 1983.

104. Pfeifer MA and Greene DA: Diabetic neuropathy current concepts, Kalamazoo, MI, 1985, The Upjohn Co.

105. Pitkanen E and others: HLA antigen distribution in juvenile diabetics with end-stage nephropathy, Am Clin Res 13:91-95, 1981.

106. Pirart J: Diabetes mellitus and its degenerative complications: a prospective study of 4,400 patients observed between 1947 and 1973, Diabetes Care 1:168-188, 1978.

107. Rabinowe SL and others: Complement-fixing antibodies to sympathetic and parasympathetic tissues in IDDM: autonomic brake index and heart-rate variation, Diabetes Care 13:1084-1088, 1990.

108. Recommended Dietary Allowances, ed 10, Washington, DC, 1989, National Research Council, National Academy Press.

109. Rettig B and Teutsch SM: The incidence of end-stage renal disease in type I and type II diabetes mellitus, Diabetic Nephropathy 3:26-27, 1984.

110. Ross DR and Varipapa RJ: Treatment of painful diabetic neuropathy with capsaicin, N Engl J Med 321:474-475, 1989.

111. Saadoun AP: Diabetes and periodontal disease: a review and update, Periodontal Abst, 28:116-139, 1980.

112. Salway JG and others: Effect of myo-inositol on peripheral-nerve function in diabetes, Lancet 2:1282-1284, 1978.

113. Saudek CD, Werns S, and Reidenberg MM: Phenytoin in the treatment of diabetic symmetrical polyneuropathy, Clin Pharmacol Ther 22:196-199, 1977.

114. Schmitz A, Gundersen HJG, and Østerby R: Glomerular morphology by light microscopy in non-insulin-dependent diabetes mellitus: lack of glomerular hypertrophy, Diabetes 37:38-43, 1988.

115. Seaquist ER and others: Familial clustering of diabetic kidney disease: evidence for genetic susceptibility to diabetic nephropathy, N Engl J Med 320:1161-1166, 1989.

116. Service FJ and others: Near normoglycemia: improved nerve conduction and vibration sensation in diabetic neuropathy, Diabetologia 28:722-727, 1985.

117. Stross JK and Harlan WR: The dissemination of new medical information, JAMA 1979; 241:2622-2624, 1979.

118. Sussman EJ, Tsiaras WG, and Soper KA: Diagnosis of diabetic eye disease, JAMA 247:3231-3234, 1982.

119. Swerdlow M: Anticonvulsant drugs and chronic pain, Clin Neuropharmacol 7:51-82, 1984.

120. Thomas PK and Brown MJ: Diabetic polyneuropathy. In Dyck PJ and others, eds: Diabetic neuropathy, Philadelphia, 1987, WB Saunders Co.

121. Vinik AI and others: Somatostatin analogue (SMS 201-995) in the management of gastroenteropancreatic tumors and diarrhea syndromes, Am J Med[], 81:23-29, 1986.

122. Virag R and others: Intracavernous self-injection of vasoactive drugs in the treatment of impotence: 8-year experience with 615 cases, J Urol 145:287-292, 1991.

123. Vlassara H, Brownlee M, and Cerami A: Nonezymatic glycosylation peripheral nerve protein in diabetes mellitus, Proc Natl Acad Sci 78:5190-5192, 1981.

124. Watts GF and others: Treatment of diabetic gastroparesis with oral domperidone, Diabetic Med 2:491-492, 1985.

125. Weinrauch LA and others: Coronary angiography and acute renal failure in diabetic azotemic nephropathy, Ann Intern Med 86:56-59, 1977.

126. Wilson J: Periodontal diseases and diabetes, Diabetes Educ 15:342-345, 1989.

127. Witkin SR and Klein R: Ophthalmologic care for persons with diabetes, JAMA 251:2534-2537, 1984.

128. Yassine MD: Diabetic nephropathy in noninsulin dependent diabetes mellitus: natural history and risk factors, PhD dissertation (Epidemiologic Science), 1990, University of Michigan.

129. Young RJ and Clarke BF: Pain relief in diabetic neuropathy: the effectivenss of imipramine and related drugs, Diabetic Med 2:363-366, 1985.

130. Zeller K and others: Effect of restricting dietary protein on the progression of renal failure in patients with insulin-dependent diabetes mellitus, N Engl J Med 324:78-84, 1991.

CHAPTER 6

Features of Macrovascular Disease of Diabetes

FRANK VINICOR

While the availability of insulin since 1922 has resulted in a decrease in death as a result of acute complications such as diabetes ketoacidosis,[16] diabetes mellitus has not been cured. Thus patients with diabetes and their health care providers today face chronic complications associated with this disorder. It is traditional to consider these chronic conditions as microvascular disorders, such as retinopathy, nephropathy, or metabolic and macrovascular disorders, such as coronary artery disease (CAD).[30] Chapter 5 focused on microvascular disorders related to diabetes. The purpose of this chapter is to discuss the importance of diabetes-associated macrovascular disease; describe why macrovascular disease is so common in persons with diabetes; address the best clinical as well as public health strategies for reducing problems associated with macrovascular disease in diabetes; and finally, discuss future therapeutic options for macrovascular disease in diabetes.

THE IMPACT OF MACROVASCULAR DISEASE
Definition

Macrovascular disease means disorders of large vessels with resultant morbidity and mortality. Pathologically, macrovascular disease in diabetes mellitus reflects atherosclerosis, the deposit of material (e.g., lipids) within the inner layer—the intima—of vessel walls, discussed later in this chapter.

Macrovascular disease underlies abnormalities in coronary, cerebral, and larger peripheral arterial vessels. Clinically, these abnormalities manifest themselves in heart disease (e.g., strokes) and vascular symptoms such as intermittent claudication. While at a cellular level there may be important pathophysiologic commonalities between microvascular and macrovascular disease, macrovascular disorders create a varied picture of a person with diabetes who exhibits exertion-associated chest pain, episodic symptoms of diz-

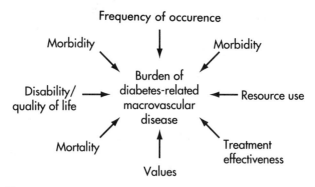

Fig. 6-1 The burden of diabetes-related macrovascular disease.

ziness and slurred speech, caused by transient ischemic attacks or exercise-related calf cramps (i.e., claudication).

This symptomatology can occur separately or concomitantly. Thus the quality and quantity of life of the person with diabetes-related macrovascular disease can be greatly affected. This burden of diease has implications not only from an individual perspective but from a clinical and public health perspective as well.

The Burden of Macrovascular Disease

The term *burden* refers to the extent to which a particular disease, or one component of that disease, is important. This importance must be measured in clinical as well as public health terms. In other words, how does one decide if a particular disease or a component of that disease is important? From a traditional clinical perspective, it is important for each individual under care for diabetes and its concomitant problems to receive the best care possible to improve quality of life. Thus, health care providers strive to reduce the individual clinical burden faced by each person with diabetes.

From a public health perspective, there are several other interrelated indicators of the impact, or burden, of a disease.[28] These are depicted in Fig. 6-1, and include the following:

1. The prevalence of the disease. Currently, the prevalence of diabetes suggests it is a significant problem for at least 8% to 10% of the population and is a problem that will become more significant in an aging society.[34,55]

2. As previously noted, from an individual perspective, the extent to which a disease affects quality of life certainly impacts the person with diabetes and the family. However, these same concerns, on a large scale, translate to the definition of burden in terms of public health, with recognition of the extent to which a disease significantly impacts mortality, morbidity, or disability. However, problems associated with morbidity and disability, such as cardiovascular disease, or amputations caused by vascular disease, suggest diabetes-related complications may

weigh heavily on public health–related concerns.[28,65]

3. The extent to which persons with diabetes use and/or stress the resources of the health care system may impact the public's perspective of how much of a burden the disease is. To that end, this perception may impact the extent to which public health resources will be channeled to accommodate the needs of those persons with diabetes.

4. The economic burden placed on the public by diabetes and its concomitant problems may impact the extent to which it is perceived as a significant problem for society. If large numbers of dollars are needed to combat the disease, it will be seen as a larger public health concern.

5. The effectiveness of the care might also influence the extent to which a disease is seen as a burden. From an individual perspective, diabetes may greatly impact daily life in terms of the therapeutic regimen and its requirements (blood glucose monitoring, dietary requirements). However, in terms of public health burden, the advances associated with management of diabetes have enabled persons with diabetes to engage in normal life activities and function as active members of society.

6. Finally, individual or societal values may impact the extent to which a disease is seen as a burden. For example, if the disease is a direct result of an individual's elected behavior (e.g., sexually transmitted diseases), the perception of burden from a public health viewpoint may be less in contrast to a disease in which the individual is viewed as an innocent "victim."

Macrovascular Disease in Diabetic and Nondiabetic Populations

Impressive data exists to support the impact of macrovascular disease as a significant burden in diabetes.* Macrovascular disease, especially CAD, is the most common cause of death in diabetes, accounting for between 40% to 60% of all causes of mortality. Over one-half of all nontraumatic lower extremity amputations, or approximately 56,000 per year,[34] in part caused by peripheral vascular disease, occur in persons with diabetes. Indeed, individuals with diabetes are 15 to 20 times more likely to have a nontraumatic amputation than their nondiabetic neighbors (see Chapter 7, Foot Care). Regrettably, about one-half of these lower extremity amputations in persons with diabetes can be prevented. The most common reasons for hospitalization among persons with diabetes are complications caused by macrovascular disease. And of the $20 billion direct and indirect costs for diabetes in the United States (most of it occurring in non–insulin-dependent diabetes mellitus [NIDDM]), macrovascular disorders are the major contributor to these costs, especially in patients over 65 years of age.[26,58,71,118]

---

*References 15, 34, 59, 82, 92, 110.

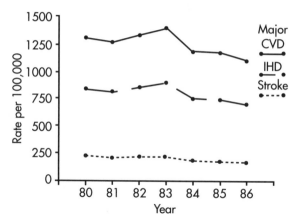

Fig. 6-2 Age-standardized mortality rates for major cardiovascular disease, ischemic heart disease, and stroke as underlying cause per 100,000 diabetic population, by year, United States, 1980 to 1986. (Adapted from Diabetes surveillance, policy, program, research: DHHS; PHS; Centers for disease control; Center for chronic disease prevention and health promotion, Atlanta, GA, 1990, Division of Diabetes Translation.)

However, it is not only epidemiologic/public health data that suggests that diabetes-related macrovascular disease is important. Clinicians and practitioners frequently see patients with diabetes in the following situations: (1) in the coronary care unit with a myocardial infarction; (2) with loss of cognitive and/or physical function as a result of a cerebral vascular accident; (3) with a lower extremity amputation caused by peripheral vascular disease (see Chapter 7, Foot Care). These are all common health problems for persons with diabetes and all too familiar clinical issues practitioners face daily.

Features of Macrovascular Disease in Diabetes

Because only about 6% to 8% of persons in the United States have diabetes,[55] *most* people with myocardial infarction or strokes, in terms of absolute numbers, do *not* have diabetes.[102] However, the *likelihood* or risk of experiencing a myocardial infarction, stroke, or lower-extremity amputation is substantially greater if one has diabetes.[61,64]

There are several special and important clinical characteristics about macrovascular disease in persons with diabetes that should receive extra notice: (1) the onset of the clinical syndromes of macrovascular disease typically occur at a relatively young age in persons with diabetes[65]; (2) mortality rates for major cardiovascular diseases in persons with diabetes appear to be declining slightly (Fig. 6-2)[34]; (3) while rates of hospital discharges for CAD were greatest in African American and white females (Fig. 6-3), mortality rates were greatest for white males (Fig. 6-4)[34]; (4) nontraumatic lower-extremity amputations appear to be more common in males and African Americans (Fig. 6-5)[34]; (5) while not supported by all studies, the general clinical experience is that with CAD or cerebrovas-

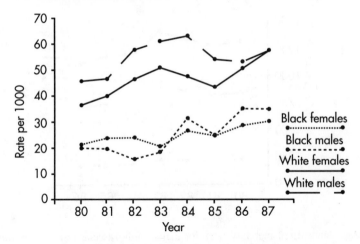

Fig. 6-3 Age-standardized rates of hospital discharges for ischemic heart disease as primary diagnosis per 1000 diabetic population, by race, sex, and year, United States, 1980 to 1987. (Adapted from Diabetes surveillance, policy, program, research: DHHS; PHS; Centers for disease control; Center for chronic disease prevention and health promotion, Atlanta, GA, 1990, Division of Diabetes Translation.)

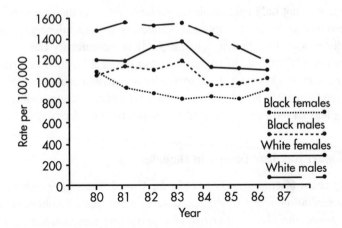

Fig. 6-4 Age-standardized mortality rates for major cardiovascular disease as underlying cause per 100,000 diabetic population, by race, sex, and year, United States, 1980 to 1986. (Adapted from Diabetes surveillance, policy, program, research: DHHS; PHS; Centers for disease control; Center for chronic disease prevention and health promotion, Atlanta, GA, 1990, Division of diabetes translation.)

cular disease, persons with diabetes are likely to experience complications of the initial clinical episode, as well as recurrence of coronary or cerebral attacks[91]; (6) features that normally "protect" one from premature macrovascular disease (e.g., female gender) do not pertain to individuals with diabetes[44]; (7) the clinical manifestations of some macrovascular events such as CAD are often (although not usually) atypical (e.g., "silent"

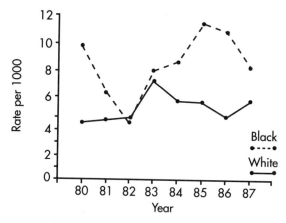

Fig. 6-5 Age-standardized rates of hospital discharges for nontraumatic lower-extremity amputation per 1000 diabetic population, by race and year, United States, 1980 to 1987. (Adapted from Diabetes surveillance, policy, program, research; DHHS; PHS; Centers for disease control; Center for chronic disease prevention and health promotion, Atlanta, GA, 1990, Division of Diabetes Translation.)

myocardial or asymptomatic infarction,[63] GI "indigestion," unexplained congestive heart failure as manifestations of atherosclerotic heart disease[62,70]); and (8) treatment modalities for macrovascular episodes (discussed in greater detail below) may be complicated by the presence of diabetes. For example, are symptoms such as weakness and dizziness a recurrent TIA or hypoglycemia? Should β-blockers be used to treat angina in patients with diabetes?

In summary, from a societal perspective, the burden of macrovascular disease in a disorder as common as diabetes mellitus is substantial, from whatever measure of burden one wants to apply. And from a clinical perspective, the challenge of preventing, recognizing, diagnosing, and treating macrovascular disease is great indeed, for the various components of large vessel disease in diabetes are subtle and often atypical, complex, and devastating.

ETIOLOGY OF MACROVASCULAR DISEASE IN DIABETES

A single, clear, and convincing explanation does not yet exist to explain why macrovascular disease is so common in diabetes. It is probable that there will be many factors and that they will be interrelated.[29,43,97] It is useful to briefly consider these various pathogenetic factors in order to understand the rationale for present and future management strategies for preventing and treating macrovascular complications of diabetes. For purposes of discussion, the reasons for macrovascular disease development can be categorized as follows: (1) factors associated with diabetes mellitus, per se; (2) the treatment of diabetes; and (3) the presence of associated conditions (see Table 6-1).

Table 6-1   Reasons for Diabetes-Associated Macrovascular Disease

Category	Examples
Diabetes	Hyperglycemia with glycoprotein formation and/or sorbitol accumulation
	Lipid abnormalities
	Microvascular abnormalities
	Neuropathy
	Clotting system dysfunction
	Genetics
	Insulin resistance/hyperinsulinemia
Diabetes treatment	Diet
	Exercise
	Oral hypoglycemic agents
	Insulin
Associated conditions	Hypertension
	Lipoprotein abnormalities
	Smoking
	Personality type

Diabetes-Specific Factors

Several abnormalities that appear to be consequences of diabetes may contribute to accelerated and premature macrovascular disease. As a result of hyperglycemia, protein glycosylation[20] and osmotic/metabolic sequela of sorbitol accumulation and/or myoinositol loss[50] may place the intima, the internal lining of large vessels, in a very vulnerable position.[19,83] Hyperlipidemia, whether primary, or secondary to the hyperglycemia of diabetes, is common and may well contribute to atherosclerosis.[100] Microvascular abnormalities, typical of diabetes, may occur and impede nutrient flow to the media and adventitia of large vessels, thus placing these vasculature layers at risk.[39]

The metabolic consequences of hyperglycemia include neuropathy, which could result in abnormal cell wall nutrition, or sympathetic/parasympathetic denervation.[79] Several components of the clotting system have been reported to be abnormal in persons with diabetes, including platelet function,[32] blood flow and viscosity,[77] and the fibrinolytic system.[62] For example, platelets appear unusually "sticky," blood flow is sluggish, and lysis of clots is impaired. Conceptually, those abnormalities could increase the likelihood of macrovascular disease in diabetic patients. The role of ethnicity and/or genetics in diabetes and macrovascular disease cannot be ignored, for it is conceivable that both conditions may be influenced by a common genetic aberration.[60]

Finally, recent concepts of the pathogenesis of macrovascular disease in diabetes suggest a primary role for insulin resistance and thereby secondary hyperinsulinemia with an associated "atherosclerotic milieu." The so-called "syndrome X," a condition in which insulin resistance, hyperinsulinemia, hyperglycemia, upper body obesity, and hypertension occur with surprising frequency in the same individual, may thus be related to the development of macrovascular disease.[66,81,99]

The Treatment of Diabetes

Diet and Exercise

As persons with diabetes are at increased risk for macrovascular disorders, one must examine the possibilities that our treatment modalities could minimize one aspect of diabetes (e.g., microvascular disorders through achievement of euglycemia), while increasing the risk for another important complication—large vessel disease (see Chapter 2 on Nutrition). For example, diet has been and remains the cornerstone of therapy for diabetes; however, the recommended *content* of that diet has changed over the years. In the past, because of primary concern for glycemic excursions with varying carbohydrate ingestion, emphasis was placed on the carbohydrate content of the diet, with relative inattention to fat ingestion.[69] Thus, to the degree that there is a relationship between fat consumption (amount and type) and atherosclerosis, it is conceivable, although not established, that past diet recommendations may not have been ideal from a macrovascular disease perspective. Such is not the case at present[6]; however, one cannot ignore the implications previous recommendations might have had with regard to current prevalence of atherosclerosis. Exercise therapy for persons with diabetes is becoming an integral part of treatment regimens, and many guidelines exist.[4,104,109] Thus careful pre-exercise evaluation is recommended.[3]

Oral sulfonylurea agents

The use of oral sulfonylurea agents remains somewhat controversial,[47] particularly because of a putative association between tolbutamide and accelerated heart disease (see Chapter 4, Pharmocologic Issues). While the University Group Diabetes Program (UGDP) results have been repeatedly questioned,[68,73] and many experienced diabetologists do not support a strong link between sulfonylurea agents and macrovascular disorders in diabetic patients,[9] one should remain cognizant of the UGDP conclusions.

Insulin

Many patients with diabetes take insulin.[5] Given the concepts of syndrome X and hyperinsulinism,[66,81,99] could the use of insulin actually contribute to macrovascular disorders? At present, while some epidemiologic studies relate insulin levels to the development of macrovascular disease[98,112,117] and concerns exist about insulin-antibody immune complexes,[35,52] such relationships must remain speculative, although worthy of continued investigation. Certainly, all the logical benefits regarding reducing macrovascular potential from appropriate insulin use—such as lowering of glucose with decreased glycoprotein formation and sorbitol accumulation,[20,50] improved lipid parameters,[95]—should not be ignored or abandoned while such studies continue.

Associated Conditions

There are several pathogenetic factors for macrovascular disease that are not unique to the person with diabetes but that also occur in the general population.[72,85,90]

Hypertension

Diabetes is a major risk factor for the development of hypertension. Specific hypotheses to explain abnormalities in blood pressure in the general population that apply as well to persons with diabetes include: autoregulatory dysfunction, renal sodium retention, abnormal cellular sodium transport, increased intracellular calcium, or acquired mechanisms. Even with the uncertainty about the pathogenesis of hypertension, several explanations can be deduced, including: (1) an increased genetic sensitivity; (2) factors that increase the cardiac output such as increased heart rate, fluid volume, or neural stimulation that may result in an increased activation of the autoregulatory process, increasing peripheral vascular resistance and thus blood pressure[36,115]; (3) the renal excretion of water and sodium that increases when blood pressure rises normally, diminishing fluid volume and returning the blood pressure to normal.

The hypertension seen in diabetes seems to be volume dependent; increased insulin concentrations stimulate sodium reabsorption and thus fluid retention. Other causes may be related to abnormalities of the sympathetic and parasympathetic systems often seen in diabetes.

Elevated blood pressure may be more prevalent in a diabetes community and at an earlier age because of the diabetes itself. Other nonmodifiable risk factors that may predispose the person with diabetes to concomitant development of hypertension include family history, with a genetic predisposition noted in African Americans. Males are at an increased risk to develop hypertension at a younger age than females and at a higher rate. Hypertension also occurs with aging, with other factors perhaps contributing to this occurrence—in particular the weight gain that sometimes accompanies aging. Modifiable factors primarily include obesity, which is also a risk factor for NIDDM, and the association of stress with hypertension development. Untreated hypertension can lead to severe cardiovascular occurrences, such as stroke or myocardial infarction.[36]

Hyperlipidemia

The presence of hyperlipidemia, also a risk factor for diabetes and hypertension, can contribute to the development of macrovascular disease in the general population as well. This metabolic abnormality (discussed in detail in Chapter 2) has a reported prevalence of 20% to 70% in patients with diabetes. The extent of hyperlipidemia depends to a great extent on glycemic control, type and severity of diabetes, age, and nutritional habits. Hyperlipidemia is a major factor in atheromatous events, and persons with diabetes have higher triglyceride levels but lower high-density lipoprotein (HDL) levels. Because HDL is inversely related to coronary risk, the person with diabetes is at a heightened risk for cardiovascular occurrences.[7]

Cigarette smoking

The occurrence of cigarette smoking in persons with diabetes is not appreciably different from that in the general population. Cigarette smoking is a major contributor to cardiovascular disease in the nondiabetic population, a risk that increases several-fold in the presence of diabetes.[85,90] In diabetes, smoking is associated with nephropathy, retinopathy, connective tissue changes, and neuropathy. Persons who already have vascular complications, pregnant women, or women using oral contraceptives are at particular risk. Stopping smoking reduces the risk of vascular morbidity and mortality in nondiabetic persons and, it is assumed, has the same beneficial effects in persons with diabetes.[54]

Other factors

Other factors that may have an impact on macrovascular disease development include obesity that predisposes to macrovascular disease, in particular obesity complicated by the tendency for a sedentary life-style. Reactions to stressful circumstance, such as seen in personality type A—the hard-driven, ambitious, time-oriented individual with hidden hostility—are also associated with development of macrovascular disease. More recently, type E personality (the hot reactor) has been described as characterizing a hypertensive, cardiovascular-risk profile in the individual who is explosive when thwarted in reaching goals. While this relationship between personality types and heart disease is controversial,[119] it is at least worth further exploration in terms of the stressful response to the requirements imposed by the regimen in the person with diabetes. Impaired glucose tolerance (IGT) is an identified risk factor for macrovascular disease in several epidemiologic studies.[60] Proteinuria is also a finding that seems to predict the subsequent development of macrovascular disease, although the significance remains unclear.

The essential feature underscoring the importance of these factors for macrovascular disease is that, in diabetes, their impact is multiplicative, not additive.[7] Given the prevalence and potency, they may contribute very significantly to the clinical and public health burden of a macrovascular disease in populations with diabetes.

TREATMENT OF MACROVASCULAR DISEASE IN DIABETES

What can be done *now* to reduce the burden of macrovascular disease in patients with diabetes, both from a public health and clinical perspective? To provide a framework, it is useful to consider three potential levels of prevention—primary, secondary, and tertiary[28] (Table 6-2).

Considering the disease, diabetes itself—one could reduce the societal and individual consequences of this condition by (1) decreasing the incidence of diabetes (i.e., *primary* prevention of new cases); (2) decreasing development of complications of diabetes by aggressive treatment of basic metabolic abnormalities associated with diabetes (i.e., *secondary* prevention through therapy for hyperglycemia or hyperlipidemia); or (3) diminish the consequences of the complications of diabetes (i.e., *tertiary* prevention through judicious use of β-blockers in the postinfarction period).

Table 6-2   Prevention Strategies

Level	Concept	Example
Primary	Decrease incidence of disease	Control weight to prevent NIDDM
Secondary	Maintain normal metabolic state to prevent/delay complications	Glucose, blood pressure, and lipid control
Tertiary	Minimize extent of damage from complications associated with disease	Beta blocker treatment after myocardial infarction to decrease incidence of sudden death

Primary Prevention

Primary prevention of diabetes, if effective, would reduce the burden of macrovascular disease in persons with diabetes to that of the nondiabetic population. In terms of primary prevention, there is (1) evidence supporting a relationship between obesity and diabetes[23,89]; (2) reason to consider prevention of NIDDM by weight control and/or obesity reduction.[93,122]; and (3) possible benefit of sustained aerobic exercise.

Obesity and diabetes mellitus

Several factors must be considered in the possible relationship between obesity and diabetes. First, while it is *logical* to relate obesity control to the prevention of NIDDM (and thereby the increased burden of macrovascular disease in this particular diabetic population), there are no large, long-term studies *at present* that convincingly support the premise that weight loss and/or minimization of weight gain will prevent or even delay the onset of NIDDM and associated macrovascular disease.

Syndrome X and macrovascular disease

Furthermore, recent data relevant to a syndrome X[66,81,99] suggest that the tendency for macrovascular disease may occur years before the onset of clinical diabetes, or even unrecognized hyperglycemia.[53,106] Studies indicate that the likelihood of CAD (and perhaps cerebral and peripheral vascular disease as well) is similar in patients with impaired glucose tolerance as in those with established NIDDM.[60] If insulin resistance/hyperinsulinemia with associated atherogenic abnormalities do occur even *decades* before onset of clinical diabetes,[53,66,81,99,106] primary prevention effects of both NIDDM, and especially macrovascular disease, will need to occur well before obesity and/or hyperglycemia have set in.

The lack of firm scientific data to assist with issues related to primary prevention of diabetes should not necessarily limit the application of weight control and exercise programs on an individual, case-by-case basis, perhaps based on such important factors as family history of vascular disorders and membership in certain ethnic groups. For example, if a strong family history for diabetes exist, weight control to possibly prevent NIDDM seems reasonable. Such an approach is logical, unlikely to do harm, and consistent with good general physical and emotional health. However, one must be somewhat guarded because of lack of clear data and established effective programs.[120] From a societal perspective, the science base regarding primary prevention of NIDDM and macrovascular disease needs to be expanded before national treatment programs should be implemented.

Secondary Prevention

Treatment of hyperglycemia, hypertension, and cigarette usage are the focus of secondary prevention efforts related to the development of macrovascular disease.

Limitation of studies in nondiabetic populations

It is important to note that most studies related to risk factors for macrovascular disease were performed in nondiabetic persons—mostly white males.[25,42,75,87,116] Thus, entry criteria were restrictive in order to emphasize a well-defined, scientifically valid study.[28] The extrapolation of the results to the larger population thus suffers. It is unclear whether the results of the extensive investigations conducted to date are relevant to females, the elderly, minority populations, or persons with diabetes. However, to repeat all studies in all subpopulations would be very demanding and certainly quite expensive. Thus, one must use logic, inference, and reason.[7,56] Particularly when risk of therapy is low, it is appropriate to apply the general recommendations of studies on lipids, blood pressure, and cigarette usage in the general population to persons with diabetes. Indeed, given the prevalence of macrovascular disease in diabetes[61,64] and the multiplicative interaction among the vascular risk factors and diabetes,[61] it may be *more* imperative to deal forcefully with these risk factors in persons with diabetes.

It is important to apply logic and inference in the absence of firm data or answers. It is fair to say that *all* strategies for risk reduction should be utilized in persons with diabetes. While there is some risk, while the goals of therapy may even be *more* rigorous than those in persons without diabetes, and while the task is even more challenging given the complexity of a diabetic regimen, the benefit may well be most substantial in persons with diabetes.[53,66,84,99]

Special considerations for secondary prevention

There may be special considerations and/or concerns regarding treatment recommendations in persons with diabetes mellitus. First, the goals for lipid and blood pressure levels may be different for the general public and for persons with diabetes. For example, at all lipid levels, including ones considered to be normal, persons with diabetes have a greater likelihood of having an adverse macrovascular event.[7,11,14,36] Similarly, while a blood pressure level of <140/90 is often stated as the goal of treatment in the general public,[114] in persons with diabetes therapeutic goals are viewed as considerably lower (e.g., <120/80) in order to minimize retinal and renal changes.[27,115] (Benefits of such blood pressure levels on macrovascular disease remains to be firmly established.) Thus, in general, one would probably treat abnormal lipid and blood pressure levels in persons with diabetes earlier, more aggressively, and with more demanding goals in mind.

Table 6-3   The Advantages and Drawbacks of Various Groups of Antihypertensive Drugs in the Treatment of Hypertension with Diabetes Mellitus

Advantages	Problems	Recommendations
Diuretics		
Monotherapy lowers high blood pressure effectively Once daily regimen Inexpensive Pathophysiologically sound (lower elevated exchangeable sodium and reduce exaggerated noradrenaline reactivity)	Impair glucose homeostasis potassium depletion, insulin receptors(?) Serum lipid alterations Increase plasma uric acid Hyperosmolar coma Erectile impotence Orthostatic hypotension	Low dose Control: potassium; glucose; lipids Potassium substitution if needed (diet, KCl, combination with potassium-sparing diuretic)
β-Blockers		
Monotherapy lowers high blood pressure effectively Once daily regimen Cardioprotection Antianginal/antiarrythmogenic properties	β_2-Blockade impairs insulin output Hypoglycaemia: prolonged by β_2-blockers; altered perception of the symptoms; hypertensive crisis (β_2-blockers) Serum lipid alterations Decrease physical exercise performance	Cardioselective (β_1-) blocker (i.e., atenolol, metoprolol, acebutolol) Low (-moderate) dose Instruction: hypoglycaemia problems Control: cardiac performance; AV conduction; serum lipoproteins
Calcium antagonists		
Monotherapy lowers high blood pressure effectively Once daily regimen possible Antianginal effects Antiarrhythmic properties (verapamil, diltiazem) Metabolic 'neutrality' (glucose, lipids, potassium) Cardioprotection (?) Antiarteriosclerotic (?) Preserve physical exercise performance Relative rarity of orthostatic and impotence problems (?)	Impair insulin secretion *in vitro;* in high doses *in vivo* (?) Headache (often transient) Flushing, ankle oedema, paradoxical angina (dihydropyridines) Constipation (verapamil)	Low to moderate dose Control: AV conduction (verapamil, diltiazem); glucose (at higher dosages)

From Trost BH: Hypertension in the diabetic patient: selection and optimum use of antihypertensive drugs, Drugs 38(4):621-633, 1989.

Table 6-3 **The Advantages and Drawbacks of Various Groups of Antihypertensive Drugs in the Treatment of Hypertension with Diabetes Mellitus—cont'd**

Advantages	Problems	Recommendations
ACE inhibitors		
Monotherapy lowers high blood pressure effectively	Proteinuria (rare)	Low to moderate dose
Once daily regimen possible	Dose adjustment with declining renal function	Control: renal function; proteinuria, plasma
Effective in heart failure	Renal failure (reversible) in renal artery stenoses	potassium
Metabolic 'neutrality' (glucose, lipids [?], no hypokalaemia)	Enhancement of hyperkalaemia in hyporeninaemic hypoaldosteronism (rare)	
Relative rarity of orthostatic and impotence problems (?)	False positive test for acetone	

Treatment of risk factors

Hyperglycemia Achieving euglycemia has remained a primary goal of therapy in diabetes care.[2] It is *logical* to expect euglycemia to result in a reduced atherogenic environment.[21,40] While there is indirect evidence that improved glucose regulation is related to decreased morbidity and mortality associated with diabetic macrovascular disease,[24] there is, at present, no clear and convincing evidence that euglycemia will reduce the risk of macrovascular disease. This does not mean that such a relationship does not exist, only that data from a systematic investigation are not yet available.

Hypertension The relationship of hypertension control and reduced risk for macrovascular events is less clear. The benefits and consequences of reducing blood pressure, especially on decreased risks for congestive heart failure, stroke, and renal failure, are well accepted.[84] Evidence that lowering blood pressure results in fewer episodes or severity of acute coronary disease is less convincing,[88] but more recent reports suggest that controlling blood pressure does affect coronary artery disease.[86]

The prevention of hypertension, as previously noted, should therefore be one of the first aims. The maintenance of ideal body weight is a primary means of achieving normal blood pressure. Nonpharmacologic measures should always be considered and discussed with the individual prior to drug therapy. Statistically, the single most important treatment for more than 50% of hypertensive persons with diabetes is to lose weight, which leads to improvement in blood pressure, diabetes, and hyperlipidemia.

Antihypertensive drug treatment in persons with diabetes is begun early because of the deleterious interaction between diabetes and hypertension.[1,36] The effect of antihypertensive drugs must be controlled, preferably together with the control of blood glucose. Adverse effects should be carefully monitored. In addition, the overall regimen should be as simple as possible in an effort to encourage adherence and, perhaps, to limit burdensome drug costs.[1,86,88]

There are four main groups of drugs used to treat hypertension in persons with diabetes: diuretics, beta blockers, calcium antagonists, and ace inhibitors. The advantages and disadvantages of each of the four main groups of drugs used in the treatment of hypertension are summarized in Table 6-3. While each of these groups has proved effectiveness in control of blood pressure, there are also untoward effects that can pose serious problems for the person with diabetes. These problems must be monitored very carefully, with routine and frequent patient contact a major priority.[1,86,88]

As evidenced by several recent reviews,* the choice of medication in hypertensive diabetic persons is complicated, both from a standpoint of side effects of drugs and ability of certain hypertensive agents to fully minimize the risk for macrovascular disease. For example, thiazide diuretics have been, and perhaps still are, the foundation for hypertensive treatment because of cost, effectiveness, and apparent safety.[114] Concern, however, exists regarding the attenuation of risk reduction efforts through decreased blood pressure by increased lipid values.[67] Similarly, other commonly used medications such as beta blockers or alpha antagonists may be associated with side effects (e.g., masking of hypoglycemia symptoms, impotence, or postural hypertension) that are particularly problematic in persons with long-term diabetes.[76] There is movement towards beginning therapy in hypertensive diabetic persons with calcium antagonists or ace inhibitors.

Hyperlipidemia   Definitive evidence is accumulating regarding the benefits of efforts to attenuate the morbidity and perhaps mortality of macrovascular disease associated with hyperlipidemia.[25,42,75,87,102,116] These data do support the view that individual clinical and public health efforts to control hyperlipidemia will result in a lower societal and, hopefully, individual burden from macrovascular disease. As noted in Chapter 2, dietary treatment of hyperlipidemia, including maintenance of ideal body weight, is critical to care from both a primary and secondary prevention perspective.

The treatment for hyperlipidemia is challenging, and it is made more so by the presence of diabetes. Consider the demands of following the diet, exercise, and drug treatment program for diabetes itself. Add to that the challenge of *additional* dietary considerations because of hyperlipidemia (e.g., restriction in amount and type of dietary fat). While one might logically think that the presence of these two serious conditions might result in *greater* effort and attention to the therapeutic regimen, the task may simply be too demanding. And how much of the hyperlipidemia is caused by poorly controlled diabetes itself (thus requiring even additional attention to blood glucose control) versus endogenous hyperlipidemia in someone who just happens to have diabetes? In addition, the question of when antilipid agents should be begun and which one should be used is critical, especially since some (e.g., niacin) may be effective in lipid reduction but have adverse effects of special significance in persons with diabetes.[45,49]

Smoking cessation   Discontinuance of cigarettes is associated with improved health, especially a decreased likelihood of macrovascular events. As summarized in the recent report of the Surgeon General[113] and other articles,[41] smoking cessation clearly decreases the risk of macrovascular disease, including heart attacks, strokes, and peripheral vascular disease.[57]

Finally, again considering the demands and complexities of a diabetic regimen, efforts to stop cigarette usage may be problematic. There are data suggesting that younger persons with diabetes smoke at a greater rate than nondiabetic persons, perhaps because

*References 1, 27, 49, 67, 76, 121.

cigarettes reflect a sense of rebelliousness in one aspect of life and balance the rigidity in another (i.e., diabetes regimen).[57,85,90]

Prevention or cessation of smoking is critical to macrovascular disease prevention. The delivery of all routine diabetes education should therefore include content related to smoking from three perspectives: prevention information, cessation strategies, and maintenance/relapse prevention.[54] This information can be presented in several phases, including:

1. Assess smoking status. The first step is to determine whether or not the individual smokes. This should be a routine part of care. If the answer is no, the health care provider should emphasize the importance of maintaining a smoke-free life-style, especially in the diagnosis of diabetes. If the individual reports smoking, a more detailed assessment, with information regarding smoking history, nicotine dependence, motivation to quit, and diabetes-specific concerns related to quitting should be addressed.

2. Determine readiness to quit. Once a person with diabetes reports smoking, several steps should be initiated to further encourage cessation, including: identifying cessation as a priority of diabetes care; building the smoker's confidence that quitting is possible; and addressing any concerns about quitting, particularly as they relate to diabetes care (e.g., weight concerns).

3. Initiate cessation interventions. The diabetes team should work together with the smoker to set a quit date within 3 weeks of visit; review the diabetic regimen and discuss issues related to short-term nicotine withdrawal; identify smoking cessation strategies; assess the need for nicotine polacrilex; determine a schedule for follow-up.

4. Follow-up. The focus of follow-up is to verify the status of patients and to assist those who may have relapsed and become smokers again. Those who are smoke-free should be praised for their tremendous efforts. Those who have relapsed need to be encouraged not to feel bad, but rather to try again, as cessation is a difficult process.

Tertiary Prevention

In the person with established diabetes *and* clinically apparent macrovascular disease (e.g., angina, recent myocardial infarction, transient ischemic attacks, and intermittent claudication), what should be our present therapeutic approach in tertiary prevention? In essence, the same strategies that are applied to the nondiabetic patient population should be utilized in persons with diabetes. Thus, medical approaches to anginal control (e.g., nitrates, calcium-channel blockers)[38,78]; use of technologically based management strategies for coronary or cerebral vascular disorders (e.g., angioplasty, bypass grafting)[10]; and very aggressive and innovative therapy for peripheral vascular disease, (e.g., laser treatment)[33,96] are all tertiary treatment options that should be used in diabetic patients when clinically appropriate.

There are, however, a few important issues to consider when applying such tertiary strategies. First, is the prognosis in persons with diabetes with active macrovascular disease significantly poorer when compared with nondiabetic persons, such that invasive and/or expensive procedures should not be considered? Some data suggest a very discouraging prognosis[91]; however, recent studies indicate that persons with diabetes can definitely benefit from tertiary treatment approaches.[105] The challenges of ensuring optimal metabolic control prior to tertiary interventions exists[103a,107] and often will be the responsibility of a nonsurgical diabetes care team.

Second, some of the components of tertiary prevention need to be carefully considered in persons with diabetes. For example, consider recommendations for aspirin therapy.[12,22,94,111] Understandable concern exists, especially in persons with diabetic retinopathy, about possible problems with bleeding secondary to aspirin therapy.[12,22] Recent reports of the Early Treatment of Diabetic Retinopathy Study indicate no excessive tendencies for retinal hemorrhage with aspirin,[37] so that if this therapy is otherwise clinically indicated it should not be denied to persons with diabetes.

Other medical recommendations for tertiary prevention may also be especially challenging in persons with diabetes. In patients with a recent myocardial infarction, beta blocker therapy is often recommended.[101] The use of beta blockers in persons with diabetes, particularly those at risk for hypoglycemia (see Table 6-3), may be problematic[31] and must be carefully considered regarding masking of hypoglycemic symptoms, with benefits associated with prevention of recurrent coronary events versus severe hypoglycemia the key issue.

Future research

Recognition of the possibility for the tendency of macrovascular disease to begin years before clinical diabetes[53,106] and the possible role of insulin resistance/hyperinsulinemia in the genesis of those macrovascular disorders[66,99] also provides a fertile intellectual framework to verify the effectiveness of primary prevention programs and begin strategies to attenuate macrovascular tendencies well before hyperglycemia begins.

Primary prevention of diabetes itself (and perhaps thereby the accompanying tendency for macrovascular disease) continues to receive attention.[93,122] Especially in high-risk populations (e.g., ethnic minorities, persons with impaired glucose tolerance, people with gestational diabetes mellitus), community- and clinic-based interventions utilizing weight control and exercise strategies are being developed.

In the meantime, what can be expected in future secondary and tertiary prevention efforts in diabetes-associated macrovascular disease? For glycemia control itself, new classes and types of glucose-lowering agents will soon be available.[78] Manipulations of the insulin molecule itself may result in compounds that achieve comparable or even greater glucose-lowering effects without any undesirable consequences (e.g., putative accelerated atherosclerosis).[18] In circumstances in which euglycemia is not achieved, pharmacologic agents to block glycoprotein formation or sorbitol accumulation/myoinositol depletion,[17,108] once safety and efficacy issues are resolved, are likely to be more widely available. Agents to reduce platelet abnormalities will also likely become part of our therapeutic armamentarium.

For hypertension and lipid abnormalities, one can anticipate many new varieties of existing classes of drugs and new classes of pharmaceuticals also. The availability of calcium-channel blockers and angiotensin-converting enzyme inhibitors has been a helpful step in managing hypertension in persons with diabetes.[27] Likewise, it is anticipated that newer and hopefully more effective antilipid agents (e.g., various HMG CoA reductase inhibitors)[51] will soon be available. This enlarging menu of agents to reduce risk elements for macrovascular disease hopefully will not result in confusion and overload for busy practitioners but will aid in targeting specific macrovascular risks with specific safe and effective pharmacologic interventions.

Finally, for all levels of prevention, the great challenge of *behavioral alteration* remains for the provider, persons with diabetes, and the public at large. Much has already been learned, but although knowledge alone is probably essential, it does not necessarily result in altered behavior.[80] Rather, other concepts (e.g., beliefs, attitudes, barriers, circumstances)[10,13,103] and programs that recognize the complexities of personal behavior are being evaluated and will likely become available in the near future. There is no simple single approach to the essential challenge of education, and multifaceted programs will be necessary. This will permit us to reduce the risk of the development of macrovascular disease in persons with diabetes with greater effectiveness and compassion.

What does the future hold regarding tertiary prevention efforts in persons who already have macrovascular disease? First, the early detection of clinically unrecognized macrovascular disease utilizing sensitive (and initially expensive) procedures (e.g., angioscopes, ultrasonography) will likely become more possible.[46,48,74] Other pharmacologic agents beyond those such as aspirin are likely to be identified that could be useful in minimizing the extent or recurrence of macrovascular disease in persons with diabetes. Likewise, technologic advances beyond presently available bypass surgery and angiopathy, such as laser therapy, will become part of the therapeutic armamentarium. The development of these innovative approaches will continue with excitement and promise. Remaining issues amidst all the enthusiasm about new approaches will be documentation of utility when compared with other treatment modalities prior to distribution within the entire health care system.

Goals of Education

While the multitude of etiologic factors provides numerous approaches to reducing the consequences of coronary, cerebral, and peripheral vascular diseases, the very breadth and scope of the possibilities may not be fully useful to the *individual* practitioner responsible for the *individual* patient with diabetes. How can one utilize all the information in developing an individualized approach for a single patient?

First, it is important to remember that because diabetes is both a complex and chronic disease, efforts over time, perhaps involving several visits, will be necessary to achieve lifelong changes. To this end, regular health care visits focusing on diabetes control and management, which allow for routine follow-up and preventive health care, are important.[103]

Table 6-4   Biochemical Indices of Metabolic Control

	Top limits (mg/dL)		
	Normal	Acceptable	Poor
Fasting plasma glucose	115	140	>200
Postprandial plasma glucose	140	200	>235
Glycosylated hemoglobin	8	10	>12
Hemoglobin A_{1c}	6	8	>10
Adjust for normal values of laboratory			
Increase limits for aged patients			
	Desirable	Borderline	High
Serum cholesterol (mg/dL)	<200	200-239	≥240
Fasting plasma triglycerides (mg/dL)	<150	150-249	≥250
Adjust for normal values of laboratory			

Second, these visits need to be structured to emphasize the importance of diabetes education that (1) makes the individual aware of the modifiable risks for macrovascular disease as it is exacerbated by diabetes; and (2) emphasizes the importance of preventive education to eliminate modifiable risk factors. As has been previously discussed, it is crucial to emphasize to persons with diabetes the risk factors for macrovascular disease and the importance of prevention.

To summarize, the critical health facts that should be consistently reviewed with the individual diabetes include the following:

1. The major goals of management of diabetes include achieving near-normal metabolic biochemical control and prevention of vascular complications. Management of diabetes strives for achieving normal biochemical indices as are cited in Table 6-4. To prevent concomitant complications that further encourage development of macrovascular disease, achievement of normal blood pressure, body weight, and elimination of modifiable risk factors, such as smoking, are stressed.

2. Diabetes is an independent risk factor for vascular disease. Women with diabetes may be at a particular risk, since they do not carry the normal protection of the female gender that is noted in their nondiabetic counterparts.[86,87]

3. Lipid abnormalities occur very commonly in persons with diabetes, from children to adults.[49]

4. Hypertension occurs frequently in diabetes and can have devastating consequences in terms of renal disease as well as macrovascular complications.[36]

5. Cigarette smoking is a major factor associated with cardiovascular disease and mortality. Prevention of smoking in those who have not started, and elimination of this risk factor in those who smoke, is crucial.[41,54,85]

6. Maintenance of ideal body weight, with an appropriate low-fat diet and adequate

physical activity, can significantly reduce the likelihood of developing[3,4,104,109] concomitant risk factors of diabetes, including hyperlipidemia and hypertension.

In summary, diabetes education regarding macrovascular disease emphasizes optimal diabetes care in the context of primary, secondary, or tertiary prevention. Assessment of the individual with diabetes as to what type of education is most critical is needed. Preventive goals of education can thus be targeted more effectively. The box below provides one such model of diabetes education.

CONCLUSIONS

Diabetes is not a single disease, and it is likely that macrovascular relationships in IDDM will not necessarily pertain to NIDDM.[59] For example, in NIDDM, the onset of hypertension often coincides with recognition of hyperglycemia; in IDDM, hypertension usually follow diabetes by years in association with onset of renal disease. Furthermore epidemiologic data and clinical experience indicate that the three main vascular systems af-

---

MACROVASCULAR DISEASE IN DIABETES
———————————— PATIENT EDUCATION ————————————

I. Primary prevention

    A. *Know your family*—History of macrovascular disease, hypertension, hyperlipidemia

    B. *Do good*—Follow good diet; keep weight under control; exercise; have blood pressure and blood lipids checked.

    C. *Do no harm*—Don't smoke.

Secondary prevention

    A. *Hypertension*—Have blood pressure checked regularly; take medicine faithfully; keep weight under control and exercise.

    B. *Hyperlipidemia*—Have blood lipid levels checked at least yearly; follow diet and, if necessary, take medicine faithfully; exercise; try to keep diabetes under control.

    C. *Cigarettes*—Don't start; stop if using cigarettes and ask for help to do this.

    D. *Hyperglycemia*—Try to keep diabetes under control, including monitoring of blood glucose, following diet and exercise program, and taking medicine faithfully.

III. Tertiary prevention

    A. *Keep track of how you feel*—your symptoms; and be sure to tell your doctor how you are doing.

    B. *Keep trying to keep risk factors for macrovascular disease under control.*

    C. *Work closely with your usual health team and new consultants.*

fected by atherosclerosis in diabetes may not be altered through the same mechanisms or to the same degree. Thus, it should not be surprising to see persons with far-advanced peripheral vascular disease without any clinical evidence of CAD. The reason(s) for these differences is not yet clear and will be the focus of important future research.

The major thrust of this discussion, however, has been to emphasize that whether dealing with an individual patient or facing a larger diabetes community, macrovascular disease is *the* major burden of diabetes, regardless of how that burden is defined. There are many factors that account for the prevalence, morbidity, disability, mortality, and cost of macrovascular disease in diabetes. It is likely that an interaction among several of these factors will be of major pathogenetic importance. It is a remarkable challenge to apply the results of population, or community, or cohort studies to the individual with diabetes who needs assistance. Societal/community/public health approaches to diabetes and macrovascular diabetes must be viewed as complimentary to the clinical management of this complication. Together, the huge burden of diabetes-associated macrovascular disease may be reduced through efforts at primary, secondary, and tertiary preventive education.

REFERENCES

1. Andrea L: General considerations in selecting antihypersensitive agents in patients with Type II diabetes mellitus and hypertension, Am J Med 87(suppl):6-39, 1987.
2. American Diabetes Association: Blood glucose control in diabetes: position statement, Diabetes Care 13:16-17, 1990.
3. American Diabetes Association: Diabetes mellitus—position paper, Diabetes Care 13:804-805, 1990.
4. American Diabetes Association: Exercise and NIDDM, Diabetes Care 13:785-789, 1990.
5. American Diabetes Association: Insulin administration: position statement, Diabetes Care 13:28-31, 1990.
6. American Diabetes Association: Nutritional recommendations and principles for individuals with diabetes mellitus, Diabetes Care 13:18-25, 1990.
7. American Diabetes Association: Role of cardiovascular risk factors in prevention and treatment of macrovascular disease in diabetes:consensus statement, Diabetes Care 12:573-579, 1989.
8. Deleted in proofs.
9. American Diabetes Association: Policy statement: the UGDP controversy, Diabetes Care 2:1-3, 1979.
10. Antman E and Braunwald E: Acute MI management in the 1990s, Hosp Pract 25:65-82, 1990.
11. Austin M: Plasma triglycerides and coronary heart disease in men, Arteriosclerosis, In press.
12. Baudoein C and others: Secondary prevention of strokes: role of platelet antiaggregant drugs in diabetic and nondiabetic patients, Diabetic Med 2:145-146, 1985.
13. Becker MH: Understanding patient compliance: the contributions of attitudes and other psychosocial factors. In Cohen SJ, ed: New directions in patient compliance, Lexington, MS, 1979, Lexington Books, AC Heath & Co.
14. Bierman EB and Brunzell J: Diet low in saturated fat and cholesterol for diabetes, Diabetes Care 12:162-163, 1989.
15. Bild D and others: Lower-extremity amputation in people with diabetes: epidemiology and prevention, Diabetes Care 12:24-31, 1989.
16. Bliss M: The discovery of insulin, Toronto, 1982, McClelland and Stewart.
17. Boulton A, Levin S, and Comstock J: A multicentre trial of the aldose-reductase inhibitor, tolrestat, in patients with symptomatic diabetic neuropathy, Diabetologia 33:431-437, 1990.
18. Brange J and others: Monomeric insulins and their experimental and clinical implications, Diabetes Care 13:923-954, 1990.
19. Brownlee N, Cerami E, and Vlassara H: Advanced glycosylation end products in tissues: biochemical basis for a new therapeutic approach to the complications of diabetes, N Engl J Med 318:1315-1321, 1988.
20. Brownlee M, Vlassara H, and Cerami A: Nonenzymatic glycosylation and the pathogenesis of diabetic complications, Ann Intern Med 101:527-537, 1984.

21. Brownlee M and Cahill G: Diabetic control and vascular complications, In Pabletti R and Gotli A, eds: Atherosclerosis Reviews, New York, 1979, Raven Press.
22. Buring J and others: Aspirin and stroke, Arch Neurol 47:1353-1354, 1990.
23. Burton B and others: Health implications of obesity: an NIH consensus development conference, Int J Obes 9:155-169, 1985.
24. Butler WJ and others: Mortality from coronary heart disease in the Tecumseh study: long-term effect of diabetes mellitus, glucose tolerance and other risk factors, Am J Epidemiol 125:541-547, 1985.
25. Casken-Hemphill L and others: Beneficial effects of colestepol-niacin on coronary atherosclerosis, JAMA 264:3013-3017, 1990.
26. Center for Economic Studies in Medicine: Direct and indirect costs of diabetes in the United States in 1987, Reston VA, 1988, Pracon Inc.
27. Christleib AR: Treatment selection considerations for the hypertensive diabetic patient, Arch Intern Med 150:1167-1174, 1990.
28. Fletcher R, Fletcher S, Wagner E, eds: Clinical epidemiology: the essentials, Baltimore, 1988, Williams & Williams Co.
29. Colwell J and Lopes-Virella M: A review of the development of large-vessel disease in diabetes mellitus: the genesis of atherosclerosis in diabetes mellitus, Am J Med 85:113-118, 1988.
30. Keen H and Jarrett J, eds: Complications of diabetes, London, 1982, Edward Arnold.
31. Cryer P, White N, and Santiago J: The relevance of glucose counterregulatory systems to patients with insulin-dependent diabetes mellitus, Endocr Rev 7:131-139, 1986.
32. Davi G and others: Thromboxane biosynthesis and platelet function in Type II diabetes mellitus, N Engl J Med 322:1769-1774, 1990.
33. DeFelice M, Gallo P, and Masotti G: Current therapy of peripheral obstructive arterial disease, the non-surgical approach, Angiology 41:1-11, 1990.
34. Diabetes Surveillance, Policy, Program, Research: DHHS; PHS; Centers for Disease Control; Center for Chronic Disease Prevention and Health Promotion, Division of Diabetes Translation, Atlanta, 1990, Centers for Disease Control.
35. DiMario V, Javicoli M, and Andreani D: Circulating immune complexes in diabetes, Diabetologia 19:89-92, 1980.
36. Dunn FL: Hypertension in diabetes mellitus, Diabetes Mellitus Rev, 6:47-61, 1990.
37. Early Treatment Diabetic Retinopathy Study Group: Early treatment diabetic retinopathy study: aspirin, Presented at Annual Meeting of the American Academy of Ophthalmology, Atlanta, GA, October 29-November 2, 1990.
38. European Stroke Prevention Study Group: European stroke prevention study, Stroke 21:1122, 1990.
39. Factor S, Okum E, and Minase T: Capillary microaneurysms in the human diabetic heart, N Engl J Med 302:384-388, 1980.
40. Feingold KR: Preventing the vascular complications of diabetes. In current concepts series, Kalamazoo, 1987, UpJohn Co.
41. Fiore M, and others: Cigarette smoking: the clinician's role in cessation, prevention, and public health, Dis Mon 36:185-242, 1990.
42. Frick M and others: Helsinki heart study: primary-prevention trial with gemfibrizole in middle-aged men with dyslipdemia: safety of treatment, changes in risk factors and incidence of coronary heart disease, N Engl J Med 317:1237-1245, 1987.
43. Ganda OP: Pathogenesis of macrovascular disease in the human diabetic, Diabetes 29:931-942, 1980.
44. Garcia M and others: Morbidity and mortality in diabetes in the Framingham population: 16-year follow-up study, Diabetes 23:105-111, 1974.
45. Garg A and Grundy S: Nicotine acid as therapy for dyslipidemia in non–insulin-dependent diabetes mellitus, JAMA 264:723-726, 1990.
46. Gehani A and others: Experimental and clinical percutaneous angioscopy experience with dynamic angioplasty, Angiology 41:809-816, 1990.
47. Gerich J: Oral hypoglycemic agents, N Engl J Med 321:1231-1245, 1989.
48. Gianrossi R and others: Cardiac fluoroscopy for the diagnosis of coronary artery disease: a meta analytic review, Am Heart J 120:1179-1188, 1990.
49. Goldberg AC: Cholesterol and diabetes: modifying risks of heart disease, Clin Diabetes, 6:84-94, 1988.

50. Greene DA, Lattimer S, and Sima A: Sorbitol, phosphoinositides and sodium-potassium-ATPase in the pathogenesis of diabetic complications, N Engl J Med 316:599-606, 1987.

51. Grundy SM: Cholesterol and coronary heart disease: future directions, JAMA 264:3053-3059, 1990.

52. Haeften TW: Clinical significance of insulin antibodies in insulin-treated diabetic patients, Diabetes Care 12:641-648, 1989.

53. Haffner S and others: Cardiovascular risk factors in confirmed prediabetic individuals, JAMA, 263:2893-2898, 1990.

54. Haire-Joshu D: Smoking cessation and the diabetic health care team, Diabetes Educ 17:54-67, 1990.

55. Harris ML and others: Prevalence of diabetes and impaired glucose tolerance and plasma glucose levels in US population aged 20-74 years, Diabetes 36:523-534, 1987.

56. Hill AB: The environment and disease, association and causation, Proc R Soc Med 58:295-300, 1965.

57. Howard B and Howard W: The compelling case for smoking cessation in diabetes, Circulation 82:299-301, 1990.

58. Huse DM and others: The economic costs of non–insulin-dependent diabetes mellitus, JAMA 262:2708, 1989.

59. Jarrett RJ: Cardiovascular disease and hypertension in diabetes mellitus: Diabetes Metab Rev 5:547-558, 1989.

60. Jarrett R: Type II (non–insulin-dependent diabetes mellitus) and coronary heart disease—chicken, egg, or neither, Diabetogia 26:99-102, 1984.

61. Kannel WB: Coronary heart disease risk factors: Framingham study update, Hosp Pract 25:119-127, 1990.

62. Kannel WB and others: Diabetes, fibrinogen and risk of cardiovascular disease, the Frammingham experience, Am Heart J 120:672-676, 1990.

63. Kannel WB: Detection and management of patients with silent myocardial eschemia, Am Heart J 117:221, 1989.

64. Kannel WB and Sytkowski PA: Atherosclerosis risk factors, Pharmacol Ther 32:207-235, 1987.

65. Kannel WB and McGee DL: Diabetes and cardiovascular risk factors: the Frammingham Study, Circulation 59:8-13, 1979.

66. Kaplan N: The deadly quartet: upper-body obesity; glucose intolerance, hypertriglycerides, and hypertension, Arch Intern Med 149:1514-1520, 1989.

67. Kaplan N, Roserstock J, and Raskin MP: A differing view of treatment of hypertension in patients with diabetes mellitus, Arch Intern Med 147:1160-1162, 1987.

68. Kilo C, Miller J, and Williamson J: The crux of UGDP: spurious results and biologically inappropriate data analysis, Diabetologia 18:179-185, 1980.

69. Kissebah A and Schectman G: Polyunsaturated and saturated fat, cholesterol, and fatty acid supplementation, Diabetes Care 11:129-142, 1988.

70. Koistinen MJ: Prevalence of asymptomatic myocardial eschaemia in diabetic subjects, Br Med J 301:92-95, 1990.

71. Laing W and Williams R: Diabetes: a model for health care management, London, 1989, Office of Health Economics.

72. Leaf A and Ryan T: Prevention of coronary artery disease: a medical imperative, N Engl J Med 323:1416-1419, 1990.

73. Lebovitz H and Melander A, eds: Sulfonylurea drugs: basic and clinical consideration. Diabetes Care 13(suppl 3):1, 1990.

74. Lefemine A and Broach J: Noninvasive imaging and frequency analysis for carotid artery diagnosis and surgical decisions, Vas Surg 24:161-166, 1990.

75. Lipid Research Clinics Program: the lipid research clinic coronary primary prevention trial results. I . Reduction in incidence of coronary heart disease, JAMA, 251:351-364, 1984.

76. Lipson L: Special problems in treatment of hypertension in the patient with diabetes mellitus, Arch Intern Med 144:1829-1831, 1984.

77. Macrury S and Lowe G: Blood rheology in diabetes mellitus, Diabetic Med 7:285-291, 1990.

78. Maseri A: Medical therapy of chronic stable angina pectoris, Circulation 82:2258-2262, 1990.

79. Mason R and others: Diabetic astronomic neuropathy and cardiovascular risk, Arch Intern Med 150:1218-1222, 1990.

80. Mazzuca S: Does patient education in chronic disease have therapeutic value? J Chron Dis 35:521-529, 1982.

81. Modan H and others: Hyperisulinemia: a link between hypertension, obesity, and glucose intolerance, J Clin Invest 75:809-817, 1985.

82. Morrish N and others: A prospective study of mortality among middle-aged diabetic patients (the London cohort of the UNO Multinational Study of Vascular Disease in Diabetics). I. Causes and death rates, Diabetologia 33:538-541, 1990.

83. Morrison A, Clements R, and Winegrad A: Effects of elevated glucose concentrations on the metabolism of the aortic wall, J Clin Invest 51:3114-3123, 1972.

84. Moser M: Suppositions and speculations—their possible effects on treatment decisions in the management of hypertension, Am Heart J 118:1362-1369, 1989.

85. Moy C and others: Insulin-dependent diabetes mellitus mortality: the risk of cigarette smoking, Circulation 82:37-43, 1990.

86. Multiple Risk Factor Intervention Trial Research Group: Mortality after 10½ years for hypertensive participants in the multiple risk factor intervention trial, Circulation 82:1616-1627, 1990.

87. Multiple Risk Factor Intervention Trial Reserach Group: Coronary heart disease death, non-fatal acute myocardial infarction and other clinical outcomes in the multiple risk factor intervention trial, Am J Cardiol 58:1-13, 1986.

88. Multiple Risk Factor Intervention Trial: Risk factor changes and mortality results, JAMA 248:1465-1477, 1982.

89. National Institute of Health Consensus Development Conference: Health implications of obesity, Ann Int Med 103:981-1077, 1985.

90. Newman J: Smoking in the diabetic population, Diabetes 39:208A, 1990.

91. Olsson T and others: Prognosis after stroke in diabetic patients. A controlled prospective study, Diabetologia 33:244-249, 1990.

92. Pecoraro R, Reiber G, and Burgess E: Pathways to diabetic limb amputation: basis for prevention, Diabetes Care 13:513-521, 1990.

93. Pederson O: The impact of obesity on the pathogenesis of non–insulin-dependent diabetes mellitus: a review of current hypothesis, Diabetes Metab Rev 5:494-509, 1989.

94. Peto R and others: Randomized trial of prophylactic daily aspirin in British male doctors, Br Med J 196:313-316, 1988.

95. Pietri A, Dunn F, and Raskin P: The effect of improved diabetic control in plasma lipid and lipoprotein levels: a comparison of conventional therapy and continuous subcutaneous insulin infusion, Diabetes 29:1001-1005, 1980.

96. Posevitz L, Greer S, and Kovacs P: Laser-assisted balloon angioplasty: analysis of 132 clinical cases, Vasc Surg 24:377-381, 1990.

97. Pyorala K, Laakso M, and Usitupa M: Diabetes and atheroclerosis: an epidemiologic view, Diabetes Metab Rev 3:463-524, 1987.

98. Pyorala K: Relationship of glucose tolerance and plasma insulin to the incidence of coronary artery disease: results from two population studies in Finland, Diabetes Care 2:131-141, 1976.

99. Reaven G: Role of insulin resistence in human disease, Diabetes 37:1595-1607, 1988.

100. Reaven GM: Abnormal lipoprotein metabolism in NIDDM, Am J Med 83(53A):31-39, 1987.

101. Report of the National Cholesterol Education Program: Expert panel on detection, evaluation, and treatment of high blood cholesterol in adults, Arch Intern Med 148:36-69, 1988.

102. Rifkin B: Cholesterol redux, JAMA 264:3060-3061, 1990.

103. Rosenstock IM: Understanding and enhancing patient compliance with diabetic regimens, Diabetes Care 8:610-616, 1985.

103a. Rosenstock J: Surgery: practical guidelines for diabetes management, Clin Diabetes 5:49-61, 1987.

104. Ruderman N and Schneider S: Exercise and the insulin-dependent diabetic, Hosp Pract 21:41-51, 1986.

105. Salomon M and others: Diabetes mellitus and coronary artery bypass: short-term and long-term prognosis, J Thorac Cardiovasc Surg 85:264-271, 1983.

106. Saudek C: When does diabetes start? JAMA 263:2934, 1990.

107. Shuman C: Management of the diabetic patient undergoing surgery, Cardiovasc Rev and Rep 3:1119-1124, 1982.

108. Sima A and others: Regeneration and repair of myelinated fibers in sural nerve biopsy specimens from patients with diabetic neuropathy treated with sorbinil, N Engl J Med 319:548-555, 1988.

109. Skarfors E, Weyerner T, and Lithell H: Physical training as treatment for Type II (non-insulin-dependent) diabetes in elderly men: a feasibility study over 2 years, Diabetologia 30:930-933, 1987.

110. Smith J, Marcus F, and Serokman R: Prognosis of patients with diabetes mellitus after acute myocardial infarction, Am J Cardiol 54:718-722, 1974.

111. Steering Committee of the Physicians' Health Study Research Group: Final report on the aspirin component of the Ongoing Physicians' Health Study, N Engl J Med 321:129-135, 1989.

112. Stout R: Insulin and atheroma: 20 year perspective, Diabetes Care 13:631-654, 1990.

113. The Health Benefits of Smoking Cessation: A report of the Surgeon General, DHHS, PHS, CDC, CCD-PHP, OSN, Pub No 90-8416, Rockville, Md, 1990, US Department of Health & Human Services.

114. The 1984 report of the Joint National Committee of Detection, Evaluation, and Treatment of High Blood Pressure, Arch Intern Med 144:1045-1057, 1984.

115. Trost BH: Hypertension in the diabetic patient. Selection and optimum use of antihypertensive drug, Drugs 38:621-633, 1989.

116. Tyroler H: Lowering plasma cholesterol levels decreases risk of coronary heart disease: an overview of clinical trials. In Steinberg D and Olefsky J, eds: Hypercholesterolemia and Atherosclerosis, New York, 1987, Churchill Livingstone, Inc.

117. Uusitupa M and others: Five year incidence of atherosclerotic vascular disease in relation to general risk factors, insulin levels, and abnormalities in lipoprotein composition in non–insulin-dependent diabetic and non-diabetic subjects, Circulation 82:27-36, 1990.

118. Weinberger M and others: Economic impact of diabetes mellitus in the elderly, Clin Geriatr Med 6:959-970, 1990.

119. Williams RB and others: Type A behavior, hostility and coronary atherosclerosis, Psychosom Med 42:539-549, 1980.

120. Wing R: Behavioral strategies for weight reduction in obese Type II diabetic patients, Diabetes Care 12:139-144, 1989.

121. Working Group on Hypertension in Diabetes: Statement on hypertension in diabetes: final report, Arch Intern Med 127:830-842, 1987.

122. Zimmit P: Primary prevention of diabetes mellitus, Diabetes Care 11:258-262, 1988.

CHAPTER 7

Foot Care and Diabetes

WILLIAM C. COLEMAN

Persons with diabetes are at significant risk for lower-extremity amputation. Such procedures are approximately 15 times more common among persons with diabetes than among those without diabetes. During the 1980s, there was an annual rate of 100,000 lower-extremity amputations in the United States. Although only about 5% of the United States population has diabetes mellitus, one-half of these amputations are performed on patients with diabetes.[55] Roughly half of these amputees will develop a limb-threatening condition of the contralateral limb within 18 months and will require amputation in 3 to 5 years.[37,45] Pecoraro and colleagues surveyed 80 consecutive diabetic foot amputations and found that an initial episode of minor trauma that resulted in cutaneous ulceration with subsequent failure to heal the wound preceded 72% of amputations.[60]

Prevention of foot problems is therefore a primary consideration for diabetes care and practice. Once problems occur, protocols to curb the rate of diabetic foot amputation must be carefully monitored. The purpose of this chapter, then, is to describe the pathology of foot problems; discuss causes of foot problems of a direct and concomitant nature; summarize procedures for assessing foot care risk; evaluate strategies for managing foot problems; and discuss the importance of preventing recurrence as it relates particularly to education and the diabetes health care team.

PATHOLOGY

Diabetes mellitus is the abnormality that produces pathologic changes associated with angiopathy and neuropathy. This process is highlighted in Fig. 7-1. Of these two secondary complications that affect the feet, three to five times as many patients are admitted as a result of painless foot trauma as for ischemic pain.[46]

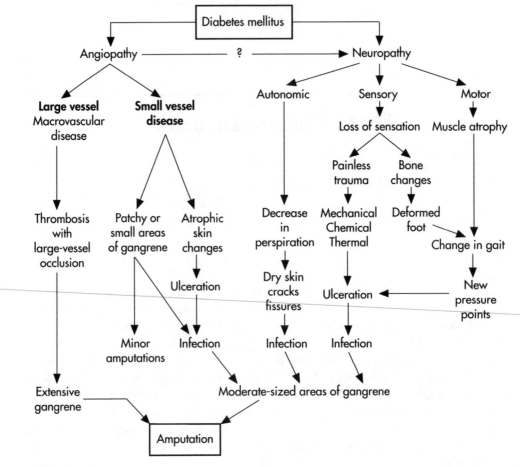

Fig. 7-1 Pathogenesis of diabetic foot lesions. (From Levin ME and O'Neal LW, eds: The diabetic foot, St Louis, 1988, CV Mosby Co.)

Angiopathy

Persons with diabetes are more likely to develop arteriosclerosis and atheromatous occlusion in the lower extremities than persons without diabetes. In addition, when arteriosclerosis develops in a person with diabetes, its progression is more rapid than that in nondiabetics and occurs at a younger age and equally in women and men. The most frequently involved vessels in diabetes are located below the knee. The result is that the normally extensive collateral circulation in the foot is compromised by the multiple complete and partial arteriosclerotic blockages of large, medium-sized, and small arteries. This results in a situation comparable to end arteries, such as the heart or kidney, becoming blocked.

Once arteriosclerotic disease is present in the small vessels in the foot, there is minimal effective means of curing the problem (see Chapter 5). Thickening of the basement membrane, increased platelet adhesion, increased viscosity of the plasma, high fibrinogen

Table 7-1 Differences in Diabetes- and Nondiabetes-Related Peripheral Vascular Disease

	Persons with diabetes	Persons without diabetes
Clinical	More common	Less common
	Younger patient	Older patient
	More rapid	Less rapid
Male/female ratio	2:1	30:1
Occlusion	Multisegmental	Single segment
Vessels adjacent to occlusion	Involved	Not involved
Collateral vessels	Involved	Usually normal
Lower extremities	Both	Unilateral
Vessels involved	Tibial artery	Aortic artery
	Perineal artery	Iliac artery
	Small vessels	Femoral artery
	Arterioles	
Gangrene	Patchy areas of foot and toes	Extensive
In-hospital mortality with amputation	Approximately 3%	Significantly less

Adapted from Levin M, and O'Neal LW: The diabetic foot, St. Louis, 1988, Mosby–Year Book.

levels, injury to the endothelium, and changes in fibrinolysis are some of the postulated causes for small-vessel disease.[39] In addition, the person with diabetes frequently has bilateral involvement, with multiple occlusions. This is different from the person without diabetes in whom the lesions are thought to be localized and unilateral (see Table 7-1).[24]

The primary signs of a decrease in blood flow include hair loss, shiny or atrophic skin changes, cold feet, feet and ankles that are darker in color than the leg, and dependent rubor. Symptoms that consistently result from decreased blood flow are summarized in the box below and include intermittent claudication or rest pain relieved by standing or walking.

SIGNS AND SYMPTOMS OF PERIPHERAL VASCULAR DISEASE

Intermittent claudication (pedal pulses usually absent)
Nocturnal and rest pain relieved with dependency
Shiny appearance of skin
Loss of hair on feet and toes
Failure of a wound to respond to appropriate treatment
Absent pulses
Blanching on elevation
Delayed venous filling after elevation

Dependent rubor
Thickened nails, often with fungal infections
Calcification of blood vessels
Gangrene
Miscellaneous
  Blue toe syndrome
  Acute vascular occlusion

Neuropathy

An individual with diabetes may not experience any pain, even with serious vascular disease, because neuropathy can diminish the feeling or perception of these symptoms. As previously noted, more diabetic patients are admitted to hospitals for neuropathic injuries than for painful ischemia.[38] (See Chapter 5 for a discussion of types of neuropathy.) For several decades, health professionals have been observing this process of injury and have been referring to it as a "trophic" change to the tissue. The term neuropathic may be more appropriate as research is yet to document the exact component of the tissue that has been adversely affected by diabetes.

Neuropathy is associated with the lack of the senses of touch and pain that provide gait protection (see box on the opposite page). Without this protection the insensate tissues break down, in part because they are subjected to stresses greater than normal. Most amputations ultimately result from this sensory loss, particularly related to pain and temperature sensations. The nerve impairment, and resulting continuous trauma, lead to ulcer development and infection, further compromising an already stressed vascular system, as is depicted in Fig. 7-1. Involvement of the autonomic nervous system also leads to foot lesions as a result of the absence of sweating, leading to dry cracking, and fissured skin and infection.

In other forms of diabetic neuropathy, individuals often experience paresthesia or burning sensations in their feet. Persons with diabetes who develop neuropathic foot ulcers, however, rarely have such feelings.[67,68]

Responses to touch and pain

In order to successfully manage the foot problems of the majority of insensate patients, the diabetes team should understand how the psychology of sensory loss affects the behavior of patients. At birth, our senses of touch and pain are our most developed senses. As the other senses become more fully developed, touch and pain become more of a background means of monitoring the environment.

Hundreds of thousands of touch and pain receptors cover the entire surface of the body. These receptors form a protective boundary between the person and the environment. Mentally a body image is established. When we are touched or when a painful stimulus penetrates this boundary, we are touched psychologically as well as physically. This effect has been demonstrated in work by Fisher and colleagues[30] that suggests that even the slightest touch alters the individual's perception of other people and their surroundings. Other work showed that touch not only affects perception but can be used to manipulate behavior as well.[41] For example, when touch accompanied a request for return of a missing coin, the likelihood of its return was almost 96% in comparison to 63% when touch did not accompany the request.

It is difficult to measure the degree to which levels of communication are lost when sensation is diminished. Portions of the body that have become insensitive appear to be

SIGNS AND SYMPTOMS OF
———————— PERIPHERAL NEUROPATHY ————————

Paresthesia
Hyperesthesia
Hypoesthesia
Loss of deep tendon reflexes
Loss of vibratory, cutaneous pressure, temperature, or position sense
Anhidrosis
Heavy callus formation over pressure points
Trophic ulcers
Foot drop
Changes in shape of foot
   Muscle atrophy
Changes in bone and joint
Radiographic signs*
   Demineralization
   Osteolysis
   Neuropathic fracture

*It may be difficult to distinguish these radiographic findings from osteomyelitis.

perceived as somewhat "disassociated" from the body. Injury to the insensitive parts become less important and less personalized to the individual since there is a loss of painful sensation. Health care providers unaccustomed to managing insensitivity often remark on their surprise at how insensate patients will have had an injury for several days or weeks prior to coming to a clinic for attention. Frequently this is because the first indication to the patient that an insensitive foot has become injured is an observed trail of blood on the floor. The patient becomes confused in trying to remember when this injury could have occurred and in most cases will not be able to recall any particular incident.

CAUSES OF FOOT PROBLEMS

The ability to characterize, localize, and identify pain is often the beginning of a process of diagnosis. Pain is an important mechanism whereby prognosis is evaluated. When the sense of pain is diminished, so is this mechanism of clinical evaluation. For example, a person in pain would be far more insistent on obtaining some form of treatment that will result in eliminating the pain than one without such a sensation. In addition, the physician will be highly motivated in reducing the pain to improve the patient's sense of well-being.

Mechanical Causes of Injury

There is a direct correlation between the amount of mechanical stress, the time the stress is applied, and the breakdown of tissue being stressed.[43,64] High pressures result in damage quickly, while lower pressures have to be applied for a longer time to damage the tissues.

In the sensate person, the inflammatory process is a part of the healing process. First, the inflammation often causes discomfort that causes the sensate injured person to limit activity at the site of inflammation. In contrast, the insensate patient will continue to use the inflamed part without restriction, further amplifying the inflammation. Ultimately, then, the inflammatory process becomes destructive to the involved tissues in the insensate person.

Second, fluids accumulate in injured feet. These fluids can be localized and infected areas can be surrounded by white cells as long as motion and pressure are kept to a minimum. One would expect limited motion in the sensate person, since it is the sense of pain that demands limited use of an injured foot.[51] Since the insensate person does not feel pain as readily, walking or other mechanical trauma continues causing pressure, forcing these fluids into previously involved tissues. This movement of fluid is further complicated by the pull of the tendons when the foot is moved. Fluids and bacteria adjacent to the tendon can be carried to new areas within the foot. A person with an injured, sensate foot "splints" the tendons, holding the joint immobile. An insensate patient will not, which increases the possibility of infection.

Based on this mechanical process of injury, Brand identified three distinct forms of injury to human soft tissues that come as a result of mechanical stress.[16]

High-pressure (penetrating wounds)
The first form of insensate foot injury from mechanical stress is the result of a very high-pressure penetrating wound. These are injuries any of us might experience by stepping on a small object of sufficient height to break through the skin, such as a piece of glass, a thumbtack, or a nail. (It takes a pressure of 600 to 900 pounds per square inch to break through the adult skin of the sole of the foot).[70]

In contrast to persons with normal sensation, those with insensitivity may not even feel the penetrating wound occur. They may continue to walk with the object imbedded in the bottom of the foot, resulting in repetitive crushing of the wound site. Each step will thus result in a constant increase of inflammation and further injury.

Low-pressure (ischemic necrosis)
Mechanical stress can cause injuries that result from very low pressure applied for a long period. This form of ulcer may result because of unrelenting low pressure (2 to 8 pounds per square inch) to the tissues for a long time (12 to 16 hours).[14] The usual causes of this type of injury would include shoes that do not fit precisely.[14] Such footwear creates pressure that pushes blood from the capillaries as the skin is compressed between the leather of the shoe and a bony prominent area of the foot. The tissues break down in a

manner similar to decubitus ulceration of immobilized patients. The low stress occludes the dermal capillaries.[14,25,47] The usual location for these ulcers are the toes, the metatarsal heads, and the styloid process at the base of the fifth metatarsal.

Moderate repetitive pressure (plantar ulceration)

The most common form of injury to insensitive feet comes as a result of the repetitive stress of walking.[15,17] Pressures generated under the foot by walking range from 20 to 80 pounds per square inch. Injury from the repetitive stress of walking usually develops when the tissues are subjected to a higher level of stress, either by walking faster or further than the tissues are used to. When normal sensation is present, a person who walks more than they have become accustomed to will have sore feet. To continue walking comfortably, this person will begin altering his or her gait and thus the way in which the foot meets the ground. The areas of the foot that are being perceived as uncomfortable can then be "rested" as the person continues to walk.

In contrast, the person with insensate feet can develop foot ulcers, since a feeling of discomfort is not perceived in the insensitive foot. The person with insensate feet has no reason to alter the way the foot meets the ground. Thus, the sore part of the foot is subjected to continuing stress with each step. The repetitive stress, the inflammatory process, and the associated accumulation of white blood cells cause tissue breakdown.[14,15] Leukocytes release lytic enzymes into severely inflamed tissues, with the accumulation of these substances eventually serving to weaken the soft-tissue structure.

Further understanding of the effects of repetitive stress are found in the work of Manly and Darby who found that an increase in repetitions resulted in earlier ulcerations.[50] They applied repetitive stress to the bottom of the feet of 45 neurectomized rats and 45 rats with nerves intact.[50] When subjected to the same levels or repetitive stress, the neuropathic feet ulcerated more easily than the normal rat feet. Subsequent to each test, the temperature of the normal feet averaged 1.2° C warmer than the feet of the rats with neurectomy. They proposed that this observation may have indicated more capillary perfusion in the feet with intact neural pathways to dilate vessels of sympathic innervation. With more perfusion, fewer metabolites, more cell debris, and less edema, fluid would remain in the tissues. In contrast, ulceration can be prevented by decreasing repetitive stress and allowing rest days.[16]

Locations of Ulcerations

Areas more likely to ulcerate are the forefoot areas of highest pressure.[5,11,51] The most frequent locations of ulcers formed as a result of repetitive walking stress are the first toe and the metatarsal heads.[26,61,66] Boulton and colleagues found patients with neuropathy develop significantly higher pressures under the metatarsal heads than normal sensate persons with or without diabetes.[29] Neuropathic subjects with limited joint motion at the subtarsal joint and the first metatarsophalangeal joint may also have much higher focal pressures. Sixty-five percent of the insensate patients with limited joint motion had a history of plantar ulceration.[14,29] Twenty percent of patients with neuropathy but normal subtalar and the first metatarsophalangeal motion had previous plantar ulceration.[29,49] Thus, limited joint mobility may predispose neuropathic feet to ulcers by concentrating pressure at susceptible sites.[22,49]

Infection and Diabetes

It is commonly reported that persons with diabetes mellitus are more susceptible to infection than cohorts with diabetes. The research on this topic is conflicting without actual evidence of impaired immunologic competence in persons with diabetes.[20] Despite the lack of specific epidemiologic evidence of increased infection, or identification of a biochemical defect, many clinicians support the use of antibiotics as important to the long-term health of the persons with diabetes.

While it is difficult to document overall increases in infection in diabetes, there are organisms to which the person with diabetes may be predisposed.[9] This predisposition may be mediated by alterations in host defenses, vascular insufficiency that limits infection fighting, and neurologic abnormalities that limit awareness of trauma or inflammation, as previously described.

Diabetic foot infections are one of the most frequent problems faced by the persons with diabetes. Bacterial and fungal infections of the skin are the most common found in persons with diabetes. The exact mechanisms, as previously noted, are unclear. Hyperglycemia per se, however, does not increase the growth rate of the pathogens.

Levin[45] characterizes patients who are at most risk for foot infections as: the elderly, those with peripheral neuropathy, and those who have neglected the infection for more than a month. In addition to the neuropathic ulcers that have been previously described, other common infections of the foot include:

Infections of the nails

Various organisms can result in nail infections, a common finding in diabetes. Not all infections are caused by fungal organisms, although various types of fungi (e.g., *Candida albicans*) are frequently associated with nail infections. Infected nails, depending upon the extent of the infection, appear discolored and can thicken or become elevated. In final stages of infection, the nail plate crumbles or is traumatically removed.[12,45]

Osteomyelitis

This is one of the most serious problems associated with care of the diabetic foot. It occurs commonly in diabetes, frequently beginning as a chronic perforating ulcer. The recurrence of such ulcers, poor tissue nutrition, and decreased antimicrobial defenses predispose to osteomyelitis. Treatment focuses on antibiotic therapy with surgery necessary in some cases to excise dead bone.[12,45]

Plantar space abscess

This is a lesion characterized by swelling and redness in the sole of the foot that may or may not be tender.[12,45]

Infected vascular gangrene

Vascular insufficiency produces necrosis of distal tissue (dry gangrene) that may be secondarily infected (wet gangrene). Clinically the lesion is often black and produces a foul odor. Amputation is generally the only form of treatment.[12,45]

Gas-forming infection

Gas gangrene is a fulminating, life-threatening infection caused by clostridia. The disease presents rapidly, generally within 3 days, and is characterized by necrotic, edematous skin. Antibiotics are supplemental to surgery.[12,45]

General Infections

Some of the other more common general infections that reportedly occur in diabetes are not directly related to foot care. However, they do compromise overall health status and provide an opportunity for spread of infection. These include the following conditions.

Urinary tract infections

Bacteriuria is 2 to 4 times more likely in women with diabetes than in controls, an incidence not apparent in males. The presence of urinary tract infections that are untreated or treated ineffectively can lead to additional problems such as pyelonephritis, perinephric abscess, and papillary necrosis. Fungal infections of the urinary tract are also commonly found. Candida leads to cystitis, pyelonephritis, or renal abscesses.[20]

Tuberculosis

Tuberculosis is more prevalent in persons with diabetes when compared with the general population. The prognosis is generally good, but poorly controlled diabetes has been associated with predisposition to reactivation of TB.

Bacterial pneumonia

This is frequently caused by staphylococcus aureus or *Klebsiella pneumoniae*. The mortality rate for such pneumonias can be high, particularly in persons with diabetes.[20]

Malignant external otitis

This infection is unique to elderly persons with diabetes. Although the cause is unclear, underlying microangiopathy is thought to be a cause, with the resultant persistent ear pain and drainage requiring surgery and long-term antibiotic therapy for treatment.[20]

In summary, there are conflicting data as to the increased prevalence of infection in general in persons with diabetes. However, what is clear is that any infection can have devastating effects, particularly if it is not identified quickly and treated aggressively. The seriousness of the infection may be underestimated because of the compromised sensory system of persons with diabetes, suggesting again the need for thorough and regular health assessments of all persons with diabetes and the critical importance of thorough patient education.

Skin Disorders

The condition of the skin provides clues to the presence of diabetes mellitus, such as frequency of infection, joint contractures, pruritis, and dryness.[24,46] The skin of the person with diabetes may have structural differences, including increased numbers of mast cells and increased capillary fragility. For this reason, persons with diabetes are prone to various skin infections more frequently than are persons without diabetes. Discussion of the diabetic foot and leg would therefore be incomplete without inclusion of the skin lesions classically seen in the lower extremity of the person with diabetes. Although not intended to be all inclusive, a review of some of the more common skin lesions found in persons with diabetes appears in Table 7-2.

ASSESSING RISK

As reported earlier, programs that incorporate patient education and early identification of injury have a major impact on the reduction of diabetic foot amputations. Through the multidisciplinary approach, members of medical organizations have the best opportunity to develop comprehensive programs of injury prevention and early treatment.

Foot Care Protocol

The best means of saving the diabetic foot involves several steps. These include: identification of the feet at risk; prevention of foot ulcers; treatment of foot ulcers; and prevention of recurrence of foot ulcers.[2,3]

The patient with peripheral vascular disease or distal symmetrical polyneuropathy, as described in Chapter 5, is at severe risk for foot problems. As was noted in the box on p. 217, signs and symptoms of vascular disease in the lower extremity should be carefully assessed at each patient visit. Examination of the feet should be routine and should include removal of shoes and socks. Thus, a systematic foot care protocol should be followed. Although foot assessment should include observation of mobility, hydration, color, swelling or edema, temperature, sensation, and nail formation as a routine diabetes care practice, the presence of structural deformities or lesions is also necessary. A sample foot assessment protocol including teaching outline appears in Appendix 7a.

Sensory assessment

Fundamental to a prevention program is a quantifiable means of testing patients for the presence or absence of protective levels of sensation.[20] Protective levels of sensation

Table 7-2 Common Skin Disorders in Diabetes Mellitus

Skin disorder	Symptoms
Primary skin disorders in diabetes mellitus	
Diabetic dermopathy	Small atrophic, red-brown, sharply circumscribed lesion; occurs on anterior skins in 50% of patients. Affects men more than women, generally after age 50.
Joint contractures	Thick, waxy skin overlying joints; noted in almost 30% of IDDM patients.
	Increased dermal collagen yields waxy texture; increased risk for microvascular disease.
Necrobiosis lipoidica	Asymptomatic plaque on unilateral or bilateral skins. Nonulcerated, yellowish, sclerotic plaque. Affects women more frequently than men, occurs in 3% of persons with diabetes.
Lipodystrophy	Mass of scar and fatty tissue caused by hypertrophy of subcutaneous fatty tissue leading to muscle hyperdevelopment. Found at site of insulin injections. Incidence low with advent of purified insulins.
Pruritis	Generalized itching, commonly affects feet and eyes. Occurs without evidence of preexisting inflammatory disease.
Bulbosis diabeticorium	Lesions of feet consisting of two types: acute superficial blister and deeper hemorrhagic type leading to skin necrosis. Mechanism for development unknown, but associated with poor diabetes control.
Insulin resistance	
Acanthosis nigricans	Hyperpigmented, evenly thickened and folded skin of flexural body regions.
Abnormal lipid levels	
Eruptive xanthomas	Multiple yellow-red and yellow-orange papules; located over joints, buttocks, and trunk; clears with good control.
Xanthelasma	Irregular plaques over eyelids.
	Most common type of xanthoma.
	Begins as pinpoint-sized yellow-orange spots that coalesce and become thicker.
Xanthochromia	Yellowish skin discoloration accompanied by increase in carotene and blood cholesterol. Rare condition, located on sole of foot.

Modified from Haire-Joshu D: Endocrine system. In Beare PG, and Myers JL, eds: Principles and practice of adult health nursing, St. Louis, 1990, Mosby–Year Book.

are defined as adequate touch and pain sensation to prevent injuries caused by sensory loss and to prevent the continued use of an injured part to a degree to cause further injury. The best means of doing this involves a procedure that uses vibration, pressure, touch, and proprioception.[46]

Vibration

A 128 cycle tuning fork touched to each toe should result in a perception of vibration for not less than 15 seconds and usually for 20 to 25 seconds.

Pressure

Semmes-Weinstein monofilaments are currently the most common form of quantifiable testing in use today. These are a set of nylon filaments similar to the bristles of a nylon brush. Each filament is the same length but varies in thickness, this difference in thickness requiring a different force to bend them. Usually a thickness of 5.07 is used. The test is performed by applying a force to one end of the filament and pressing the other end against the patient's skin. The patient is requested by the tester to report when the pressure from the filament is felt. By not touching the patient with a filament every time, by varying the rate at which the filaments are applied, and by not following a regular pattern of sites to be tested, reliability can be increased.[65]

Touch

This is a simple modification of the traditional pinprick test. The end of a cotton swab is used to evaluate sensitivity to blunt touch. The cotton end is used to evaluate blunt touch and the sharp point for sharp perception.

Proprioception

For this test, the toes are moved up and down. Patients with significant neuropathy will be unable to determine position in space. In addition, delayed venous or capillary filling time can be measured by having the patient lie supine with feet elevated to a 45 degree angle until one or both feet blanch. The patient then sits upright with the feet dependent until the color returns to normal, which should occur in 15 seconds or less. A filling time longer than this indicates moderate to severe ischemia.

Risk Categories

Once protective sensory loss can be identified, diabetic patients can then be categorized according to their risk of being injured. In this way, resources can be assigned to focus attention on the "at risk" patients. Such a program has been evolving at the Hansen's Disease Center in Carville, Louisiana for almost 10 years.[20] The risk categories used by the team at Carville are noted in Table 7-3 and described below.

Risk category zero

Patients assigned to risk category 0 have a disease process, such as diabetes, that has the potential to result in sensory loss. These patients have not yet lost protective sensation. They should have their sensory status evaluated each year and be educated concerning sensory loss, footwear selection, smoking, diabetes control, and other possible risk factors. The need for proper footwear selection is discussed with these patients at every visit, (e.g., for women, do not wear high heels). However, an overemphasis of proper footwear at this relatively low-risk time can also result in the person with diabetes resisting footwear changes at a later time when the risk from shoe injuries is much greater. For example, when educating women who are in category 0, some of them may respond better to a gradual change from tapered toes and high heels.[20]

Table 7-3   Risk Categories and Associated Footwear Guidelines

	Clinical findings	Footwear changes
Category 0	Has protective sensation	Education on proper footwear
Category 1	Has lost protective sensation	Add a soft insole to a shoe of proper contour and fit
Category 2	Has lost protective sensation and has a foot deformity	Depth footwear or custom shoe for severe deformity, molded insoles
Category 3	Has lost protective sensation and has a history of foot ulcer	Inspect the type and condition of footwear and insoles at every visit

Risk category one

Patients in category 1 differ from category 0 patients by demonstrating loss of protective levels of sensation. With their higher risk, footwear is examined much more carefully. The shape of the shoes should be compared with the shape of the foot. If there is adequate room inside the shoe, a thin soft insole can help protect the bottom of the foot. Category 1 patients should break in new shoes gradually until the upper leather parts conform to the shape of the foot. They are educated in foot inspection and early wound care. An appointment for foot examination is arranged every 6 months to assist the patient by looking for skin temperature changes or changes in foot morphology.

Risk category two

Category 2 patients have not only lost sensation but have limited joint mobility or deformity that creates focal points of pressure under the foot. Footwear and shoe inserts become even more important at this level of risk. Most of these patients require custom inserts and prescription footwear. In some cases, shoes custom-made for the foot are needed only in cases of severe foot deformity or partial foot amputation. Surgical correction of deformity may be considered to lower the patient's risk of injury. Clinical foot inspections are performed with footwear evaluation every 3 months.[20]

Risk category three

Patients in category 3 are at highest risk of developing skin ulcers and have a history of previous ulceration. These patients should be in molded inserts for their shoes and if they also have foot deformity in prescription shoes. The condition of the shoes and inserts need to be inspected by a health team member trained in footwear form and function at every visit. Often the shoes of insensate patients wear down and threaten the foot if not kept in proper repair. Their return appointments come every 1 to 2 months to prevent recurrence of ulcers.[20]

EDUCATION AND PREVENTION OF FOOT ULCERS
Guidelines for Teaching

Patients with diabetes must learn how to protect their feet. By identifying level of risk, education can be tailored to meet the particular needs of the person with diabetes. These

_____ **PATIENT INSTRUCTIONS FOR DIABETIC FOOT CARE** _____

Foot care

Do not use tobacco.

Inspect your feet daily for blisters, cuts, and scratches.

Use a mirror to see the bottom of the feet. Always check between the toes for dryness, redness, tenderness, and localized areas that rub (hot spots).

Inspect the inside of your shoes daily for foreign objects, nail points, torn linings, and rough areas.

Wash feet daily. Dry carefully, especially between the toes.

Avoid temperature extremes. Test water with elbow before bathing.

Soak feet only if specifically prescribed by your health care provider. For dry feet, use a very thin coat of lubricating cream or oil. Apply this after bathing and drying the feet. Do not put the oil or cream between the toes.

If feet are cold at night, wear socks to bed. Do not apply hot water bottles or heating pads or soak feet in hot water.

Cut nails in contour with the toes. Do not cut deep down the sides or corners.

Do not use chemical agents for the removal of corns and calluses. Do not use corn plasters.

Do not cut corns and calluses. These should be treated regularly by an experienced health care provider.

Do not use adhesive tape on your feet.

If your vision is impaired, have a family member or friend inspect your feet and shoes daily or assist with foot care.

Footwear

Avoid walking barefoot or in thongs or sandals if your feet are insensitive.

Avoid wearing open-toed shoes or sandals unless specifically prescribed by a health care provider.

principles of education fall into three categories: general foot care principles, knowledge of types of footwear, and preventive care instructions, including involvement with the health care provider. An example of a foot care assessment protocol appears in Appendix 7a. A teaching outline, which addresses critical components to be included by the educator in any foot care program appears in Appendix 7b. Specific care instructions for the patient appear in the box above.

Finally, the time with the patient should be used to explore various methods of encouraging foot care as a diabetes management priority.[2,33,37,46] This includes the use of various educational methods, such as those addressed in Chapter 15.

Footwear

As previously noted, insensate patients should always wear footwear with a sole thick enough to absorb the potential penetrating object. This would mean that footwear should

_____ **PATIENT INSTRUCTIONS FOR DIABETIC FOOT CARE**—cont'd _____

Preventive care instructions

Never walk barefoot on surfaces such as hot sandy beaches or on the cement or asphalt around swimming pools that are often hot; you may not be able to feel the increased temperature.

Wear clean and properly fitting socks or stocking at all times with your shoes. Avoid wearing mended socks or stockings with seams.

Avoid wearing garters, elastic bands on socks, and/or rolling hose.

Avoid crossing your legs; this can cause pressure on nerves and blood vessels.

Shoes should be properly measured and should fit at the time of purchase. Shoes should be made of material that breathes, such as leather.

Avoid pointed toes or high-heeled shoes.

If your feet have decreased sensation, rotate your shoes 3 to 4 times/day. Before putting on your shoes, check the insides of the shoes by hand to ensure that there are no rough surfaces (e.g., nail heads) and no small objects (e.g., pebbles, coins) in your shoes.

Wear appropriate shoes for the weather. In winter, take special precautions such as wearing wool socks and protective foot gear, e.g., fleece-lined boots.

Stay in contact with your healthcare provider

See your physician or podiatrist regularly and be sure that your feet are examined at each visit.

Notify your health care provider at once if you develop a blister, sore, or crack in the skin of your feet.

---

be worn around the household, in the yard, or any time the patient is walking. Depth footwear has extra vertical space within the shoe. A wide variety of these types of footwear are now available "off-the-shelf" to make room for contracted toes or thicker insoles. However, neuropathy can result in loss of motor control as well as sensory pathology. The most common early sign of motor involvement is claw-toe deformity resulting from intrinsic muscle paralysis. This deformity requires extra room in the shoe to prevent toe ulcers.[6,7]

The option of therapeutic footwear should be explored with persons with diabetes in general and, more specifically, those at high risk for foot problems. Footwear is one of the most critically important components of preventing injury to insensate feet. In a survey of previously ulcerated diabetic patients, Edmonds and associates found that among people who continued to wear special shoes, 26% had reulcerated their feet. Of those who reverted to using their former shoes, 83% reulcerated.[27]

Since plantar forefoot ulceration caused by repetitive stress is the most common form of insensate foot injury, outer shoe sole modifications[53,61] such as a curved roller or single fulcrum rocker 5 are being incorporated into the shoe design to reduce walking pressures under the forefoot. Inserts molded to the shape of the plantar aspect of the foot help to reduce focal pressures by increasing the areas of weight bearing over more of the foot. The need and availability of special footwear should be carefully examined with the podiatrist or physician. Criteria for therapeutic shoe design are summarized in the box below.

MANAGEMENT OF FOOT PROBLEMS

The identification of foot problems is a direct result of the assessment process. These data should then be used to identify treatment guidelines for the various foot problems commonly associated with diabetes. General guidelines for treatment appear in Appendix 7a. More specific aspects of treatment, especially related to ulcer care, are as follows.

Grading Ulcers

Despite education, 15% of all people with diabetes mellitus will develop foot ulcers.[58] Wagner and associates developed a system of classifying skin ulcers on diabetic feet that is used worldwide[66] (see Table 7-4). Briefly, grade 0 described feet that are not ulcerated but may have skeletal deformities, while a grade 1 lesion is an ulcer involving first the epidermis, exposing the dermis with either a necrotic or a viable base. Grade 2 ulcers penetrate to bone, tendons, or a joint, while a grade 3 lesion involves abscess or osteomyelitis. Some part of the toes or forefoot are gangrenous with grade 4. Grade 5 is a generally gangrenous foot requiring amputation.

When an ulcer is encountered, the would should be classified according to Wagners criteria. The circumference and depth should be recorded, perhaps be recording the ulcer on film. Look for evidence of purulence, necrosis, odor, edema, cellulitis, or abscess.

_____ **CRITERIA FOR THERAPEUTIC SHOE DESIGN** _____

Critical conditions
Insensitivity
Multiple hammertoes, claw foot, cocked-toe deformity
Charcot feet
Bunions, calluses, and other deformities
Previously ulcerated or partially amputated feet
Accommodations
Shoe shape matching foot shape
Adequate shoe depth
Shock absorption
Adjustability by lace or straps
Breathability, softness, flexible material for uppers
Changes for gait and limb-length disorders
Ability to subsequently modify the shoe

Table 7-4   Wagner's Grades of Foot Lesions

Grade	Criteria
0	Skin intact (all of the risk categories are included here)
1	Localized superficial ulcer of the skin
2	Ulcer extending deeper to tendon, bone, ligament or joint
3	Foot contains abscess or osteomyelitis
4	Gangrene present on or by one or more toes
5	Whole foot involved with gangrene

From Wagner FW: A classification and treatment program for diabetic, neuropathic, and dysvascular foot problems, AAOS 27:143, 1979.

Assess for systemic signs of infection, keeping in mind that body temperature and white blood cell count can be normal in the presence of serious systemic infection.[3] Radiographs may be required to rule out subcutaneous gas or foreign body and assess the nature of bone involvement. Frank destruction of bone is likely to be diagnostic of osteomyelitis.

Diagnosis and treatment of foot ulcers

Diabetic patients with infected ulcers should be hospitalized.[31] The majority of amputations are performed on patients with a history of infectious complications.[60] However, it is quite possible that some evaluations, such as bone scans, have been recently overemphasized in their ability to provide pure diagnostic information. Bone scans may be positive when no osteomyelitis is present and so should not be used as an absolute diagnosis.[3,63] Three-phase bone scans may offer some increased specificity. Radioactive uptake in the entire bone may also be specific. Indium-labeled white blood cell scintigraphy has shown uptake at simple fracture sites. Scans can be helpful in showing the extent of osteomyelitis but bone biopsy remains the only definitive means of the diagnosis of osteomyelitis.[1]

Debridement

All infected abscesses should be incised and drained.[3] Necrosis and callouses should be completely excised. Cultures should be taken at the time of debridement. Aerobic and anaerobic organisms must be cultured precisely. Surface debridement followed by some form of curettage most accurately represent the mixture of pathogens. Infections are often polymicrobial suggesting that broad-spectrum coverage may be needed initially. The precise to antibiotic therapy should be carefully monitored and antibiotics changed as necessary.

Wound Care

There are no adequately controlled studies of topical agents for diabetic wound care.[3] The role of foot soaks and topical agents therefore remain controversial. The closest consensus today would include the use of normal sterile saline as a wound flush or in wet-to-dry dressings.[32] The selection of a dressing is dependent upon several factors. According to Christensen and associates,[18] treatment options and dressing selections are dependent upon: type of tissue (red versus yellow or black), presence of infection or swelling, amount of drainage, size and depth of wound, location and whether bone or tendon is exposed, condition surrounding the skin, and the ease, frequency, and cost of dressing changes.

Flushing of the wounds is an important aspect of care since it allows for the loosening and removal of debris. A dry wound is not conducive to healing, since dehydration results in scab formation. This can become a mechanical barrier to epidermal cell migration.

Monitoring Mechanical Stress

When ulcers are found under forefoot or midfoot, the most successful forms of management address both the cause or ulceration (repetitive stress or walking) and mechanical factors that can make it worse. Denervation of the skin does not affect epithelialization of superficial wounds.[57] On insensate feet, healing is usually delayed by continuing injury and motion at the wound site. Therefore weight bearing should be restricted. Modification of weight bearing can include crutches, shoe insets, special shoes, bedrest with elevation of legs, and total-contact casting.

Recent studies indicate that total-contact casting is a very reliable means of healing these wounds in a timely fashion.[36] The casting technique was first used and developed for healing ulcers on the feet of leprosy patients.[16] Mooney and Wagner[54] have called it the most effective means of controlling lower extremity edema. Total contact coating casting prevents excessive compression of the wound site by weight bearing, controls edema, immobilizes the joints and tendons, and eliminates inflammation at the wound site. The technique of this form of casting has been described several times.[13,19,42] It is a weight bearing, below-the-knee cast with the toes enclosed and an inner plaster layer contoured exactly to the foot and leg, with little interior padding to shift and alter the support.

The results of the first controlled clinical trial on total-contact casting were published in 1989.[56] A group of physical therapists followed the wounds of 40 diabetic patients, 21 of whom were casted versus 19 who were given traditional wound dressings. These were wet-to-dry saline dressings changed 2 to 3 times a day. Ninety percent of the ulcers on casted feet healed in a mean time of 42 days. Thirty-two percent of the traditionally treated ulcers healed in a mean time of 65 days.

Metabolic Control

Infection may result in fluctuations of blood glucose. Prompt and thorough treatment of foot ulcers or infections therefore encourage good blood glucose levels. In contrast, persons in poor control may be hindered in their recovery. Therefore, attention to metabolic control is necessary.

Surgical Intervention

Persons with poor circulatory status may be candidates for surgical intervention. Referral to a vascular surgeon may yield positive results with regard to improved blood flow. However, careful evaluation by the diabetes team is needed prior to surgical intervention, and requires thorough and comprehensive communication among the team members as well as thorough education of the patient and family.

PREVENTION OF RECURRENCE OF FOOT ULCERS

Any patient with a history of diabetic foot ulcers is at high risk for future ulcers. An extensive education program emphasizing the principles suggested in the box on pp. 228–229 is needed. In addition, frequent follow-up should be stressed with referral to a specialist, such as a pedorthist, recommended as needed.

DIABETIC OSTEOARTHROPATHY

As previously noted, diabetic osteoarthropathy, often referred to as Charcots joint, is a relatively painless, progressive, and quite destructive disorder found most commonly in the feet of persons with long-term diabetes. The term osteoarthropathy more appropriately attributes this joint disorder to an underlying neuropathic disease process. The use of the terms *Charcots joint* or *neuroarthropathy* are often misnomers in that the fractures often do not involve a joint at all.[34] A neuropathic fracture is unique from other forms of fracture mostly because there is no feeling in the limb and the person thus continues to destroy the bone by walking on the unfelt fracture.[3] Denervation alone does not predispose the bone to fracture. In fact, most denervated joints function normally for a lifetime.[28]

Diabetic osteoarthropathy has a high incidence in those patients with a duration of diabetes over 12 years, regardless of age. In most cases only one foot is affected, although an 18% bilateral incidence has been reported in some studies. Two essential factors can be implicated in the development of neuropathic fracture: neuropathy and trauma. This results in further instability of the joint, and degeneration, further perpetuating the destructive process as is depicted in Fig. 7-2. Neuropathic fractures are also commonly seen after an inflammatory condition or casting has resulted in demineralization.[59] Increased blood flow has been implicated or a major factor in the development of neuropathic fractures.[10,71] The increased flow results in rarefaction of bone, making the area more prone to injury.[69]

In most cases, a neuropathic fracture probably begins as an unfelt microtrauma.[34,40] A small fracture, sprain, or ligamentous tear occurs and goes unnoticed because of in-

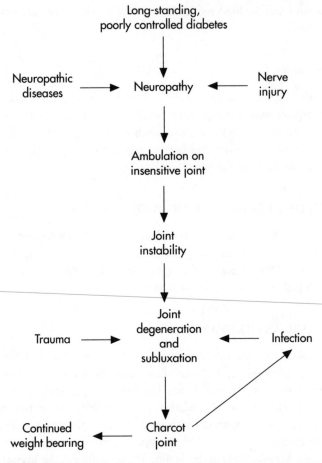

Fig. 7-2. Pathogenesis of the diabetic Charcots joint. (From Frykberg RG and Kozak GP: Neuropathic arthropathy in the diabetic foot, Am Fam Physician 17:105-112, 1978.)

sensitivity. The insensate patient may notice instability, hear sounds of popping, or feel "rubbing" in the foot as an early symptom of fracture. However, there is no pain and because the person is unaware of the injury, he or she continues to walk. With each step the inflammation increases. The inflammation creates hyperemia. The hyperemia results in local bone absorption that further weakens the structure. The characteristic destruction of neuropathic fracture develops as the insensitive patient continues to use the foot as though no injury were present.[59] Small fragments of bone are separated and spread through adjacent soft tissue by joint motion. The cartilage can become destroyed and, with the force of weight bearing and joint motion, the bones grind into one another. The redness created by the inflammatory process frequently leads to a diagnosis of infection.

Diagnosing Osteoarthropathy

Diabetic neuroarthropathy often eludes prompt diagnosis, despite increasing reports in the literature. This is most likely attributable to the clinician's lack of awareness or suspicion for the disorder. The possibility of fracture is not considered because of the absence of pain.

Differential diagnosis for neuropathic fracture is frequently necessary. Swelling, erythema, deformity, or symptoms may be absent. A history of injury or misstep is rarely encountered.[68] For acute dislocation there may be some pain or aching, but markedly less than might be expected. Usually, the foot and ankle show a marked deformity, are grossly swollen, and may have a "fallen arch." The foot is very erythematous, warm, and anhidrotic with bounding pulses. These findings, in association with mild to absent pain, contribute significantly to a diagnosis of Charcots joint.

As previously reviewed, a lot of attention has been directed to various forms of bone scans to differentiate osteomyelitis from Charcots joints.[1,52] Bone scans most reliably identify the presence of inflammation. Thermometry (temperature evaluation) will perform a similar task in less time and at much less expense. Virtually all structures in the foot are close to the surface. This makes thermometry an indispensable tool for early detection of injury on an insensate foot. Surface skin temperature is the key early sign that indicates the presence of fracture in an insensate foot.[8] With no skin ulcer present or a recent history of ulceration, an area of skin on a foot 3° C warmer than the rest of the foot, or the same location on the other foot, should be treated as a fracture until the temperature equalizes or another cause for the difference is identified.[34,38]

Treatment

For most neuropathic fractures the first form of treatment should arrest the possibility of continued use and breakdown. Progressive destruction can be halted if recognized early.[34,48] Hospitalization may be necessary to ensure that the individual's foot is kept absolutely non–weight-bearing and elevated. During this time diabetes control treatment for recurrent ulcerations and infections can take place. In addition, this allows time for the gross edema to subside.

Once the edema has subsided or is under control, below-the-knee casting remains the most effective form of immediate immobilization of the fracture sites. Surface skin temperatures can be measured at each cast change to monitor the inflammation. As the area of fracture cools to temperatures of those on the unfractured foot, less restrictive forms of support can be used to begin the rehabilitation back to footwear. The process of rehabilitation can take from 12 weeks to 1 year.[14,27]

If there is little fragmentation, reduction and surgical fusion may be indicated.[44] Surgery may also be useful when skin ulceration cannot be prevented by footwear or bracing.[35] In the case of very flail ankle or midfoot fractures of long duration and cool surface skin temperature, amputation is often the only recourse.

Education

Many of the same principles for foot care education apply to the individual with osteoarthropathy. Emphasis on preventive education is critical. Frequent, regular follow-up needs to be emphasized. These individuals should be treated by the diabetes team, as high risk for future foot care problems. As such, this aspect of diabetes care should assume a major focus. Daily foot assessments should be carefully stressed, while follow-up should be frequent by the health care provider (see box on pp. 228–229).

THE ROLE OF THE DIABETES HEALTH CARE TEAM IN FOOT CARE

The involvement of many disciplines from the diabetes health care team is necessary not only to promote optimal diabetes care in general but also to decrease the morbidity common among persons with diabetes. Models of the effectiveness of diabetes education with regard to impact on foot care are impressive. During the early 1970s, Grady Memorial Hospital in Atlanta developed a diabetes team that included nurses, clinicians, and a considerable amount of patient education in emphasizing the need for every health care professional to examine the feet of patients with diabetes. Included in this protocol was the utilization of the services of podiatrists when foot pathology was identified as well as the need for daily foot inspection by patients. Within a few years, the annual rate of lower-extremity amputations had been diminished by almost 50%.[21]

Later in the same decade, the County Health Department of Memphis, Tennessee, transferred 800 patients from the centrally located outpatient clinic to the patient's small neighborhood clinics where nurse practitioners were specially trained in new conservative management and foot inspection protocols. Over a 2-year period, a 68% reduction in hospital days and amputations was obtained.[62] At the University Hospital of Geneva, a similar program of patient education and staff training in foot care resulted in an 85% reduction in below-the-knee amputations.[4]

Multidisciplinary members of the diabetes team can have particular impact regarding the care of the person with diabetes in the prevention or treatment of foot problems. These members range from the nurse as a primary source of education for the patient; the podiatrist, whose education spans functional biomechanics of the foot, recognition of early deformity, and management of foot problems; the physical therapist, who can educate or aid in the development of exercise programs that minimize mechanical trauma to the foot; the neurologist who can verify diagnosis of neuropathy; the vascular or orthopedic surgeon who may be required to treat various deformities; and the social worker, who can assist in job-related problems that may occur as a result of foot problems. The involvement of all disciplines is critical to the care of the patient with diabetes in general, but in particular as it relates to foot problems.

REFERENCES

1. Al-Sheikh W and others: Subacute and chronic bone infections: diagnosis using In-lll, Ga-67 and Tc-99mMDP bone scintigraphy and radiology, Radiology 155:501, 1985.

2. American Diabetes Association: Clinical practice recommendations, Diabetes Care 14(suppl 2):14, 1991.
3. American Diabetes Association: Diabetic foot care, Alexandria, VA, 1990, American Diabetes Association.
4. Assal JP and others: Patient education as the basis for diabetic foot care in clinical practice, Diabetologia 28:602, 1985.
5. Barton AA and Barton M: Plantar ulcers occurring after neurectomy: light and electron microscope study, Aust J Exp Biol Med Sci 46:155, 1968.
6. Bauman JH, Girling JP, and Brand PW: Plantar pressures and trophic ulceration, and evaluation of foot wear, J Bone Joint Surg 45B:652, 1963.
7. Bauman JH and Brand PW: Measurement of pressure between foot and shoe, Lancet 1:629, 1963.
8. Bergtholdt HT: Thermography on insensitive limbs. In Uematsu S, ed: Medical thermography, theory and clinical applications, Los Angeles, 1976, Brentwood Publishing Corp.
9. Bessman AN and Sapico FL: Infectious complications: a multifactorial problem, Diabetes Spect, 4:68, 1991.
10. Boulton AJM, Scarpello JWB, and Ward JD: Venous oxygenation in the diabetic neurotrophic foot: evidence of arteriovenous shunting? Diabetologia, 22:6, 1982.
11. Boulton AJM and others: Dynamic foot pressure and other studies as diagnostic aids in diabetic neuropathy, Diabetes Care 6:26, 1983.
12. Brenner MA: Management of the diabetic foot, Baltimore, 1987, Williams & Wilkins.
13. Burnett O: Total contact cast, Clin Podiatr Med Surg, 4:471, 1987.
14. Brand PW: Pressure sores, the problem. In Kenedi RM, Cowden JM, and Scales JT, eds: Bedsore biomechanics, London, 1976, MacMillian.
15. Brand PW: Management of the insensitive limb, Phys Ther 59:8, 1979.
16. Brand PW: The insensitive foot (including leprosy). In Jahss MH, ed: Disorders of the foot, vol 2, Philadelphia, 1982, WB Saunders Co.
17. Brand PW: The diabetic foot. In Ellenberg M and Rifkin H, eds: Diabetes mellitus, theory and practice, New Hyde Park, New York, 1983, Medical Examination Publishers.
18. Christiansen MH and others: How to care for the diabetic foot, Am J Nurs March, pp. 50-56, 1991.
19. Coleman WC, Brand PW, and Birke J: The total contact cast: a therapy for plantar ulceration on insensitive feet, J Am Podiatr Med Assoc 11:548, 1987.
20. Cooper R: Infection and diabetes. In Marble A and others, eds: Joslin Diabetes Mellitus, ed 12, Philadelphia, 1986, Lea and Febiger.
21. Davidson JK and others: Assessment of program effectiveness at Grady Memorial Hospital—Atlanta. In Steiner G and Lawrence PA, eds: Educating diabetic patients, New York, 1981, Springer-Verlag.
22. Delbridge L and others: Limited joint mobility in the diabetic foot: relationship to neuropathic ulceration, Diabetes Med, 5:333, 1988.
23. Deleted in proofs.
24. Donovon JC and Rowbotham JL: Foot lesions in diabetic patients: Cause, prevention and treatment. In Marble A and others, eds: Joslins diabetes mellitus, ed 12, Philadelphia, 1986, Lea and Febiger.
25. Dinsdale SM: Decubitus ulcers in swine: light and electron microscopy study of pathogenesis, Arch Phys Med Rehab 54:51, 1973.
26. Duckworth T and others: Plantar pressure measurements and the prevention of ulceration in the diabetic foot, J Bone Joint Surg, 67:79, 1985.
27. Edmonds ME and others: Improved survival of the diabetic foot: the role of a specialized foot clinic, J Med 232:763,1986.
28. Eloesser L: On the nature of neuropathic affections of the joints, Ann Surg 66:201, 1947.
29. Fernando DJS and others: Relationship of limited joint mobility to abnormal foot pressures and diabetic foot ulceration, Diabetes Care 14:8, 1991.
30. Fisher JD, Rytting M, and Heslin R: Hands touching hands: affective and evaluative effects of an interpersonal touch, Sociometry 39:416, 1976.
31. Gibbons GW and Eliopoulos GM: Infection of the diabetic feet. In Kozak GP and others, eds: Management of diabetic foot problems, Philadelphia, 1984, WB Saunders.
32. Goodson WH and Hunt TK: Wound healing and the diabetic patient, Surg Gynecol Obstet 149:600, 1979.
33. Haire-Joshu D: Endocrine system. In Beare P and Meyer J, eds: Principles and practice of adult health nursing, St Louis, 1990, Mosby–Year Book.
34. Harris JR and Brand PW: Patterns of disintegration of the tarsus in the anesthetic foot, J Bone Joint Surg 48B:4, 1966.

35. Heiple KG and Chammarn MR: Diabetic neuroarthropathy with spontaneous peritalar fracture dislocation, J Bone Joint Surg 48B:1177, 1966.

36. Heim PA, Walker SC, and Pullium G: Total contact casting in diabetic patients with neuropathic foot ulcers, Arch Phys Med Rehab 65:691, 1984.

37. Herman WM, ed: The prevention and treatment of complications of diabetes mellitus. A guide for primary care practitioner, Atlanta, 1990, Department of Health and Human Services, Public Health Service, Centers for Disease Control.

38. Jacobs E: Observations of neuropathic mellitus, J Bone Joint Surg, 40A:1043, 1958.

39. Jauw-Tjen L and Brown AL: Normal structure of the vascular system and general reactive changes of the arteries. In Fairbairn JF, Juergens JL, and Spittell JA, eds: Peripheral vascular diseases, Philadelphia, 1972, WB Saunders Co.

40. Karat S, Karat ABA, and Foster R: Radiological changes in bones of the limbs in leprosy, Lepr Rev 39:147, 1968.

41. Kleinke CL: Compliance to requests made by gazing and touching experimenters in filed settings, J Exp Social Psych 13:218, 1977.

42. Kominsky SJ: The ambulatory total contact cast. In Frykberg RG, ed: The high risk foot in diabetes mellitus, New York, 1991, Churchill Livingstone.

43. Kosiak M: Etiology and pathology of ischemic ulcers, Arch Phys Med Rehab 40:62, 1969.

44. Lesco P and Maurer RC: Talonavicular dislocations and midfoot arthropathy in neuropathic diabetic feet: natural course and principles of treatment, Clin Orthop 240:226, 1989.

45. Levin ME and O'Neal LW: The diabetic foot: pathophysiology evaluation and treatment. In Levin ME and O'Neal LW, eds: The diabetic foot, St Louis, 1988, CV Mosby Co.

46. Levin ME, Poucher RL and Stavosky JW: Neuropathic ulcers and the diabetic foot. Treatment of chronic wounds, Number 1 of series, 1991, Curative Technologies.

47. Lindan O: Etiology of decubitus ulcers: experimental study, Arch Phys Med Rehab 42:774, 1961.

48. Lippman HI, Perotto A, and Farrar R: The neuropathic foot of the diabetic, Bull NY Acad Med 52:1159, 1976.

49. Lithner F and Tornblom N: Gangrene localized to the lower limbs in diabetics, Acta Med Scand 208:315, 1980.

50. Manley MT and Darby T: Repetitive mechanical stress and denervation in plantar ulcer pathogenesis in rats, Arch Phys Med Rehab 61:171, 1980.

51. Masson EA and others, eds: Abnormal pressure alone does not cause foot ulceration, Diabetic Med 6:424, 1989.

52. Merkel K and others: Comparison of indium-labeled leukocyte imaging with sequential technetium gallium scanning in the diagnosis of low grade musculoskeletal sepsis, J Bone Joint Surg 67A:465, 1985.

53. Milgram JE: Office measures for relief of the painful foot, J Bone Joint Surg 46:1095, 1964.

54. Mooney V and Wagner FW: Neurocirculatory disorders of the foot, Clin Orthop 122:53, 1977.

55. Most RS and Sinnock P: The epidemiology of lower-extremity amputations in diabetic individuals, Diabetes Care 6:87, 1983.

56. Mueller MJ and others: Total contact casting in treatment of diabetic plantar ulcers, Diabetes Care 12:384, 1989.

57. Muren A and Zederfeldt B: Delayed effect of denervation on healing of superficial sin defects in rabbits, Acta Chir Scand 132:618, 1966.

58. Palumbo PJ and Melton LJ: Peripheral vascular disease in diabetes. In: Diabetes in America: diabetes data compiled in 1984, NIH publ no 85-1468, Washington, DC, 1985, US Government Printing Office.

59. Paterson DE and Job CK: Bone changes and absorption in leprosy. In Cochrane RG and Davey TF, eds: Leprosy in theory and practice, ed 2, Briston, England, 1964, John Wright & Sons, Ltd.

60. Pecoraro RE, Reiber GE, and Burgess EM: Pathways to diabetic limb amputation, Diabetes Care 13:513, 1990.

61. Price EW: Studies on plantar ulceration in leprosy. VI. The management of plantar ulcers, Lepr Rev 31:159, 1960.

62. Runyan JW: The Memphis chronic disease program, JAMA 231:264, 1975.

63. Shih WJ and others: Malunion of a femoral fracture mimicking osteomyelitis in three phase bone imaging, Clin Nucl Med 13:38, 1988.

64. Soames RW and others: Measurement of pressure under the foot during function, Med Biol Eng Comput 20:489, 1982.

65. Vissre HJ and others: The use of differential scintigraphy in the clinical diagnosis of osseous and soft tissue changes affecting the diabetic foot, J Foot Surg 23:74,1984.

66. Wagner FW: A classification and treatment program for diabetic, neuropathic, and dysvascular foot problems, AAOS Instruct Course Lect, 27:143, 1979.

67. Ward JD and others: Pain in the diabetic leg, Pharmatherpeutica 2:642, 1981.

68. Warren G: Tarsal bone disintegration in leprosy, J Bone Joint Surg 53B:688, 1971.

69. Watkins PJ and Edmonds ME: Sympathetic nerve failure in diabetes, Diabetologia 25:73, 1983.

70. Yamada H: Strength of biological materials, Baltimore, 1970, Williams & Wilkins.

71. Young RJ and others: Variable relationship between peripheral somatic and autonomic neuropathy in patients with different syndromes of diabetic polyneuropathy, Diabetes 35:192,1986.

_____

Foot Care Protocol*

Foot care for the individual with diabetes required a two-step process involving thorough assessment and treatment. This foot care protocol utilizes such a process. Section I requests information related to completing a foot assessment. Section II uses the responses from this information, and suggests treatment recommendations based on these responses.

I. FOOT ASSESSMENT

1. Mobility (CIRCLE ONE)
   a. Walks without assistance   b. Walks with help of equipment   c. Does not walk, uses wheelchair   d. Bedfast   e. Amputation

	(CIRCLE ONE)	
2. Ask, Does the condition of your feet or legs limit your activity in any way?_____	Y	N
3. Ask to walk 10 feet. Any gait disturbance?	Y	N
4. Are the feet clean?	Y	N
5. Shoes and socks clean and in repair?	Y	N
6. Shoes and socks well fitting?	Y	N
7. Ask, Do you do anything special when you choose your shoes?_____	Y	N
8. Hydration		
a. Dry skin present on the feet?	Y	N
b. Do the feet perspire excessively?	Y	N
c. Ask, What do you do about the (dryness or perspiration)?_____		

_____

*Adapted from King PA, et al: Diabetes foot care project, Ann Arbor, 1990, University of Michigan Department of Public Health Foot Care Project.

9. Color

                                                               If yes, which?

a. Feet red or blue when dependent?	Y	N	Rt.	Lt.
b. Feet blanched when elevated?	Y	N	Rt.	Lt.
c. Do the feet have a brownish discoloration?	Y	N	Rt.	Lt.

10. Edema

a. Is edema present?	Y	N	Rt.	Lt.

    b. Ask, What do you do when your feet
       swell?_____

11. Temperature (CHECK WITH THE BACK OF YOUR HAND)

                                                  If no, which
                                                  are cool?

a. Feet warm to the touch bilaterally?	Y	N	Rt.	Lt.

    b. Ask, What do you do to keep your feet
       warm?_____

12. Sensation

                                                  If no, not
                                                intact in:

a. Sense of touch intact?	Y	N	Rt.	Lt.
b. Pain?	Y	N	Rt.	Lt.
c. Position?	Y	N	Rt.	Lt.
d. Hot and cold?	Y	N	Rt.	Lt.

    e. If no, ask, Do you take any special
       precautions since your feet are not very
       sensitive?

13. Toenails

                                                  If yes, which
                                                foot?

a. Ingrown	Y	N	Rt.	Lt.
b. Overgrown	Y	N	Rt.	Lt.
c. Thickened	Y	N	Rt.	Lt.
d. Discolored (DESCRIBE)	Y	N	Rt.	Lt.

    e. Ask, Who cuts your toenails?_____

14. Circulation

                                                Not palpable

a. Dorsalis pedis present bilaterally? (USE THREE FINGERS ON DORSUM OF FOOT USUALLY JUST LATERAL TO EXTENSOR TENDON)	Y	N	Rt.	Lt

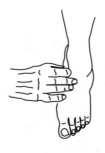

b. Posterior tibial present bilaterally?   Y   N   Rt.   Lt
   (CURVE YOUR FINGERS BEHIND
   AND SLIGHTLY BELOW THE
   MEDIAL MALLEOLUS)

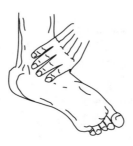

c. Capillary refill of great toe less   Y   N   Rt.   Lt
   than two seconds?

15. Structural deformities
   a. Hallux valgus (bunion)   Y   N   Rt.   Lt
   b. Hammer toes   Y   N   Rt.   Lt.
   c. Overlapping digits   Y   N   Rt.   Lt.
   d. Ask, What do you do to manage these
      conditions?
16. Lesions (CIRCLE IF PRESENT, MARK PICTURE WITH LETTER.)
   a. Fissures between toes   h. Gangrene (DESCRIBE)
   b. Fissures on the heel
   c. Ulcers (DESCRIBE)   _____
                                  i. Celullitis (local redness, warmth,
   _____   swelling)
   d. Corns   j. Blisters
   e. Calloused areas   k. Ask, What do you do to treat
   f. Plantar wart   these problems?_____
   g. Redness over pressure points
                                  _____

Lateral right   Lateral left

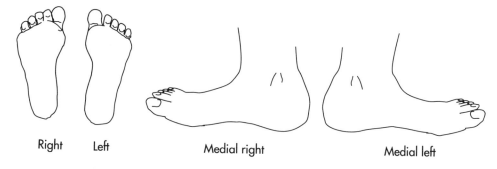

Right   Left   Medial right   Medial left

Summary of Risk Factors (CIRCLE IF PRESENT)

a. Previous amputations because disease and/or circulation problem
b. Previous foot ulcers
c. Chronic illness for 10 years or more (e.g., diabetes mellitus, circulation problems, arthritis, heart disease, kidney disease, gout, hypertension, other)
d. Age forty or over
e. Smokes
f. Poor compliance with diet or diabetes not well controlled
g. Reduced ability to care for own feet because of physical or cognitive impairment
h. Poor general hygiene of feet
i. Decreased circulation to feet (poor color, cold to touch, decreased palpable pulses)
j. Decreased sensation in feet
k. Existing lesions or structural deformities of the feet
l. Language/communication difficulty

Plan

a. Continued monitoring and assessing
b. Teaching by nurse/therapist/dietitian
c. Treatment by nurse/therapist
d. Referral to physician and/or podiatrist
e. Foot care prescription
f. Scheduled follow-up

II. GUIDELINES FOR TREATMENT OF FOOT PROBLEMS

Mobility	1.	
	2. Y	Refer to orthotic specialist or podiatrist for gait problems.
	3. Y	
Hygiene	4. N	Wash feet daily with nondrying soap and water.

Shoes	5. N 6. N	Teach regarding need to wear natural fiber shoes that protect the feet. Wear shoes with 1/2 to 3/4 inch toe room. Wear socks that allow feet to breathe. Avoid tight socks or those with holes or repairs.
	7.	Teach to buy new shoes in the afternoon when feet are a little swollen and to break in slowly (1 to 2 hours a day).
Hydration	8a. Y 8b. Y 8c.	Apply nondrying lotion one to two times a day. Apply powder or cornstarch and teach to wear absorbent socks. Teach that dry skin may lead to openings in the skin and damp skin is prone to breakdown and fungal infections.
Color	9a. Y 9b. Y 9c. Y	Assist in maintaining a position which avoids dependent feet or obstructed blood flow. Teach
Edema	10a. Y	• to avoid trauma and wear protective shoes as much as possible
		• to wear wool socks to keep feet warm
Temp	11a. N 11b.	• signs of infection and that if a lesion develops, to wash with water, cover with bandage or sterile dressing, and notify a health care professional if it does not begin to heal within 3 days.
Edema	10b.	Teach to elevate feet as much as possible and to use powder or nylon stockings under support stockings to avoid skin trauma when putting on.
Sensation	12a. N 12b. N 12c. N 12d. N 12e.	Provide trauma-free environment. Teach to • avoid heating pads, sunlamps, temperature extremes • wear wool socks to keep feet warm • avoid going barefoot when there is a potential for foot injury • wear protective shoes as much as possible • inspect feet daily. If unable to see well, have another person do it. • wear shows that allow 1/2 to 3/4 inch toe room • examine shoes for possible causes of injury before putting on. If feet are very insensitive, refer to orthotic specialist or podiatrist for footwear.
Toenails	13a. Y	Pad edge with cotton or lamb's wool and refer to foot specialist for surgical removal.
	13b. Y 13c. Y	Reduce with pumice stone or other instrument and soften before cutting.
	13d. Y	Refer to physician for possible fungal infection.
	13e.	Use of selected instrument should be demonstrated until

adequate skill is achieved. Trim nails to follow the natural curve of the toe. Refer to foot specialist for trimming if very thick.

Circulation	14a. N	Teach to
	14b. N	• avoid heating pads, sunlamps, temperature extremes
	14c. N	• wear wool socks to keep feet warm

• avoid going barefoot when there is a potential for foot injury
• align extremities when sitting to avoid cutting off circulation (for those with very restricted blood flow)
• wear protective shoes as much as possible
• inspect feet daily. If unable to see well, have another person do it.
• wear shoes that allow 1/2 to 3/4 inch toe room
• examine shoes for possible causes of injury before putting them on
• recognize signs of infection. If a lesion develops, wash with water, cover with a bandage or sterile dressing, and notify a health care professional if it does not begin to heal within 3 days.

Assist in maintaining position that avoids dependent feet or obstructed blood flow

Structural deformities	15a. Y	Reduce pressure through use of pads, lamb's wool. If feet
	15b. Y	are very insensitive, refer to orthotic specialist or podiatrist
	15c. Y	for footwear.

Fissures	16a. Y	*Wound care*
	16b. Y	Clean open wounds

• Clean with normal saline or tap water (no soap)

Ulcers	16c. Y	• Hydrotherapy to increase circulation and clean wound surfaces

• Maintain a moist environment (moist gauze, dressings, OpSite, Duoderm)
• Carrington gel to stimulate fibroblasts

Infected open or necrotic wounds
• Evaluation of process for causative organism, extent of infection
• Debride necrotic tissue
• Clean with normal saline or tap water (no soap)
• Hydrotherapy to increase circulation and clean wound surface
• Maintain a moist environment

Teach wound care as necessary

Corns	16d. Y	⎱ Mechanical reduction or removal with pumice stone or
Calluses	16e. Y	electric instrument. Refer to foot specialist if extensive
Plantar wart	16f. Y	⎰ treatment needed.
Redness from pressure	16g. Y	Teach regarding use of a pumice stone or similar device to debride calluses and corns, how to relieve pressure from bunions, corns, calluses using various padding techniques, and the role of the foot specialist in diabetes foot care.

Gangrene   16h. Y   Dry gangrene
- Keep dry and clean
- Maintain activity as tolerated

Wet gangrene
- IV antibiotics
- Surgery

Cellulitis	16i. Y	Bedrest and antibiotics
Other	16j. Y	⎱ Teach regarding care of specific lesion and how to prevent
	16k.	⎰ further foot trauma.

Foot Care Teaching Outline: For Health Care Providers*

B efore beginning a foot care training program, the development of an educational plan is essential. The plan needs to include both the information to be communicated and the mechanism to provide the information and the needed skills. An example of such a plan that includes the steps for skill acquisition is as follows:

- Explanation—includes the importance and steps for the skills.
- Experience—includes observing and then practicing with the skills.
- Debriefing—includes a discussion of the persons reactions to the skill and their beliefs about their ability to carry it out.
- Application—includes assisting the person to incorporate foot care into their lifestyle and care practices.

TEACHING OUTLINE

A. Explanation
  1. Benefits of carrying out the treatment program. This includes patients' being better able to recognize problems early when treatment can be most effective or to care for those problems at home as he/she is able.
  2. Risk factors that put the patient at greater risk for foot problems and specific steps that the patient can take to reduce the risks.
  3. Explanation of each step to take was provided as it was demonstrated to the patients.
B. Experience
  1. Remove shoes and socks. The instructor should also remove shoes to demonstrate procedures.
  2. Inspect shoes for proper fit. Shoes that allow for ½- to ¾-inch of toe room are generally best. Shoes should be fitted by a competent sales person. For best results, buy shoes in the middle of the day, after feet have become somewhat swollen, but not as much as by the end of the day. Patients with loss of sensation

---

*Adapted from King PH et al: Diabetes foot care project, Ann Arbor, 1990, University of Michigan Diabetes Foot Care Project.

caused by neuropathy can draw an outline of their feet on heavy paper and put that into the shoe as a test for fit.

3. Shoes should be made of natural fibers, either leather or canvas, that allow feet to breathe. Avoid thongs and plastic shoes. Use common sense about sandals and bare feet.

4. Feel inside shoes for foreign objects, wrinkled insoles or breaks in the shoes that can cause lesions. Shake shoes out before putting them on each time.

5. Look at your socks. Socks should be made of natural fibers (wool or as much cotton as you can buy are best as these allow the feet to breathe). Socks do not have to be white.

6. Socks should fit well and be free of darns or holes.

7. For women, stocking should also fit well and not decrease circulation. Knee-high stocking with a wider elastic band usually will decrease blood flow less than a narrow band. Avoid tight-fitting garters and rubber bands to hold up stockings.

8. Inspect feet. First look at the tops of the feet. Be sure to look at both feet every day. Is the skin dry or damp? If dry, use a lotion that does not contain alcohol. If damp, use talcum powder. Show samples of lotions and powders that are appropriate. Avoid soaking the feet as this can lead to dryness.

9. Look for areas of redness caused by shoes and corns, callouses, or lesions. If shoes are causing red areas, they do not fit correctly and may need to be replaced.

10. Corns should be treated by padding the area. Show samples of products that are widely available. Corns can also be debrided slowly with a pumice stone or similar device. Show examples. Avoid cutting the corn with a razor blade or other device. Avoid using caustic products to remove corns, as these can burn the skin.

11. Calluses can be debrided each day using a pumice stone or similar device. Show examples. Pumice stones should be used daily to gently rub the area. Avoid rubbing hard and damaging skin. After a bath, while feet are damp is a good time to debride areas.

12. Look for any areas of cracking or fissures in the skin. These can easily become infected. These are often caused by dry skin and can be treated with lotion.

13. Bunions can be padded to increase comfort. Demonstrate technique and products.

14. Look at the toenails. Nails should be cut to follow the curve of the toe and be even with the end of the toe. Nails that are split and cracked can be treated with oil. Nails should be clean. Nails that have fungal infections can be treated by a podiatrist.

15. Look at the bottoms of both feet. If you can't see the bottoms of your feet, use a full length mirror on the wall or a mirror that you can place on the floor. Pass around a mirror, so that participants can look at their feet. This should also be done each day, looking for areas that have callouses, corns, or ulcers. Ulcers should be treated promptly.

CHAPTER **8**

Special Issues in Diabetes Management

NEIL H. WHITE AND DOUGLAS N. HENRY

In this chapter, we review special issues in the management of diabetes mellitus. Many of these issues may affect diabetes and its treatment across the entire lifespan. Some can affect the control of diabetes at any age and stage of development, regardless of the type of diabetes or its underlying etiology. Other issues might be limited to subjects with one type of diabetes or only at certain times of life. These issues include management of diabetes during severe or persistent metabolic decompensation (diabetic ketoacidosis; hyperosmolar, nonketotic coma syndrome; hypoglycemia; "brittle diabetes") and during intercurrent events (surgery, sick days). We will also review some of the inherent and external factors that contribute to ease of establishing diabetic control, and alternative forms of insulin delivery that may help deal with some of these. The specifics of therapy at different stages of life are discussed in more detail elsewhere in this text.

DIABETIC KETOACIDOSIS

Diabetic ketoacidosis (DKA) is the most serious metabolic disturbance of insulin-dependent, or type I, diabetes mellitus (IDDM).[62,92] DKA is identified in approximately 40% of patients with newly diagnosed IDDM and is responsible for more than 160,000 hospital admissions each year.[58] The highest rates of DKA are found in teenagers and the elderly. A precipitating cause can be identified in about 80% of cases of DKA. DKA should always be considered a medical emergency and requires immediate medical attention. The majority of the morbidity and mortality associated with DKA is preventable by appropriate treatment and careful monitoring. Prevention of DKA is a primary goal in the long-term management of IDDM, and many would consider the development of DKA in a known diabetic subject as a treatment failure.

Ketoacidosis is a state of severe metabolic decompensation manifested by the over-production of ketone bodies and ketoacids resulting in metabolic acidosis.[62,92,104] Diabetic ketoacidosis (DKA) is the occurrence of ketoacidosis secondary to diabetes mellitus. During DKA, disturbances of protein, fat, and carbohydrate metabolism are all present. Although DKA is primarily a state of absolute or relative insulin deficiency, counterregulatory hormone, particularly glucagon, excess appears to play an important role in the development of DKA (Fig. 8-1). In DKA, elevations of the counterregulatory hormones (glucagon, catecholamines, cortisol, and growth hormone) antagonize the effects of insulin. The elevated counterregulatory hormones increase lipolysis and ketogenesis. Inhibition of glucagon release by an infusion of somatostatin markedly slows the development of ketosis and DKA during acute insulin withdrawal from subjects with IDDM.[68] Ketoacidosis is best defined based on the presence of metabolic acidosis secondary to ketosis and not simply hyperglycemia. The hallmark features of DKA are ketosis and ketonuria, metabolic acidosis (low serum bicarbonate), and dehydration. In addition, since elevated counterregulatory hormones, accompanied by insulin deficiency, stimulate glucose production from glycogenolysis and gluconeogenesis, blood glucose is usually elevated (>

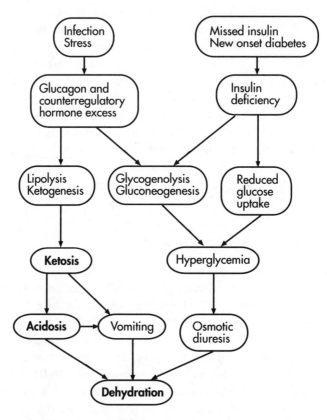

Fig. 8-1 Pathophysiology of diabetic ketoacidosis (DKA).

250 mg/dL) in subjects with DKA. The ketosis and metabolic acidosis result in electrolyte disturbances and vomiting. Hyperglycemia results in an osmotic diuresis. Together with reduced fluid intake and vomiting, this results in dehydration.

Ketoacidosis can occur in association with conditions other than diabetes. If a person not known to have diabetes is seen with ketoacidosis without hyperglycemia, other diagnoses need to be considered. These include alcoholic ketoacidosis, starvation, and certain inborn errors of metabolism. However, diabetes is by far the most common cause of ketoacidosis. DKA is almost always associated with hyperglycemia (plasma glucose > 250 mg/dL), although normoglycemia does not rule out DKA.[106] DKA without hyperglycemia can be seen in pregnancy, partially treated cases, or in those with prolonged vomiting and little carbohydrate intake for many days before presentation.

The diagnosis of DKA should be considered in any known diabetic subject who is seen with abdominal pain, vomiting, dehydration, rapid or deep breathing (Kussmaul breathing), or altered mental status. It should also be considered in any child with new onset of these symptoms, especially if classic diabetes symptoms have been present. DKA can be confused with many other medical conditions, including gastroenteritis, urinary tract infection or pyelonephritis, appendicitis, and pneumonitis. Precipitating factors in the development of DKA include the new diagnosis of IDDM, deliberate or inadvertent omission of insulin, infection (e.g., pneumonia, gastroenteritis, influenza, otitis media, meningitis, appendicitis), pancreatitis, trauma, psychologic and emotional stresses (especially in adolescents), and myocardial infarction or stroke in older persons. A search for precipitating factors should be initiated.

The classical signs and symptoms of DKA include polyuria, polydipsia, hyperventilation, and dehydration. Dehydration is usually apparent as dry mucus membranes, absent tearing, poor skin turgor, acute weight loss, and poor perfusion. A fruity odor to the breath can often be appreciated as a result of exhaled ketone bodies. Abdominal pain, which can be severe enough to suggest an acute surgical abdomen, as well as tenderness to palpation, diminished or absent bowel sounds, and guarding, can be seen as a result of DKA alone. However, a surgical consultation may be indicated in some cases if appendicitis, bowel perforation, or infarction are suspected. Extreme thirst, tachycardia, nausea, vomiting, hypotension, weakness, anorexia, dehydration, warm dry skin, visual disturbances, hyperventilation, somnolence, hypothermia, hyporeflexia, and impaired consciousness can all be present in DKA.

The common laboratory findings in DKA include metabolic acidosis, ketonemia and ketouria, elevated anion gap from ketoacids and lactate, hyperglycemia, leukocytosis, hyponatremia, hypophosphatemia, and, in some cases, hyperosmolarity and elevated amylase. Serum potassium can be high, low, or normal. In mild cases of DKA or simple ketosis, the serum bicarbonate and pH may be normal or only slightly reduced. In severe cases, arterial pH is usually less than 7.2, plasma bicarbonate is less than 15 mEq/L, and ketones are present in both blood and urine. Shock or coma can be present, although these are uncommon in children and in otherwise healthy young adults with uncomplicated diabetes. Although the blood glucose concentration is usually markedly elevated, a blood glucose level below 300 mg/dL (16.6 mM) and even one within the normal range does not exclude DKA.[106] In the presence of hyperglycemia, marked apparent hyponatremia can be seen; the serum sodium will be decreased by 1.6 mEq/L for each 100 mg/dL glucose increase above a plasma glucose concentration of 100 mg/dL. Serum potassium can be normal, elevated, or decreased. Regardless of the serum potassium, however, total body potassium depletion is nearly always present as a result of urinary and/or gastrointestinal losses. An elevation of the peripheral white blood cell count is often seen in DKA and is an unreliable indicator of infection. However, the white blood cell count normalizes quickly with treatment, and persistent elevations may indicate underlying infection. Underlying infection should be considered in any patient with DKA of unidentified etiology. An ECG should be performed in all adult patients to rule out myocardial infarction. The ECG can also be used as a rapid assessment of a critically low or high potassium. Hypokalemia results in flattened or inverted T waves, a depressed S-T segment, a prolonged Q-T interval, and the presence of U waves. Hypokalemia results in peaked T waves, a widened QRS interval, depressed P waves, or A-V dissociation.

When the individual is brought to a hospital or clinic with known or suspected DKA, he or she should be considered a critically ill patient until proved otherwise. Sufficient support services must be available to deal with the patient's needs. Monitoring of vital signs, blood gas analysis, bedside blood glucose monitoring, skilled nursing care, and serum electrolyte analysis must all be readily and rapidly available. If adequate support is not available, the patient should be transferred to a facility where these services are available as soon as possible. Mild cases of DKA can sometimes be managed at home or with only very short stays in the emergency room setting (see "Sick Day Management" for discussion of managing mild DKA). In cases of severe DKA, hospitalization is necessary, and access to a medical or pediatric intensive care unit would be advisable.

Goals of Treatment

The general goals in the treatment of DKA are to: (1) correct the fluid and electrolyte imbalance, (2) correct the metabolic acidosis, (3) provide adequate insulin to prevent ketosis and lower plasma glucose, and (4) prevent and monitor for complications of treatment. Initial therapy of severe DKA should be directed at correcting life-threatening abnormalities and stabilization of the patient. Adequate ventilation should be established, if necessary. Shock should be corrected with vigorous fluid resuscitation. Comatose patients should have nasogastric (NG) drainage to prevent aspiration. Intravenous access should be established as soon as possible and laboratory studies sent to confirm the diagnosis and the severity of the condition. A medical history, physical examination, and additional laboratory studies should be performed, as necessary, to rule out any precipitating causes and other underlying medical conditions. After initial stabilization and evaluation, the mainstays in the therapy of DKA are correction of dehydration and interruption of the metabolic imbalance (ketosis, acidosis, and hyperglycemia). The former is accomplished with intravenous fluid therapy; the latter is accomplished with insulin administration.

Management Protocols

Insulin hormone replacement, fluid therapy, correction of electrolytes, and treatment of any underlying disorders will direct initial therapy.[98] A comprehensive flow sheet should be kept to follow intake and output, weight, fluids, insulin, ketones, and electrolytes. Patients with hyperglycemia and simple ketosis who are alert and not vomiting can often be rehydrated orally. Intravenous hydration is required in patients with vomiting, inability to drink, or severe acidosis. Good intravenous (IV) access with a relatively large catheter should be established. Initially, volume expansion should be given as 10 to 20 ml/kg of isotonic (0.9%) saline over 30 to 60 minutes. Subsequently, maintenance requirements, ongoing excessive fluid losses (vomiting, osmotic diuresis), and replacement of dehydration need to be considered in fluid therapy. If fluid deficits are not known, an estimated fluid deficit of 10% or greater should be assumed. Maintenance fluid needs can be calculated at 1500 to 2000 ml/M^2 per day or higher if fever is present. Ongoing losses can be minimized by keeping blood glucose below or near renal threshold (150 to 200 mg/dL). After the initial volume expansion, fluid replacement can usually be accomplished using 0.45% saline. If severe hyponatremia (serum sodium below what can be accounted for by hyperglycemia), extreme hyperosmolarity (serum sodium normal despite marked hyperglycemia), hypotension, or shock are present, it may be appropriate to continue hydration with 0.9% saline. It is essential to accurately monitor intake and output. Bladder catheterization may be indicated in very severe cases, especially if documentation of urine output is difficult and hydration status uncertain.

In nearly all cases of DKA, total body potassium depletion exists despite a normal or even elevated serum potassium level. Potassium depletion occurs secondary to urinary loss from polyuria, acidosis, catabolic state, and vomiting or diarrhea. Correction of potassium depletion requires cautious and timely intervention. Potassium replacement should begin immediately after the initial fluid bolus unless renal failure is suspected. If serum potassium is so low as to endanger the patient (generally serum potassium <2.5 mEq/L or ECG changes suggestive of hypokalemia), potassium should be started sooner. If renal failure (acute or chronic) is suspected and potassium is high (>5.5 mEq/L), then potassium administration should be delayed until the serum potassium begins to fall. The potassium maintenance and replacement should be added to the intravenous fluid. Generally, the potassium concentration in the IV fluid is 30 to 40 mEq/L or 0.1 to 0.5 mEq/kg/hour. Potassium salts can be added as potassium chloride, potassium acetate, and/or potassium phosphate. Serum phosphate should be measured and if low, phosphate should be given. Some physicians routinely use some potassium phosphate in therapy. Without the use of any phosphate during the therapy of DKA, hypophosphatemia is common, although the clinical significance of this is unknown.[87,162] However, administration of potassium phosphate should not exceed 1.5 mEq/kg/24 hours because of the danger of hypocalcemia. The exclusive use of potassium chloride can result in a hyperchloremic acidosis, especially in children, but the clinical significance of this is likewise unknown. Serum potassium levels should be monitored closely (at least every 2 hours) until stable, and then every 4 to 6 hours while intravenous fluid and insulin therapy continue. The rate of potassium administration can be adjusted accordingly, as necessary, based on the serum potassium concentrations. EKG monitoring can also serve as a guide to potassium status (see above).

All patients with DKA have an absolute or relative insulin deficiency.[62,92,104] Therefore, exogenous insulin must be provided. Insulin suppresses ketone body and ketoacid formation and interrupts the production of excess acid and acidosis. Insulin also will reverse the catabolic state of protein breakdown and lipolysis. Once lipolysis, proteolysis, and ketogenesis are halted, IV fluids and rehydration will remove ketone bodies and ketoacids from the circulation and correct the acidosis. Insulin will lower blood glucose by inhibiting glycogenolysis and gluconeogenesis, and stimulating glucose uptake and oxidation.

Insulin can be administered by different routes during the treatment of DKA. The choice of the route of insulin administration depends upon the clinical picture. In mild DKA, especially that in which intravenous fluids may not be necessary, subcutaneous insulin can certainly be used (see "Sick Day Management" later in this chapter for discussion of managing mild DKA). Preferably, these patients will seek medical assistance early in the course of their illness before severe DKA is present. In cases of severe DKA, intravenous insulin is usually the preferred route of administration, although subcutaneous or intramuscular insulin can be used. In cases complicated by shock, only intravenous insulin should be used, since, coupled with poor peripheral perfusion, absorption of insulin given subcutaneously or intramuscularly may be reduced or delayed. Regular (fast-acting) insulin is the primary insulin preparation used in the management of DKA and is the only insulin that should be given intravenously or intramuscularly.

Intravenous insulin therapy for DKA is most commonly given as a "continuous low-dose insulin infusion."[56,150] This should begin with a bolus of regular insulin equivalent to 0.1 to 0.15 U/kg (rarely is more than 5 to 7 U necessary), followed by an infusion of regular insulin at 0.1 U/kg/hr (rarely is more than 5 to 7 U/hr necessary). Insulin should be mixed in normal saline and the IV tubing should be flushed with about 50 ml of insulin solution to saturate binding sites on the IV tubing before administration. Failure to do this could result in diminished insulin delivery over the first few hours. The insulin infusion can be "piggy-backed" into the existing IV line and should be controlled by a pump. After initiation of IV insulin therapy, if there is no improvement in blood pH, anion gap, bicarbonate, or plasma glucose is seen by two to three hours, the insulin infusion rate can be doubled. If these measures fail to improve acidosis, then consider other underlying problems, such as sepsis, meningitis, myocardial infarction, or pneumonia, and consultation with a diabetologist should be undertaken.

Often the blood glucose will normalize more quickly than acidosis. After the initial volume expansion phase, adequate insulin administration should decrease the blood glucose concentration by about 1 to 2 mg/dL/min (60 to 120 mg/dL/hr). Attempts should be made to stabilize the plasma glucose near the renal threshold, that is, in the range of 150 to 200 mg/dL. This will minimize urinary fluid losses from osmotic diuresis and avoid the occurrence of hypoglycemia, which would trigger a counterregulatory hormone response.

Therefore, when blood glucose approaches 250 mg/dL, 5% dextrose should be added to the IV fluid. A 5% dextrose solution at the rate commonly used for rehydration in DKA, delivers 3 to 5 mg/kg/min of dextrose. If this fails to stabilize the glucose, higher concentrations of dextrose infusion can be used or the insulin infusion rate can be reduced. However, the insulin infusion rate should not be reduced if acidosis is not correcting and should not be reduced to below 0.05 U/kg/hr. In general, IV insulin should be continued until the patient can take oral fluids well, electrolyte abnormalities are correcting, serum bicarbonate is greater than 15 mEq/L, and acidosis has resolved. Because of the short half-life of IV insulin (about 7 to 10 minutes), IV insulin infusion should not be discontinued until approximately 30 minutes after subcutaneous insulin has been given. In patients known to have IDDM, the usual insulin dose can be resumed. In patients with new-onset of IDDM, subcutaneous insulin should be started as discussed elsewhere.

Following patients with DKA requires careful attention to every detail. Clinical status, including neurologic condition, should be assessed frequently (at least every 1 to 2 hours) for at least the first 6 to 12 hours. An accurate record of intake and output should be maintained, and blood glucose should be monitored using bedside monitoring techniques hourly. Serum electrolytes should be monitored at least every 2 to 6 hours, with serum potassium, bicarbonate and pH more frequently in severe cases. Unexpected changes in clinical status, mental status, or laboratory results should be promptly investigated and the therapy should be changed appropriately. The vast majority of subjects with DKA do quite well, unless it is complicated by a significant underlying medical or surgical condition. Most uncomplicated cases of DKA that do poorly are a result of a lack of appropriate evaluation, monitoring, and attention.

Complications of Treatment

Complications associated with the treatment of DKA include hypoglycemia, aspiration, fluid overload with congestive heart failure, and cerebral edema. The first three of these can usually be avoided by careful attention to all aspects of the therapy. Cerebral edema as a complication of DKA and its treatment occurs primarily in children.[91,121] Its etiology is unclear but it may relate to too rapid correction of osmolality, acidosis, and/or hyperglycemia. Too rapid a rate of hydration should be avoided. Bolus doses of bicarbonate should be avoided, and, when bicarbonate is used, it should be done only with great caution. A bicarbonate infusion of 1 to 2 mEq/kg over 2 hours can be given if the arterial pH is less than 7.0 to 7.1. This should rarely be continued beyond the first 2 to 3 hours. The benefits of bicarbonate infusion are not proven. Unexpected alteration in mental state or the development of neurologic signs, bradycardia, or hypertension could indicate developing cerebral edema. Although the incidence of clinically significant cerebral edema is low (probably about 1%), the outcome after its development is poor. Cerebral edema remains a leading cause of death in diabetic children, accounting for about 31% of deaths associated with DKA and 20% of the overall mortality in children with diabetes. Therefore, cerebral edema warrants prompt and aggressive treatment with IV mannitol (0.5 to 1.0 g/kg), hyperventilation, and perhaps dexamethasone.

HYPEROSMOLAR NONKETOTIC COMA SYNDROME

Hyperosmolar nonketotic coma syndrome (HNKC) is the most common severe metabolic derangement in non–insulin-dependent type II diabetes mellitus. As is the case with DKA, HNKC is usually a life-threatening medical emergency. The mortality rate for HNKC is higher than that for DKA, primarily because these patients are older and frequently have significant other medical problems that either precipitate or are precipitated by HNKC. Factors associated with HNKC are shown in Table 8-1. Approximately half of those who are seen with HNKC are known to have type II diabetes, whereas the other half are newly diagnosed when they present with HNKC.

Persons with HNKC present with markedly elevated blood glucose, extreme hyperosmolality, and severe dehydration without significant ketosis and often with minimal acidosis. They often present with neurologic manifestations such as severe obtundation, seizure, coma, or focal neurologic findings suggestive of a stroke. Plasma glucose is over 600 mg/dL and is usually between 1000 and 2000 mg/dL. Marked hyperosmolality is present with serum osmolality in excess of 340 mOsm/L of water and BUN over 60. Dehydration is usually 10% to 15%. Serum and urine ketones are absent or only slight.

The general principles for the management of HNKC are similar to those for DKA; that is: (1) to correct the fluid and electrolyte imbalance, (2) to provide adequate insulin to lower plasma glucose, (3) to prevent and monitor for complications of treatment, and (4) to treat any underlying medical conditions. Initial therapy of HNKC should be directed at correcting life-threatening abnormalities and stabilization of the patient. Adequate ventilation should be established if necessary. Shock should be corrected with vigorous fluid resuscitation. Comatose patients should have nasogastric (NG) drainage to prevent aspiration. Intravenous access should be established as soon as possible and laboratory studies sent to confirm the diagnosis and the severity of the condition. A medical history, physical examination, and additional laboratory studies should be performed as necessary, to

Table 8-1   Factors Associated with Nonketotic Hyperosmolar Coma Syndrome

Therapeutic agents	Therapeutic procedures	Chronic illness	Acute illness
Glucocorticoids	Peritoneal dialysis	Renal disease	Infection
Diuretics	Hemodialysis	Heart disease	Gangrene
Diphenylhydantoin	Hyperosmolar alimentation	Hypertension	Urinary tract infection
β-adrenergic blocking agents	Surgical stress	Previous stroke	Burns
L-asparaginase		Alcoholism	GI bleeding
Immunosuppressive agents		Psychiatric	Myocardial infarction
Chlorpromazine		Loss of thirst	Pancreatitis
Diazoxide			Stroke

Adapted from Physician's guide to non–insulin-dependent (Type II) diabetes: diagnosis and treatment, Alexandria, VA, 1988, American Diabetes Association, Inc.

rule out any precipitating causes and underlying other medical conditions. After initial stabilization and evaluation, the mainstays in the therapy of HNKC are correction of dehydration and interruption of the metabolic imbalance (hyperglycemia). The former is accomplished with intravenous fluid therapy, the latter with insulin administration.

After the initial volume expansion phase using isotonic saline, additional isotonic saline or colloid containing solutions are used only if the patient is hypotensive or in shock. Subsequently, rehydration is usually accomplished using 0.45% saline with appropriate addition of potassium, phosphate, and other anions. Large amounts of potassium supplementation with EKG monitoring are usually necessary. Careful and frequent (at least every 1 to 2 hours) assessment of fluid and electrolyte status is essential, especially if acute or chronic renal failure complicates the course. Close monitoring of vital signs and neurologic status is also indicated. Therapy and monitoring should always be done in an ICU setting.

Although there have been reports of successful treatment of HNKC without insulin, insulin administration is certainly recommended as part of its therapy. The insulin regimen used is similar to that used in DKA (0.1 U regular insulin/kg/hr), except that the insulin can be stopped when the plasma glucose nears 200 to 250 mg/dL; there is no need to continue insulin therapy to interrupt ketosis and prevent recurrent acidosis. Because of the severe dehydration and marked volume depletion associated with HNKC, plasma glucose may fall rapidly even without insulin administration. Although cerebral edema is much less common in adults with HNKC than in children with DKA, it is probably advisable to limit the decline of plasma glucose to 1 to 2 mg/dL/min.

Identification and treatment of underlying illnesses or intercurrent events during the management of HNKC should be aggressive. Even though cerebral edema is less common than in DKA, the mortality associated with HNKC is greater and is probably in the range of 10% to 40%.

RECOGNITION AND TREATMENT OF HYPOGLYCEMIA

Hypoglycemia is a common feature of insulin-treated diabetes mellitus and can also be seen in subjects treated with oral agents. Hypoglycemia occurs as a result of a mismatch in the timing or amount of insulin in the circulation, physical activity, and exogenous availability of carbohydrate. Consumption of ethanol can also precipitate hypoglycemia. The signs and symptoms of hypoglycemia and the plasma glucose level at which they are noted will vary from person to person, but the hypoglycemic symptoms and signs are generally divided into two major categories, adrenergic and neuroglycopenic (Table 8-2).

The adrenergic symptoms and signs of hypoglycemia are those associated with a rising epinephrine. These include shakiness, irritability, nervousness, tachycardia, headache, hunger, and tremulousness. Paresthesias and pallor can also occur. Diaphoresis is usually considered along with the adrenergic symptoms of hypoglycemia, even though it is not mediated via adrenergic nerve endings. These symptoms are usually present when the circulating plasma epinephrine concentration is above approximately 150 pg/ml.[35] Increments in plasma epinephrine to this level occur not only during hypoglycemia, but also

Table 8-2   Symptoms and Signs of Hypoglycemia

Adrenergic	Neuroglycopenic
Shakiness	Headache
Irritability	Mental dullness
Nervousness	Inability to concentrate
Tachycardia/palpitations	Slurred speech
Tremor	Blurred vision
Hunger	Confusion
Diaphoresis	Irrational behavior
Pallor	Amnesia
Paresthesias	Severe lethargy
	Loss of consciousness
	Seizure
	Coma
	Death

during rapid decrements in blood glucose concentration from a hyperglycemic (200 mg/dL or 11.1 mM) to a nonhypoglycemic (100 mg/dL or 5.6 mM) level.[123] This occurs in the experimental setting and probably also occurs as a clinical event in some poorly controlled diabetic subjects with persistent hyperglycemia who report experiencing adrenergic symptoms of hypoglycemia even when blood glucose is not low.[29,133] Adrenergic symptoms can also occur during other stressful or anxiety provoking events.

The neuroglycopenic signs of hypoglycemia are those associated with lack of glucose availability to the brain and the resultant cerebral dysfunction. The neuroglycopenic manifestations of hypoglycemia include headache, inability to concentrate, slurred speech, blurred vision, confusion or irrational behavior, severe lethargy, seizure, coma, and death. Occasionally, transient focal neurologic findings can be seen in association with severe hypoglycemia.[149] Lesser degrees of neuroglycopenia can occur in the form of altered cognitive functioning[17,50,80,116] as measured by increased reaction time and response time,[17] and increased latency of the P300 wave on auditory[50] or visual[17] evoked response testing. Neuroglycopenia occurs as a result of low plasma glucose concentration and diminished availability of glucose to the central nervous system and is rarely, if ever, observed during falling plasma glucose that is still within or above the normal range. Recognizable neuroglycopenia rarely occurs until the glucose concentrations is below about 45 mg/dL (2.5 mM).[29,133] However, subtle alterations in cerebral function (increased reaction time and P300 waves) can be documented in persons with diabetes with glucose levels only as low as about 60 mg/dL (2.2 mM)[17,50] and even at higher values in children or poorly controlled persons with diabetes.

Clinically, hypoglycemia in persons with diabetes is usually divided into mild and severe. Mild hypoglycemia is that which is recognized and appropriately treated by the individual. The symptoms of mild hypoglycemia are usually primarily adrenergic (shaky, sweaty, hungry, tachycardia or palpitations, nervousness). The treatment of mild hypoglycemia should be with the oral ingestion of rapidly absorbed carbohydrate, either in the form of food or drink, or as glucose from one of the many commercially available sources to treat hypoglycemia (glucose tablets, Monojel, and others). The use of these preparations is convenient but not essential, as carbohydrate intake in the form of juice, milk, crackers, or hard candies is equally effective if taken in the appropriate quantity. Usually, 5 to 15 g of carbohydrate are adequate to treat mild hypoglycemia. This carbohydrate can be obtained from one to three glucose tablets, three to eight Life Savers candies, or two to six ounces of juice (see Chapter 2).

Severe hypoglycemia is that which results in the inability of the subject to recognize or treat himself or herself. Severe hypoglycemia usually presents with neuroglycopenic signs and can result in loss of consciousness, seizure, or coma. Severe hypoglycemia can occur as a complication of treatment in any insulin-treated subject but, fortunately, is uncommon according to most reports. Data in the literature suggest that severe hypoglycemia occurs in between 6.5% and 26% of adults with IDDM and between 4% and 9.8% of children.[12,72,105] The definition and documentation of severe hypoglycemia vary from study to study, and ascertainment bias is likely; therefore, these estimates vary considerably and may be inaccurate. The frequency of severe hypoglycemia appears to be higher in those suffering from hypoglycemia unawareness, defective glucose counterregulation, or autonomic neuropathy, as well as in those using intensive insulin therapy (see appropriate sections below).

During severe hypoglycemia, the individual is unable to treat himself or herself. This can be the result of lack of recognition, confusion, or inability to treat. Treatment, therefore, must be implemented by an outside party. If the individual is alert and awake, ingestion of oral carbohydrate (10 to 15 g) should be used. If the person will not allow oral carbohydrate to be used or is not fully alert and conscious (convulsing, postictal, unarousable, comatose), then treatment should consist of either parenteral glucose or glucagon. Glucose should be given intravenously (either as 50% dextrose or 25% dextrose) if the setting allows, since this is the most rapid way to raise the blood glucose concentration. The usually recommended dose is 10 to 25 grams of dextrose given over 1 to 2 minutes, followed by an infusion of a 5% dextrose solution at 5 to 10 grams per hour (3 to 5 mg/kg/min in children). If intravenous dextrose is not immediately available for administration and the patient is unable to safely ingest oral carbohydrate, then an injection of glucagon (1 mg for adults and children over 30 kg; 0.5 mg for children below 30 kg) should be given. Even though glucagon is effective in the majority of subjects, it is usually advisable to seek medical assistance after its administration in case hypoglycemia recurs (the effect of glucagon is relatively transient), vomiting occurs preventing oral intake of carbohydrate (vomiting is common after glucagon), or the subject's mental status does not improve. After glucagon administration, the patient should ingest oral carbohydrate or a meal to assure that the blood glucose does not once again fall to the hypoglycemic range. After resolution of a severe hypoglycemic event, the patient and health care team should try to identify the cause and patient education related to prevention should occur.

Clinical hypoglycemia can occur at any time of day or night but seems to occur most commonly during exercise, 8 to 24 hours after strenuous exercise (late postexercise hypoglycemia),[100] and in the middle of the night (see later discussions of the Dawn phenomenon and Somogyi phenomenon). Nocturnal hypoglycemia[78,96,135] has been reported to occur in 7% to 56% of adults with IDDM and in 10% to 26% of children. Reported percentages vary depending on the definition and the methods of ascertainment. Late postexercise hypoglycemia[100] refers to the occurrence of clinically significant, and sometimes severe, hypoglycemia 8 to 24 hours after strenuous exercise; usually this occurs overnight or early the following morning. The pathophysiology of late postexercise hypoglycemia is poorly understood. It does not occur in all subjects with diabetes, but it does represent a significant problem for some. Late postexercise hypoglycemia is best managed by monitoring blood glucose more frequently after strenuous exercise and using extra carbohydrate-containing snacks if the blood glucose is falling rapidly or falls to below the target range (see Chapter 3).

THE GLUCOSE COUNTERREGULATORY HORMONES

Insulin is the primary hormone resulting in lowering of blood glucose. However, there is a redundancy of the hormonal mechanisms for raising blood glucose.[37,39] The hormones that work to raise the blood glucose are generally referred to as the glucose counterregulatory hormones. Redundancy in the glucose counterregulatory hormone system seems appropriate because of the potential significant dangers associated with even brief periods of hypoglycemia. The central nervous system is the largest consumer of glucose. The brain utilizes glucose as its primary fuel, rarely using other substrates. Even brief periods of hypoglycemia can cause cerebral dysfunction,[17,50,80] brain damage, or death.

The glucose counterregulatory hormones include glucagon, catecholamines (epinephrine and norepinephrine), cortisol, and growth hormone. These hormones play an important role in regulation carbohydrate metabolism in subjects with, as well as those without, diabetes mellitus.[37,39] These hormones increase in the circulation during hypoglycemia and exercise and play an important role in bringing the blood glucose up to normal after hypoglycemia and preventing the occurrence of hypoglycemia during fasting and exercise.

Glucagon

Glucagon is a polypeptide hormone of molecular weight 3500 kD. It is synthesized in the α-cells of the pancreatic islets and is secreted into the portal venous circulation where it circulates directly to the liver. Glucagon acts on plasma membrane receptors of hepatic parenchymal cells to activate a G protein–dependent process resulting in stimulation of glycogenolysis, gluconeogenesis, and ketogenesis. The actions of glucagon are relatively transient, and it is thought that changes (increases) in glucagon concentration and the glucagon-to-insulin ratio in the portal vein may be more important determinants of its action than the absolute glucagon concentration. In nondiabetic individuals, plasma glucagon concentration increases in response to hypoglycemia or stress. However, subjects with type I diabetes mellitus develop α-cell dysfunction starting during the first few years of diabetes.[13,20] This α-cell dysfunction results in a failure of glucagon to be released in response to hypoglycemia or a rapidly falling glucose despite normal or perhaps even an exaggerated glucagon response to stress and other stimuli. The etiology of this α-cell dysfunction is poorly understood. However, after the first few years of diabetes, it is clear that increments in endogenously released circulating glucagon play little, if any, role in hypoglycemic counterregulation, despite its important role in stress-induced hyperglycemia and ketosis.

Epinephrine

Epinephrine (also known as adrenaline) is synthesized in the adrenal medulla and norepinephrine in the preganglionic sympathetic and parasympathetic neurons. Together, epinephrine and norepinephrine are referred to as catecholamines. The catecholamines act on the α- and β-adrenergic receptors to cause peripheral vasoconstriction, tachycardia, and the typical adrenergic symptoms of irritability, shakiness, tremor, hunger, and diaphoresis. It should be noted that although diaphoresis is usually categorized as "adrenergic," it is probably mediated by stimulation of cholinergic nerve fibers in the skin. In addition to producing these well-known adrenergic symptoms, the catecholamines serve as glucose counterregulatory hormones. By activation of β-adrenergic receptors, epinephrine and norepinephrine stimulate gluconeogenesis and lipolysis from muscle and perhaps liver resulting in an increase in glucose production and a rising blood glucose concentration.[49,115] Epinephrine also inhibits the release and action of insulin. This latter effect contributes to its glucose counterregulatory potential in diabetes. The catecholamines are released in both diabetic and nondiabetic individuals in response to stress, exercise, or hypoglycemia. However, some persons with diabetes develop a diminished or absent release of epinephrine in response to hypoglycemia or falling blood sugar. This blunted epinephrine response can be seen in subjects with neuropathy[81] and in those with the syndromes of defective glucose counterregulation[20,40,128,158] and hypoglycemia unawareness[84] (see below).

Cortisol

Cortisol is the major steroid, glucocorticoid hormone of the human. Cortisol is synthesized in the adrenal cortex via a series of enzymatic reactions starting from the precursor cholesterol. Cortisol is released into the circulation in a diurnal pattern, with cortisol release and circulating cortisol concentration increasing during the early morning hours and in response to stress or hypoglycemia. Although cortisol acts as a glucose counterregulatory hormone, its effects are primarily long-term in the form of causing some resistance to insulin action. Although subjects with cortisol deficiency (Addison's disease, congenital adrenal hyperplasia, hypopituitarism adrenalectomy) can be seen with hypoglycemia, cortisol seems to have little effect on raising blood glucose concentration quickly after insulin-induced hypoglycemia.[37]

Growth Hormone

Growth hormone is a 22,000 kD molecular weight polypeptide hormone produced and secreted by the anterior pituitary gland. Growth hormone exerts its effects on growth through modulation of growth factors, primarily insulin-like growth factor-1/somatomedin-C (IGF-1). Growth hormone also exerts effects on carbohydrate metabolism that are not mediated through IGF-1. The effect of growth hormone on carbohydrate metabolism appears to be biphasic.[101] The initial response, which occurs within 1 to 2 hours after growth hormone administration or increments in endogenous growth hormone, is "insulin-like"; hepatic glucose production is diminished and blood glucose concentration falls. This effect is short-lived, and after about 4 hours, growth hormone blunts insulin-mediated glucose uptake and oxidation. As with cortisol, growth hormone increases in response to hypoglycemia but probably has little effect on fluctuations in blood sugar over short periods.[37] Growth hormone is likely to play a role in the diurnal variation of blood glucose (see discussion of Dawn phenomenon below).

Regulation of blood glucose within the narrow normal range depends on the rapid modulation of insulin and the counterregulatory hormones (glucagon, catecholamines, cortisol, growth hormone). In the nondiabetic individual, the fluctuations of these hormones are closely timed so that blood glucose remains in the narrow range of about 70 to 140 mg/dL (3.9 to 7.8 mM). Individuals with overproduction of insulin (hyperinsulinism) or underproduction of counterregulatory hormones (adrenalectomy, autonomic dysfunction, Addison's disease, hypopituitarism) can experience hypoglycemia as a manifestation of their disorder. Persons with diabetes have poorly timed insulin action either as a result of exogenous absorption (as in IDDM) or inappropriate secretion/action (as in (NIDDM). This loss of glucose regulation by insulin makes glucose counterregulation by the counterregulatory hormones even more critical in maintaining a stable blood glucose.

GLUCOSE COUNTERREGULATION IN NONDIABETIC PERSONS

The works of Cryer and colleagues,[37,39] Gerich and associates,[20,49] and other investigators have clearly shown redundancy of the glucose counterregulatory mechanisms, with a hierarchical effect of the various hormones. Maintenance of euglycemia during fasting (in adults), exercise, and recovery from insulin-induced hypoglycemia all follow a similar pattern. Dissipation of insulin is a primary factor in preventing or recovering from hypoglycemia. Glucagon plays a primary role in the recovery from hypoglycemia. Epinephrine is not essential but can compensate for glucagon and becomes essential in its absence. Cortisol and growth hormone have counterregulatory effects, but these effects are not rapid and are not sufficiently potent to compensate for a diminished or absent glucagon and epinephrine response accompanied by mild hyperinsulinemia. Likewise, other substrate effects and hepatic glucose autoregulation,[24,75] though present, are weak.

In the absence of epinephrine release (such as after bilateral adrenalectomy) or action (such as during continuous α- and β-adrenergic blockade), glucose counterregulation during insulin-induced hypoglycemia occurs normally as a result of glucagon release.[37] In the absence of an incremental glucagon response during insulin-induced hypoglycemia, glucose counterregulation is essentially within normal limits, though slightly delayed. In the absence of a glucagon response and epinephrine secretion or action, glucose counter-regulation fails to occur. Therefore, epinephrine, though not essential for normal glucose counterregulation in the presence of normal glucagon secretion, becomes critical in the absence of glucagon. The combined effects of other glucose counterregulatory factors (cortisol, growth hormone, hepatic autoregulation) are insufficient to cause significant glucose counterregulation during insulin-induced hypoglycemia in the absence of gluca-gon and epinephrine secretion or action. These concepts are summarized in Fig. 8-2. In the presence of growth hormone deficiency *(panel C)* or epinephrine deficiency *(panel D)*, the glucose counterregulatory response is normal. Glucagon deficiency alone *(panel B)* and in combination with growth hormone deficiency blunts, but does not eliminate, the

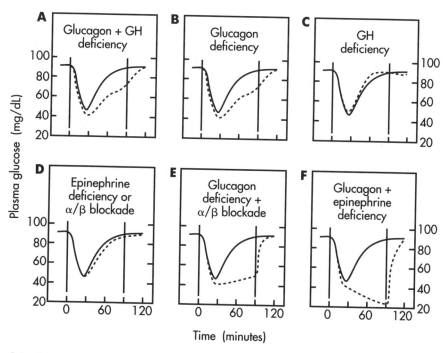

Fig. 8-2 Summary of the experimental evidence leading to the current views about the physiology of glucose counterregulation in normal man. The plasma glucose following an IV injection of insu-lin without other intervention is shown in the solid lines, and that following insulin along with the indicated intervention is shown in the broken line. **A,** Somatostatin infusion (glucagon + growth-hormone deficiency). **B,** Somatostatin infusion with growth-hormone replacement (glucagon defi-ciency). **C,** Somatostatin infusion with glucagon replacement (growth-hormone deficiency). **D,** Epi-nephrine deficiency or combined α/β-blockade with intact glucagon response. **E,** Glucagon defi-ciency and α/β-blockade. **F,** Glucagon and epinephrine deficiency. Note the complete absence of glucose counterregulation in **E** and **F.** (Adapted from Cryer PE: Glucose counterregulation in man, Diabetes 30:261-264, 1981.)

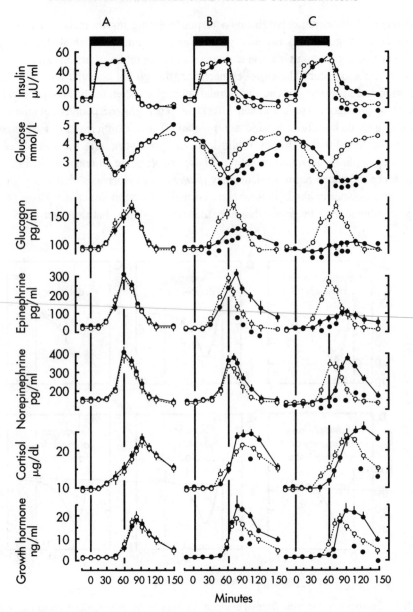

Fig. 8-3 Glucagon responses to insulin-induced hypoglycemia in IDDM. **Left,** Counterregulatory hormone response (mean±SEM) to insulin-induced hypoglycemia in diabetic subjects *(closed circles/solid lines)* and 10 nondiabetic controls *(open circles/broken lines).* Insulin infusion was 28 mU/M²/min from 0 to 60 minutes. **A,** IDDM less than 1 month; *N* = 5. **B,** IDDM 1 to 5 years; *N* = 11. **C,** IDDM 14 to 31 years; *N* = 5. **Right,** Correlation between the maximal incremental glucagon response to insulin-induced hypoglycemia and duration of IDDM. (Adapted from Bolli G and others: Abnormal glucose counterregulation in insulin dependent diabetes mellitus: interaction of anti-insulin antibodies and impaired glucagon and epinephrine secretion, Diabetes 32:134-141, 1983.)

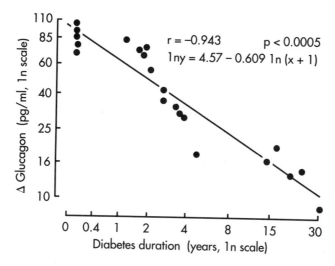

$r = -0.943 \qquad p < 0.0005$

$\ln y = 4.57 - 0.609 \ln (x + 1)$

Fig. 8-3 cont'd. For legend see opposite page.

counterregulatory response. Combined glucagon and epinephrine deficiency *(panels E and F)* results in the absence of glucose counterregulation.

GLUCOSE COUNTERREGULATION IN PERSONS WITH IDDM

The physiologic and pathophysiologic concepts related to glucose counterregulation noted above are similar for subjects with diabetes mellitus.[39] However, as can be seen in Fig. 8-3, after 4 to 5 years of diabetes, subjects with type I diabetes fail to secrete glucagon in response to hypoglycemia or decrements of blood glucose.[13,26] Subsequently, they would be dependent on epinephrine as their primary counterregulatory hormone for defense against hypoglycemia. In the absence of an epinephrine response, subjects with diabetes would be essentially defenseless against the occurrence of significant hypoglycemia during even the slight hyperinsulinemia of day-to-day therapy; cortisol and growth hormone increments and hepatic autoregulation are not sufficiently potent to protect against the development of significant hypoglycemia. Individuals with diabetes who develop an absent or blunted epinephrine response to decrements in plasma glucose or absolute hypoglycemia are seen with the syndromes referred to as "hypoglycemia unawareness"[84] or defective glucose counterregulation[39,40,128,158] (see below). In such subjects, hypoglycemia often becomes the rate-limiting factor in maintaining good glycemic control.[23,38,39,128,158]

MANIFESTATIONS OF NORMAL OR ALTERED GLUCOSE COUNTERREGULATORY SYSTEMS IN DIABETES
Hypoglycemia Unawareness

Hypoglycemia unawareness refers to the syndrome in which persons with diabetes are unaware that they are hypoglycemic and therefore do not initiate treatment. Persons with hypoglycemia unawareness have a blunted epinephrine response to hypoglycemia[84] (Fig. 8-4). Note that subjects with fewer recognizable symptoms of hypoglycemia (low hypoglycemic index) have reduced peak epinephrine responses to hypoglycemia. As a result, they tend to lack the adrenergic symptoms of hypoglycemia, and often develop neuroglycopenic symptoms and severe hypoglycemia without previous warning. Some subjects have adrenergic signs, which are observed by others but not recognized by themselves, preceding the development of neuroglycopenia. The etiology of this latter phenomenon is unclear, but individualized reeducation about the symptoms of hypoglycemia may diminish the frequency of severe hypoglycemia in these individuals.

There has been some concern that the use of β-adrenergic blockade medications, such as propranolol and metaprolol, could cause hypoglycemia unawareness and blunt the counterregulatory effects of the catecholamines in diabetic subjects since adrenergic symptoms of hypoglycemia are primarily mediated via the β-adrenergic receptor.[49,88,115] Therefore, many physicians recommend that these drugs not be used in diabetic subjects unless absolutely necessary. Some consider intensive insulin therapy aimed at normalization of blood glucose to be contraindicated in subjects using β-adrenergic blockade medications.[51] There is little in the literature, however, to directly address this problem, and recent reports suggest that β-adrenergic blockade in individuals with diabetes may not present a significant clinical problem.

Persons with diabetes and hypoglycemia unawareness are more likely to have epi-

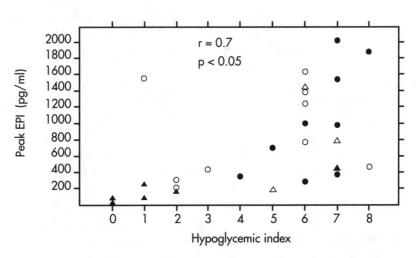

Fig. 8-4 Correlation between peak epinephrine (EPI) concentration during hypoglycemia and hypoglycemia symptom score. *Closed circles,* Healthy controls. *Open circles,* IDDM without autonomic neuropathy. *Closed triangles,* IDDM with autonomic neuropathy and hypoglycemia unawareness. *Open triangles,* IDDM without hypoglycemia unawareness. Note the low peak EPI response in those with hypoglycemia unawareness compared with those without hypoglycemia unawareness. (Adapted from Hoeldke RD and others: Reduced epinephrine secretion and hypoglycemia unawareness in diabetic autonomic neuropathy, Ann Intern Med 96:459-462, 1982.)

sodes of severe hypoglycemia.[84] Extensive discussion about the problem and reeducation about hypoglycemia, along with increased monitoring and vigilance, seem to be the best way to minimize severe hypoglycemia. In other persons symptoms related to hypoglycemia may change (usually diminish) over time, and the patient or family may need guidance in recognizing subtle symptoms of hypoglycemia. In other persons with hypoglycemia unawareness, raising the glycemic target may be necessary to prevent repeated episodes of severe hypoglycemia.

Defective Glucose Counterregulation

As discussed above, the rapid defense against insulin-induced hypoglycemia is primarily dependent on glucagon and epinephrine.[37,39] In persons with and without diabetes, cortisol, growth hormone, and hepatic autoregulation[24,75] are insufficiently potent to prevent significant hypoglycemia in the absence of decrements of insulin and increments of glucagon and epinephrine. Despite the fact that most persons with diabetes (after the first few years of diabetes) have a deficient glucagon response to hypoglycemia,[13,20] most have adequate glucose counterregulation because their epinephrine secretory response is normal or perhaps exaggerated. In association with mild overinsulinization, these persons will often maintain a stable plasma glucose in the mild hypoglycemia range for as long as 30 to 60 minutes.[158] This should give adequate time for the recognition of adrenergic symptoms and the treatment of hypoglycemia before it becomes severe.

Some individuals with diabetes, however, lose their incremental epinephrine response (mean peak epinephrine response, 115 pg/ml) to glucose decrements or hypoglycemia as compared with normal controls (mean peak epinephrine, 234 pg/ml) and responsive subjects with IDDM (mean peak epinephrine, 344 pg/ml)[128,158] (Fig. 8-5). This rarely occurs before 10 to 15 years of diabetes[20] and may be associated with the development of autonomic neuropathy. These subjects are said to have defective glucose counterregulation.[158] In subjects with defective glucose counterregulation, combined deficiencies of increments in both glucagon and epinephrine in response to hypoglycemia result in the inability to interrupt a falling plasma glucose during insulin infusion.

In addition, since the epinephrine response is blunted, defective glucose counterregulation is often accompanied by hypoglycemia unawareness. Therefore, severe hypoglycemia can develop quickly and without warning. Persons with defective glucose counterregulation have a markedly increased risk of developing severe hypoglycemia, especially during the use of intensive insulin therapy, when the risk has been reported to be as high as 25 times that of subjects with adequate glucose counterregulation[23,38,158] (Table 8-3).

Defective glucose counterregulation can occur in association with autonomic neuropathy[81] but can also occur in subjects without other signs or symptoms of peripheral or autonomic neuropathy. However, some investigators feel that defective glucose counterregulation that develops after 10 to 15 years of diabetes is a manifestation of autonomic neuropathy even when no other manifestations of neuropathic involvement are present.[61] This speculation is based on the observation that persons with defective glucose counterregulation have an absent pancreatic polypeptide response to hypoglycemia.[61,81,99,151,152]

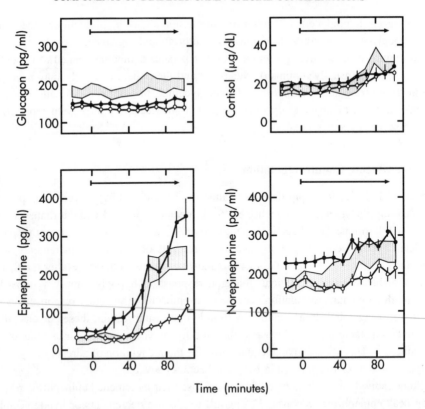

Fig. 8-5 Counterregulatory hormone responses to insulin infusion in controls and IDDM subjects with adequate or defective glucose counterregulation. Plasma glucagon, epinephrine, norepinephrine, and cortisol concentration (mean± SEM) during insulin infusion (40 mU/kg/hr) in 10 normal controls *(stippled area)*, 13 IDDM subjects with adequate counterregulation *(closed circles)*, and 9 IDDM subjects with defective counterregulation *(open circles)*. Note the deficient glucagon response in both diabetic groups and the blunted epinephrine response in those with defective counterregulation. (Adapted from White NH and others: Identification of type I diabetic patients at increased risk for hypoglycemia during intensive therapy, N Engl J Med 308:485-491, 1983.)

Because the pancreatic polypeptide response to insulin-induced hypoglycemia is generally felt to be a marker for parasympathetic function,[81,99] the epinephrine response, which correlates well with the pancreatic polypeptide response, seems likely to be a marker for sympathetic function.

   In addition to occurring spontaneously as an isolated finding or in association with neuropathic complications, a form of defective glucose counterregulation has been reported to occur as a result of improving glycemic control using intensive insulin therapy.[4,6] In this form of defective glucose counterregulation, the hormonal response to hypoglycemia occurs in the same general pattern as in patients with normal counterregulation (epinephrine, cortisol, and growth hormone all rise), but the threshold to trigger the counterregulatory hormone response (usually about 60 mg/dL or 3.3 mm) is lowered; neuroglycopenia

Table 8-3 Incidence and Event Rate of Severe Hypoglycemia During Intensive Insulin Therapy in Patients with IDDM with Adequate (+CR) and Defective (−CR) Glucose Counterregulation as Determined by an Insulin Infusion Test

	Number of subjects	Severe hypoglycemia	
		Incidence (number of subjects)	Event rate (events/patient/year)
Cohort #1			
Total	22	9	1.2
+CR	13	1	0.1
−CR	9	8	2.5
Cohort #2 (includes Cohort #1)			
Total	37	14	—
+CR	24	2	—
−CR	13	12	—

Cohort #1 adapted from White NH, et al: Identification of Type I diabetic patients at increased risk for hypoglycemia during intensive therapy, N Engl J Med 308:485-491, 1983.

may precede the appearance of significant adrenergic symptoms. These persons may be at increased risk for severe hypoglycemia during IIT despite having adequate counterregulation when beginning IIT. Improved glycemic control, or the use of IIT, does not normalize the counterregulatory hormone response in diabetic persons with defective glucose counterregulation.[13,21] Persons with defective glucose counterregulation may require similar educational interventions or adjustment of glycemic target to that of those with hypoglycemia unawareness.

The Dawn Phenomenon

For persons with IDDM, maintenance of good glycemic control presents as much of a problem overnight as at any other time of day. Hypoglycemia occurring between 1 and 4 AM is common,[78,96,135] and hyperglycemia before breakfast is also common. Diurnal variation in the counterregulatory hormones may play a significant role in glucose homeostasis overnight, especially in diabetic subjects. However, a cause-and-effect relationship between nocturnal hypoglycemia and morning hyperglycemia remains controversial. The controversy continues as to the relative importance of the *dawn phenomenon (DP)* and the *Somogyi phenomenon* in the development of morning hyperglycemia.[38] The dawn phenomenon refers to an early-morning (4 to 8 AM) rise in blood glucose concentration without antecedent nocturnal hypoglycemia. The Somogyi phenomenon refers to morning hyperglycemia occurring as a result of "rebound" from preceding nocturnal hypoglycemia.

The DP was first observed as early as the 1920s when it was described as a paradoxic rise in blood glucose, sometimes causing morning fasting hyperglycemia. The term *dawn phenomenon* was first used to describe this event by Schmidt and associates[132] in a 1981 paper reporting 24-hour glucose profiles in diabetic subjects. A prebreakfast, dawn-time rise of blood glucose was a common observation. This rise averaged 30 to 50 mg/dL (1.7 to 2.8 mM) between 5 AM and 8 AM before breakfast. The authors attributed this rise to the waning activity of the previous day's insulin, resulting in early morning insulin deficiency.

It soon became apparent, however, that the DP represented more than simply a waning of the previous day's insulin. Insulin deficiency alone appears not to be the sole cause of the rising blood glucose concentration during the dawn period. Even during continuous insulin infusions, blood glucose tended to rise during the dawn period. This was seen in studies using the Biostator[34] as well as during continuous subcutaneous insulin infusion (CSII). Although the initial recognition and descriptions of the DP were in those with IDDM, it is now clear that this phenomenon is also present in those with NIDDM[25] and probably in nondiabetic subjects as well,[22] in whom insulin availability is not a problem.

The most concise definition of the DP is that of Bolli and Gerich[25] from their 1984 paper. They define the DP as "an abrupt increase in plasma glucose concentration or insulin requirements or both between 5 AM and 9 AM in the absence of antecedent hypoglycemia." For example, during constant insulin infusion, the DP is seen as a rising blood glucose between 5 AM and 8 AM after a stable period without hypoglycemia between about midnight and 5 AM. During variable-rate insulin delivery, the DP is seen as increasing doses of insulin required during the dawn period to maintain a stable, not rising, blood glucose concentration (Fig. 8-6).

A number of possible causes for the DP have been suggested. These include waning of the previous day's insulin,[132] diurnal variation of insulin clearance,[54,55,138,139] diurnal variation of insulin sensitivity,[22] and diurnal variation of counterregulatory hormones.[34] The latter could exert their effect through variations in either insulin clearance, insulin sensitivity, or both.

After the initial descriptions of the DP by Schmidt and associates[132] and Clarke and associates,[34] the diurnal variation of plasma cortisol seemed a likely candidate for its cause because of the temporal relationship between the rising insulin requirements and the early morning cortisol rise. However, Skor and associates[139] demonstrated that the rising cortisol appears not to be a significant factor in the etiology of the DP. During Skor's study,[139] it was also observed that despite a 30% to 50% higher insulin infusion rate during the dawn period, the plasma-free insulin concentrations were identical to those seen earlier in the night. This raised the possibility that there may be some diurnal variation of insulin clearance as a contributor to the DP.

Follow-up studies of Skor and associates[138] and Dux and colleagues[54,55] were able to show that insulin clearance was higher during the dawn period than during the earlier nighttime hours. This higher clearance is most pronounced at physiologic rates of insulin delivery. Despite some criticism of the methods used in some of these studies,[32] insulin clearance does appear to play some role in the etiology of the DP. However, other factors are probably also important.

Many glucose counterregulatory hormones have been studied as possibly contributing

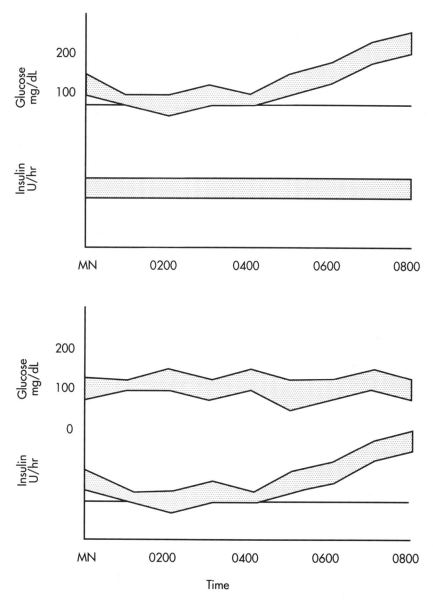

Fig. 8-6 Schematic representation of the dawn phenomenon. **Top,** During constant-rate overnight insulin infusion, blood glucose is stable from midnight to 4 AM and rises during the dawn period (4 AM to 8 AM). **Bottom,** During feedback-controlled overnight insulin infusion to maintain a stable blood glucose, insulin requirements increase during the dawn period.

to the DP. There is general consensus, based on data in the literature, that cortisol,[139] glucagon,[40] and the catecholamines[35,40] play little or no role in the DP. Initial studies suggested that growth hormone played little role in the DP,[137] but subsequent investigations are suggestive that diurnal variation in growth-hormone secretion may be a key determinant of the DP.[30] There are three lines of evidence in support of this hypothesis. First, somatostatin with glucagon replacement eliminates nocturnal growth-hormone spikes and blunts the DP.[31] Second, blunting growth-hormone spikes by cholinergic blockade blunted the DP in two separate studies.[7,43] Third, Boyle and associates[28] showed that the DP was absent in a group of five growth-hormone–deficient persons with IDDM.

In a report by Campbell and associates[30] persons with IDDM were studied overnight on 3 nights—a control night, a growth-hormone–deficient night using somatostatin with glucagon replacement, and a growth-hormone–replacement night using somatostatin with replacement of both glucagon and growth hormone. The absence of growth hormone markedly blunted the overnight rise in blood glucose. The authors attributed this to blunting of the DP, but reduction of the nighttime insulin requirements without elimination of the DP might be another explanation.[10] Skor and others,[137] using a very similar study design but slightly higher rates of insulin replacement, came to different conclusions. Elimination of nocturnal growth-hormone spikes with long-acting somatostatin analog[31] or anticholinergic agents[7,43] appears to blunt the DP.

Recent data reported by Boyle and associates[28] appear to tie together the growth hormone hypothesis and the insulin clearance hypothesis for the DP. Boyle and colleagues[28] studied the DP and insulin clearance in five growth-hormone–deficient persons with IDDM and compared them with persons with IDDM but without growth hormone deficiency. The control subjects with IDDM demonstrated the DP as expected, whereas the growth-hormone–deficient subjects with IDDM did not. In addition, the control persons with diabetes showed a higher prebreakfast insulin clearance, whereas those with growth-hormone deficiency had a stable clearance throughout the night. This suggests that growth hormone does play a role in the DP and that its role may be, at least in part, causing changes in insulin clearance. Despite conflicting reports, it is the prevailing current opinion that growth hormone does play some role in the DP and is perhaps the primary determinant of the DP.

With growth hormone as a strong candidate for the etiology of the DP, questions related to mechanism have been asked. Growth-hormone spikes are known to occur during early hours of sleep. Growth hormone is known to have an insulin-like effect within the first few hours after a spike,[101] followed by an insulin-antagonistic effect subsequently. Blackard and associates[16] have suggested that the DP is not a "dawn phenomenon" at all, but rather a "sleep phenomenon." The observation of increasing early morning insulin requirements could indeed be explained by a lowering of basal insulin requirements earlier in the night, possibly as a result of the insulin-like effects of the sleep-related growth-hormone spikes, with a return to normal insulin sensitivity or clearance during the dawn period. This hypothesis appears to be consistent with all the previous observations related to the DP and warrants further study.

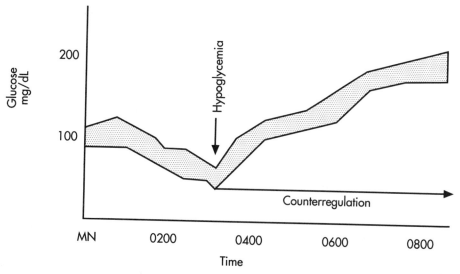

Fig. 8-7 Schematic representation of the Somogyi phenomenon. Nocturnal hypoglycemia causes stimulation of glucose counterregulation, which results in morning hyperglycemia (posthypoglycemic hyperglycemia, or rebound hyperglycemia.)

The Somogyi Phenomenon

The *Somogyi phenomenon (SP)* has been defined as a morning rise of blood glucose to hyperglycemic levels following an episode of nocturnal hypoglycemia and a counterregulatory hormone response (Fig. 8-7).

The SP is named for Dr. Michael Somogyi, who, in 1938, stated: "We obtained evidence to the effect that the extreme fluctuations in the blood sugar level and the progressively increasing unstability of diabetic patients are the direct results of the administration of excessive amounts of insulin. . . . In the past, we failed to recognize the cause and effect relationship between hypoglycemia and hyperglycemia, and by administering insulin doses sufficiently large to cause hypoglycemias, we produced more severe hyperglycemias."[144] Dr. Somogyi's statement has been interpreted in various ways. The most widely used interpretation has been that of rebound hyperglycemia, or posthypoglycemic hyperglycemia.

The SP has been implicated as a common cause for fasting, morning hyperglycemia. The hypothesis is that nocturnal hypoglycemia is followed by a glucose counterregulatory hormone response which, in turn, is followed by a rising plasma glucose and rebound hyperglycemia. This chain of events seems quite logical in theory and probably does occur in certain experimental settings.[26] However, in practice, it appears to be a very rare occurrence during day-to-day management of diabetes. Numerous studies have now confirmed this fact.*

*References 67,78,83,111,118,135,146,147.

Havlin and Cryer[78] evaluated 216 nighttime blood glucose profiles to determine if nocturnal hypoglycemia were followed by rebound morning hyperglycemia while patients with diabetes received their usual insulin therapy. They found that 2 AM blood glucose values below 100 mg/dL (5.5 mM) and below 50 mg/dL (2.8 mM) were associated with lower, not higher, glucose concentrations the following morning. In the 15 persons who experienced nocturnal hypoglycemia (2 AM blood glucose below 50 mg/dL), none had a fasting morning glucose concentration above 200 mg/dL (11.1 mM). In addition, following nocturnal hypoglycemia a substantial rise in blood glucose between 2 and 7 AM was seen only in those 12 who had received carbohydrate treatment for their nocturnal hypoglycemia. The three persons whose nocturnal hypoglycemia was not treated had little or no rise in the blood glucose concentration between 2 AM and breakfast (Fig. 8-8). Lerman and Wolfsdorf[96] reported similar results and extended the findings to show that blood glucose concentrations later in the day on the day following nocturnal hypoglycemia were similar to those on days not following nocturnal hypoglycemia.

Shalwitz and associates,[135] studying children, found similar results. From 388 nights during 166 elective routine hospitalizations of 135 diabetic children ages 6 to 18 years, nocturnal hypoglycemia (blood glucose <60 mg/dL or 3.3 mM) occurred 70 times (18% of the nights). Only 3 of these, or 4.3%, were followed by a morning fasting glucose concentration above 200 mg/dL (11.1 mM). In addition, blood glucose concentrations throughout the remainder of the day following nocturnal hypoglycemia were no higher than they were in the same children on a day not following nocturnal hypoglycemia.

Three studies[83,111,147] in which nocturnal hypoglycemia was induced overnight and compared with nonhypoglycemic nights have likewise shown that morning fasting hyperglycemia does not necessarily follow insulin-induced nocturnal hypoglycemia. Tordjman and colleagues[147] studied 10 persons with IDDM on 3 separate nights, 1 as a control, 1 in which hypoglycemia was prevented by IV dextrose, if necessary, and 1 in which nocturnal hypoglycemia was induced with IV insulin. Nocturnal hypoglycemia did not cause rebound hyperglycemia. Overall, morning plasma glucose concentration was not higher after the hypoglycemic nights than it was after the control or prevention nights. When a higher morning plasma glucose concentration was observed, these patients had been treated for their symptomatic nocturnal hypoglycemia.

Perriello and associates[111] reported the only study in which nocturnal hypoglycemia was followed by hyperglycemia in a predictable way. They found slightly higher morning glucose concentration following insulin-induced nocturnal hypoglycemia. However, the difference was only 13 mg/dL (0.7 mM), of uncertain clinical significance. Perriello and colleagues[111] did, however, find substantially higher postbreakfast blood sugars following nocturnal hypoglycemia, suggesting rebound hyperglycemia as a cause of daytime postprandial hyperglycemia. Hirsch and associates,[83] however, were unable to confirm this finding, and found that blood glucose concentrations over the entire day following insulin-induced nocturnal hypoglycemia were similar to those following the control and prevention night (Fig. 8-9). They also found that the increment of glucose between 2 AM and 8 AM was directly, not inversely, correlated with the glucose nadir (i.e., the lower the nocturnal nadir glucose concentration, the lower the rebound observed). These data would

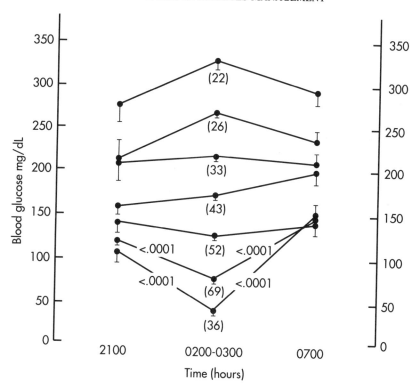

Fig. 8-8 Blood glucose concentrations from overnight profiles in patients with IDDM. Blood glucose concentration (mean± SEM) at 2100 hours, 0200 to 0300 hours, and 0700 hours from 281 profiles in 66 IDDM patients. Profiles are separated based on 0200 to 0300 hours blood glucose into 50 mg/dL intervals. Numbers in parentheses refer to number of profiles in each group. Note that nocturnal hypoglyemia is not followed by morning fasting hyperglycemia. (Adapted from Lerman IG and Wolfsdorf JI: Relationship of nocturnal hypoglycemia to daytime glycemia in IDDM, Diabetes Care 11:639, 1988.)

be in good agreement with Gale's observation[67] that the morning glucose concentration following nocturnal hypoglycemia was inversely correlated with the free insulin concentration, not the nadir glucose concentration (Fig. 8-10). In other words, high morning sugars following nocturnal hypoglycemia are a result of absolute or relative insulin deficiency, or the dawn phenomenon, and not excessive glucose counterregulation, the so-called Somogyi phenomenon. The recent studies of Stephenson and Schernthaner[146] would support this conclusion.

Taken together, these studies suggest that nocturnal hypoglycemia does not cause, or rarely causes, morning fasting hyperglycemia in patients with IDDM using their usual therapeutic regimens. Likewise, nocturnal hypoglycemia rarely causes postprandial hyperglycemia the following day. Morning hyperglycemia is more likely to be a result of absolute or relative underinsulinization during the dawn period than of excessive glucose counterregulation earlier in the night. This is not to say that overinsulinization cannot lead

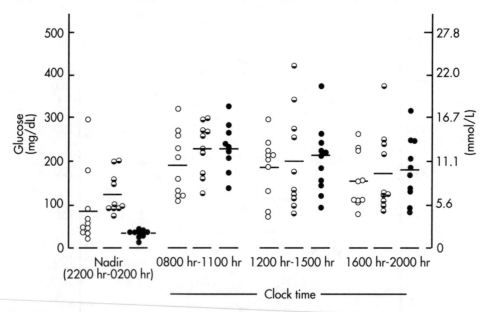

Fig. 8-9   Blood glucose concentration throughout the day following induction and prevention of nocturnal hypoglycemia. Blood glucose concentration during the morning (0800 to 1100 hours), afternoon (1200 to 1500 hours), and evening (1600 to 2000 hours) following a night of sampling only *(open circles)*, insulin-induced nocturnal hypoglycemia *(closed circles)*, and prevention of hypoglycemia with intravenous dextrose *(half-closed circles)*. Patients were maintained on their usual doses of insulin and dietary regimen. Note the similar blood glucose concentrations throughout the following day regardless of whether or not nocturnal hypoglycemia occurred. (Adapted from Hirsch IB and others: Failure of nocturnal hypoglycemia to cause daytime hyperglycemia, Diabetes Care 13:133-142, 1990.)

to poor control through a mechanism of recurrent hypoglycemia, leading to sustained increases in counterregulatory hormone concentrations and insulin resistance. If poor control is associated with high doses of insulin and recurrent hypoglycemia, attempts at lowering or redistributing the insulin dose should be made. However, in the absence of recognized hypoglycemia and in the presence of morning hyperglycemia, lowering the insulin dose should not necessarily be the first course of action.

Implications of the Dawn and Somogyi Phenomena in the Management of Morning Fasting Hyperglycemia in Persons with Diabetes

The evaluation and management of morning hyperglycemia in persons with IDDM requires considerable monitoring, discussion and patient education. First, it is important to be sure that the bedtime snack is taken regularly and is adequate. Too small or missed snacks are likely to result in nocturnal hypoglycemia; too large a snack could contribute to hyperglycemia throughout the night and into the next morning (see Chapter 2). Second,

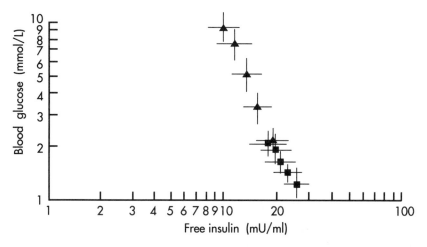

Fig. 8-10 Relationship between fasting blood glucose and plasma-free insulin after spontaneous nocturnal hypoglycemia. Correlation between fasting blood glucose and plasma-free insulin (mean ± SEM) following nocturnal hypoglycemia. Patients with fasting hyperglycemia had lower and falling free insulin concentrations as compared with those with lower morning glucose values. Fasting hyperglycemia after nocturnal hypoglycemia seemed to correlate with lower circulating insulin levels. (Adapted from Gale E, Kurtz A, and Tattersall R: In search of the Somogyi effect, Lancet 2:279, 1980.)

individuals and their family members should be carefully questioned for symptoms and signs of nocturnal hypoglycemia such as tremors, night sweats, nightmares, restlessness, nocturnal awakening, early morning headaches, or stomachaches. Third, whenever seriously trying to evaluate and manage morning hyperglycemia, blood glucose monitoring should be instituted at bedtime, morning, and, perhaps, at 2 to 3 AM. If the bedtime and/or 2 AM glucose is low, or if signs or symptoms of nocturnal hypoglycemia are present, the appropriate insulin dose should be reduced. Nocturnal hypoglycemia should be avoided even though it is not likely to be the primary cause of morning hyperglycemia. However, lowering the insulin dose is not likely to bring down the morning blood glucose concentration. If the 2 AM blood glucose concentration is normal or high, the appropriate dose of insulin should be increased. If satisfactory control of 2 AM and morning blood glucose concentration cannot be achieved using a split-mixed regimen of regular and NPH/Lente insulin twice daily, then alternative regimens should be considered.

Recommended Regimens

A number of alternative therapeutic regimens have been suggested for dealing with unacceptable glycemic control as a result of either the DP or the SP. First, since normalization of the blood glucose may not be possible for all patients with IDDM, consideration should be given to tolerating some degree of morning hyperglycemia, especially in very young children or toddlers, and especially if glucose control during the rest of the day is satisfactory and the glycosylated hemoglobin is in an acceptable range. Occasional monitoring of blood glucose at 2 AM to 3 AM may be necessary to guide therapy. If the 2 AM to 3 AM blood glucose is low, the suppertime dose of NPH should be reduced. If control is not considered acceptable, and there is no evidence of nocturnal hypoglycemia, the first approach should be to increase the suppertime dose of NPH or Lente insulin in hopes of providing better insulin coverage throughout the entire night and bringing the morning blood glucose concentration down.

If both higher and lower doses of NPH fail, or if nocturnal hypoglycemia becomes a problem after increasing the dose, the NPH or Lente dose can be moved to bedtime. By doing this, its peak action occurs closer to the dawn period when there are increasing insulin requirements, and there is less insulin action between 2 and 4 AM when hypoglycemia is likely. A trial of IIT (see below), especially CSII with multiple basal infusion rates, might be appropriate for some patients.

Finally, consideration should be given to an approach recently investigated by Johnson and associates[85] at Indiana University. Humulin Ultralente (Eli Lilly and Company) was substituted for NPH as part of a split-mixed insulin regimen in hopes of achieving more insulin action during the dawn period. The 36 patients studied were between 5 and 20 years old with IDDM and an early morning blood glucose rise of at least 50 mg/dL (2.8 mM). They were randomized to either continue on their usual regimen of regular and Lente insulin or be switched to regular and Ultralente twice a day. In the group receiving Ultralente, the mean early morning rise of glucose was only 7 mg/dL (0.4 mM) as compared with 46 mg/dL (2.6 mM) for the control subjects remaining on Lente. Unexpectedly, the blood glucose values throughout the rest of the day, including the afternoon, were not higher on the Ultralente regimen than the Lente regimen, and the HbA_{1c} was similar. The fasting blood glucose concentration was lower (188 mg/dL or 10.4 mM versus 222 mg/dL or 12.3 mM) on the Ultralente regimen, and blood glucose before lunch, supper, bedtime, and at 3 AM were similar.

BRITTLE DIABETES

Most individuals with diabetes can be expected to successfully maintain a relatively normal lifestyle aside from the certain requirements and restrictions related to carrying out their complex medical regimen on a daily basis. Children with diabetes can be expected to attend and perform normally in school, grow and develop normally, and maintain a normal social life. Adults with diabetes can perform well at most careers, unless diabetes complications diminish their capabilities. Most subjects with diabetes rarely develop diabetic ketoacidosis or significant ketosis except during intercurrent medical illnesses. However, a minority of subjects with diabetes are unable to participate in the normal activities of daily living because of recurrent episodes of severe metabolic decompensation. These subjects are said to suffer from brittle diabetes.[113]

The term *brittle diabetes* should be reserved for those cases in which diabetic instability is manifest by recurrent episodes of ketosis or ketoacidosis, or severe hypoglycemia, or both, and is significant enough to result in an inability to maintain a normal life style or to endanger life.[113] It is not appropriate to use the term to describe patients with stable diabetes who maintain a relatively normal life-style despite less than optimal glycemic control with persistently elevated or widely fluctuating blood glucose. Rather, persons with brittle diabetes are frequently absent from school or the workplace and are often visiting emergency rooms or are hospitalized.

Brittle diabetes is almost exclusively limited to subjects with IDDM and is rarely seen in subjects with NIDDM. It occurs more commonly among females than males[69,114,156] and usually presents during the teenage or young adult years. It rarely presents before puberty and usually does not persist into adulthood. Brittle diabetes presents during this phase of life regardless of duration of diabetes.[156] For example, brittle diabetes will present after only 1 or 2 years of diabetes in a girl whose onset of diabetes occurred at age 10 to 12 years, whereas it may present after 8 to 10 years if the onset was during the preschool years (Fig. 8-11). The reason why brittle diabetes presents primarily in teenage girls is not completely understood but probably relates to a combination of physiologic changes (insulin resistance, hormonal changes, menarche) and psychosocial and developmental events.

True brittle diabetes occurs in about 5% to 10% of the population seen in tertiary care subspecialty diabetes clinics.[69,114,156] Since it is presumed that the majority of persons with brittle diabetes are referred to specialists for care, whereas many stable persons with diabetes are not, the true prevalence of brittle diabetes is probably less than 5%. However, the greatest majority of emergency room visits and hospital admissions for patients with diabetes to pediatric or adolescent medical services, other than those for newly diagnosed subjects, are in this small group of patients. These persons consume a substantial portion of the time and effort of the staff at most pediatric diabetes units. It has been estimated that hospital bills for patients with brittle diabetes can be as high as $30,000 to $80,000 per patient per year.

The causes of brittle, or unstable, diabetes are often difficult to sort out. Most patients have little, if any, endogenous insulin reserve. Brittle diabetes rarely occurs during the honeymoon period. However, in addition to a low endogenous insulin reserve, other factors are necessary to cause brittle diabetes. Cases of brittle diabetes have been described to be secondary to overinsulinization, underinsulinization, defective glucose counterregulation, erratic insulin absorption,[110] excessive insulin degradation,[64,110,126] recurrent or persistent infection or inflammation, insulin antibodies, and true insulin resistance. Multiple factors may contribute in one person. Underinsulinization is frequently one of the many factors contributing to recurrent episodes of DKA in teenagers, especially teenage girls. The dogma that total daily doses above 1.0 U/kg/day represent overinsulinization is incorrect. Puberty is associated with a degree of insulin resistance,[5,19] and teenagers will often require insulin doses of 1.0 to 1.5 U/kg/day, especially during their peak growth spurt and immediately preceding menarche.

However, the majority of cases of brittle diabetes are caused, at least in part, by psychologic or psychiatric problems.[69,156] Noncompliance with the prescribed regimen is

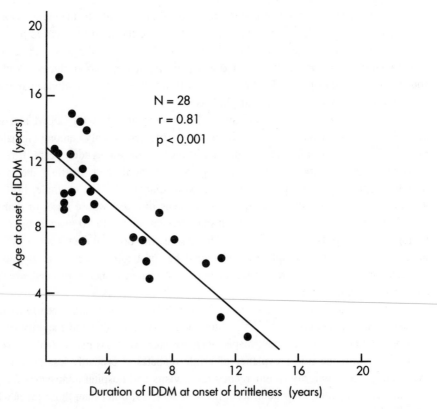

Fig. 8-11 Comparison of age at onset of IDDM and duration of IDDM at onset of brittle diabetes. Correlation between age at onset of IDDM and disease duration at onset of brittleness in 28 persons with brittle diabetes evaluated at St. Louis Children's Hospital from 1978 to 1985. Note that brittleness begins at the age of puberty, regardless of how long the patient has had IDDM. (Adapted from White HN and Santiago JV: Clinical features and natural history of brittle diabetes in childhood. In Pickup JC, ed: Brittle diabetes, Oxford, 1985, Blackwell Scientific Publications.)

common, including missed insulin doses,[70,108] surreptitious insulin administration,[107] failure of adequate monitoring, and even fabrication of monitoring results. Eating disorders,[15] such as anorexia nervosa and bulimia, as well as the behavior known as *induced glycosuria,* which is considered to be a variation on an eating disorder, will precipitate brittle diabetes. Severe family problems, child abuse or neglect, school problems or phobias, and drug or alcohol abuse can also be associated with a picture of brittle diabetes. Certainly more than half,[156] and some believe nearly all,[70,130] cases of brittle diabetes are the result of emotional, family, or psychiatric disturbance, and cases that have an entirely physiologic basis are infrequent. Therefore, whenever dealing with a case of brittle diabetes, aggressive psychosocial and/or psychiatric evaluation is essential.[73,76,131,153]

Management of Brittle Diabetes

When dealing with any case of brittle diabetes, a comprehensive multidisciplinary evaluation is required.[73,131] This often needs to take place over many visits, as all issues can rarely be addressed during one visit, and it is necessary to establish a close working relationship with the patient and the family before all the issues can be openly and adequately addressed. Involvement of health care professionals, such as nurses, nutritionists, social workers, and psychologists or psychiatrists, are important.[79] During an initial visit, the goals of therapy should be reviewed and modified so that the primary goals are the avoidance of ketosis, ketoacidosis, and severe hypoglycemia, maintenance or establishment of normal growth, and the resumption of normal participation in school, employment, and day-to-day life. Initially, blood glucose targets should be loose or, perhaps, abandoned altogether. Realistic goals should be established. The entire diabetes care regimen should be reviewed by many members of the team to determine its appropriateness for the patient and the family in light of the established goals. Psychosocial parameters should be assessed, including compliance, behavior, school performance, family functioning, and cognitive function.[153] Health beliefs should be examined to determine their consistency with the established goals. The regimen should be modified as necessary to achieve these goals.

If brittle diabetes continues despite modification of the goals and the therapeutic regimen, more extensive evaluation and intensive intervention is required. It may be necessary to implement an increased amount of parental supervision, including in some cases parental responsibility for giving all insulin injections. This has proven to be helpful in some cases, even when missed injections cannot be documented. Reduced parental support has been associated with worsening of metabolic control in teenagers.[86] If increased parental responsibility for diabetes care–related events fails to correct the problem, inhospital evaluation is indicated.

Inpatient evaluation for recurrent ketoacidosis or brittle diabetes should include a formal psychiatric evaluation.[76,131] All diabetes care (i.e., insulin injections, monitoring) should be performed, or at least very closely supervised, by the nursing staff. The regimen should be adjusted in the hospital to achieve the established goals. If control cannot be maintained despite all care being administered by the staff, then physiologic causes of brittleness should be sought. This should include a search for persistent, recurrent, or occult infection or inflammation, erratic insulin absorption or degradation,[64,126] and insulin resistance. These are rarely found, however, and when they are not and brittle diabetes continues, admission to a psychiatric facility is often indicated.[70] This is also true if in-hospital care results in adequate control but outpatient management consistently fails. In some cases, management at home consistently fails to avoid DKA. In these cases, evidence of abuse or neglect should be sought, and, if found, placement in a residential care facility or foster placement should be considered.

Persons with brittle diabetes rarely respond to intensification of the regimen using multiple daily injections or CSII unless erratic insulin absorption appears to be a major contributing factor. However, aggressive use of extra doses of regular insulin (a "sliding-scale" regimen), especially during ketosis or sick days, to prevent progression to diabetic ketoacidosis can be helpful. The addition of an extra 10% to 20% of the total daily dose given as regular insulin every 4 to 6 hours when urine ketones are high will reduce the frequency of hospital visits, if implemented regularly. Since the overall daily insulin dose for many teenage girls needs to be 1.0 to 1.5 U/kg/day, an additional 5 to 15 U may be needed in some cases (see below, "Sick Day Management").

STABLE INSULIN-DEPENDENT DIABETES

Some persons with IDDM seem exceptionally easy to control and can achieve all the stated goals with minimal effort and often very little insulin. These individuals fall into three main categories, but endogenous insulin reserve is a common feature. The three situations likely to result in stable diabetes are the honeymoon period of IDDM, NIDDM of youth, and diabetes with a long duration of continued endogenous insulin release.

The honeymoon period occurs shortly after the diagnosis of IDDM. During the honeymoon period there is a temporary recrudescence of β-cell function, resulting in near normalization of blood glucose despite diminishing doses of exogenous insulin.[142] Some small children may appear to be insulin independent during the honeymoon phase, although most physicians elect to continue very low–dose insulin therapy during this time. The use of diluted insulin (U-10 or U-25) may be needed. The honeymoon usually starts during the first few weeks after diagnosis and can last anywhere from a few weeks to a year. The honeymoon rarely lasts beyond a year, although cases of an apparent prolonged honeymoon have been observed. Even if a true honeymoon does not occur, residual endogenous insulin reserve (measured as circulating C-peptide) will result in stable, easy-to-control diabetes. Adults tend to have a less rapid decline of C-peptide than do young children[47] and therefore may remain stable for longer periods.

Some cases of long-lasting stable diabetes in children could be the result of relatively rare causes of diabetes mellitus, which are not typical IDDM. These include maturity-onset diabetes of youth (MODY),[59] the diabetes unique to black Americans who present with DKA but subsequently respond similarly to NIDDM,[163] and genetic mutations of the insulin molecule, such as hereditary hyperproinsulinemia and biologically defective insulin.[145]

GROWTH FAILURE IN DIABETES AND MAURIAC'S SYNDROME

Most diabetic children grow within the normal percentiles for age and sex, although some studies suggest that they are slightly shorter than expected. Our examination of a large cohort of diabetic children,[154] for example, showed that the final adult height and the corrected height of diabetic children fall at about the fortieth percentile. This is about 1 to 2 cm below the median for the general population. Most of this reduced height is likely the result of poor glycemic control; subjects in good or fair glycemic control (HbA$_{1c}$ <11.0%) grow at an annualized growth velocity that was normal for age, whereas those in poor control (HbA$_{1c}$ >11.0%) grow approximately 0.5 cm per year less than expected.

However, despite these minor alterations in growth, major growth disturbance as a result of diabetes mellitus is unusual. Short stature or reduced growth velocity in children with diabetes should be investigated using the same guidelines and with the same vigor as in those without diabetes. Thyroid function tests and plasma cortisol should be measured, especially since hypothyroidism and Addison's disease are more common in subjects with IDDM. Celiac disease (gluten-sensitive enteropathy) may also be more common in type I subjects. Growth-hormone testing is rarely indicated, and measurement of somatomedin-C/IGF-1 may not be helpful since it is often low in poorly controlled diabetes.

Markedly diminished growth can be seen as a result of the Mauriac's syndrome.[95] Mauriac's syndrome is poor diabetic control in association with the combination of reduced growth, delayed sexual maturation, hepatomegaly, hypertriglyceridemia and, often, a cushingoid appearance of truncal obesity and peripheral muscle wasting. The etiology of the Mauriac's syndrome is unknown, but poor control is probably only one component, as not all poorly controlled diabetic children will manifest this constellation of findings.

Whenever growth failure or Mauriac's syndrome occurs in a child with diabetes and no other etiology for growth failure is identified, aggressive efforts at establishing better diabetic control are indicated. Careful nutritional assessment is essential, and higher doses of insulin are usually needed. Teenagers may require 1.0 to 1.5 U/kg/day of insulin to maintain adequate control for the maintenance of normal growth and development. Increased parental involvement may be necessary, and an evaluation for possible psychosocial dwarfism should be considered. IIT should be utilized if other attempts to normalize growth fail. Improvement of glycemic control will usually result in a better growth velocity, or even catch-up growth (Fig. 8-12). However, during the catch-up growth phase of treating Mauriac's syndrome, careful surveillance for diabetic microvascular complications should be performed because an apparent rapid progression of retinopathy and nephropathy[57] has been observed within the first few months of IIT in these subjects.

SICK DAY MANAGEMENT

The primary goal for the management of diabetes during any illness is to prevent the need for hospitalization. Of course individuals can and do develop other medical illnesses as well, and if these are serious enough to warrant hospitalization, the patient with diabetes will be hospitalized regardless of his or her ability to deal with diabetes. However, in most cases, early intervention in consultation with an experienced health care team can prevent the development of severe DKA, severe hypoglycemia, or dehydration requiring hospitalization. It is imperative that every person with diabetes and his or her family have an experienced health care team available to help during times of illness. Without rapid intervention, illnesses that might be relatively insignificant for the person without diabetes can develop into a major medical emergency in persons with diabetes, particularly IDDM. In addition, diabetes itself, or its complications, can mimic other serious health problems.

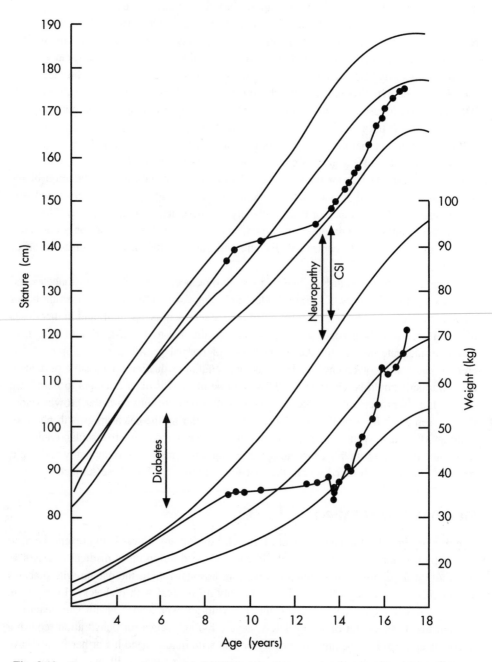

Fig. 8-12 Growth curve of a boy with IDDM and marked growth failure. IDDM was diagnosed at 6 years old. Growth failure started at about 9 years old and continued until aggressive insulin therapy and eventually CSII was started at 13 years old. Catch-up growth followed the initiation of intensive insulin therapy. Growth curve shows the fifth, fiftieth, and ninety-fifth percentile.

Common illnesses, even those as simple as a cold or the flu, can affect the control of diabetes in three ways. First, illness or stress raise the counterregulatory hormones (glucagon, catecholamines, growth hormone, cortisol), and these hormones will act to cause hyperglycemia (by stimulating gluconeogenesis and inhibiting insulin action) and ketosis (by stimulating lipolysis and ketogenesis). Second, since it may be difficult to eat during illness, hypoglycemia can occur. Third, illness, especially gastrointestinal illness, can cause vomiting and an inability to take fluids, resulting in dehydration. The problem of dehydration is worsened by the glucose-induced osmotic diuresis and acidosis accompanying DKA. Dehydration and acidosis combine to cause significant electrolyte imbalance. During the management of any sick day, the combination of ketosis and dehydration requires immediate and aggressive action. Likewise, the presence of hypoglycemia in a subject who is unable to eat or drink requires immediate and aggressive action.

Home management of sick days is best accomplished by a well-informed and highly motivated patient. If the patient is too young to care for himself or herself or is temporarily incapacitated by the illness, it is important that the assistance and supervision from a family member or friend is available at times of intercurrent illness. Occasionally, hospitalization may become necessary for a relatively mild illness because of the lack of family support and motivation. However, if this happens repeatedly, other action needs to be taken, including the possibility of obtaining outside help for the family (see discussion under "Brittle Diabetes").

Management of Sick Days

Guidelines for the management of sick days[97] should be established and discussed early in the relationship between the patient and health care team. Whenever possible, specific individualized guidelines should be discussed with each patient and should be reviewed and updated regularly. General guidelines that all persons with diabetes should follow as a part of sick day management, as discussed in Chapter 2, include: (1) never omiting insulin, (2) always monitoring blood glucose and urine ketones at least every 2 to 4 hours, (3) always providing plenty of fluids, (4) using supplemental insulin, if necessary, to break ketosis, and (5) contacting the health care team or see a physician if there is a fever, persistent vomiting, persistent presence of large ketones or symptoms of DKA, or the presence of other severe symptoms suggesting a significant underlying medical problem (see box on p. 286). The physician should be available to evaluate the patient for underlying illnesses and provide rapid treatment, as indicated by the patient's condition and course. If the person's own physician is not readily available, a visit to an emergency clinic or hospital emergency room is in order.

Monitoring is an essential part of the management of diabetes, and this is even more important during an intercurrent illness. Whenever a person with diabetes is ill, regardless of the symptoms or the blood glucose, urine ketones should be monitored. Likewise, whenever the blood glucose is unexpectedly high (>240 mg/dL), urine ketones should be monitored regardless of whether their are any symptoms. Ketones indicate insulin deficiency and/or stress-related insulin resistance, and is nearly always an indication for an

---

SICK DAY MANAGEMENT: WHEN TO SEEK MEDICAL ASSISTANCE

Seek immediate medical assistance if any of the following occur:
 Shortness of breath, or respiratory difficulty
 Severe abdominal pain
 Persistent vomiting
 Chest pain
 Severe dehydration
 Acute visual loss
Seek medical attention if any of the following persist:
 Elevated preprandial blood glucose (>250 mg/dL) that is not responding to changes
 Ketonuria
 Persistent diarrhea
 Fever above 100° F
 Other unexplained symptoms

---

additional insulin dose. A large amount of urinary ketones is usually accompanied by hyperglycemia; however, even if the blood glucose is only slightly elevated, large ketonuria warrants the use of sick day guidelines.

Fluids are an essential part of managing diabetes during a sick day (for further discussion see Chapter 2). It is usually recommended that a teenager or young adult attempt to take 6 to 8 ounces of fluid each hour, if possible. If not possible, careful monitoring for the presence or development of dehydration should be implemented. More frequent ingestion of small quantities of fluid (3 to 4 ounces every half hour) is usually better tolerated by people with gastrointestinal illness than less frequent ingestion of larger quantities. Young children, of course, should take proportionately less (perhaps 3 to 6 ounces every hour). Ingestion of food is not essential during the few-day course of a brief illness, but an inability to take fluids by mouth is a clear indication for intravenous therapy. If meals are not being taken, carbohydrate-containing fluids should be taken to compensate for the carbohydrate intake of the usual meal plan. Additional fluids should be carbohydrate-free as long as hyperglycemia is present. However, once the blood glucose falls to below the 150 to 200 mg/dL range, additional fluids should contain carbohydrates. In some cases, even dehydrated patients can be managed without hospitalization if oral intake is good and close follow-up is ensured. However, when developing a plan to rehydrate a patient at home, it is helpful to have the patient obtain a weight and follow weight changes, as well as blood sugar and urinary ketones, throughout treatment. As the patient feels better and vomiting resolves, gradual resumption of the usual meal plan can begin.

In the presence of ketonuria, supplemental doses of insulin are usually required. If intravenous therapy is not indicated, supplemental insulin should be subcutaneous short-acting regular insulin. A dose equivalent to approximately 10% of the total daily dose is usually recommended; this should be repeated every 2 to 4 hours until ketosis is clearing. If hyperglycemia is absent or minimal in conjunction with significant ketones, supplemental insulin should be given anyway, and additional sugar, in the form of carbohydrate-containing beverages, are used to prevent hypoglycemia. Ketosis accompanied by an inability to take oral fluids, especially if the blood glucose drops to below 150 to 200 mg/dL before successful oral intake can be reestablished, is a clear indication for intravenous fluid therapy. If intravenous fluids and insulin are indicated, it is best to follow the guidelines similar to those reviewed for the treatment of severe DKA (see above).

During any sick day, it is imperative that blood glucose, urine ketones, hydration status, and patient symptoms and well-being be monitored at least every few hours. Any deterioration should be promptly reported to the health care team and consideration should be given to having the patient seen by the physician for evaluation. Maintaining a flowsheet of the individual's status is often helpful in following response to therapy. If the individual demonstrates resolution of ketones, improvement of hydration status, and resolution of the symptoms, it is appropriate to continue the sick-day regimen at home and resume the customary insulin dose and meal plan when they are ready to resume eating meals. However, should vomiting persist, symptoms worsen, or signs of severe DKA occur, a medical evaluation should be performed without delay.

Diabetes itself, or its complications, can mimic other serious health problems. Any underlying illness must be addressed. Laboratory studies should include electrolytes, BUN, creatinine, and assessment of acidosis, as well as other studies necessary to help rule out underlying causes. However, other serious health problems need to be considered if the history and/or examination is suggestive. Symptomatic treatment for mild illness, such as with analgesics, decongestants, or antihistamines, is appropriate, unless contraindicated because of diabetes complications or other medical problems. However, antiemetics should be used only with great caution and after evaluation by a physician. Many nonprescription medications can be used by people with diabetes without major effects on blood glucose. However, patients should be instructed to read the label for warnings. Aspirin and acetaminophen (Tylenol)—the mainstays in treating minor illnesses—are generally well tolerated and safe, except in persons allergic to them. In commonly used doses, they do not interfere with blood or urine sugar or with monitoring of glucose or ketones. Of course, many pediatricians advise parents not to use aspirin in children with flulike or viral illnesses because of the association with Reye's syndrome.

Persons with diabetes should use over-the-counter cold medications—particularly those containing decongestants—with caution. Some contain substances that not only raise blood glucose but create symptoms mimicking hypoglycemia. Other nonprescription drugs, such as cough syrups, may contain sugar and alcohol, although in limited quantities; the effects on diabetes is usually negligible. In general, the effects of these over-the-counter medications on blood glucose are small and can be easily compensated for by the changes in insulin therapy made during sick day management. Use of decongestant medications may also be inadvisable in persons with hypertension or heart disease.

SURGERY IN THE PATIENT WITH DIABETES MELLITUS

It has been estimated that a patient with diabetes has a 50% chance of undergoing surgery sometime during his or her lifetime.[2] The risk associated with surgery and anesthesia may be increased in diabetic patients as compared with healthy individuals, especially if diabetic control is poor or diabetic complications are present. Poor metabolic control is associated with impaired response to infection, poor wound healing, increased protein breakdown, and electrolyte imbalance. The risk of hypoglycemia in the surgical patient and in the patient recovering from anesthesia is increased, especially since he or she may not be unable to sense or communicate symptoms and needs. Insulin requirements often increase in response to the stress of illness and/or surgery. In addition, stress can precipitate ketosis or DKA. DKA can mimic other conditions, including an abdominal examination suggesting a need for surgical intervention.

The metabolic effects of surgery and anesthesia are principally those of the stress response. Catecholamines, cortisol, glucagon, and growth hormone all increase, leading to increased glycogenolysis and gluconeogenesis, protein catabolism, and lipolysis. Insulin resistance also occurs. The net effect of this response is the development of hyperglycemia, protein breakdown, lipolysis, and ketogenesis. Insulin is necessary to overcome this stress hormone response and prevent the intraoperative development of a catabolic and ketotic state. In general, the response to surgery itself is greater than the response to anesthesia, and the magnitude of the metabolic response relates to the severity of the surgery and underlying illness. The response to general anesthesia is greater than the response to local or spinal anesthesia, which has a minimal effect on metabolism.

The primary goals of management for the persons with diabetes undergoing surgery are to avoid hypoglycemia, marked hyperglycemia, ketoacidosis, and fluid and electrolyte imbalance. Normalization of blood glucose during surgery and the immediate postoperative period is not essential and may not even be desirable. Mild hyperglycemia is preferable to unrecognized hypoglycemia. The regimens used to reach the goals should minimize the possibility of error and be widely applicable to the variety of conditions that pertain to surgical wards and operating theaters.

Elective surgery offers the greatest opportunity to anticipate and identify problems. Persons with diabetes requiring elective surgery should be in the best possible metabolic control before admission. If acceptable metabolic control cannot be achieved before elective surgery, it may be warranted to hospitalize the patient for 2 to 3 days to establish good control. Elective surgery should be postponed in the presence of ketosis. Screening for diabetic complications should be done before elective surgery; this should include testing for renal, cardiovascular, neuropathic, and retinal disease as directed by the age and duration of disease of the patient. Surgery should be scheduled as early as possible in the day to avoid prolonged fasting. Short-acting (regular) and intermediate-acting (NPH or Lente) doses of insulin should be altered on the day of surgery. Long-acting (Ultralente) insulin should be reduced 1 or 2 days before surgery, if possible, and supplemental regular insulin given as needed to control hyperglycemia. Oral hypoglycemic agents should be held for 1 or 2 days before surgery.

In general, insulin should be used in all patients with diabetes (whether insulin-treated or not) during major surgery or any surgery requiring general anesthesia. In some cases of minor surgery under local or spinal anesthesia, no change in therapy is warranted, except as dictated by change in dietary intake. If surgery is relatively minor and will not involve prolonged periods without oral intake, the use of subcutaneous insulin during the perioperative period seems appropriate. The simplest regimen seems to be using a reduced dose of intermediate-acting insulin alone (one-half to two-thirds of the usual morning dose of NPH or Lente) before surgery and then dextrose-containing intravenous fluids. Together, these should be adjusted to maintain the blood glucose between 150 and 200 mg/dL. These adjustments can be made based on readings from a reflectance meter. A small amount of regular insulin can be added if marked hyperglycemia is present. If ketosis is present, it is probably best to postpone elective surgical procedures.

The operative and postoperative health care teams must understand the management objectives during surgery in patients with diabetes (see box below). The clinician should

---

GUIDELINES FOR THE MANAGEMENT OF PATIENTS WITH DIABETES MELLITUS DURING SURGERY

General goals of perioperative therapy

Prevent hypoglycemia, ketoacidosis, electrolyte and fluid imbalance

Control hyperglycemia; blood glucose 115 to 140 mg/dL is ideal; 150 to 200 mg/dL is acceptable in most settings

Resume oral intake as soon as possible

Use human insulin when insulin required in patient who is not usually treated with insulin

Schedule surgery early in the morning

Specific guidelines

Stabilize glucose before surgery, whenever possible

    Use insulin during surgery for:
        (1) All insulin-requiring patients
        (2) All major surgical procedures
        (3) Procedures requiring general anesthesia
        (4) Minor surgery, if hyperglycemia or ketosis are present

For type II patients managed on diet and/or oral hypoglycemic agents alone:
        (1) Hold oral agent for 1 to 2 days before surgery, if possible
        (2) No specific therapy on day of surgery if:
            Surgery minor
            Local or spinal anesthesia
            Fasting blood glucose less than 125 mg/dL
            No ketones

Adapted from Albert KGMM, Gill GV, and Elliot MS: Insulin delivery during surgery in the diabetic patient, Diabetes Care 5(suppl 1):65-77, 1982; and from Physicians guide to non–insulin-dependent (type II) diabetes: diagnosis and treatment, Alexandria, VA, 1988, American Diabetes Association, Inc.

learn specific techniques and plan the preoperative, intraoperative, and postoperative management of these patients before the surgery actually takes place. The management technique should be individualized to meet the specific needs of the patient and his or her situation; one regimen will not be applicable to all situations. The reader is referred to the bibliography for a more detailed description of various regimens.[2,82,148]

If surgery will require prolonged periods of general anesthesia, if hypoperfusion, shock, or electrolyte imbalance are likely during surgery, or if ketosis is present and surgery cannot be postponed, then it is best to use intravenous insulin and dextrose. Serum electrolytes, BUN, creatinine, urine ketones, and hydration status should be determined before surgery and monitored during surgery. Omit the usual subcutaneous insulin on the day of surgery. Insulin should be administered at 0.05 to 0.1 U/kg/hr, and IV fluid begun with a 5% to 10% dextrose solution to give approximately 5 mg/kg/min. Potassium can be added to the IV fluid as necessary to prevent hypokalemia. Blood glucose should be monitored by meter every 4 hours before surgery, hourly during surgery, and at least every 2 to 4 hours after surgery until well into the recovery phase. Blood glucose should be kept in the 150 to 200 mg/dL range. Intravenous infusions should be continued until it is appropriate to resume subcutaneous insulin.

After surgery, meals, or at least oral fluids, should be resumed as quickly as possible. If the patient cannot eat or drink for more than 1 day, intravenous insulin and dextrose should be continued or regular insulin given every 4 hours throughout that time. Blood glucose monitoring should be performed every 1 to 4 hours. Adults typically require IV dextrose at 150 to 200 g/day and children about 2 to 4 gm/kg/day. When meals are fully tolerated, the patient's customary insulin regimen should be resumed along with supplemental regular insulin to compensate for elevated blood glucose and ketones.

Emergency surgery may not permit sufficient time to stabilize the patient. In persons who require emergency surgery and are in DKA, treatment of DKA must begin without delay (see the section on treatment of DKA) and should be continued vigorously throughout surgery and into the postoperative period until DKA has resolved. Careful monitoring of electrolytes, blood glucose, rehydration, and urine output are essential throughout surgery. Intravenous regular insulin should be used in all cases of emergency surgery accompanied by DKA. If possible, surgery should be delayed until the acidosis is beginning to improve. Whenever possible, emergency surgery in a patient in DKA should be performed at a center with appropriate medical and surgical intensive care available.

Individuals with diabetes undergoing local anesthesia (such as dental or spinal anesthesia) should be scheduled as early in the day as possible to avoid prolonged fasting. Oral hypoglycemic agents should be held for 1 to 2 days before surgery and on the morning of surgery. Insulin should be decreased on the morning of surgery. Depending on the length of surgery, regular insulin can be decreased or omitted. Often one-half to two-thirds of the usual dose of intermediate insulin dose can be given. Careful monitoring of blood glucose by meter should be performed before, during, and after surgery as outlined above. Blood glucose in excess of 240 mg/dL can be treated with supplemental regular insulin and low blood glucose (<70 mg/dL) can be treated with intravenous dextrose or oral carbohydrate, as tolerated. Typically, the usual insulin or oral hypoglycemic agent regimen and meal plan can be resumed with the first scheduled postoperative dose of insulin or meal. In cases of extensive dental work, soft foods or liquids containing carbohydrates should be given until oral feeding is reestablished. Careful monitoring of blood glucose and urine ketones should occur as with general anesthesia.

ALTERNATIVE METHODS OF INSULIN ADMINISTRATION

Essentially all persons with IDDM receive insulin subcutaneously. The intraperitoneal route of administration from implantable infusion pumps should be considered experimental at the present time, although these devices have met with some recent success. Success has been achieved with rectal or nasal administration of insulin, but neither of these routes have become popular.

Subcutaneous insulin is most commonly given in the form of injection. The use of portable infusion pumps to deliver insulin is discussed below. Numerous injection aids are available. These facilitate the insertion of the needle through the skin and may be particularly applicable for young children. Forced-air (or jet) injectors are also available for insulin delivery.[134] These are effective but are relatively expensive and offer little advantage for most young people with IDDM. A recent summary of injection aids and other diabetes care–related devices and supplies is available.[3] The available supplies and devices on the market change rapidly.

INTENSIVE INSULIN THERAPY

Insulin is the primary hormonal regulator of carbohydrate metabolism and an important regulator of protein and fat metabolism as well. For the individual without diabetes, insulin is secreted by the β-cells of the islet into the portal vein where it circulates to the liver and subsequently to the rest of the body. The modulation of pancreatic insulin release is under numerous mechanisms of control, including the ambient glucose concentration, autonomic nervous system input, gut hormonal stimulatory factors, and the hormonal milieu. The hormonal factors include circulating endocrine effects as well as intraislet paracrine effects. As a result of these factors, insulin release by the pancreas and the circulating insulin concentration is modulated to produce the rapid changes necessary to normalize carbohydrate metabolism and maintain blood glucose in the very narrow range of 70 to 140 mg/dL (3.9 to 7.8 mM).

A consistent pattern of insulin release, measured as circulating plasma insulin concentration, is reproduced with each meal. With the ingestion of each meal, the circulating insulin concentration rises 10- to 15-fold, from a baseline concentration of 5 to 10 μU/ml to a peak of 50 to 150 μU/ml. This peak insulin concentration is reached about 1 hour after ingestion of the meal, and the insulin concentration then rapidly declines returning to its baseline level after about 4 to 6 hours. This pattern repeats itself with the ingestion of the next meal. During the postabsorptive and fasting states, the circulating insulin concen-

Schade DS and others: Intensive insulin therapy, Princeton, 1983, Excerpta Medica.

tration remains low but is not absent. This low level of insulin is required to prevent hyperglycemia from unchecked glycogenolysis and gluconeogenesis.

As discussed elsewhere, the rapid decline in circulating insulin after its postprandial peak is a key component of glucose counterregulation during the postprandial period; that is, the prevention of postprandial hypoglycemia. Likewise, the rapid rise of insulin during the first hour postprandial is a key component in preventing postprandial hyperglycemia. This can be demonstrated by the postprandial hyperglycemia associated with the blunted or delayed first-phase insulin release seen in persons with early IDDM and in some persons with NIDDM. In addition, in insulin-deficient persons, a 15-minute delay in the administration of an intravenous dose of insulin that would otherwise normalize blood glucose results in postprandial hyperglycemia.[33] Therefore, the maintenance of blood glucose within the narrow normal range throughout the day is dependent on rapid modulation of insulin release and circulating insulin concentration.

The exogenous administration of insulin as one or two injections per day of fast-acting regular and/or intermediate-acting NPH or Lente insulin does not result in the rapid modulation of circulated insulin concentrations necessary to normalize carbohydrate metabolism and blood glucose. Instead, conventional insulin therapy results in a slow rise, followed by gradual decline, of circulating insulin and relatively constant hyperinsulinemia throughout most of the day, with declining insulin overnight. Along with this highly unphysiologic pattern of insulinemia, it is not unexpected that glycemic control is less than perfect. In addition, meal, snack, and exercise timing are relatively inflexible.

Intensive insulin therapy (IIT) is the term used to describe therapeutic regimens of insulin delivery that are designed to mimic physiologic insulin release and normalize blood glucose. Before launching into a discussion of insulin administration in IIT, it is essential to point out that any diabetes care regimen, whether it be conventional or intensive, is more than simply insulin administration. Meal planning, exercise, and monitoring are important components of any diabetes care regimen, and no diabetes care plan can succeed without the proper implementation of all these.

Approaches to Insulin Replacement

There are four basic approaches to insulin replacement therapy aimed at mimicking physiologic insulinemia and normalizing blood glucose. These include: (1) pancreas or islet cell transplantation, (2) the "closed loop," feedback-controlled artificial pancreas,[124] (3) continuous subcutaneous insulin infusion (CSII),[127] and (4) multiple daily insulin injections (MDII). CSII and MDII are discussed here.

All IIT regimens must combine two components of insulin delivery. The first is rapid rise of insulin followed by a rapid decline back toward baseline following each meal. In CSII and MDII regimens, this is accomplished by what is called the mealtime bolus, or simply bolus, dose. Because of the desired timing of the postprandial insulin needs, the bolus must be given in the form of rapidly acting insulin or regular insulin. Even when giving subcutaneous regular insulin (the use of intravenous insulin as part of an IIT regimen is not discussed here), the peak action does not correspond to the desired time of 1 hour postprandial, but rather occurs 2 to 3 hours later. Optimal benefit can, therefore, be obtained by administering the dose 30 to 45 minutes before the meal. At least three studies have demonstrated benefit to such a delay.[53,90,164] With any IIT regimen, mealtime bolus doses are given before each meal. The specific dose and timing may vary depending on current blood glucose, time of day, site of injection, planned carbohydrate intake, and anticipated exercise or activity.

The second component of insulin delivery in an IIT regimen is referred to as the basal insulin. The basal insulin is a slow, relatively continuous supply of insulin throughout the day and night which provides a low, but present, insulin concentration necessary to balance glucose consumption (glucose uptake and oxidation) and glucose production (glycogenolysis and gluconeogenesis). Basal insulin needs are usually about 10 to 15 mU/kg/hr and account for 30% to 50% of the total daily insulin needs. However, considerable individual variation is seen. In addition, basal insulin needs may vary from one time of day to another, especially as part of the dawn phenomenon (see above).

The implementation of IIT using continuous subcutaneous insulin infusion (CSII) involves the use of an externally worn portable infusion pump.[102,124,127] The reservoir or syringe of the pump is filled with regular insulin, which is infused continuously through a catheter that is placed subcutaneously. The catheter is not permanent and is replaced every 1 to 3 days. The pump is preprogrammed to infuse insulin continuously at a constant, or variable, basal rate throughout the day and night. The infusion rates are predetermined and adjusted as necessary. The pump is instructed to rapidly (over a few minutes) administer a bolus dose of regular insulin before each meal. Each of these mealtime bolus doses is under the control of the patient. Over the years, numerous devices for CSII have been available.[3]

IIT using multiple daily insulin injections (MDII) usually involves three or more injections of insulin per day. Regular insulin is injected before each meal. Basal insulin is provided using various combinations of intermediate- or long-acting insulin. The most popular MDII regimens are NPH or Lente at bedtime or Ultralente once or twice a day. When bedtime NPH or Lente is used to provide overnight basal insulin needs, basal insulin (NPH or Lente) is usually not necessary throughout the waking hours if mealtime bolus doses are given at least every 4 to 6 hours. Beef/pork Ultralente is usually divided and given twice daily but can be given once daily in some persons. Human Ultralente, however, has a shorter duration of action and nearly always needs to be given twice a day (breakfast and supper, or breakfast and bed). It has been observed that some subjects using MDII appear to require much higher basal insulin doses (>50% of the total dose) than expected. The reason for this is not clear.

The choice of CSII versus MDII as the method for implementation of IIT is usually an individual one. One regimen has not been consistently shown to be better than the other. Although some subjects might respond better to CSII than MDII or vice versa, most persons respond equally well to either mode.

Regardless of whether CSII or MDII is chosen as the means of implementing IIT, mealtime bolus doses need to be regularly adjusted based on measured blood glucose and anticipated dietary intake and exercise. Breakfast bolus doses are usually higher (for equivalent carbohydrate intake) than are lunchtime or suppertime doses. Occasionally, bolus doses may be required before snacks, especially if the snack is large. However, snacks become a less essential part of the regimen. Algorithms for adjustment of insulin doses during IIT have been developed by many investigators.[140] Similar algorithms have been developed for use with conventional insulin regimens.[141]

Initiation of an intensive insulin therapy regimen is often done in an inpatient setting in which extensive education and close monitoring can be performed. This is especially true when starting CSII therapy. Insulin requirements during IIT may be considerably different from those used during conventional therapy. Basal insulin doses are often calculated as 30% to 50% of the usual daily insulin dose, but this can only be done if the total daily dose the patient is receiving is thought to be appropriate. Alternatively the basal needs can be estimated using a variable rate intravenous infusion based on hourly blood glucose measurements, as described by White and associates.[159] Basal insulin requirements are usually 10 to 15 mU/kg/hr. However, for those with a significant DP, lower insulin delivery rates of 8 to 12 mU/kg/hr may be adequate during the early night, whereas higher rates of 15 to 20 mU/kg/hr may be needed during the dawn or prebreakfast period.

Mealtime bolus doses will vary considerably from person to person. Although results calculated from intravenous infusions or taken from artificial pancreas use (Biostator GCIIS, Miles Laboratories, Elkhart, IN) can be used effectively to determine mealtime bolus doses, this is rarely necessary. In most cases, the breakfast dose is 0.15 to 0.30 U/kg, the lunchtime dose 0.10 to 0.20 U/kg, and the suppertime dose 0.15 to 0.25 U/kg. Snacks are not always covered with a bolus dose, but can be covered with about 0.05 U/kg. Of course, the mealtime bolus doses are adjusted based on blood glucose, anticipated activity, and planned carbohydrate intake. Many algorithms, such as those of Skyler and associates,[140,141] have been developed for this purpose. After initiation of IIT, changes in both the basal and bolus insulin doses and insulin adjustment algorithms are made based on self-monitored blood glucose determinations and individually determined goals. Monitoring usually needs to be done four times each day with additional readings taken overnight a few times each week in order to most safely and effectively make the necessary adjustments.

Although the goals of IIT in the Diabetes Control and Complications Trial (DCCT) are for preprandial glucoses between 70 and 120 mg/dL, postprandial glucoses below 180 mg/dL, and a glycated hemoglobin (HbA$_{1c}$) within two standard deviations of the nondiabetic mean,[51] this target may not be achievable for all persons.[48] Goals must be individualized. In some cases, goals related to flexibility of life-style may be primary and blood sugar targets less rigid.

Benefits and Risks of IIT

All the benefits and risks of IIT have not yet been fully defined.[45] Potential benefits include: (1) increased flexibility of life-style, (2) better glycemic control resulting in reduced prevalence, delayed onset, slowed progression, or reversal of diabetic complications, (3) better glycemic control during pregnancy with better fetal outcome, and (4) an increased feeling of well being and control. The increased flexibility comes as a result of using premeal bolus doses instead of twice a day "split-mixed" insulin for IIT. Insulin doses are given and timed based on planned meals and activities, whereas in a conventional insulin regimen, meals and activities need to be planned and timed around the insulin doses. Snacks are often an essential part of any conventional therapy regimen because of the peaking insulin action between meals and during periods of activity. With IIT, inappropriately timed peaks of insulin action are not usually present and many of these snacks are no longer essential. Exercise snacks may still be needed, especially for strenuous or prolonged exercise. A bedtime snack is still recommended as protection against nocturnal hypoglycemia.

The effectiveness of IIT and normalization of blood glucose in preventing, slowing, or reversing diabetic complications remains controversial. Although many retrospective analyses have suggested poorer glycemic control as a primary risk factor in the development of diabetic retinopathy, nephropathy, and neuropathy, prospective studies and controlled clinical trials have given conflicting results.[45] IIT does not reverse diabetes complications at its later stages, and can result in transient worsening at earlier stages.[57] IIT can reverse some early subclinical measures associated with complications.[119,125,157,160,161] Studies have so far failed to show that IIT slows the progression of clinically manifest diabetes complications.[41,93] However, we must await the results of ongoing studies, especially the Diabetes Control and Complications Trial (DCCT),[44-46,48] before the important questions related to diabetes control and complications can be answered with any degree of certainty.

The potential risks[102] of IIT include: (1) an increased rate of severe hypoglycemia, (2) an increased rate of mild hypoglycemia, (3) excessive weight gain, and (4) the possibility of life-threatening DKA or hypoglycemia as a result of pump malfunction in those using CSII. This latter complication is now unusual using modern pump technology and well-educated, conscientious patients. However, severe hypoglycemia continues to be a major concern.[27,158] IIT is associated with a two- to three-fold increased risk for severe hypoglycemia,[44,48] and this could worsen with the development of autonomic neuropathy, hypoglycemia unawareness, or defective glucose counterregulation (see discussion above). IIT does not reverse existing abnormalities of glucose counterregulation,[13,21] and may indeed lower the threshold for triggering a counterregulatoy hormone response.[4,6] Mild hypoglycemia is also more frequent,[48] but this is not usually thought of as a major risk unless hypoglycemia unawareness develops or hypoglycemia is frequent enough to interfere with maintenance of a normal life-style. IIT is often associated with a 5- to 10-pound weight gain.[44]

Until the results of the DCCT are known, IIT should not be considered the treatment of choice for all diabetic subjects. Experience with IIT in young children is minimal, and experience in teenagers is mixed,[136] though usually poor.[11] Many would consider poor growth secondary to IDDM as an indication for IIT when other methods have failed. Many consider IIT the treatment of choice during pregnancy and preconception planning.[63,65] In general, other than during pregnancy, IIT should be reserved for the highly motivated, conscientious young adult or adult patient who desires the improved control and/or increased flexibility that IIT can offer and is willing to put forth added effort to obtain these benefits. IIT should also be strongly considered for patients who have undergone renal transplantation because of end-stage diabetic nephropathy. IIT as a primary therapeutic option in NIDDM or in brittle IDDM requires further study. Compliance problems cannot be improved by making the regimen more complex, and, indeed, complexity usually worsens compliance problems.

The decision to implement IIT should be made only after careful consideration of the risks and benefits by a team of health care professionals experienced in the care of persons with diabetes. The patient's level of education and motivation, as well as support systems, need to be considered. A health care team familiar with the patient and knowledgeable and experienced in IIT should be available at all times.

AGE-RELATED CONSIDERATIONS: INFANTS AND CHILDREN

IDDM is by far the most common cause of diabetes in infants and children. Prompt diagnosis and treatment of new-onset IDDM in infants and young children is of critical importance because delay may result in increased morbidity and mortality. A delay in diagnosis can be caused by the nonspecific nature of symptoms in this age group. Vomiting, dehydration, irritability, fever, and frequent urination can commonly be seen in infants and children with illness other than IDDM. Kussmaul breathing in an infant or young child may be confused with a respiratory disorder such as asthma or pneumonitis. Metabolic acidosis, and even ketoacidosis, can occur in certain inborn errors of metabolism. During infancy, a high degree of suspicion is necessary to lead one to screen for IDDM by measuring urine glucose and ketones. Of course, establishing a definite diagnosis of diabetes requires measurement of blood glucose; diagnosis of diabetes mellitus should never be made using urine glucose alone.

The medical history should focus on the classic signs and symptoms of diabetes mellitus, including increased urination, extreme thirst, and weight loss. Parents may report that the child's urine has become "sticky" as a result of glycosuria. Parents often describe that their child will "drink anything and everything," including water from toilets, pets' bowls, the bath, or watering cans for plants. Diabetes insipidus can also be mistaken for diabetes mellitus in this age group.

Hyperglycemia or diabetes presenting in the first few days of life is quite rare. Although IDDM can be present very early in life, other types of diabetes need to be considered if hyperglycemia presents within the first week of life. Disorders that need to be considered in this setting include agenesis of the pancreas, genetic mutations of the insulin gene (biologically defective insulin or hereditary hyperproinsulinemia[145]) or insulin receptor, or transient neonatal diabetes mellitus (TNDM).[14,109] TNDM is a rare and unusual disorder manifested by neonatal onset of extreme hyperglycemia without ketosis but associated with severe failure to thrive. The condition lasts between 1 and 18 months and subsequently resolves with no residual identifiable abnormality of carbohydrate metabolism. However, during the period of abnormality, treatment with low doses of insulin is essential to establish normal growth[18] and prevent marked hyperglycemia. The etiology of TNDM is unknown but may represent a process of pancreatic islet cell dysmaturity.[109]

Luckily, IDDM is uncommon during infancy. The initial management of IDDM in infants and children is a therapeutic challenge that can be overwhelming for even the most capable of families[74] (see Chapters 11 and 12). After the diagnosis of IDDM has been made in an infant or toddler, the family should be referred to a center with a multidisciplinary diabetes health care team experienced in the management of children with diabetes.[94] The goals of treating an infant or toddler with IDDM should differ from those in treating older patients. The major goals should be: (1) avoidance of hypoglycemia, (2) maintenance of normal growth and development, (3) avoidance of DKA, (4) maintenance of emotional well-being, and (5) freedom from persistent symptoms. Euglycemia and normalization of glycated hemoglobin are not primary goals in these patients because the risk of severe hypoglycemia may be too great. In 1961, Ack and associates[1] reported lower IQ scores in children with IDDM diagnosed before the age of 5 years. Both EEG abnormalities and deficits of cognitive function have been reported in children diagnosed before 4 years of age and in children who have had previous bouts of severe hypoglycemia.[77,122,143]

Initiating Therapy

Hospitalization is necessary for most infants and toddlers with new-onset IDDM. In this environment, initiation of insulin hormone replacement therapy, family education, and close monitoring of the patient and progress of the parents in learning diabetes care skills can be carefully followed. Most infants and toddlers will require an initial insulin dose of about 0.5 U/kg/day. Though not universal, some pediatric endocrinologists feel that pork insulin is preferable to human insulin in infants and toddlers because of its longer time course of action. However, most pediatric endocrinologists initiate therapy using human insulin at all ages. Most patients are begun on intermediate-acting insulin (NPH or Lente) alone, or a split-mixed regimen, with doses before breakfast and supper. Changes of insulin doses should be made as indicated by blood glucose monitoring after observing 1 or 2 days of blood glucose values. It can be anticipated that the child's activity and appetite in the hospital environment will not be equivalent to what it will be at home. It is often necessary to decrease insulin dose after discharge from the hospital when the child's activity is greater and as the honeymoon phase begins.[142] Intensive insulin therapy is unproven in this age group and should not be employed until it has been studied further.

Management Strategies

For children who weigh less than 10 kg and require less than 5 U of insulin per day, it is often necessary to adjust insulin by fractions of a unit.[71,74] Since doses this small are difficult to precisely measure using U-100 insulin, a diluted insulin (usually U-10) can be used. Diluent is available from most insulin manufacturers. Diluted insulin should be clearly labeled and each vial should usually not be used for longer than 1 month. Despite the recent literature suggesting that some of the variability of insulin absorption and blood sugars can be reduced by using the same anatomic site[9] (i.e., not rotating), rotation of injection sites continues to be important in infants and young children. Because of the relatively small area for injection at each anatomic site, lipodystrophy may develop if injection sites are not rotated. In addition, parents are rarely comfortable using the abdominal injection sites in infants and toddlers, although these sites can be used.

It is normal for children to be frightened of shots and for the parents to harbor much anxiety about giving injections. Many parents feel that they are hurting their child both physically and emotionally when they give injections. Injections should be given quickly and without a need to firmly restrain the child. Discussion and debate with the child about his or her receiving injections usually prolongs the anticipated concern related to the injection for both patient and parents and usually increases the anxiety. Most often the young child forgets the discomfort of the injection shortly after the injection is given. The child (and parent) need to be reassured about their fear of injections. Most young children become quickly acclimated to receiving injections and blood glucose monitoring when the parents express less anxiety about it. Infants and toddlers are obviously too young to give their own injections, although some school-aged children can learn to help with parts of the procedure. Forced-air or jet insulin injectors are not usually recommended for infants and young children with IDDM as they are designed for use in older patients, are not necessarily without pain, and do not obviate the anxiety related to insulin administration. Other injection aids are often useful.

Nutritional planning for the infant or young child with IDDM is also uniquely different from that of older patients.[71] Children under 4 years of age are usually unpredictable in their eating habits. Infants are fed around the clock and on demand. Behaviors typical of the "terrible twos" can certainly last more than just 1 year. A specific, rigid meal plan may not be a reasonable goal at this age. The child should be offered a well-balanced diet usually consisting of 4 to 6 feedings a day for infants and 3 meals and 3 snacks a day for toddlers. Avoidance of concentrated sweets should be encouraged. A pediatric nutritionist with experience in the treatment of infants and young children with IDDM should be consulted initially and should be available to the family to help answer questions and solve problems. Force feeding of the child who refuses to eat should be discouraged. Rather, a reduction of insulin dose of 10% to 20% and looser blood sugar goals should be used. Variability of blood sugars is to be expected, since variability in dietary intake and activity is unavoidable. Avoidance of hypoglycemia should be a primary goal in this age group.

Normal growth is also of utmost importance. Growth and development of the child should be determined and plotted on standard growth curves at each visit. Most diabetic children grow within the normal percentiles of the appropriate growth curve when taking into account parental height. However, children with poor diabetic control grow slightly slower[154] and can develop growth failure[95] (see discussion above under "Growth Failure in Diabetes and Mauriac's Syndrome"). A decline in growth velocity or poor weight gain may indicate underinsulinization, undernutrition, hypothyroidism, or other chronic medical illness. Excessive weight gain is uncommon in toddlers with IDDM but may reflect overinsulinization and/or overfeeding.

The question remains as to what the optimal degree of metabolic control is for infants and toddlers with IDDM.[36] Parents tend to be anxious about diabetes complications and their relationship with blood glucose control. This relationship is not well established for young children, however, and the risks related to hypoglycemia are well established. Many investigators have recently suggested that the postpubertal duration of IDDM is a more accurate determinant of the development of microvascular complications than total duration, suggesting that the contribution of the prepubertal years of diabetes to the development of long-term complications may be minimal.[8,42,89,120,155] To prevent severe hypoglycemia, preprandial blood glucose values of 80 to 150 mg/dL (4.5 to 8.4 mM) are generally recommended.

Self-monitoring of blood glucose

Parents of all children with IDDM should be instructed in self-monitoring of blood glucose (SMBG). Urine glucose monitoring is unreliable and will not detect low blood glucose. Collection of urine can be difficult to obtain when needed. At least two preprandial blood glucose determinations each day should be requested in this age group. Parents should check the child's glucose if hypoglycemia is suspected. Urinary ketones should be checked whenever blood glucose is unexpectedly greater that 240 mg/dL (13.4 mM) or if the child is ill. Urine can often be obtained from diapers or bedding. glycated hemoglobin determinations should be obtained every 3 to 4 months at routine visits. Before 6 to 9 months of life, determinations of glycated hemoglobin need to be performed by a method in which hemoglobin F does not interfere, such as a total glycated hemoglobin by affinity chromatography.

Hypoglycemia

Hypoglycemia in the infant and toddler deserves special consideration because these children have a limited repertoire in how they can respond to low blood glucose, and their response is easily confused with other needs. Early recognition and treatment of hypoglycemia is important and families should be taught, before the patient's discharge from the hospital, how to recognize and treat both mild and severe insulin reactions. In the infant, hypoglycemia may present as fussiness, irritability, crying, pallor, somnolence, unconsciousness, or convulsion. In the toddler, hypoglycemia may present as night terrors, temper tantrums, voracious appetite, moodiness, sweating, shaking, staring, or seizure. It has been suggested that severe hypoglycemic reactions during the period of neurologic development may be a cause of cognitive deficits later in life.[1,77,122,143] Unrecognized nocturnal hypoglycemia is of great concern to these families. Restlessness during sleep, night terrors, and sweating may be signs of nocturnal hypoglycemia. Blood glucose determinations during the night at the time of peak action of the evening NPH or Lente insulin may help detect unrecognized nocturnal hypoglycemia. These blood glucose determinations are often suggested soon after discharge from the hospital, when increases in the evening insulin dose are recommended, and when symptoms suggestive of hypoglycemia are occurring during sleep.

Treatment of severe hypoglycemia should not await confirmation by blood glucose determination (see Chapters 11 and 12). Mild reactions can be confirmed by the blood glucose meter. Mild insulin reactions in a conscious child can be treated with 2 to 4 ounces of fruit juice or nondietary soft drink. Glucose paste or cake frosting in tubes are good alternatives that can be easily carried out of the home. Glucose tablets and candy present a risk of aspiration in this age group and are not recommended. Severe insulin reactions should be treated immediately with glucagon. Administration of glucagon should not be delayed until the child is unconscious or convulsing but may be given when the risk of aspiration or ability to drink is in question.

Glucagon is available in a standard 1 mg vial with 1 ml of diluent. Children less than 30 kg should receive 0.5 mg (0.5 ml) of glucagon, and children heavier than 30 kg should receive 1 mg (1 ml). Nausea and vomiting are not infrequently seen after glucagon administration. When glucagon is administered, the family should be instructed to contact the child's physician without delay. If vomiting should occur, the child should be taken to an emergency room so intravenous dextrose can be administered. After the occurrence of severe hypoglycemia, a precipitating cause should be sought. In infants and toddlers, if no cause is found, the insulin dose should empirically be reduced by 10% to 20%.

Psychosocial Considerations

Emotional growth and well-being present particular difficulties for the preschool-aged child with IDDM and his or her parents. The young child's limited cognitive ability to cope with the stress of diabetes and its management may lead to other coping strategies such as aggression, noncompliance, withdrawal, and psychosomatic complaints. A child's resolution of separation anxiety and development of self-confidence may be impeded by life with IDDM. These concerns may contribute to risk of developing general adjustment difficulties to the behavioral demands of IDDM.[165] It is easy to understand how many parents feel overwhelmed by the responsibility of daily care for their child with IDDM. It is important that both parents learn daily diabetes care together and share the responsibilities of home management for their child. Equally important is the involvement of the diabetes health care team and primary care physician in helping to problem solve and provide psychosocial support to the family. More detailed discussion of care for the infant and young child is addressed in Chapters 11 and 12.

AGE-RELATED CONSIDERATIONS: ADOLESCENCE TO ADULTHOOD

Another very difficult period of life for diabetes management is that of adolescence and the transition to adulthood (see Chapters 13 and 14). Deterioration of glycemic control at the time of adolescence is multifactorial, including psychosocial, physiologic, emotional, and developmental factors. Puberty is associated with a component of insulin resistance. This can be demonstrated in nondiabetic adolescents as higher insulin levels during an oral glucose tolerance test[19] and in teenagers with and without diabetes by using glucose clamp studies.[5] The cause of this insulin resistance is not known but probably relates to the normally occurring hormonal changes of puberty. Because of this relative insulin resistance, many teenagers require as much as 1.0-1.5 U/kg/day of insulin. Furthermore, it is becoming increasingly apparent that puberty is a risk factor for the initial development of complications in patients with IDDM.[8,42,89,120,155] The period of adolescent development begins with both physical and behavioral changes. It is during this period of development that independence from dependent relationships (family and parents) begins and peer acceptance gains more importance. Body awareness and physical appearance become paramount, and independent cognitive, biophysical, psychologic, social, and sexual identity develops. Diabetes self-care requires balancing many metabolic and life-style factors, and each person must make many diabetes-related choices each day. Problem-solving on these new constructs sets the stage for rebellion and anxiety as self-esteem and confidence fluctuate on a daily basis.

Diabetes Education

The challenge of diabetes education during adolescence is to provide a transition of care from the parents to the child that not only addresses metabolic control of the disease but empowers the developing young adult to gain understanding of diabetes self-care and the consequences based on his or her own goals and choices. Few adolescents will accept complete parental control of their diabetes, but many will do poorly without some continued parental support.[86] This challenges the drive for independence and peer acceptance. Empowerment is a process by which people gain mastery over their own affairs.[117] Empowerment places emphasis on the whole person (biopsychosocial). Components of empowerment include: (1) finding personal strengths rather than shortcomings, (2) identifying the learning needs of the patient, (3) negotiating common goals, (4) transferring decision making to the patient, (5) encouraging self-generation of solutions to problems, (6) analyzing failure to achieve goals as a problem to solve rather than as personal failure, (7) encouraging use of support networks, (8) promoting the patient's inherent drive toward health and wellness, and (9) recognizing behavior change as an achievement.[66] The physician and other health care providers should be willing to compromise on almost all aspects of the diabetes care in meeting the personal goals of the patient as he or she learns self-care. Even the slightest acceptance of self-care should be encouraged, and failure of an agreed treatment goal must be evaluated as a problem to solve and not as a personal deficit. Health care providers should act as a resource and objective sounding board for the patient so as to not be viewed as a surrogate parent by the patient.

During office or clinic visits, the adolescent should be seen alone and a summary session held with the parents at the end of the visit. This promotes a relationship between health care provider and patient, yet keeps parents informed and provides them with an opportunity to discuss areas of concern with the clinician and their child. Treatment regimens and goals should be kept as simple as possible. SMBG and record keeping seem to be particularly difficult tasks for adolescents to perform. Patients who refuse to perform self-care should not be abandoned, and any agreement to perform monitoring should be praised. Health care providers should be willing and ready to make major alterations in diabetes self-care expectations. The health care provider needs to remember that the transition from surrogate care to self-care is a long process; patient empowerment should ultimately promote this process.

Risk Behaviors

Important issues to adolescents, such as alcohol, recreational drug use, dating, sex, pregnancy planning, driving, employment, college, sports, and chronic complications from IDDM, must be openly discussed in an objective and nonjudgemental manner. Emphasis should be placed upon how drugs and alcohol can affect blood glucose levels. Smoking should be strongly discouraged. Patients should be informed about how to prevent unwanted pregnancy and sexually transmitted disease. Ready access to birth control counseling should be made available to the patient. Those patients planning a pregnancy should be informed of the importance of acheiving excellent metabolic control before conceiving and maintaining it throughout pregnancy[63,65] and should also be referred to expert obstetric care. Often genetic counseling is helpful for these patients to answer questions about probability of their child developing IDDM. Medic alert badges should be worn by all persons with IDDM operating a motor vehicle. Hypoglycemia and unrecognized low blood glucose is an important issue to address when discussing driving. Adolescents with IDDM can participate safely in all types of sports and activities as long as they are taught how to adjust food or insulin in relation to their activity. A carbohydrate source to treat insulin reactions should be available during and after exercise. Exercise snacks are often necessary. The potential benefit of regular physical activity should be explained.

As the adolescent makes transition to young adulthood, the option of IIT should be discussed. Even though all the risks and benefits of IIT have yet to be fully understood, the life-style considerations make IIT a preferred mode of treatment for many young adults with IDDM. IIT can be particularly helpful in negotiating new work or school schedules that may not be as predictable as desired. IIT also provides an opportunity to master the schedules of adult life and more independence in self-care without sacrificing any degree of diabetic control.

AGE-RELATED CONSIDERATIONS: THE ELDERLY

The elderly person with diabetes also faces special considerations and has special needs (see Chapter 15). As a person becomes older, he or she faces physiologic, cognitive, financial, and personal changes over which he or she may have little control. These developmental changes can include changes in cognitive functioning, alterations in sensory systems, decreased visual and auditory acuity, and declining dexterity, mobility, and physical strength. In addition, elderly persons may be faced with the loss of a spouse or loved one and the loss of financial self-determination.

The diagnosis of diabetes mellitus often brings with it the initiation of a treatment program that is likely to dictate changes in life-style. This may be particularly difficult for an elderly person, especially if spousal or family support is lacking. Dietary and exercise habits are already well ingrained and difficult to change. Initiation of an exercise program may be complicated by the presence of other medical conditions, disabilities, or diabetic complications. Insulin injections and blood or urine monitoring may be difficult when there is declining vision and dexterity. Devices developed to help the visually impaired persons with diabetes (such as auditory additions to blood glucose meters, special syringes and magnifiers, and jet injectors) may help in some cases.

Factors related to economic and social support may become paramount. Loss of income and health benefits often results in an inability of the elderly patient to obtain appropriate and consistent medical care and the necessary medical supplies. Public assistance (such as Social Security or Medicare) often falls short of meeting all the needs. Loss of the spouse and unavailability of consistent help and support by family and friends also impair ability to manage diabetes and receive continued medical care. Many elderly persons with diabetes will not have the physical and mental capability and family and financial support to continue with an independent life-style. Adult foster care or nursing home placement may be necessary, but diabetes care may be suboptimal and very expensive in these settings.

Careful assessment of patient ability and available resources is essential. The health care team needs to be prepared to assist the individual in obtaining appropriate help with management of diabetes. This help needs to include diabetes education appropriate for age and cognitive abilities and appropriate financial and social support (e.g., supplies, transportation, in-home assistance). The diabetes care regimen needs to be designed to meet the patient's needs and to be within the patient's capabilities. Development and implementation of such regimens requires the involvement of a multidisciplinary team of experienced health care professionals, including physicians, nurse clinicians and nurse educators, a nutritionist, a social worker, and perhaps a psychologist. The reader is referred to the bibliography[52] and to Chapter 15 of this text for more specific guidelines related to managing diabetes mellitus in elderly persons.

REFERENCES

1. Ack M, Miller I, and Weil WB: Intelligence of children with diabetes mellitus, Pediatrics 28:764-770, 1961.
2. Alberti KGMM, Gill GV, and Elliot MJ: Insulin delivery during surgery in the diabetic patient, Diabetes Care 5(suppl 1):65-77, 1982.
3. American Diabetes Association, Inc: 1991 Buyer's guide to diabetes products, Diabetes Forecast 43:33-74, 1990.
4. Amiel SA and others: Effect of intensive insulin therapy on glycemic thresholds for counterregulatory hormone release, Diabetes 37:901-907, 1988.
5. Amiel S and others: Impaired insulin action in puberty: a contributing factor to poor glycemic control in adolescent diabetics, N Engl J Med 315:215-219, 1986.
6. Amiel SA and others: Defective glucose counterregulation after strict glycemic control of insulin-dependent diabetes mellitus, N Engl J Med 316:1376-1383, 1987.
7. Atiea JA and others: Early morning hyperglycemia in IDDM: acute effects of cholinergic blockade, Diabetes Care 12:443-448, 1989.

8. Bach LA and Jerums G: Effect of puberty on initial kidney growth and rise in kidney IGF1 in diabetic rats, Diabetes 39:557-562, 1990.

9. Bantle JP and others: Rotation of the anatomic regions used for insulin injections and day-to-day variability of plasma glucose in type I diabetic subjects, JAMA 263:1802-1806, 1990.

10. Beaufrere B and others: Dawn phenomenon in type 1 (insulin-dependent) diabetic adolescents: influence of nocturnal growth hormone secretion, Diabetologia 31:607-611, 1988.

11. Becker DJ and others: Current status of pump therapy in childhood, Acta Paediatrica Japonica 26:347-358, 1984.

12. Bergada I and others: Severe hypoglycemia in IDDM children, Diabetes Care 12:239-244, 1989.

13. Bergenstal RM and others: Lack of glucagon response to hypoglycemia in type I diabetes after long-term optimal therapy with a continuous subcutaneous insulin infusion pump, Diabetes 32:398-402, 1983.

14. Bilginturan AN and Jackson RV: Transient hyperglycemia in infancy and childhood, Clini Pediatr 17:338-342, 1978.

15. Birk R and Spencer ML: The prevalence of anorexia nervosa, buliminia, and induced glycosuria in IDDM females, Diabetes Educ 15:336-341, 1989.

16. Blackard WG and others: Morning insulin requirements: critique of dawn and meal phenomena, Diabetes 38:273-277, 1989.

17. Blackman JD and others: Hypoglycemic thresholds for cognitive dysfunction in humans, Diabetes 39:828-835, 1990.

18. Blethen SL and others: Plasma somatomedins, endogenous insulin secretion, and growth in transient neonatal diabetes mellitus, J Clin Endocrinol Metab 52:144-147, 1981.

19. Bloch C, Clemons P, and Sperling MA: Puberty decreases insulin sensitivity, J Pediatr 110:481-487, 1987.

20. Bolli GB and others: Abnormal glucose counterregulation in insulin dependent diabetes mellitus: interaction of anti-insulin antibodies and impaired glucagon and epinephrine secretion, Diabetes 32:134-141,1983.

21. Bolli GB and others: Effects of long-term optimization and short-term deterioration of glycemia control on glucose counterregulation in type I diabetes mellitus, Diabetes 33:394-400, 1984.

22. Bolli GB and others: Demonstration of a dawn phenomenon in normal human volunteers, Diabetes 33:1150-1153, 1984.

23. Bolli GB and others: A reliable and reproducible test for adequate glucose counterregulation in type I (insulin-dependent) diabetes mellitus, Diabetes 33:732-737, 1984.

24. Bolli GB and others: Role of hepatic autoregulation in defense against hypoglycemia in humans, J Clin Invest 75:1623-1631, 1985.

25. Bolli GB and Gerich JE: The "dawn phenomenon"—a common occurrence in both non–insulin-dependent and insulin-dependent diabetes mellitus, N Engl J Med 310:746-750, 1984.

26. Bolli GB and others: Glucose counterregulation and waning of insulin in the Somogyi phenomenon (posthypoglycemic hyperglycemia), N Engl J Med 311:1214-1219, 1984.

27. Bolli GB and others: Defective glucose counterregulation after subcutaneous insulin in noninsulin dependent diabetes mellitus, J Clin Invest 73:1532-1541, 1984.

28. Boyle PJ and others: Absence of the dawn phenomenon and abnormal lipolysis in growth hormone deficient IDDM's, Diabetes 38(suppl 2):3A, 1989.

29. Boyle PJ and others: Plasma glucose concentrations at the onset of hypoglycemic symptoms in patients with poorly controlled diabetes and in nondiabetics, N Engl J Med 318:1487-1492, 1988.

30. Campbell P and others: Pathogenesis of the dawn phenomenon in insulin-dependent diabetes mellitus: accelerated glucose production and impaired glucose utilization due to nocturnal surges in growth hormone secretion, N Engl J Med 312:1473-1479, 1985.

31. Campbell PJ, Bolli GB, and Gerich JE: Prevention of the dawn phenomenon (early morning hyperglycemia) in insulin-dependent diabetes mellitus by bedtime intranasal administration of a long-acting somatostatin analog, Metabolism 37:34-37, 1988.

32. Campbell PJ and Gerich JE: Occurrence of dawn phenomenon without change in insulin clearance in patients with insulin-dependent diabetes mellitus, Diabetes 35:749-752, 1986.

33. Chisholm DJ and others: Programming of insulin delivery with meals during subcutaneous insulin infusion, Diabetes Care 4:265-268, 1981.

34. Clarke WL, Haymond MW, and Santiago JV: Overnight basal insulin requirements in fasting insulin-dependent diabetics, Diabetes 29:78-80,1980.

35. Clutter WE and others: Epinephrine plasma metabolic clearance rates and physiologic thresholds for metabolic and hemodynamic actions in man, J Clin Invest 66:94-101,1980.
36. Copeland KE: Too uptight about tight control? Diabetes Care 13:1089-1091, 1990.
37. Cryer PE: Glucose counterregulation in man, Diabetes 30:261-264, 1981.
38. Cryer PE and others: Conference summary: hypoglycemia is IDDM, Diabetes 38:1193-1199, 1989.
39. Cryer PE and Gerich JE: Glucose counterregulation, hypoglycemia and intensive insulin therapy in diabetes mellitus, N Engl J Med 313:232-239.1985.
40. Cryer PE, White NH, and Santiago JV: The relevance of glucose counterregulation systems to patients with insulin dependent diabetes, Endocrine Rev 7:131-139, 1986.
41. Dahl-Jorgenson K and others: Effect of near normoglycemia for two years on progression of early diabetic retinopathy, nephropathy and neuropathy: the Oslo Study, Br Med J 293:1185-1189, 1986.
42. Dahlquist G and Rudberg S: The prevalence of microalbuminuria in diabetic children and adolescents and its relation to puberty, Acta Paediatr Scand 76:795-800, 1987.
43. Davidson MB and others: Suppression of sleep-induced growth hormone secretion by anticholinergic agent abolishes dawn phenomenon, Diabetes 37:166-171, 1988.
44. The DCCT Research Group: The diabetes control and complications trial (DCCT): an update, Diabetes Care 13:427-433, 1990.
45. The DCCT Research Group: Are continuing studies of metabolic control and microvascular complications in IDDM justified? The diabetes control and complications trial (DCCT), N Engl J Med 318:246-250, 188.
46. The DCCT Research Group: The diabetes control and complications trial (DCCT): design and methodological considerations for the feasibility phase, Diabetes 35:530-545, 1986.
47. The DCCT Research Group: Effects of age, duration and treatment of IDDM on b-cell function: observations during eligibility testing for the diabetes control and complications trial (DCCT), J Clin Endocrinol Metab 65:30-36, 1987.
48. The DCCT Research Group: The diabetes control and complications trial: results of the feasibility study (phase II), Diabetes Care 10:1-19, 1987.
49. DeFeo P and others: The adrenergic contribution to glucose counterregulation in type I diabetes mellitus: dependency on A cell function and medication through beta$_2$ adrenoreceptors, Diabetes 32:887-893,1983.
50. DeFeo P and others: Modest decrements in plasma glucose concentration cause early impairment in cognitive function and later activation of glucose counterregulation in the absence of hypoglycemic symptoms in normal man, J Clin Invest 82:436-444, 1988.
51. The Diabetes Control and Complications Trial (Full-scale Clinical Trial-Phase III) Protocol, NIH, Pub No 88-2951, Washington, DC, 1987, U.S. Government Printing Office.
52. Halter JB and Christensen NJ, eds: Diabetes mellitus in elderly people, Diabetes Care 13(suppl 2):1-98, 1990.
53. Dimitriadis GD and Gerich JE: Importance of timing of preprandial subcutaneous insulin administration in the management of diabetes mellitus, Diabetes Care 6:374-377, 1983.
54. Dux S, White NH, and Santiago JV: The dawn phenomenon: an increased insulin clearance rate during the prebreakfast period in diabetic and nondiabetic subjects, J Pediatr Endocrinol 1:171-176, 1985.
55. Dux S and others: Insulin clearance contributes to the variability of nocturnal insulin requirements in insulin-dependent diabetes, Diabetes 34:1260-1265, 1985.
56. Edwards GA and others: Effectiveness of low-dose continuous intravenous insulin infusion is diabetic ketoacidosis, J Pediatr 91:701-705, 1977.
57. Ellis D and others: Diabetic nephropathy in adolescence: appearance during improved glycemic control, Pediatrics 71:824-829, 1983.
58. Faich GA, Fishbein HA, and Ellis SE: The epidemiology of diabetic acidosis: A population-based study, Am J Epidemiol 117:551, 1983.
59. Fajans SS: Scope and heterogeneous nature of MODY, Diabetes Care 13:49-64, 1990.
60. Floyd JC and others: An insulin infusion test as a predictor of metabolic events during continuous subcutaneous infusion of insulin in type I diabetes mellitus, Diabetes Res Clin Pract Suppl 1:S171, 1985.
61. Floyd JC and others: Prevalences of impaired secretion of pancreatic polypeptide and of cardiovascular neural signs as indicators of autonomic neuropathy in type I diabetes, Diabetes 36(supp 1)86A, 1987.
62. Foster DW and McGarry JD: The metabolic derangement and treatment of diabetic ketoacidosis, N Engl J Med 309:159-169, 1983.
63. Freinkel N, Dooley SL, and Metzger BE: Care of the pregnant woman with insulin-dependent diabetes mellitus, N Engl J Med 313:96-101, 1985.

64. Friedenberg GR and others: Diabetes responsive to intravenous but not subcutaneous insulin: effectiveness of aprotinin, N Engl J Med, 305:363-368, 1981.

65. Fuhrmann K and others: Prevention of congenital malformations in infant of insulin-dependent diabetic mothers, Diabetes Care 6:219-223, 1983.

66. Funnell MM and others: Empowerment: an idea who's time has come in diabetes education, Diabetes Ed 17:37-41, 1991.

67. Gale E, Kurtz A, and Tattersall R: In search of the Somogyi effect, Lancet 2:279-282, 1980.

68. Gerich JE and others: Prevention of diabetic ketoacidosis by somatostatin: evidence for an essential role of glucagon, N Engl J Med 292:985-989, 1975.

69. Gill GV and others: Clinical features of brittle diabetes. In Pickup JC, ed: Brittle diabetes, Oxford, 1985, Blackwell Scientific Publications.

70. Golden M, Herrold A, and Orr D: An approach to prevention of recurrent diabetic ketoacidosis in the pediatric population, J Pediatr 107:195-200, 1985.

71. Golden MP and others: Management of diabetes mellitus in children younger than five years of age, Am J Dis 139:448-452, 1985.

72. Goldgewicht C and others: Hypoglycaemic reactions in 172 type 1 (insulin-dependent) diabetic patients, Diabetologia 24:95-99, 1983.

73. Gray DL and others: Chronic poor metabolic control in the pediatric population: a stepwise intervention program, Diabetes Educ 14:516-520, 1988.

74. Grunt JA and others: Problems in the care of the infant diabetic patient, Clin Pediatr 17:772-774,1978.

75. Hansen I and others: The role of autoregulation of hepatic glucose production in man: response to a physiologic decrement in plasma glucose, Diabetes 35:186-191, 1986.

76. Hanson CL, Henggeler SW, and Burghen GA: Race and sex differences in metabolic control of adolescents with IDDM: a function of psychosocial variables? Diabetes Care 10:313-318, 1987.

77. Haumont D, Dorchy H, and Pelc S: EEG abnormalities in diabetic children: influence of hypoglycemia and vascular complications, Clin Pediatr 18:750-753, 1979.

78. Havlin CE and Cryer PE: Nocturnal hypoglycemia does not commonly result in major morning hyperglycemia in patients with diabetes mellitus, Diabetes Care 10:141-147, 1987.

79. Henderson G: The psychosocial treatment of recurrent diabetic ketoacidosis: an interdisciplinary team approach, Diabetes Educ 17:119-123, 1991.

80. Herold KC and others: Variable deterioration in cortical function during insulin-induced hypoglycemia, Diabetes 34:677-685, 1985.

81. Hilsted J and others: No response of pancreatic hormones to hypoglycemia in diabetic autonomic neuropathy, J Clin Endocrinol Metab 54:815-819, 1982.

82. Hirsch IB and others: Role of insulin in management of surgical patients with diabetes mellitus, Diabetes Care 13:980-991, 1990.

83. Hirsch IB and others: Failure of nocturnal hypoglycemia to cause daytime hyperglycemia in patients with IDDM, Diabetes Care 13:133-142, 1990.

84. Hoeldtke RD and others: Reduced epinephrine secretion and hypoglycemia unawareness in diabetic autonomic neuropathy, Ann Intern Med 96:459-462, 1982.

85. Johnson NB and others: Use of Humulin Ultralente in selected IDDM patients with morning fasting hyperglycemia, Diabetes 39(suppl 1):111A, 1990.

86. Johnson PD and others: Nonsupportive maternal behaviors are associated with poorer glycemic control in adolescents with type I diabetes (IDDM), Diabetes 39(suppl 1):163A, 1990.

87. Keller U and Berger W: Prevention of hypophosphatemia by phosphate infusion during treatment of diabetic ketoacidosis and hyperosmolar coma, Diabetes 29:87-95, 1980.

88. Kleinbaum J and Shamoon H: Effect of propranolol on delayed glucose recovery after insulin-induced hypoglycemia in normal and diabetic subjects, Diabetes Care 7:155-162, 1984.

89. Kostraba JN and others: Contribution of diabetes duration before puberty to development of microvascular complications of IDDM, Diabetes Care 12:686-693, 1989.

90. Kraegen EW, Chrisholm DJ, and McNamara ME: Timing of insulin delivery with meals, Horm Metab Res 13:365-367, 1981.

91. Krane EJ and others: Subclinical brain swelling in children during treatment of diabetic ketoacidosis, N Engl J Med 312:1147-1151, 1985.

92. Kreisberg RA: Diabetic ketoacidosis: new concepts and trends in pathogenesis and treatment, Ann Intern Med 88:681-695, 1978.

93. The Kroc Collaborative Study: Blood glucose control and the evolution of diabetic retinopathy and albuminuria: a preliminary multicenter trial, N Engl J Med 311:365-372, 1984.

94. Kushion W and others: Issues in the care of infants and toddlers with insulin-dependent diabetes mellitus, Diabetes Educ 17:107-110, 1991.

95. Lee RGL and Bode HH: Stunted growth and hepatomegaly in diabetes mellitus, J Pediatr 91:82-84, 1977.

96. Lerman IG and Wolfsdorf JI: Relationship of nocturnal hypoglycemia to daytime glycemia in IDDM, Diabetes Care 11:636-642, 1988.

97. Levandoski LA, White NH, and Santiago JV: How to weather the sick-day season, Diabetes Forecast 36:30-33, 1983.

98. Levine SN and Loewenstein JE: Treatment of diabetic ketoacidosis, Arch Intern Med 141:713-715, 1981.

99. Levitt NS and others: Impaired pancreatic polypeptide responses to insulin induced hypoglycemia in diabetic autonomic neuropathy, J Clin Endocrinol Metab 50:445-449, 1980.

100. MacDonald MJ: Postexercise late-onset hypoglycemia in insulin-dependent diabetic patients, Diabetes Care 10:584-588, 1987.

101. MacGorman LR, Rizza RA, and Gerich JE: Physiological concentrations of growth hormone exert insulin-like and insulin antagonistic effects on both hepatic and exaahepatic tissues in man, J Clin Endocrinol Met 53:556-559, 1981.

102. Mecklenburg RS and others: Clinical use of the insulin infusion pump in 100 patients with type I diabetes, N Engl J Med 307 513-518, 1982.

103. Meyers EF, Alberts D, and Gordon MO: Perioperative control of blood glucose in diabetic patients: a two-step protocol, Diabetes Care 9:40-45, 1986.

104. Miles JM and others: Effects of acute insulin deficiency of glucose and ketone body turnover in man: evidence for the primacy of overproduction of glucose and ketones bodies in the genesis of diabetic ketoacidosis, Diabetes 29:926-930, 1980.

105. Muhlhauser I and others: Incidence and management of severe hypoglycemia in 434 adults with insulin-dependent diabetes mellitus, Diabetes Care 8:268-273, 1985.

106. Munro JF and others: Euglycaemic diabetic ketoacidosis, Br Med J 2:578-580, 1973.

107. Orr DP and others: Surreptitious insulin administration in adolescents with insulin-dependent diabetes mellitus, JAMA 256:3227-3230, 1986.

108. Orr DP and others: Characteristics of adolescents with poorly controlled diabetes referred to a tertiary care center, Diabetes Care 6:170-175, 1983.

109. Paglira AS, Karl IE, and Kipnis DB: Transient neonatal diabetes: delayed maturation of the pancreatic beta cell, J Pediatr 82:97-101, 1973.

110. Paulsen EP, Courtney JW, Duckworth WC: Insulin resistance caused by massive degradation of subcutaneous insulin, Diabetes 28:640, 1979.

111. Perriello G and others: The effect of asymptomatic nocturnal hypoglycemia on glycemic control in diabetes mellitus, N Engl J Med 319:1233-1239, 1988.

112. Pezzarossa A and others: Perioperative management of diabetic subjects: subcutaneous versus intravenous insulin administration during glucose-potassium infusion, Diabetes Care 11:52-58, 1988.

113. Pickup JC: Preface. In Pickup JC, ed: Brittle diabetes, Oxford, England, 1985, Blackwell Scientific Publications.

114. Pickup JC: Clinical features of patients unresponsive to continuous subcutaneous insulin infusion. In Pickup JC, ed: Brittle diabetes, Oxford, 1985, Blackwell Scientific Publications.

115. Popp DA, Shah SD, and Cryer PE: The role of epinephrine mediated B-adrenergic mechanisms in hpoglycemic glucose counterregulation and posthypoglycemic hyperglycemia in insulin dependent diabetes mellitus, J Clin Invest 69:315-326, 1982.

116. Pramming S and others: Cognitive function during hypoglycemia in type 1 diabetes mellitus, Br Med J 292:647-650, 1986.

117. Rappaport J: Terms of empowerment/exemplars of prevention: toward a theory for community psychology, Am J Commun Psychol 15:121-148, 1987.

118. Raskin P: The Somogyi phenomenon: sacred cow or bull, Arch Intern Med 144:781-787, 1984.

119. Raskin P and others: The effect of diabetic control on the width of skeletal-muscle capillary basement membrane in patients with type I diabetes mellitus, N Engl J Med 309:1546-1550, 1983.

120. Rogers DG and others: The effect of puberty on the development of early diabetic microvascular disease in insulin-dependent diabetes, Diabetes Res Clin Pract 3:39-44, 1987.

121. Rosenbloom AL and others: Cerebral edema complicating diabetic ketoacidosis in childhood, J Pediatr 96:357-361, 1980.

122. Ryan C, Vega A, and Drash A: Cognitive deficits in adolescents who developed diabetes early in life, Pediatrics 75:921-927, 1985.

123. Santiago JV and others: Epinephrine, norepinephrine, glucagon, and growth hormone release in association with physiologic decrements in the plasma glucose concentration in normal and diabetic man, J Clin Endocrinol Metab 51:877-883, 1980.

124. Santiago JV and others: Closed-loop and open-loop devices for blood glucose control in normal and diabetic subjects, Diabetes 28:71-84, 1979.

125. Santiago JV and others: Ocular fluorophotometry: studies in experimental and human diabetes. In Irsigler K and others, eds: New approaches to insulin therapy, Lancaster, England, 1981, MTP Press.

126. Santiago JV, Sargeant DT, and White NH: The syndrome of excessive degradation of subcutaneously injected insulin: treatment with aprotinin. In Irsigler K, ed: New approaches to insulin therapy, Lancaster, England, 1981, MTP Press.

127. Santiago JV, White NH, and Skor DA: Mechanical devices for insulin delivery. In Santiago J and Natrass M, eds: Recent advances in diabetes, Edinburgh, 1984, Churchill Livingstone.

128. Santiago JV and others: Defective glucose counterregulation limits intensive therapy of diabetes mellitus, Am J Physiol 247:E215-E220, 1984.

129. Schade DS: Surgery and diabetes, Med Clin North Am 72:1531-1543, 1988.

130. Schade DS and others: The etiology of incapacitating brittle diabetes, Diabetes Care 8:12-20, 1985.

131. Shade DS and others: A clinical algorithm to determine the etiology of brittle diabetes, Diabetes Care 8:5-11, 1985.

132. Schmidt MI and others: Fasting early morning rise in peripheral insulin: evidence of the dawn phenomenon in nondiabetics, Diabetes Care 7:32-35, 1984.

133. Schwartz NS and others: Glycemic thresholds for activation of glucose counterregulatory systems are higher than the threshold for symptoms, J Clin Invest 79:777-781, 1987.

134. Selam J-L and Charles MA: Devices for insulin adminstration, Diabetes Care 13:955-979, 1990.

135. Shalwitz RA and others: Prevalence and consequences of nocturnal hypoglycemia among conventionally treated children with diabetes mellitus, J Pediat 116:686-689, 1990.

136. Shiffrin AD and others: Intensified insulin therapy in the type I diabetic adolescent: a controlled trial, Diabetes Care 7:107-113, 1984.

137. Skor DA and others: Influence of growth hormone on overnight insulin requirements in insulin-dependent diabetics, Diabetes 34:135-139, 1985.

138. Skor DA and others: Relative roles of insulin clearance and insulin sensitivity in the prebreakfast increases in insulin requirements in insulin dependent diabetic patients, Diabetes 33:60-63, 1984.

139. Skor DA and others: Examination of the role of the pituitary-adrenocortical axis, counterregulatory hormones, and insulin clearance in variable nocturnal insulin requirements in insulin-dependent diabetes, Diabetes 32:403-407, 1983.

140. Skyler JS, Seigler DE, and Reeves, ML: Optimizing pumped insulin delivery, Diaetes Care 5:135-147, 1982.

141. Skyler JS and others: Algorithms for adjustment of insulin dosage by patients who monitor blood glucose, Diabetes Care 4:311-318, 1981.

142. Sochett EB and others: Factors affecting and patterns of residual insulin secretion during the first year of type I (insulin-dependent) diabetes mellitus in children, Diabetologia 30:453-459, 1987.

143. Soltesz G and Acsadi G: Association between diabetes, severe hypoglycemia and electroencephalographic abnormalities, Arch Dis Child 64:992-996, 1989.

144. Somogyi M: Exacerbation of diabetes by excess insulin action, Am J Med 26:169-91, 1959.

145. Steiner DF and others: Lessons learned from molecular biology of insulin gene mutations, Diabetes Care 13:600-609, 1990.

146. Stephenson JM and Schernthaner G: Dawn phenomenon and Somogyi effect in IDDM, Diabetes Care 12:245-251, 1989.

147. Tordjman KM and others: Failure of nocturnal hypoglycemia to cause fasting hyperglycemia in patients with insulin-dependent diabetes mellitus, N Engl J Med 317:1552-1559, 1987.

148. Watts NB and others: Postoperative management of diabetes mellitus: steady-state glucose control with bedside algorithm for insulin adjustment, Diabetes Care 10:722-728, 1987.

149. Wayne EA and others: Focal neurologic deficits associated with hypoglycemia in children with diabetes, J Pediatr 117:575-577, 1990.

150. Weber ME and Abbassi V: Continuous intravenous insulin therapy in severe diabetic ketoacidosis: variations in dosage requirements, J Pediatr 91:755-756, 1977.

151. White N and others: Plasma pancreatic polypeptide measurements as a marker for defective glucose counterregulation in insulin-dependent diabetes, Diabetes Res Clin Pract Suppl l:S601, 1985.

152. White NH and others: Plasma pancreatic polypeptide response to insulin induced hypoglycemia as a marker for defective glucose counterregulation in insulin-dependent diabetes mellitus, Diabetes 34:870-875, 1985.

153. White K and others: Unstable diabetes and unstable families: a psychosocial evaluation of diabetic children with recurrent ketoacidosis, Pediatrics 73:749-755, 1984.

154. White NH and Robinson GH: Impaired growth in children with poorly controlled type I diabetes (IDDM), Pediatr Res 21:349A, 1987.

155. White NH and others: Puberty as a risk factor for complications of diabetes mellitus (IDDM), Pediatr Res 25(part 2):204A, 1989.

156. White NH and Santiago JV: Clinical features and natural history of brittle diabetes in childhood. In Pickup JC, ed: Brittle diabetes, Oxford, 1985, Blackwell Scientific Publication.

157. White NH and Santiago JV: What can be achieved with and what are the complications of the insulin pump? In Raptis S and Church J, eds: Diabetes mellitus: achievements and scepticism, London, 1984, Royal Society of Medicine.

158. White NH and others: Identification of Type I diabetic patients at increased risk for hypoglycemia during intensive therapy, N Engl J Med 308:485-491, 1983.

159. White NH, Skor D, and Santiago JV: A practical closed loop insulin delivery system for the maintenance of overnight euglycemia and the calculation of basal insulin requirements in insulin-dependent diabetics, Ann Intern Med 97:210-213, 1982.

160. White NH and others: Comparison of long-term intensive conventional therapy and pumped subcutaneous insulin on diabetic control, ocular fluorophotometry and nerve conduction velocities. In Brunetti P and others, eds: Artificial systems for insulin delivery, New York, 1983, Raven Press.

161. White NH and others: Reversal of abnormalities in ocular fluorophotometry in insulin-dependent diabetes after five to nine months of improved metabolic control, Diabetes 31:80-85, 1982.

162. Wilson HK and others: Phosphate therapy in diabetic ketoacidosis, Arch Intern Med 142:517-520, 1982.

163. Winter WE and others: Maturity-onset diabetes of youth in black Americans, N Engl J Med 316:285-291, 1987.

164. Witt MF, White NH, and Santiago JV: Roles of site and timing of the morning insulin injection in type I diabetes, J Pediatr 103:528-533, 1983.

165. Wysocki T and others:: Adjustment to diabetes mellitus in preschoolers and their mothers, Diabetes Care 12:524-529, 1989.

CHAPTER 9

Diabetes and Pregnancy

PRISCILLA HOLLANDER

Prior to the introduction of insulin as a therapy in 1923, pregnant women with insulin-dependent, type I diabetes (IDDM) were at high risk for maternal mortality and even a higher risk for perinatal mortality.[43,61] Once insulin was available, maternal mortality fell dramatically from 45% to 2% for all pregnancies over the following decade.[60] Perinatal mortality also improved, but more slowly, dropping from 60% to 20% for all pregnancies by midcentury. But this was still rather high when compared with the rate in the nondiabetic pregnancy[60,96] (Fig. 9-1). Not until the role of meticulous blood glucose control during pregnancy was understood and emphasized did the perinatal mortality rate reach its present level of 3% to 5%. The linear relationship between blood glucose level and perinatal mortality was demonstrated in a landmark study published by Karlsson and Kjellmer[67] in 1972. Numerous other studies have supported their findings* (Fig. 9-2). In addition to the emphasis on blood glucose control, advances in the obstetric care of women with high-risk pregnancies have also contributed to the successful outcome of the pregnancy complicated by diabetes.[23,51]

There are still, however, some problems associated with the pregnancy complicated by diabetes. One of the major concerns is the high rate of congenital malformation, which ranges anywhere from 4% to 12% in various studies.[39] The risks of pregnancy for the woman with pregestational diabetes also includes a higher incidence of maternal complications such as toxemia, premature labor and delivery by cesarean section and neonatal complications such as respiratory distress syndrome, macrosomia, hyperbilirubinemia, and hypoglycemia.† There is also a small but significantly higher incidence of stillbirth.[15]

The concept of pregnancy complicated by gestational diabetes ("glucose intolerance occurring during pregnancy that disappears following delivery") was formulated as re-

---

*References 42, 43, 53, 61, 62, 67.
†References 43, 59, 68, 81, 113, 126.

cently as 1952; however, studies prior to then and many since that time have shown an association between glucose intolerance diagnosed during pregnancy and maternal and neonatal morbidity.[10,57,91] How to optimally define, diagnose, and treat gestational diabetes continues to be a matter of some controversy.

Not all the questions about diabetes and pregnancy have been answered. Nevertheless, based on present knowledge and the current approach to treatment of the pregnancy complicated by diabetes, it is possible to assure the pregnant woman with pregestational diabetes or with gestational diabetes that her chances for a successful pregnancy are very close to those of the woman without diabetes.

The purpose of this chapter then, is to: compare management of pregnancy as complicated by pregestational and gestational diabetes; address issues related to the physiology of pregnancy and diabetes; identify necessary components of care including the diabetes team approach; discuss complications associated with diabetes treatment during

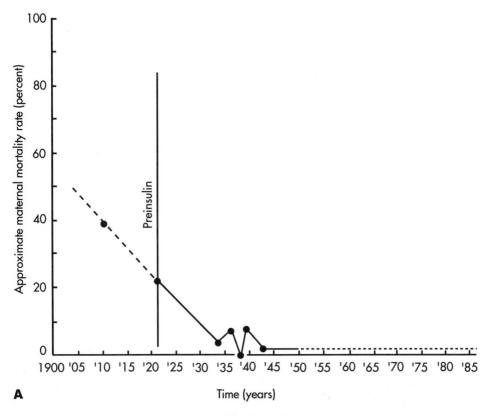

A

Fig. 9-1 A, Maternal mortality before and after the discovery of insulin. Although a decline in perinatal death was observed, this decline was gradual over time. **B,** Maternal mortality before and after the discovery of insulin. A precipitous decline in maternal deaths is depicted shortly after the discovery and use of insulin. (From Reece E: The history of diabetes. Diabetes and pregnancy, principles and practices, New York, 1989, Churchill Livingstone, Inc.)   *Continued.*

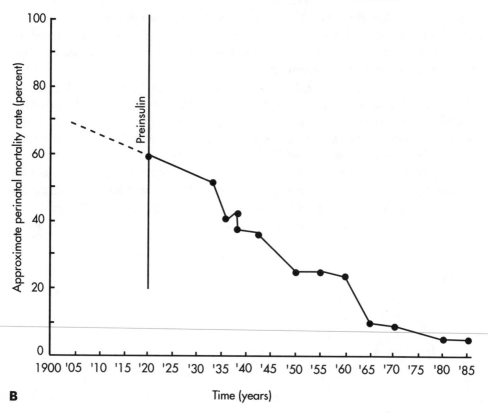

Fig. 9-1 cont'd. For legend see pg. 311.

pregnancy; discuss the relationship of vascular disease in diabetes and pregnancy; describe outcome measures as they relate to maternal, prenatal, and neonatal complications; and describe management of diabetes as complicated by pregestational and gestational diabetes.

Physiology of Pregnancy

The condition of pregnancy is characterized by major physiologic changes in the woman without diabetes. In fact, every aspect of intermediary metabolism will be affected. Thus, it is not surprising that the combination of pregnancy and diabetes can provide the setting for the development of major metabolic dysfunction with marked effect on the integrity of the fetus and the health of the mother. Since the goal of the optimal treatment of diabetes during pregnancy is to establish a normal or near-normal metabolic milieu for the fetus, an understanding of fetal and maternal metabolism in both the nondiabetic and diabetic woman is important for implementing the best approach.

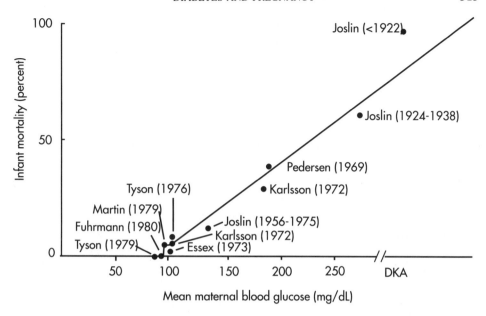

Fig. 9-2 Relationship of perinatal mortality rate to mean plasma glucose levels over the past 60 years. (Jovanovic L and Peterson CM: Management of the pregnant, insulin-dependent diabetic woman, Diabetes Care 3:63, 1980.)

Maternal metabolism

The metabolic state in pregnancy has been characterized as one of accelerated starvation. What does this phrase mean? To maintain blood glucose within accepted bounds in the fasting and postabsorptive state, the balance depends on the production and utilization of glucose. In the fasting state, glucose availability depends upon the liver. The major hormonal signal regulating production of the glucose by the liver is the fall in circulating insulin levels that takes place in a fasting condition. In pregnancy, as early as perhaps the fourteenth week of gestation, it is noted that fasting blood glucose levels are at 15% to 20% mg/dL—lower than in the nonpregnant state.[33] Because of this fall in blood glucose levels, the fasting insulin concentration may fall, and in turn this may lead to an exaggeration of what is called starvation ketosis—that is, more fat tissue will be metabolized leading to increased blood levels of ketones including beta-hydroxybutyric acid and acetoacetic acid. Factors that contribute to the lower fasting blood glucose are thought to be increasing glucose utilization by the fetus and an increase in the volume of glucose distribution.

In the nongravid woman, when nutrients are ingested they are rapidly assimilated and utilized for fuel, replacement of tissue, and/or as storage in the form of glycogen or triglycerides. Ingestion of food is followed rapidly by an increase in insulin that facilitates the utilization of the nutrients. Because of this system, blood glucose excursions are somewhat limited, and blood glucose levels during the day for a nonpregnant, nondiabetic individual are maintained within a very narrow range, from 60 to 160 mg/dL.

During pregnancy, several characteristic metabolic responses occur in response to feeding. Increases in insulin response, blood glucose levels, and triglyceride levels as compared with the nonpregnant state are seen.[36,115] There also is a diminished sensitivity to insulin leading to increased plasma insulin levels in pregnancy. The hyperinsulinemic effect is most noted in the third trimester. In fact, during the pregnancy the amount of insulin produced by the pancreas may increase by two- to threefold.[16] Studies have indicated that tissue sensitivity may be reduced by as much as 80% in pregnancy. This insulin resistance in pregnancy is thought to be related to the increased production of the hormones of pregnancy including the human placental lactogen, progesterone, and estrogen.[58,66,112] Another factor that may be related to increasing insulin resistance during pregnancy is increase in both maternal weight and the weight of the fetus and the placenta.

Because of the decreased responsiveness of maternal tissues to insulin during normal pregnancy, an exaggerated rise in plasma glucose concentration may be seen following a meal compared with the nonpregnant state. For individuals who may have an inherited defect in beta cell function, the secretion of insulin by the mother may fail to keep up with the insulin demands of the pregnancy. If this is the case, an increase in blood glucose levels may occur, resulting in the appearance of overt diabetes, that is, the condition termed *gestational diabetes*.

Fetal metabolism

The fuel requirements of the developing fetus are met mainly by glucose.[6] The level of glucose in fetal blood is generally 10 to 20 mg/dL below that in the maternal circulation.[7] Therefore diffusion favors the movement of glucose from the mother to the fetus. In contrast to the movement of glucose to the fetus, maternal insulin and glucagon do not traverse the placenta.[34] Therefore fetal glucose utilization is not directly dependent on maternal insulin availability.

Fetal insulin is thought to play an important role in the growth of the fetus. Insulin has been shown to be present as early as nine weeks of gestation.[78] Not only glucose is transferred across the placenta, but also amino acids are actively transported from the maternal to the fetal circulation. Transfer of free fatty acids from the maternal to the fetal circulation is limited to the provision of essential fatty acids.[34] Unfortunately ketones such as beta-hydroxybutyrate and acetoacetate are also readily transferred to the fetus through a diffusion process.[109]

Since the volume of glucose transferred across the placenta is related to the level of maternal blood glucose in a pregnancy complicated by diabetes, the level of glucose available to the fetus could vary enormously. At times adequate substrate might not be available, but, more often, there may be excess glucose delivery. Certainly the effects of high concentrations of glucose have been observed in animal experiments.[111] If a continuously high level of glucose is presented to the fetus, fetal insulin production will increase and hyperinsulinemia will result. According to the Pederson hypothesis, increased levels of insulin in the fetus lead to increased fat deposition and macrosomia.[97] As ke-

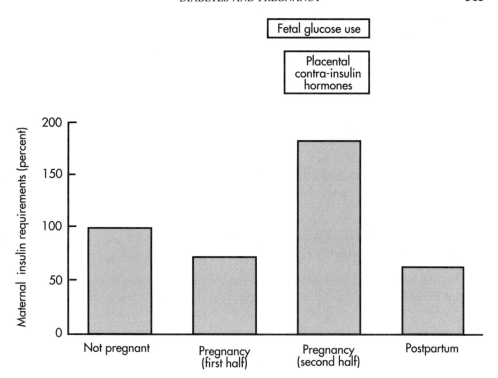

Fig. 9-3 Influence of pregnancy on insulin requirements in pregnancy. The prepregnancy insulin dose is shown as 100% prepregnancy. (Modified from Felig P and Coustan C: Diabetes mellitus. In Burrows G and Ferris F: Medical complications during pregnancy, Philadelphia, 1987, WB Saunders Co.)

tones are also transferred across the placenta, high blood levels of ketones present in the mother could be present in the fetus.

Overview of insulin requirements during pregnancy

Fig. 9-3 illustrates the relationship of maternal insulin requirements to the changes in glucose metabolism. During the early stages of pregnancy, the main factor influencing carbohydrate metabolism is the transfer of glucose and amino acids to the fetus. This transfer may result in symptomatic hypoglycemia in the mother. Some women may actually need reduction of insulin dosage during the first trimester.[126] The increased risk for hypoglycemia may prevail for up to 12 to 18 weeks, but this will vary with the individual pregnancy.

During the second half of the pregnancy, the diabetogenic actions of the placental hormones start to become increasingly evident, and their effect will outweigh the use of maternal glucose by the fetus. Insulin requirements may increase rapidly and insulin dose needs to be changed frequently. With the increase in insulin resistance that occurs during this phase, ketogenesis may be more active in some women.

During the last 3 to 4 weeks of pregnancy, insulin requirements may plateau, or, in some women, decrease. Episodes of moderate or even severe hypoglycemia may occur. Why insulin requirements may fall toward the end of the pregnancy is unclear. Placental detachment or decreasing placental activity may underlie this phenomena.

Following delivery, the concentrations of the placental lactogen hormone, estrogen, and progesterone fall rapidly.[14] In fact, within hours the insulin requirements are rapidly reduced to prepregnancy needs or below. No insulin may be required on the day of delivery and for up to 24 to 48 hours thereafter. Insulin requirements will generally return to prepregnancy levels within 4 to 8 weeks. Special dietary needs such as increased caloric intake for nursing or decreased caloric intake for weight loss may also play a role in determining postpregnancy insulin requirements.

MANAGEMENT OF THE PREGNANCY COMPLICATED BY PREGESTATIONAL DIABETES

First and foremost of the goals of treatment for the pregnancy complicated by pregestational diabetes is strict metabolic control. Support for this goal has been outlined earlier in the chapter. Although the importance of blood glucose control has been widely advocated, what blood glucose goals should be sought has led to some discussion. Pregnant women without diabetes have fasting plasma glucose values averaging 74 to 88 mg/dL and postprandial mean values at one hour of 90 to 100 mg/dL[63] (Fig. 9-4). It is rare in such a woman for plasma glucose to exceed 130 mg/dL.

As early as 1972, Karlsson and Kjellmer[67] reported perinatal mortality rates of 3.6% if average blood glucose level was kept below 100 mg/dL, in a study of pregnancy complicated by diabetes. Other research studies have also demonstrated that the best outcomes are achieved when blood glucose profiles approximate those seen in the pregnant woman without diabetes. At the present time or until other data are available, target goals for the pregnancy complicated by diabetes should include fasting plasma glucoses in the range of 60 to 90 mg/dL and one-hour postprandial blood glucoses in the range of 100 to 120 mg/dL. Glycated hemoglobin goals should be well within the normal range of the assay used for monitoring.

Components of Care

Setting the optimal blood glucose goals is important for the treatment of the pregnancy complicated by diabetes, but the challenge comes in helping the woman with diabetes achieve these goals. A well structured treatment program with a number of different care components is needed for success.

Team approach

Many high-risk pregnancy treatment centers have found the most effective way to treat diabetes and pregnancy is to use a team consisting of an obstetrician who specializes in high-risk pregnancy, a diabetologist, a nurse educator, and a nutritionist. In some cen-

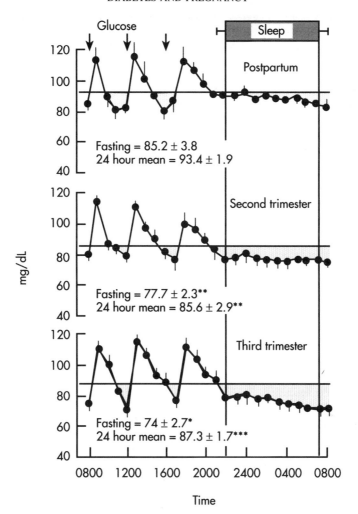

Fig. 9-4 Excursion of plasma glucose during a 24-hour blood glucose profile in six normal pregnant women during the second and third trimesters of pregnancy and 6 to 11 weeks' postpartum. Meals are indicated by ↓ . Data points reflect +/− SEM. Horizontal lines represent the 24-hour mean. *p < 0.05; **p < 0.01; ***p < 0.005. (Cousins L, and others: The 24-hour excursion and diurnal rhythm of glucose, insulin, and C-peptides in normal pregnancy, Am J Obstet Gynecol 136:483, 1980.)

ters, the perinatologist may also be part of the team. Often a psychologist or social worker is of benefit as well. The team members should know and understand their responsibilities and communication should be open. In some cases, the physical location of the team members may be different with the diabetes team located in one area and the obstetrical team in another. Such physical separations may be overcome by preset guidelines for written and/or oral communication.

The most important member of the team is the woman with diabetes. She must un-

—————————————— **BASELINE ASSESSMENT** ——————————————

Endocrinologist

1. Discuss diabetes and pregnancy; risks for mother and child
2. Discuss the importance of blood glucose control during the pregnancy and outline blood glucose goals
3. Assess current insulin regimen and past history of blood glucose control
4. Medical history
    a. General health
    b. Risk factors
    c. OB/GYN history
    d. Current medications
    e. Smoking/alcohol use
5. Physical examination
    a. Height, weight, blood pressure
    b. HEENT
        (1) Assess retinopathy
        (2) Assess thyroidmegaly
    c. Cardiac/lung/abdomen
    d. Extremities
        (1) Edema
        (2) Pulses
        (3) Neurologic status

Diabetes nurse specialist

1. Explain team concept
2. Blood glucose monitoring
    a. Discuss rationale for capillary monitoring
    b. Teach or assess motivation technique
    c. Assess meter reliability
    d. Review frequency of/monitoring and recording of results
3. Blood glucose goals
4. Urine ketone testing
    a. Review or teach technique
    b. Instruct on appropriate times for testing

dertake the major responsibilities of carrying out the day to day regimen. If she does not accept and understand the goals of the program, the risk for complications of the pregnancy will increase.

The responsibilities of the diabetes management team once the woman is pregnant include an initial assessment of the pregnant woman's current diabetes regimen and setting up a plan for consistent and routine follow-up (see accompanying boxes).

Appointments for the pregnant woman should be frequent. In some centers these appointments are set up every 2 weeks with both the obstetrician and the diabetes manage-

———————————— **BASELINE ASSESSMENT—cont'd** ————————————

Diabetes nurse specialist—cont'd

5. Hypoglycemia
   a. Assess knowledge of symptoms and treatment
   b. Review or teach appropriate treatment
   c. Review or teach use of glucagon follow-ups

Diabetes nutrition specialist

1. Diet recall
2. Assess nutrient adequacy of diet and recommend changes or additions
3. Describe goals of diet for pregnancy diabetes and make recommendation for mother's diet
4. Write a meal plan for appropriate weight gain such as alcohol and caffeine
5. Discuss nutrition factors to consider during pregnancy such as caffeine and alcohol

Laboratory evaluation

1. Glycated hemoglobin
2. Thyroid studies
3. Hemoglobin
4. Urine analysis
5. Creatinine/potassium (history of renal disease/hypertension)
   Routine follow-up (visits every 2 weeks) ·

———————————— **ROUTINE FOLLOW-UP APPOINTMENTS** ————————————

Endocrinologist

1. Discuss blood glucose results
2. Make recommendations for changes in insulin
3. Discuss weight/blood pressure
4. Intercurrent/illness/concerns
5. Brief physical exam to include eyes, thyroid, extremities

Diabetes nurse specialist

1. Phone consultation 1-2 times a week for insulin adjustment
2. Review SMBG technique at periodic intervals
3. See patient every other visit

Diabetes nutrition specialist

1. See patient every other visit
2. If concerns with weight or blood glucose problems, see more frequently
3. Review meal plans and adjust accordingly

ment team. Some appointment schedules will need to be individualized, and initially the patient may need to see the diabetes team more often with more frequent obstetric appointments as the pregnancy proceeds.

Automatic hospitalization of a pregnant woman with IDDM or non–insulin-dependent diabetes mellitus (NIDDM) to achieve metabolic control is not necessary in most cases. If glucose control is poor and factors such as intellect, compliance, and/or social situations make achieving diabetes control on an outpatient basis difficult, then it is best to hospitalize the individual for 5 to 7 days. For women with diabetic complications such as poorly controlled hypertension, renal disease, neuropathies, or a history of severe hypoglycemia, the goal of treatment whether through inpatient or outpatient programs, is to bring the blood glucose levels into the target range within one to two weeks. The hospital may be the proper setting to help them achieve blood glucose control.

Self-monitoring of blood glucose

The development of the technology for self-monitoring of blood glucose (SMBG) has been a major advance in the ability to treat diabetes and has been especially beneficial for the monitoring of blood glucose during pregnancy. By using the technique of SMBG, capillary glucose values can be measured on a day to day basis and insulin adjustments made in a timely manner.

SMBG can be of great value in pregnancy, but to use it well its limitations must be understood. Falsification of data, both by pregnant and nonpregnant individuals with diabetes, has been documented.[75,82] Memory reflectance meters can be helpful for detecting this problem. Poor technique can also result in either falsely low or high readings. Meter technique and meter reliability should be assessed at the beginning of the pregnancy and reviewed periodically. Most of the commonly used blood glucose reflectance meters are hematocrit dependent, and a low hematocrit may lead to falsely high blood glucose levels.[5] Some women will develop anemia during pregnancy that if severe enough, could affect the validity of the capillary glucose readings.

During pregnancy, blood glucose testing ideally should be done four to seven times a day. How often it is done may vary depending upon the viewpoint of the managing team; however, premeal tests should be done routinely. Many programs would advocate one-hour or two-hour postprandial tests as well. If there are problems with fasting blood glucose levels, 2 AM or 3 AM blood tests should be done to help determine why the fasting blood glucose level is not in the target zone.

For adequate monitoring of blood glucose control during pregnancy, SMBG should not be the exclusive measure of blood glucose. Glycated hemoglobin, although not useful on a day-to-day basis, is very helpful in confirming overall blood glucose control. In utilizing this test, remember that blood glucose levels may improve within days, but it takes longer for the glycated hemoglobin to reflect this fall. However, there should be a downward trend, and once blood glucose control has been stable over a period of 6 to 8 weeks, the blood glucose levels should match the glycated hemoglobin. Discrepancy between the glycated hemoglobin and the blood glucose values at this point can be a sign of problems with falsification of data. Glycated hemoglobin is done every 2 weeks in some programs and monthly in others.

The fructosamine test is a blood test that reflects blood glucose control over a period of 2 to 3 weeks. This shorter measurement interval may make it a better test in pregnancy than glycated hemoglobin, as was suggested in a study by Roberts and associates.[107] If the test is available to the health care team, it may be a helpful adjunct for monitoring blood glucose during pregnancy.

Diet

Diet plays major role in the management of diabetes in any individual, as is described in Chapter 2, but it is possibly even more important in managing diabetes in pregnancy. In planning a meal plan for pregnancy, three factors should be taken into consideration: optimal caloric intake to achieve blood glucose control, appropriate weight gain, and prevention of starvation ketosis. Severe calorie restriction and weight reduction programs during pregnancy are strongly condemned. Present dietary guides emphasize avoidance of calorie restriction as well as prevention of excess weight gain.[12,120]

The Recommended Dietary Allowances (RDAs) for pregnancy in 1980 advised an additional food intake of 300 calories per day above basal requirements during the second and third trimesters, 30 g additional protein per day (1.3 g protein per kg body weight), 30 to 60 mg of elemental supplemental iron, and a diet or vitamin supplement that would provide for additional amounts of all vitamins and minerals including an additional 400 mg of calcium and 400 mg of folacin. These guidelines and the 1979 American Dietetic Association recommendations have provided the basis for nutritional counseling of the pregnant woman with diabetes during the past decade.[12] In 1989 the RDAs were revised and estimates of requirements for pregnancy lowered for several nutrients.[89] The recommended increment in protein was reduced from 30 to 10 g per day, and iron from 30 to 60 mg to 15 mg per day. Total allowances are 50% lower for all adults with 80 mg per day recommended for non-pregnant women and 400 mg per day during pregnancy. Recommendations for calcium and calorie intake remained the same.

Nutritional and caloric needs during pregnancy continue to be reevaluated. In assessing calorie requirements during pregnancy, the RDA guidelines do not address or take cognizance of pregestational weight and of optimal weight gain in that regard. In a recent publication, Nutrition During Pregnancy, the Subcommittee on Nutritional Status and Weight Gain During Pregnancy recommended new guidelines in regard to desirable weight gain ranges for pregnancy based on a woman's prepregnancy body mass index [119] (Table 9-1). These guidelines were predicated in regard to women delivering term babies weighing between 3 and 4 kg. These are general guidelines for pregnancy that can serve as a framework for looking at desirable weight gain in the pregnancy complicated by diabetes.

In light of new guidelines for weight gain, studies have indicated that 300 calories per day above basal caloric requirement during the second and third trimester may not be optimal. Recommendations of no extra calories during the first trimester and 150 calories in the second and third trimester have been made.[27]

Table 9-1   Recommended Weight Gain for Pregnant Women Based on Prepregnancy Body Mass Index (BMI)

Weight-for-height category	Recommended weight gain	
	kg	Pounds
Low (BMI* < 19.8)	12.5-18	28-40
Normal (BMI of 19.8 to 26)	11.5-16	25-35
High (BMI > 26 to 29)	7.0-11.5	15-25
Obese (BMI > 29)	>6	>15

Modified from Subcommittee on Nutritional Status and Weight Gain During Pregnancy, Food and Nutrition Board, National Academy of Science: Nutrition during pregnancy, Washington DC, 1990, National Academy Press.
*BMI-weight/(height)^2; weight in kg; height in meters.

Calorie intake for most individuals should be divided into six times of food intake per day, including breakfast, midmorning snack, lunch, midafternoon snack, evening meal, and bedtime snack. Routine and consistency of food intake should be stressed.

An important consideration in planning an adequate diet for the pregnant woman with diabetes is the problem of starvation ketosis. This type of ketosis does not carry the major risk of diabetic ketoacidosis; however, urinary ketones may be a sign of inadequate insulin and/or inadequate calories, especially carbohydrate calories. Most commonly, starvation ketosis will manifest itself in the morning. This problem can be avoided by increasing the number of calories in the evening snack and, if needed, by increasing overnight insulin.

There are certain aspects of the pregnancy complicated by diabetes that can make planning an appropriate diet and evaluating weight gain difficult. True weight gain can be difficult to assess, especially during the last trimester since the diabetic pregnancy is more often complicated by toxemia, hydramnios, and increased fluid retention.

Early in the pregnancy hyperemesis may cause problems. Often insulin may need to be adjusted to allow for minimal caloric intake at various times of day, most often in the morning. Some women may have gastroparesis with symptoms of fullness, nausea, and vomiting, which may persist throughout the pregnancy.

Women with poor blood glucose control prior to pregnancy may have been eating excess calories but not gaining weight because of glycosuria. Instead of increasing calories, these women may need to actually decrease their calorie intake, in some cases substantially, to prevent excess weight gain during pregnancy.

Another problem is weight gain related to hypoglycemia. If a woman is having frequent hypoglycemia and treats it with too many extra calories, problems with additional weight gain may ensue.

Exercise

Exercise and/or physical activity can play an important role in determining the level of blood glucose. Physical activity results in the utilization of glucose and in many instances can cause a decrease in blood glucose level. Exercise, however, can exacerbate problems with blood glucose control, as is discussed in Chapter 3.

If exercise is ill-timed, hypoglycemia can occur. Overtreatment of the hypoglycemia can lead to hyperglycemia. Exercise needs to be carefully controlled and timed for an optimal effect on blood glucose level during pregnancy. The best time to exercise may be after meals rather than before meals. By testing blood glucose before and after activity, insulin and food can be adjusted to help maintain stable blood glucose levels.

Mild exercise is encouraged during pregnancy, whereas vigorous exercise is not.[2] Walking and swimming are suitable for pregnant women, whereas high impact aerobics, running, and contact sports are not recommended. For women with complications of pregnancy such as toxemia and preterm labor, physical activity may need to be extremely limited.

Insulin treatment

Insulin is the treatment of choice as a blood glucose–lowering agent in diabetes and pregnancy. Oral hypoglycemic agents have previously been used in pregnancy, but their effect on the fetus has not been adequately evaluated.[11,80,127] It is possible they may cross the placenta and stimulate fetal insulin secretion. *Patients with NIDDM on oral agents should be changed to insulin treatment if they are planning pregnancy or if they become pregnant.*

The principal goal of insulin replacement in the treatment of the pregnant woman with diabetes is to achieve normal daily blood glucose profiles. The most optimal insulin regimen is one which best mimics the function of the normal pancreas. This regimen can not generally be accomplished on less than two shots of insulin a day. In most instances, it will take three or four injections of insulin per day to maximize blood glucose control. Besides multiple daily injections, another method of insulin delivery that has been used during pregnancy is that of continuous subcutaneous insulin infusion (CSII). This method employs an insulin pump that can be programmed to deliver low basal rates of insulin and also deliver boluses of insulin prior to meals.[20]

Over the years a number of different insulin programs for pregnancy have been recommended. Jovanvic and Peterson reported excellent results for blood glucose control and perinatal outcomes with a multi-injection regimen of regular and NPH insulin.[62] Insulin intensification programs in general have used a number of different regimens (Table 9-2). In the Diabetes Control and Complications Trial, over 39 different insulin regimens have been used with patients.[98] Whether CSII or MDII (multiple daily insulin injections) is more advantageous in pregnancy was studied by Coustan and associates in a randomized trial. No difference between the two groups of women was found in regard to glycated hemoglobin, fetal outcome, or adverse effects such as hypoglycemia.[20]

Is there one right approach to insulin therapy in pregnancy? The most optimal insulin program for any patient may depend upon the individual's present regimen and the experience and preference of the diabetes team. For the woman already on an intensified program with either MDII or CSII, no fundamental changes may be needed. If an individual is on a basic program such as an injection of regular and NPH at breakfast and dinner, an

Table 9-2   Insulin Regimens in Pregnancy

Breakfast	Lunch	Supper	Bedtime
R/I*	—	R/I	—
R/I	—	R	I
R/I	R	R/I	—
R/I	R	R	I
R	R	R	I
R/UL*	R	R/UL	—
R/UL	R	R	—
R	R	R/UL	—
R	R	R	UL

*R, Regular; I, NPH or lente; UL, ultralente.

initial change would be to split the dinner injection to regular insulin at dinner and NPH insulin at bedtime. A new insulin program can be constructed for any woman, using her initial insulin regimen as a foundation. There are two key points in constructing a new regimen: (1) the guide for changes should be the target preprandial and postprandial blood glucose levels, and (2) changes must be made in a timely and expeditous manner. The level of blood glucose control at the time the woman is seen by the diabetes team will determine the need for a change in insulin regimen.

All insulin regimens may not be equal. There are certain characteristics of available insulins that make them more or less desirable for use during pregnancy. For instance, the long half-life of nonhuman Ultralente insulins can be a problem in making timely changes in insulin. Control of the morning blood glucose value is also sometimes difficult with this insulin as a basal or background insulin. Human Ultralente insulins may have an unpredictable peaking effect leading to unexpected hypoglycemia. NPH or Lente may be a better choice for background insulin during pregnancy, as their time course and peak effect are usually more consistent and predictable.

Insulin administration

One important aspect of using multiple injections of regular insulin during pregnancy is the timing of injections. In general, injections should be given 30 minutes before a meal; however, the rate of insulin absorption may vary from patient to patient. Establishing the right timing for the injection is essential because of its effect on postprandial blood glucose control and the occurrence of hypoglycemia. Optimal individual absorption rates may vary anywhere from 15 minutes to an hour. A recent study has indicated that absorption was more routine and reliable when injections were given at one site.[4] Certainly if problems with control arise, the use of one site during pregnancy may be important. Many pregnant women give injections in the abdomen.

Insulin preparation

Human insulin is recommended for new patients starting on insulin and for patients who may be having problems with insulin antibodies, lipoatrophy, hypertrophy, and al-

Table 9-3   Algorithms for Compensatory Insulin Adjustments*

Premeal blood glucose	Adjustment
<70 mg/dl	Reduce regular insulin by 1 to 2 units
71-120	Take prescribed regular insulin
121-150	Increase regular insulin by 1 unit
151-200	Increase regular insulin by 2 units
201-250	Increase regular insulin by 3 units
>250	Increase regular insulin by 4 units

*Do not use these algorithms at bedtime.

lergies. At the present time there is no general recommendation that all individuals with diabetes on nonhuman insulins be changed to human insulin.

Should all women seeking pregnancy and those who are already pregnant be changed to human insulin? There have been theoretic concerns that maternal insulin antibodies in women treated with nonhuman insulins may pass to the fetus and in some way be harmful. Such antibodies may stimulate insulin production in the fetus and play a role in the development of macrosomia. A recent study demonstrated that insulin antibodies do apparently pass through the placenta; however, a definite link between maternal insulin antibodies and fetal risk has not been established.[83] At the present time the choice of species of insulin for treatment during pregnancy will in most instances depend on the decision of the health care team and the patient.

Adjustment of insulin dosage

Self-adjustment of insulin is a key part of an intensified insulin program in pregnancy. Without this component it is almost impossible to achieve targeted blood glucose goals. Each woman should be provided with an individualized set of algorithms to help her adjust her insulin on a day-to-day basis.

Self-adjustment of insulin usually refers to changing the dose of regular insulin. Insulin changes can be based on a number of different parameters. The three most common are blood glucose levels, anticipated activity, and changes in diet. Table 9-3 illustrates fairly simple algorithms set up on the basis of blood glucose levels. For example, a woman is on a basic insulin regimen of 20 units of NPH and 5 units of regular insulin before breakfast, 4 units of regular insulin before lunch, 6 units of regular insulin at dinner, and 20 units of NPH at bedtime. If her blood glucose is 150 mg/dL before lunch, according to the algorithms she would add 3 units of regular insulin to the usual 4 units of regular insulin dose, in anticipation of bringing the next premeal blood glucose level into the target range. This is a very simple algorithm; some women have different scales for each meal. More complicated algorithms may be used if the woman wishes to vary exercise. Some women will be able to master a fairly complicated supplemental scale, whereas others may be able to use only a very simple scale.

Algorithms are generally based on experience, and, as the pregnancy progresses, the algorithm may need to change. Insulin supplements given for extra food also need to be worked out on an individual basis. During pregnancy, however, too much flexibility in diet is discouraged because it makes achieving target blood glucose levels more difficult and also because of the concern about weight gain.

Complications of Diabetes Treatment During Pregnancy

Ketoacidosis

Ketoacidosis is associated with up to a 50% rate of fetal death and was the major contributor to both fetal and maternal mortality prior to the introduction of insulin.[26,79] At the present time ketoacidosis usually occurs during pregnancy in a setting of an intercurrent illness, such as influenza or urinary tract infection, and is also more likely to occur in women whose diabetes control during pregnancy is poor. The diabetogenic effect of pregnancy and the increased level of ketones produced during pregnancy can set the stage for mild intercurrent illness to cause ketoacidosis in the woman with poor diabetes control.

Routine monitoring for ketones is important to help identify ketosis associated with poor blood glucose control and also to identify starvation ketosis. Many protocols suggest that women check for urinary ketones every morning. Ketoacidosis has also been described in pregnancy with fairly mild elevations of blood glucose level, so testing for ketones whenever the blood glucose test is above 200 mg/dL is very important. To help minimize the incidence of ketoacidosis, all women should have protocols that include guidelines for insulin use and diet changes when ill. Women should be instructed to call their health provider fairly early in the course of an illness if blood glucose levels are not in the target range or if moderate to large ketones are present in the urine.

Hypoglycemia

The main concern in seeking strict blood glucose goals during pregnancy is maternal hypoglycemia because of its effect on the mother and its possible effects on the fetus. Studies in nongravid women and men treated with intensified insulin programs have found a higher rate of hypoglycemia than that seen in individuals on conventional insulin therapy.[124,125] Coustan reported that both MDII and CSII were associated with a high frequency of both symptomatic and biochemical hypoglycemia in pregnancy. In this group, 3 of 11 patients on CSII and 5 out of 11 MDII patients had a total of 31 episodes of severe hypoglycemia. Not all reviews show such a high incidence of severe hypoglycemia, but it is a risk in individuals pursuing normal blood glucose goals.[20]

Studies are few, so at the present time there is minimal evidence that severe hypoglycemia has an adverse effect on perinatal mortality or upon subsequent mental and motor function of offspring of mothers with diabetes.[20,108] An interesting study was done by Rovergi and associates in which insulin doses were increased until the patient manifested symptoms of hypoglycemia. The doses were than decreased slightly and the patients were maintained through pregnancy on the brink of symptomatic hypoglycemia. Perinatal mortality rate in this study was approximately 2.7% when congenital anomalies incompatible with life were excluded.[108]

Risk to the mother from hypoglycemia is unclear. Maternal deaths from hypoglycemia have been reported, although they are rare.[44] At the present time possible links between severe hypoglycemia and neurobehavioral damage are being monitored in the Diabetes Control and Complications Trial.[124] If results from that trial show a relationship between hypoglycemia and neurobehavioral morbidity, it is possible that a reassessment of blood glucose goals during pregnancy may be needed.

Present evidence would indicate that risk from maternal hypoglycemia to the fetus is small and that prolonged hyperglycemia is a much greater danger. Maternal risk from hypoglycemia appears to be low and not above that seen for individuals on intensified insulin regimens. One group of women, those with a history of severe hypoglycemia and/or hypoglycemic unawareness, may need to have blood glucose goals set at a higher level than those for other women with diabetes.

Severe hypoglycemia can be characterized in a number of ways. Its strictest definition is hypoglycemia requiring hospitalization, an emergency room visit, or a paramedic visit with intravenous administration of glucose or intramuscular administration of glucagon. This definition is often expanded to mean any episode of hypoglycemia that cannot be self-treated.

The best approach to avoiding maternal hypoglycemia is a treatment plan that combines the appropriate insulin regimen with a consistent routine of diet and activity. The patient must also always be on guard for the possible occurrence of hypoglycemia. Unusual changes in schedule or activity should be avoided. Deleting food from the meal plan, especially dropping the evening snack, can be a major cause of hypoglycemia.

At the beginning of the pregnancy the patient and her family members' knowledge of the recognition and treatment of hypoglycemia should be evaluated. Such an assessment is important even for women who appear knowledgeable about hypoglycemia. An episode of severe hypoglycemia during pregnancy should not be the stimulus for a belated educational effort about this problem.

The optimal treatment of hypoglycemia, including mild, moderate and severe hypoglycemia, should be reviewed with the pregnant woman and her family at the beginning of the pregnancy (see Chapter 2 for treatment guidelines). Overtreatment, especially for mild to moderate episodes, should be avoided. The recommended treatment for mild to moderate hypoglycemia for the typical individual patient with diabetes can be applied in pregnancy. Tablets of glucose are especially useful for treating a reaction with the right amount of carbohydrate. With regard to severe hypoglycemia, the woman's family and possibly co-workers should be trained in the administration of glucagon and the appropriate time to use it.

Vascular Disease

Concern about the effect of diabetic vascular disease on pregnancy outcomes in women with diabetes has long been evident. In the past perinatal mortality rates were significantly higher among patients with diabetic vascular complications. Because of this relationship, a classification system of perinatal outcome related to the extent and severity of the mother's diabetic complications were set up by Dr. P. White, an early pioneer in the care of the pregnancy complicated by diabetes[133] (see accompanying box). Because of recent advances in assessment and treatment of diabetic complications and improved obstetric care, this classification has not been as helpful or useful as in the past. Women with vascular complications who may have been previously advised against pregnancy may now consider it.

The fear that pregnancy will aggravate existing vascular complications or promote the development of future problems has also been a major concern. Studies on the effect of pregnancy on diabetic vascular complications are still somewhat limited, but available evidence indicates the effect of pregnancy, at least in individuals with mild to moderate diabetic vascular complications, is minimal.

Retinopathy

Fears about the effect of pregnancy on the progression of retinopathy initially arose from reports of individual cases. Early formal studies of this question did not look at control groups of nonpregnant woman, and their results are inconclusive and contradictory.[114,117]

More recently it has been shown that the institution of tight blood glucose control may cause progression of diabetic retinopathy.[125] Thus, progression of retinopathy in an individual woman during pregnancy may relate to rapid improvement in blood glucose control rather than the pregnancy itself.

In a recent population study on retinopathy, Klein and associates found a small increase in the incidence of advanced retinopathy in women with a history of pregnancy as

---

_____ **REVISED WHITE CLASSIFICATION (1980)** _____

Gestational diabetes

Abnormal GTT, but euglycemia maintained by diet alone
Diet alone insufficient; insulin required

Diabetes diagnosed before pregnancy

Class A Treatment with diet alone; any duration or onset age
Class B Onset age 20 years or older, duration less than 10 years
Class C Onset age 10-19 yr or duration 10-19 years
Class D Onset under 10 years, duration over 20 years, background retinopathy, or hypertension (not preeclampsia)
Class R Proliferative retinopathy or vitreous hemorrhage
Class F Nephropathy with over 500 mg/day proteinuria
Class RF Criteria for both classes R and F
Class H Arteriosclerotic heart disease clinically evident
Class T Previous renal transplantation

Modified from Hare J, and White P: Gestational diabetes and the White classification, Diabetes Care 3:394, 1980.

compared with the general population of women with diabetes.[72] These data did not show a relationship between number of pregnancies and worsening retinopathy.[71]

At the present time the presence of retinopathy, unless it is unstable proliferative retinopathy, should not stop a woman from considering pregnancy. All women who are pregnant should have an eye exam early in the pregnancy and further exams scheduled as needed. Assessment and treatment of retinopathy during pregnancy do not differ from treatment of the nongravid woman with diabetes.

Nephropathy

Nephropathy can affect the outcome of pregnancy. An increased incidence of intra-uterine fetal growth retardation, preterm delivery, stillbirth, and poorer perinatal survival has been seen in pregnancy with kidney disease, as described by Kitzmiller and associates. They combined the results of several studies on pregnancy and renal disease and showed a 91.2% perinatal survival in diabetic pregnancies complicated by renal disease versus a 97% perinatal survival for diabetic pregnancies not complicated by nephropathy.[69,105] Pregnancy for a woman with nephropathy is accompanied by a higher risk for maternal and fetal morbidity and in the woman with advanced disease, a higher risk for perinatal mortality is also present. Pregnancy for a woman with advanced renal disease is not advisable.

Can pregnancy affect the course of renal disease? Kitzmiller and others have looked at available data and concluded that pregnancy in women with early renal disease does not contribute to increased progressive loss of function.[69]

Neuropathy

Peripheral diabetic neuropathy does not appear to be aggravated or worsened in a permanent way by pregnancy, although there is a paucity of data in this area. Carpal tunnel syndrome, which is more common in pregnancy and in people with diabetes, certainly may get worse or appear during pregnancy. Symptoms improve or disappear following delivery.

Macrovascular disease

The major macrovascular complication of concern in diabetic pregnancy is heart disease. Although it is unusual for a woman of childbearing age to have known coronary artery disease, it does occur and with greater frequency in women with diabetes.[111] Pregnancy is therefore not advisable for a woman with a history of cardiovascular disease.

Outcome Measures

There has been a dramatic improvement in both maternal and fetal outcomes in the pregnancy complicated by diabetes, but it is still characterized by a variety of complications that affect both the mother and the fetus. Fetal mortality, at least in tertiary care centers, has been reduced to the range of 3% to 5%; however, there are still isolated areas where fetal mortality rates are higher.[69]

Maternal Complications

Hypertensive disorders of pregnancy

Hypertensive disorders are more commonly seen in pregnancies complicated by diabetes than in nondiabetic pregnancies. Their increased incidence is thought to be related to underlying diabetic vasculopathy. Somewhat inconsistent definitions of preeclampsia make it difficult to give exact rates of occurrence, but an incidence of 10% to 15% of all diabetic pregnancies has been frequently reported.[59,81] Some women with pregestational diabetes will already have a diagnosis of either essential hypertension or hypertension related to diabetic nephropathy.

Treatment of preeclampsia in the pregnancy complicated by diabetes does not differ from the approach in the nondiabetic pregnancy. Most of the newer medications used in the treatment of essential or diabetes-related hypertension, such as calcium channel blockers, have not been well tested in human pregnancy, and their effect is unknown. Capoten, an ace inhibitor, has been shown to have detrimental effects on the fetus in animal experiments,[9] although the calcium channel blocker, nifedipine, has been used to treat toxemia during labor[128] with no apparent problems. Beta blockers such as atenolol have been tested in pregnancy and have not been associated with increased neonatal or perinatal morbidity or mortality.[129] Because of their ability to block the adrenaline-induced symptoms of hypoglycemia in some individuals, their use in the woman with diabetes is not recommended. Both aldomet and hydralazine are regarded as safe and effective drugs for treatment of preexisting hypertension in the pregnant woman with diabetes.[103] The use of diuretics is discouraged but may be necessary for blood pressure control in some women.[45] If a woman is planning pregnancy and is being treated with one of the newer drugs, switching treatment to a drug like aldomet may be the best approach.

Hydramnios

Hydramnios has been historically associated with diabetes mellitus in pregnancy, but its true incidence is difficult to document, and a detrimental effect on perinatal mortality has not been shown. Its incidence has been reported at around 15% to 16% in diabetic pregnancy.[68]

Pyelonephritis

Pyelonephritis has been reported in up to 4% of all pregnancies complicated by diabetes[68] and may be more common in individuals with severe diabetes. A urine culture should be done for a baseline and once a trimester. Additional cultures should be done if there are symptoms of a urinary tract infection.

Preterm labor

Different studies have found varying incidences of preterm labor in the pregnancy complicated by diabetes. Reports have ranged from preterm labor being present in 6.1% to 9.2% of women with diabetes compared with 3.9% for the nondiabetic pregnancy.[68,79] A number of agents are available for treatment of this problem such as the beta-agonists.[3] Vasodilan and Brethine can be very effective for individual patients but have been associated with deterioration of blood glucose control.[3] If a woman is started on oral medication as an outpatient, she may need major insulin adjustments to control blood glucose. If preterm labor is so severe that hospitalization for treatment with intravenous magnesium sulfate or terbutaline is necessary, intravenous insulin infusions may be needed to maintain blood glucose control.

Cesarean section

One of the more common problems of the pregnancy complicated by diabetes is the increased rate of cesarean section. Early studies indicated anywhere from a 40% to 60% rate of cesarean section in women with pregestational diabetes as compared with a norm of 20%.[32,68,126] At the present time more emphasis is being placed on achieving a vaginal delivery. This is especially true in individuals with diabetes of shorter duration and in women with minimal problems during the pregnancy. One major contributor to this approach has been the improvement in monitoring and assessment of fetal status.

Maternal mortality

The ultimate obstetric complication is maternal death, which was a reality before the availability of insulin. Up to 50% of pregnancies resulted in death. The present maternal mortality rate is approximately 0.5%. However, this rate is still about 10 times that seen in women without diabetes.[13] Leading causes of mortality include sepsis, hemorrhage, ketoacidosis, hypoglycemia, cardiac arrest, and myocardial infarction.[44]

Perinatal and Neonatal Complications

Intrauterine fetal death

Remarkable improvement has occurred in the perinatal mortality rate among pregnant women with diabetes. In 1975, the fetal death rate was about 4% to 12%, which was 3 to 8 times higher than stillbirth rates in the general population.[35] Recently, stillbirth rates have been reported ranging anywhere from 1% to 4%.[113] This dramatic decline can be attributed to: the emphasis on improved glycemic control, decreased incidence of ketoacidosis, improvement of antepartum monitoring, and the ability to determine the best time to deliver the fetus.

Neonatal mortality

Another success story has been the reduction in neonatal mortality rates, now at about 1% to 5%.[113] Respiratory distress syndrome (RDS) was a major cause of neonatal mortality. The incidence of RDS has been reduced from 25% to 35% to rates of about 3% to 10%.[41,113] Deaths from this problem are becoming so rare that the current major cause of neonatal mortality is congenital anomalies.

Congenital anomalies

Major congenital anomalies continue to affect from 4% to 12% of all infants of mothers with diabetes.[39,46,86,87,110] Congenital heart defects are the most common defects, and their incidence is increased fivefold over that of the general population. Neural tube defects are also common.[104] Since organogenesis occurs during the first 3 to 8 weeks after conception, attention has focused on hyperglycemia during this period as a major factor in development of anomalies. A number of studies, both retrospective and prospective, have shown a link between hyperglycemia and incidence of congenital malformation.[86,87,116] More recently, the reports of several studies have indicated that preconceptual control of blood glucose can lower the incidence of malformation to that seen in the nondiabetic pregnancy.[53,70,116]

The question is, what level of glycemia is necessary to achieve these results? It appears that the major link between glycemia and malformation is strongest in mothers who have markedly elevated blood glucose levels during the first weeks of pregnancy. In a recent Swedish study the cutoff point appeared to be at a hemoglobin A_{1c} 7 to 10 standard deviations above the mean of the normal level.[53] Kiztmiller and associates in a recent study established a cutoff point of hemoglobin A_{1c} 1.7 times that of the mean.[66]

The Diabetes in Early Pregnancy Study (DIEP) was initiated in 1980 to look at the high rate of congenital anomalies in pregnancy complicated by diabetes.[87] Three groups of patients were enrolled: 347 women were entered early in pregnancy (within three weeks of the diagnosis of pregnancy), a second group of 279 women were entered later in pregnancy, and 389 pregnant nondiabetic women were in the control group.[83] Major malformations occurred in the infants of 2.1% of the control group, 4.1% of the early entry subjects, and 9% of the late entry diabetic woman. This study also supports a link between markedly elevated hemoglobin A_{1c} and increased malformation rate. The rate of anomalies for the early entry group was significantly elevated when compared with a rate for the control group of nondiabetic pregnancies even though average hemoglobin A_{1c} was low. This discrepancy may relate to the fact that a number of the women in the early entry group were already three weeks' pregnant when they entered the study, and overall glycemic control may not have approached the level seen in the previously cited studies.

There is substantial evidence that blood glucose control is important in preventing congenital anomalies but that euglycemia is not absolutely necessary to prevent the problem. If presenting glycated hemoblogin is within the normal range or 1 to 1.5 units above the top of this range, risk for congenital malformation appears to be similar to the rate seen in the pregnancy not complicated by diabetes.

Respiratory distress syndrome

Respiratory distress syndrome has been a major contributor to neonatal death. The ability to do in utero tests for pulmonary maturity has helped bring the dramatic decrease in its incidence.[41,113] These tests include the lecithin/sphingomyelin (L/S) ratio and the phosphatidylinositol test. Recently the reliability of the mature ratio for predicting the absence of RDS in offspring of mothers with diabetes has been questioned.[85] The cause of the increased incidence of RDS in infants of women with diabetes continues to be unclear, but is probably multifactorial. Delays in fetal lung maturation may be secondary to fetal hyperglycemia and hyperinsulinemia. The fetus in a diabetic pregnancy is often delivered prematurely, and this may also contribute to the increased incidence of RDS.

Macrosomia and microsomia

Excessive fetal size for gestational age, or fetal macrosomia, has long been recognized as a common complication of the pregnancy associated with diabetes.[43] The infant will have a characteristic body habitus including a round, puffy face and an increased length, which may be proportionate to their weight.

The increase in body weight is related to an increase in body fat, mainly of the viscera; non–insulin-sensitive tissues such as the brain are generally not enlarged.[29] Fetal macrosomia can be explained by the Pederson hypothesis that maternal hyperglycemia leads to fetal hyperglycemia.[97] In response to the hyperglycemia, the fetal pancreas produces increased amounts of insulin. This hyperinsulinemia is thought to stimulate growth in utero. This hypothesis has been supported by animal experiments.[120] Large infants result in an increased rate of cesarean section and also can cause complications for vaginal delivery, including shoulder dystocia.

On the opposite end of the spectrum is the fetus that is small for date of delivery. This condition is often seen in women with known advanced vascular complications and may be related to vascular disease in the uterine vessels that leads to decreased availability of nutrients despite maternal hyperglycemia. There has also been speculation that poor blood glucose control may also lead to infants who are small for date of delivery.

Hypoglycemia

Neonatal hypoglycemia is considered to be a common finding in infants of mothers with diabetes, occurring in up to 20% to 60% of such infants.[68] The definition of hypoglycemia in the newborn is a blood glucose level that drops below 30 mg/dL and 20 mg/dL in a premature neonate. Endogenous insulin levels are generally high in the fetus of the mother with diabetes and may remain so after delivery. Since maternal glucose delivery has stopped and the glucagon system of the infant may be inhibited, glucose production by the neonate may not increase or may even be reduced during the immediate post-delivery period. Hypoglycemia may be prolonged in some infants, lasting up to 48 to 72 hours. Hypoglycemia in the neonate is usually asymptomatic, but if severe and prolonged, it may be accompanied by tremors, apnea, or cyanosis.[54] Long-term consequences of neonatal hypoglycemia have not been established. The best approach to avoiding neonatal hypoglycemia is strict control of maternal blood glucose levels during the pregnancy and labor.

Hypocalcemia

This complication has been seen variably in infants of the mother with diabetes. Studies indicate anywhere from 8% to 22% of offspring may have hypocalcemia.[68] Its etiology is unclear, but may be related to maternal hyperparathyroidism.

Hyperbilirubinemia

Neonatal jaundice can be seen in any infant. Its incidence has been reported to be as high as 20% in the infants of mothers with diabetes.[68,123] Prematurity is thought to contribute to this incidence.

Obstetric Treatment

The importance of comprehensive obstetric monitoring of the pregnancy complicated by diabetes cannot be overemphasized. Most high-risk obstetricians will have their own approach; however, in general, the routine diabetic pregnancy should be followed every 2 weeks initially, once a week at the seventh month, and then biweekly at 34 weeks. The actual timing and frequency of visits will depend, of course, on the needs of the individual woman.

All usual testing done in the nondiabetic pregnancy should be performed in the pregnancy complicated by diabetes. This includes a baseline evaluation of the mother at the first office visit. Biochemical evaluation of the fetus starts at 16 to 17 weeks of gestation in the form of a maternal serum alpha-feto protein screen for neural tube defects.

Ultrasound evaluation of the fetus should be done at 16 to 18 weeks for assessment of major congenital anomalies. If there is concern about viability of the pregnancy, such as poor heart tones, an ultrasound examination may be done earlier at 10 to 12 weeks of gestation. Another ultrasound may not be done until the third trimester at 34 weeks. If there is concern about a large-for-gestational-age infant, an ultrasound may be performed later in the pregnancy to help determine the optimal method of delivery. Some programs suggest ultrasound evaluations at 4-week intervals until delivery. This protocol allows for better and earlier detection of polyhydramnios or oligohydramnios, abnormal fetal growth, or late-onset abnormalities.[106]

At one point maternal estrogen levels were used to help manage a high-risk pregnancy. Dooley and associates, in a major review, concluded this assay is of little value in the management of the pregnancy and may even contribute to inappropriate deliveries.[25]

The mainstay of antepartum monitoring at the present time is biophysical assessment. The nonstress test (NST), which is based on the presence or absence of fetal heart accelerations associated with fetal movement, is a key component of this assessment. A major collaborative study published in 1970 showed significantly increased morbidity/mortality during pregnancy in the presence of a nonreactive NST.[37] The study also evaluated the oxytocin challenge test (OCT), which was found to be a more sensitive test than the NST but is more expensive and on occasion may induce labor.[38] The most common approach is to do either weekly or twice weekly nonstress tests and to follow up with an OCT if the NST is suspicious or nonreactive. This testing should begin at 30 to 32 weeks; however, it may be started earlier in some women.

Another aspect of the biophysical assessment is the biophysical profile (BPP). While both the NST and OCT are nonphysiologic, the BPP is physiologic in that it evaluates the status of the fetus in the absence of uterine contractions. The battery is made up of the NST, fetal breathing movements, a quantitative amniotic fluid volume, gross body movement, and fetal tone. Each of these parameters is given a score. A score of 8 to 10 is generally indicative of fetal well-being. A score of 4 or less may indicate that the fetus is seriously compromised and delivery needs to be imminent.[50]

Additional important measures of fetal maturity can be obtained by measuring the lecithin/sphingomyelin ratio in amniotic fluid plus a variety of other tests of amniotic fluid, which allow accurate evaluation of pulmonary maturity.

Timing and management of delivery

Historically, the timing of delivery in a pregnancy complicated by diabetes was usually at 36 weeks of gestation. Clearly delivery was a compromise between the increasing incidence of stillbirth seen beyond 36 weeks and the risk of developing respiratory distress syndrome if delivery was too early. The development of better methods of assessing the maturity of the fetus has allowed many deliveries to be delayed to at least 38 weeks and longer if the cervix is not ripe. Arbitrary early delivery is no longer mandatory in women with diabetes.[21] The longer the delivery can be delayed, the more likely chance of a vaginal delivery. Moreover, maternal diabetes does not have to be a primary indication for cesarean section. The decision for such a delivery should be made on the basis of general obstetric indications. There may be some exceptions to this rule, such as the case of the woman who has or develops active retinopathy during the pregnancy. There is the possibility that active labor could aggravate her eye disease.

Diabetes management during delivery

The goal in management of diabetes during labor is to achieve and maintain euglycemia. Administration of excess glucose during labor can lead to maternal hyperglycemia and contribute to neonatal hypoglycemia. Recent data have shown that many women with diabetes may not need exogenous insulin during labor to maintain blood glucose control.[49,64] The current approach for the woman who has been in good metabolic control during the pregnancy is to make sure that the day prior to induction she follows her usual routine, assuring that fasting blood glucose level is within the 60 to 100 mg/dL range. On induction morning, insulin and breakfast should be withheld, and an infusion of D5 dextrose initiated at a rate of 75 to 100 ml per hour. Capillary glucose measurement can be done at bedside every one to two hours. In most cases the patient can do her own measurements, or, if that is not possible, a trained nurse or technician can do the measurement. If blood glucose does exceed target levels of 60 to 120 mg/dl, an insulin infusion should be started at one unit per hour. The insulin dosage and intravenous glucose can be adjusted on the basis of the blood glucose values.

If an elective cesarean section is planned, the patient should also follow her usual meal and insulin regimen on the day prior to the procedure. The cesarean section should be planned for very early in the morning. An intravenous line with normal saline can be started. If the procedure is done quickly and expeditiously, the patient may not need glucose or insulin.

If the woman does not present with euglycemia on the morning of induction or cesarean section, an insulin infusion and glucose infusion may need to be started immediately.

For a woman with a known history of poor blood glucose control, hospitalization prior to delivery may be necessary to optimize control.

In the postdelivery period, there is a rapid fall-off in insulin resistance and often a fall in blood glucose levels. Hypoglycemia is not uncommon. Frequent monitoring of blood glucose after delivery is necessary to avoid such problems. Until the trend of blood glucose level is ascertained, insulin should not be given. Women who have injected an intermediate- or long-acting insulin shortly before an unexpected delivery, that is one related to spontaneous labor with vaginal delivery or an unplanned cesarean section, may have special problems with postdelivery hypoglycemia and should be monitored very closely. Many women may not need insulin for up to 24 to 48 hours after delivery.

When restarting a daily insulin regimen, a cautious approach should be taken. Insulin requirements in most women will have dropped substantially below the predelivery requirement. Often the question will arise as to what type of insulin regimen should be started. Most women will have been on an intensified regimen during the pregnancy, whereas some will have been on a conventional insulin regimen prior to becoming pregnant and will want to return to that regimen.

Long-Term Outcome of Infants of Mothers with Diabetes

The role of heredity in the determination of IDDM and NIDDM has long been recognized. Epidemiologic studies done in the past allow the prediction of the risk of development of IDDM in the offspring of parents with diabetes. For children of a mother with IDDM, the rate of development of diabetes is approximately 1.2%. The rate is substantially higher for children of a father with IDDM, reaching 6%.[130] If both parents have IDDM, the chances of the child developing diabetes increases significantly to 20% to 30%.[130]

HLA typing of the offspring can be done to identify the child with a high-risk profile for developing IDDM.[48] If such identification is made, the question becomes how closely the child should be monitored for the development of diabetes. Islet cell antibodies may precede the development of IDDM by a number of years; however, there is currently no successful intervention or preventive therapy available for treating these individuals.[48]

Heredity plays a more important role in determination of NIDDM than IDDM. NIDDM is probabiy inherited as a dominant trait but with incomplete penetrance. Thus 50% of offspring could inherit the predisposition for this disease. Identical twins may have 100% concordance for NIDDM.[122] The chances of inheriting NIDDM appears to be equal in terms of paternal versus maternal diabetes. If both mother and father had NIDDM, the risk for the offspring could be much higher than 50%.[122]

Besides genetic concerns, many questions have been asked about the effect of maternal environment in causing long-term problems for the infant. Children of mothers with diabetes may have an increased risk for obesity as has been shown in studies in the Pima Indian population.[100] Studies in other populations, including one from the Joslin Clinic, have supported these findings.[132] Excess obesity seen in offspring of women with diabetes may not be inevitable and can be prevented if the child is of normal birth weight and is placed on a carefully controlled diet.[30]

A study on the Pima Indian population indicated that the maternal blood glucose environment may also have an effect on the development of glucose intolerance in offspring.[10] They found the rate of diabetes was higher in offspring of women with onset of diabetes before pregnancy than in the offspring of women who did not have diabetes at the time of the pregnancy, but who developed it later.

Some studies have looked at the effect of diabetes in the mother during the pregnancy on subsequent neurologic development and IQ. Most of these studies have found no difference in neurologic outcome between the children of women with diabetes and the children of women without diabetes.[52,99]

Prepregnancy Counseling

All women with pregestational diabetes who are capable of childbearing should be well informed about pregnancy and diabetes (see accompanying box). The problems and con-

---

_____ **EDUCATION PRINCIPLES: PREGESTATIONAL DIABETES** _____

Emphasize the importance of prepregnancy care.

Work with the patient, her partner, her family, and other health care providers to improve the patient's nutrition, exercise program, and blood glucose control.

Recommend that conception be delayed until the patient's blood glucose control is excellent and the glycated hemoglobin level is normal or near normal.

Explain the risks of birth defects and adverse perinatal outcomes and the need for fetal surveillance.

Recommend that the patient's vascular condition be thoroughly evaluated before she becomes pregnant. Explain that pregnancy may exacerbate advanced diabetic retinopathy but generally does not permanently worsen diabetic nephropathy.

Explain that, overall, pregnancy does not shorten the life expectancy of a woman with diabetes but does increase her risk for hypoglycemia and ketoacidosis and for associated mortality.

Inform patients with coronary atherosclerosis that their risks for morbidity or mortality may be greater during pregnancy.

Discuss the emotional and financial demands of pregnancy with the patient, her partner, and her family.

Inform patients about life-style elements—such as drinking alcoholic beverages and smoking—that increase the risk for a poor outcome of pregnancy. Emphasize that patients will need to modify such behaviors before becoming pregnant.

Department of Health and Human Services Public Health Service: Prevention and treatment of complications of diabetes: a guide for primary care practitioners, Atlanta, 1991, Centers for Disease Control, Center for Chronic Disease Prevention and Health Promotion, Division of Diabetes Translation.

cerns of the pregnancy must be understood, as well as the excellent chances for a successful pregnancy if a treatment program is followed. Careful patient teaching regarding prepregnancy planning needs to be carefully followed. Involvement of the entire diabetes team is critical to optimal patient education. The importance of optimal blood glucose control at the time of conception and during the pregnancy should be stressed.

The question of initial poor blood glucose control on the outcome of a pregnancy can be a difficult one. Some women find themselves unexpectedly pregnant, and are not sure they wish to continue the pregnancy. They may want definite answers about the risk for congenital abnormalities and other problems for themselves and the fetus. As discussed previously in this chapter, there is now available information as to the relative risk of maternal blood glucose level during the first trimester and the incidence of congenital anomalies.

Many women also have concerns about the effect the vascular complications of diabetes on the success of a pregnancy and, conversely, the effect of pregnancy on vascular complications such as retinopathy and nephropathy. These questions need to be covered thoroughly in prepregnancy counseling.

Counseling on birth control should also be part of the routine care for all women who are capable of childbearing. This includes women not only in the age range of 20 to 40 years but also teenagers.

Many educational materials about diabetes and pregnancy are now available and can be utilized either as handouts or for interactive sessions between the prospective mother and the health care provider. Some diabetes centers have participated in programs that actively seek out women with diabetes who are interested in pregnancy to enroll them in an education program that addresses the problems of a pregnancy complicated by diabetes. A recent study showed that such interventions led to a decrease in congenital anomalies and pregnancy problems.[66]

If a woman is seeking pregnancy, her diabetes control should be assessed and, if not adequate, a program for achieving optimal blood glucose control can be instituted. How long the patient has to be in optimal blood glucose control before conception is unclear. Many programs advise at least 3 to 6 months prior to attempting to achieve pregnancy.

Pregestational Diabetes and Pregnancy: Conclusion

The present approach to treatment has made successful pregnancy a real possibility for the vast majority of women with diabetes who desire children. The key to success is a treatment program that utilizes a number of components, including preconceptual counseling, intensive efforts at tight blood glucose control before and during the pregnancy, frequent evaluations by the diabetes team and the high-risk obstetrics team, regular noninvasive measurements of fetal integrity, appropriate timing of delivery, and the provision of neonatal care.

MANAGEMENT OF PREGNANCY COMPLICATED BY GESTATIONAL DIABETES

Up to 5% of all pregnant women experience gestational diabetes, making it one of the most common complications of pregnancy.[1] Gestational diabetes is defined by the Second International Workshop Conference on Gestational Diabetes Mellitus as carbohydrate intolerance of variable severity with onset at first recognition during the present pregnancy.[102] This definition does not depend on the need for or use of insulin, nor does it preclude the possibility that the condition existed before the present pregnancy and that it may be permanent. For the vast majority of women, the condition will disappear at the end of pregnancy. In fact, statistics indicate that in 97% of women with gestational diabetes, glucose tolerance returns to normal after delivery.[92,101]

Gestational diabetes has been associated with increased fetal and maternal morbidity.[17,41,91,131] Therefore, careful management of this condition is crucial. Over the past decade, increased awareness of the problems of gestational diabetes has led to a reevaluation of treatment programs and exploration of new approaches. Questions include: how tightly controlled blood glucose levels should be to ensure optimal outcome for both mother and child, how should the diagnosis be made, and at what risk for subsequent diabetes are women with gestational diabetes?

Physiology

As discussed earlier in this chapter, during pregnancy insulin resistance increases and insulin requirements rise steeply. In some women, possibly because of genetic factors, the production of insulin by the beta cells appears to be limited. In these women, at some point in the pregnancy, insulin demand exceeds supply and hyperglycemia will occur. Since insulin requirements start to rise sharply around the twenty-fourth to twenty-eighth week of gestation, gestational diabetes is most likely to manifest itself at that time. Once delivery occurs, insulin requirements drop dramatically, generally within a matter of hours.

Screening

In the past, most health care providers have screened pregnant women for diabetes on the basis of certain risk factors. Research has shown, however, that screening on this basis alone will detect only 50% of all cases of gestational diabetes.[24] This has led the American Diabetes Association to recommend that all pregnant women be screened for abnormal glucose metabolism between the twenty-fourth and twenty-eighth week of gestation. Screening prior to 24 weeks might also be recommended if the presence of risk factors dictates. Risk factors that have been considered important for the development of gestational diabetes include a history of stillbirth or abortion, a family history of diabetes, previous delivery of an infant weighing over 9 pounds, previous gestational diabetes, a his-

Table 9-4   Criteria for 100 g Oral Glucose Tolerance Test in Pregnancy

Time	O'Sullivan*	NDDG Adaption†
Preglucose	90‡	105
1 hour	165	190
2 hours	145	165
3 hours	125	145

*O'Sullivan JB and Mahan CM: Criteria for the oral glucose tolerance test in pregnancy, Diabetes 13:278, 1964.
†National Diabetes Data Group: Classification and diagnosis of diabetes mellitus and other categories of glucose intolerance, Diabetes 28:1039-1051, 1979.
‡mg/dL.

tory of toxemia, urinary tract infections, hydramnios, advanced maternal age, glycosuria, and obesity. Interestingly, the incidence of gestational diabetes is significantly higher in pregnancies complicated by twins.[28]

The recommended screening method for gestational diabetes is the glucose challenge test. A 50 g oral glucose load is given regardless of previous meal or time of day. Venous plasma glucose level is measured 1 hour later. If this level is 140 mg/dL or above, a full 3-hour 100 g oral glucose tolerance test is recommended.[90] In this test, 100 g of oral glucose in at least 400 ml of liquid is given in the morning after an overnight fast. An unrestricted diet containing at least 150 g of carbohydrate should be eaten on the day prior to the test. The venous plasma glucose level is measured after fasting and at 1, 2, and 3 hours after glucose loading during which the patient remains seated and does not smoke. The current criteria for a definitive diagnosis is two or more blood glucose values in excess of the following: fasting blood glucose 105 mg/dL, 1-hour 190 mg/dL, 2-hour 165 mg/dL, 3-hour 145 mg/dL (Table 9-4). If only one of the above values is elevated or the woman has a clinical history suspicious of glucose intolerance, the glucose tolerance test is repeated at 32 weeks. If an individual has a previous history of gestational diabetes, it is often recommended that they be screened earlier than the 24- to 28-week period. Testing at 18 to 20 weeks has been suggested. If the screen is negative, a retest should be done at the 24 to 28 week period.

Because of discrepancies between capillary blood glucose and whole venous blood glucose levels, the use of capillary blood glucose determinations is not recommended by the ADA for the initial glucose challenge test.[65,74] The glycated hemoglobin also should not be used for the diagnosis of gestational diabetes as it is not sensitive enough to catch the changing glucose intolerance in gestational diabetes.[15]

Currently the 3-hour oral glucose tolerance test that is based on long-term studies by O'Sullivan and Mahan is regarded as the gold standard of diagnosis in gestational diabetes. Questions have been raised as to whether the present criteria allow enough specificity not to miss cases of gestational diabetes as defined by perinatal morbidity. Much of this concern has related to the individual with only one abnormal blood glucose level on the test. Langer and Masse followed women with only one abnormal test and found increased macrosomia.[77] Even more interestingly, Tallargo and co-workers studied the relationship of 2-hour plasma glucose levels on an oral glucose tolerance test to fetal and maternal morbidity. They found that women with 2-hour levels in the range of 120 to 160 mg/dL, values which would be called normal by present accepted criteria for the oral glucose tolerance test, had an increased incidence of macrosomia, toxemia, and cesarean section.[121] Obviously there should be ongoing evaluation and reassessment of methods of screening and diagnosis in gestational diabetes. The current recommendations from the ADA would be to screen all pregnant women for gestational diabetes and to diagnose it on the basis of the O'Sullivan criteria.

Morbidity and Mortality

Studies have shown the infant of a mother with gestational diabetes to be at an increased risk for a number of different conditions including hypoglycemia, polycythemia, hyperbilirubinemia, and respiratory distress syndrome. The incidence of intrauterine death, premature delivery, and neonatal mortality is also increased.[17,41,131] Macrosomia is more common in gestational diabetes and can lead to difficulties in delivery that may affect the infant and the mother.[16] Not only are there increased problems with complications in the infant in gestational diabetes, there is also increased risk for maternal complications. These include pregnancy-induced hypertension, hydramnios, and an increased incidence of cesarean section.[18] Two recent studies have shown that the average cesarean rate for patients with gestational diabetes approximates 30%.[19,55]

Management of Gestational Diabetes

A pregnancy complicated by gestational diabetes must be considered a high-risk pregnancy. Once the diagnosis is made, the mother and fetus should be under close scrutiny. Some gestational diabetes programs emphasize the team approach to management with the involvement of a diabetologist and an obstetrician specializing in high-risk pregnancy. Other professionals who are important for an effective treatment program are a nurse educator and dietitian. Involvement of a psychologist or a counselor can be helpful in many cases. The diagnosis of gestational diabetes may create severe anxiety and concern on the part of the pregnant woman. Her major fears usually focus on risk for the fetus and future maternal risk for permanent diabetes. Concerns may be especially pronounced in a woman with a family history of diabetes.

Approaches to Therapy in Gestational Diabetes

Traditionally, therapy for gestational diabetes has been based on the results of a 3-hour oral glucose tolerance test. If a woman presented with a fasting blood glucose level greater than 105 mg/dL, she was started on a program of insulin and diet therapy. A woman with a fasting blood glucose level less than 105 mg/dL, but with abnormal post-glucose challenge values, is usually started on diet therapy alone. Metabolic goals for those women are fasting blood glucose levels of less than 105 mg/dL, 1-hour postprandial blood glucose levels less than 140 mg/dL, and 2-hour postprandial blood glucose levels less that 120 mg/dL.[102]

Blood glucose goals in gestational diabetes are currently being reevaluated in light of blood glucose levels found in the nondiabetic pregnancy. The blood glucose values seen in a nondiabetic pregnancy are lower than traditionally accepted treatment goals for gestational diabetes. In fact, in the third trimester of a nondiabetic pregnancy, fasting blood glucose levels generally range from 50 to 90 mg/dL and 1-hour postprandial levels from 80 to 120 mg/dL.[31] Langer and Masse found that a treatment program based on blood glucose values compatible with those seen in the nondiabetic pregnant woman brought about a marked lowering in perinatal complications in a group of women with gestational diabetes.[76] This result was also shown by Hollander and associates.[55]

Monitoring

An important aspect of any treatment program for gestational diabetes is ongoing monitoring of blood glucose. In the traditional approach to treatment of gestational diabetes, women may visit their physician's office once or twice a week for pre- and postprandial blood glucose values. This frequency of monitoring does not give adequate information to make decisions on therapy in a timely manner. Glycated hemoglobin is also not helpful in monitoring gestational diabetes as it is not sensitive enough to detect the degree of maternal hyperglycemia that needs treatment.

SMBG done on a daily basis can provide the necessary data to implement the current, more intensive treatment programs in gestational diabetes. Most investigators suggest that both premeal and postmeal blood glucose levels be checked. Such a program involves testing at least 4 to 6 times a day, including 1- or 2-hour postprandial values.[55,76] For SMBG to be useful, technique and machine reliability must also be consistently evaluated.

Diet therapy

Diet therapy is a key part of treatment for gestational diabetes, whether used alone or with insulin therapy. The basic goals in regard to calorie planning are the maintenance of euglycemia, that is, blood glucose levels within the target range, and appropriate weight gain. Goals for weight gain are the same for both pregnancy complicated by pregestational diabetes and for gestational diabetes. See the discussion of caloric intake and weight gain earlier in the chapter. There are certain aspects of diet therapy for gestational diabetes that are challenging. First a disproportionate number of obese women develop gestational diabetes, and at diagnosis many women have already gained excess weight.

Diet counseling in a gestational diabetes program should begin with a meeting between the woman and the dietitian. A diet with a specific calorie goal should be set based on her prepregnancy weight and desired weight gain during the pregnancy.

Weight and calorie intake must be monitored closely throughout the program. Some women make extreme calorie cuts to control blood glucose level to avoid insulin therapy and may not achieve proper weight gain. Many women are eating excess carbohydrate in the form of simple sugars such as sodas, ice cream, and other desserts. Often the elimination of these simple sugars can make a significant difference in blood glucose control. It is not unusual to see a plateau in weight gain for 1 or 2 weeks in most women after starting their new diet.[55] However, if subsequent weight gain is not appropriate, calorie level may need to be increased.

Insulin Therapy

Insulin therapy should be started if blood glucose goals are not met on diet treatment alone. As in pregestational diabetes, oral hypoglycemic agents are not recommended for treatment of gestational diabetes.[80] A number of different insulin regimens have been used for the treatment of gestational diabetes. Although it has been suggested that all women with gestational diabetes should be treated with insulin, most current gestational programs initiate insulin therapy on the basis of maintaining blood glucose goals.[8,19,55,76]

Coustan described a program of insulin treatment in which women are treated initially with a dose of 30 units of insulin per day, 20 units of NPH and 10 units of regular insulin in the morning.[22] If hyperglycemia persists, adjustments are made in the specific components based on the blood glucose pattern. Board and associates[8] describe a program of insulin therapy for gestational diabetes similar to an intensive program for women with pregestational diabetes; that is, a four-shot regimen that uses both NPH and regular insulin. A mixed injection of regular and NPH insulin given before breakfast and dinner has been described by Hollander and colleagues.[56] In this regimen a high ratio of regular insulin to NPH is used to control postprandial blood glucose excursion. All these groups have shown good outcomes with insulin treatment.

For most women with gestational diabetes, insulin can be started on an outpatient basis. Arrangements should be made so that insulin can be adjusted quickly and consistently. This goal can be accomplished by frequent contact with the diabetes management team, such as telephone calls twice a week, and by weekly appointments. Simple algorithms for self-adjustment of insulin by the patient can also be helpful. If a woman initially presents with markedly elevated blood glucose levels and ketones, hospitalization is mandated. Human insulin is the insulin of choice in the treatment of gestational diabetes. Since these women have not been exposed to nonhuman insulins, using human insulin will significantly decrease the chance of the development of insulin antibodies during the pregnancy. This may be important for the subset of women who will develop diabetes in the future and will require insulin. Although severe hypoglycemia is rare in insulin-treated gestational diabetes, mild episodes are not uncommon. The patients should be taught to recognize the symptoms of hypoglycemia and how to treat it effectively.

Obstetric Care and Fetal Evaluation

A key aspect of any gestational diabetes treatment program is antepartum monitoring. Once the diagnosis of pregnancy is made the woman should have close follow-up by her obstetrician. Increased frequency of antenatal monitoring of the fetus is necessary, especially in the insulin-treated mother. In women in whom blood glucose control is not optimal or who have a history of maternal complications such as pregnancy-induced hypertension, this monitoring should begin early. Thirty-four weeks has been suggested, and certainly by 36 weeks all fetuses should be monitored quite closely. This assessment may consist of a weekly NST followed by an OCT if necessary. Biophysical profiles may also be helpful.[73] Generally it is not desirable to let delivery go beyond term.

Postpartum Follow-Up

At the present time most women are tested with a 75 g oral glucose tolerance test at 6 weeks' postpartum.[88] Whether this test is optimal or necessary is currently being questioned. For instance, if the women who have overt diabetes immediately following delivery are eliminated, glucose tolerance will be normal in 99% of the women tested.[92] Other methods of testing for diabetes, such as a fasting blood glucose or glycated hemoglobin, are simpler, more reliable, and less expensive. Besides being inappropriate for diagnosis, the relevance of an oral glucose tolerance test in a nonpregnant woman as a predictor of future diabetes must be questioned.

Another approach to postpartum evaluation of glucose intolerance is to continue capillary blood testing for individuals whose anticipated risk for the development of diabetes in the postpartum period is high. Women who present with elevated fasting blood glucose levels or elevated glycated hemoglobin during pregnancy are the best candidates for this approach.

Long-Term Outcomes

What are the long-term outcomes for women with gestational diabetes? Most women are concerned about the chance of recurrent gestational diabetes with future pregnancies as well as the possibilities of developing clinical diabetes at some point in their life. Because of these fears, discussion of potential future problems with the woman is essential. If gestational diabetes has occurred once, the chances of recurrence in a subsequent pregnancy are fairly high, although not inevitable. For most women, recurrent gestational diabetes should not be a major factor in the decision for or against another pregnancy as repeat episodes of gestational diabetes do not appear to contribute to a greater incidence of future diabetes.[93]

The development of clinical diabetes later in life should be a major concern. Twenty percent of nonobese and about 60% of obese women with gestational diabetes will develop clinical diabetes within 15 years of pregnancy[94] (Fig. 9-5). Women with a history of gestational diabetes have also been shown to exhibit an increased mortality rate and a higher incidence of cardiovascular disease than the general population of women.[95]

In the past, gestational diabetes was thought to be a predictor of NIDDM. However, recent studies indicate that some women with gestational diabetes will eventually develop

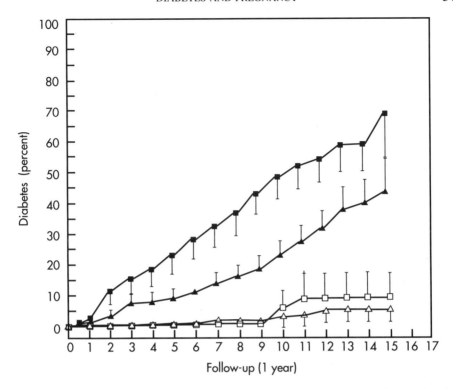

Fig. 9-5 Cumulative incidence of diabetes in overweight *(black squares)* and normal weight women *(black triangles)* gestational diabetes; overweight *(white squares)* and normal weight *(white triangles)* controls. Percentage +/≥ SE. (O'Sullivan JB: Body weight and subsequent diabetes mellitus, JAMA 248:949, 1982.)

IDDM. Studies of islet cell antibody levels and determination of HLA antigens in several populations of women with gestational diabetes have identified a number of women who present with profiles characteristic of pre-IDDM individuals.[40,118] In some women with gestational diabetes, ICA positivity may be as high as 30% to 48%.[47]

About 3% of all women with gestational diabetes will remain diabetic following delivery.[92] According to Metzger and associates, if fasting hyperglycemia is identified during pregnancy, diabetes is more likely to persist after delivery. In his series, women with fasting blood glucose levels of 105 to 130 mg/dL had a 43% chance of remaining diabetic. If fasting blood glucose exceeded 130 mg/dL, this probability rose to 83%.[84]

In essence, gestational diabetes is one of the most reliable predictors of future clinical diabetes mellitus. Most women will develop NIDDM, whereas a minority will develop IDDM. A woman with a history of gestational diabetes should be screened periodically for diabetes. Once a year testing should be a minimal requirement. Since obesity is a risk factor for NIDDM, some women may be able to delay or even prevent its onset by controlling their weight.

_____ EDUCATION PRINCIPLES: GESTATIONAL DIABETES _____

For women with gestational diabetes

Work with the patient, her partner, her family, and other health care providers to improve the patient's nutrition, exercise program, and blood glucose control.

Explain the risks of adverse perinatal outcomes and the need for fetal surveillance.

Inform patients that they are at increased risk both for developing gestational diabetes during future pregnancies and for developing overt diabetes later in life.

Encourage physical activity and postpartum weight loss to decrease the likelihood of developing diabetes later in life.

Recommend a postpartum evaluation at 6 to 8 weeks and annually thereafter for detecting the development of diabetes.

For women with a history of gestational diabetes

Recommend screening for overt diabetes before subsequent pregnancies.

Recommend early screening for the onset of carbohydrate intolerance during subsequent pregnancies.

Department of Health and Human Services Public Health Service: Prevention and treatment of complications of diabetes: a guide for primary care practitioners, Atlanta, 1991, Centers for Disease Control, Center for Chronic Disease Prevention and Health Promotion, Division of Diabetes Translation

Gestational Diabetes and Pregnancy: Conclusion

The importance of patient education for all women with gestational diabetes, as well as those with a positive history of risk for gestational diabetes, is imperative (see accompanying box). The diabetes health care team is crucial to a positive outcome for both the woman with diabetes and her child. As has been previously addressed, close monitoring before conception, as well as during and after pregnancy, is related to optimal outcomes for mother and child. Patient education principles that guide the health care team in caring for the woman with gestational diabetes need to be carefully administered. Careful documentation of care is also necessary with follow-up and progress comprehensively recorded.

REFERENCES

1. American Diabetes Association Workshop-Conference on Gestational Diabetes: Summary and recommendations, Diabetes Care 3:499-501, 1980.
2. American College of Obstetricians and Gynecologists (ACOG): Technical bulletin: exercise during pregnancy and the postnatal period, Washington, DC, 1985, American College of Obstetricians and Gynecologists.
3. Angel J and others: Carbohydrate intolerance in patients receiving oral tocolytics, Am J Obstet Gynecol 159:762, 1988.
4. Bantle JP and others: Rotation of the anatomic regions used for insulin injections and day-to-day variability of plasma glucose in type I diabetes, JAMA 263:1802, 1990.
5. Barreau P and Buttery J: The effect of the haematocrit value on the determination of glucose levels by reagent strip methods, Med J Aust 147:286, 1987.

6. Battaglia FC and Meschia G: Principal substrates of fetal metabolism, Physiol Rev 58:499, 1978.
7. Beard A and others: Neonatal hypoglycemia: a discussion, J Pediatr 79:314, 1971.
8. Board PJ and others: Gestational diabetes: definition, diagnosis and treatment strategies, Pract Diabetol 5:1, 1986.
9. Broughton-Pipkin F, Symonels E, and Turner S: The effect of captopril on the mother and fetus in the chronically cannulated ewe and pregnant rabbit, J Physiol 323:415, 1982.
10. Carrington ER, Shuman CR, and Reardon H: Evaluation of the prediabetic state during pregnancy, Obstet Gynecol 9:664, 1957.
11. Coetzee EJ and Jackson WPU: Metformin in management of pregnant insulin-dependent diabetics, Diabetologia 16:241, 1979.
12. Committee on Dietary Allowances, Food and Nutrition Board, National Academy of Sciences: Recommended dietary allowances, ed 9, Washington, DC, 1980, US Government Printing Office.
13. Corwin RS: Pregnancy complicated by diabetes mellitus in private practice: a review of ten years, Am J Obstet Gynecol 134:156, 1979.
14. Costrini NV and Kalkhoff RK: Relative effects of pregnancy, estradiol, and progesterone on plasma insulin and pancreatic islet insulin secretion, J Clin Invest 50:992, 1971.
15. Cousins L and others: Glycosylated hemoglobin as a screening test for carbohydrate intolerance in pregnancy, Am J Obstet Gynecol 150:455, 1984.
16. Cousins L: Pregnancy complications among diabetic women: review 1965-1985, Obstet Gynecol Surv 42:140, 1987.
17. Cousins L and Jacoby J: Infant and maternal outcomes in gestational diabetes mellitus: a prospective control study, Diabetes 36 (suppl 1):818A, 1987.
18. Coustan D, Berkowitz RL, and Hobbins JC: Tight metabolic control of overt diabetes in pregnancy, Am J Med 68:845, 1980.
19. Coustan D and Imarah J: Prophylactic insulin treatment of gestational diabetes reduces the incidence of macrosomia, operative delivery, and birth trauma, Am J Obstet Gynecol 150:836-842, 1984.
20. Coustan D and others: A randomized clinical trial of the insulin pump vs. intensive conventional therapy in diabetic pregnancies, JAMA 255:631, 1986.
21. Coustan D: Delivery timing, mode, and management. In Reece E and Coustan D, ed: Diabetes mellitus in pregnancy: principles and practice, New York, 1988, Churchill Livingstone.
22. Coustan D: Management of gestational diabetes. In Reece E and Coustan D, eds: Diabetes mellitus in pregnancy principles and practices, New York, 1988, Churchill Livingstone.
23. Coustan D: Obstetrical complications. In Reece E and Coustan D, eds: Diabetes mellitis in pregnancy: practices and principles, New York, 1988, Churchill Livingstone.
24. Davin JP, Jr: Screening of high-risk and general populations for gestational diabetes: clinical application and cost analysis, Diabetes 34(suppl 2):24, 1985.
25. Dooley S and others: Urinary estriols in diabetic pregnancy: a reappraisal, Obstet Gynecol 64:469, 1984.
26. Drury MI, Greene AT, and Strong JM: Pregnancy complicated by clinical diabetes mellitus: A study of 600 pregnancies, Obstet Gynecol 49:519, 1977.
27. Durin J: Energy requirements of pregnancy: an integration of the longitudinal data from the five-county study, Lancet 2:1131, 1987.
28. Dwyer PL and others: Glucose tolerance in twin pregnancy. Aust/New Z J Obstet Gynecol 22:131, 1982.
29. Enzi G and others: Development of adipose tissue in newborns of gestational-diabetic and insulin-dependent diabetic mothers, Diabetes 29:100, 1980.
30. Enzi G and others: Postnatal development of adipose tissue in normal children on strictly controlled calorie intake, Metabolism 31:1029, 1982.
31. Espinosa de los Monteros AM and others: Periprandial blood glucose and insulin values during the third trimester of normal pregnancies, Diabetes Care 7:180, 1984.
32. Fadel H and Hammond S: Diabetes mellitus and pregnancy: management and results, J Reprod Med 27:56, 1982.
33. Felig P and Lynch V: starvation in human pregnancy: hypoglycemia, hypoinsulinemia, and hyperketonemia, Science 170:990, 1970.
34. Felig P: Body fuel metabolism and diabetes mellitus in pregnancy, Med Clin North Am 66:43, 1977.
35. Felig P and Coustan D: Diabetes mellitus. In Burnow A and Ferris T, eds: Complications of pregnancy, ed 2, Philadelphia, 1982, WB Saunders.

36. Fisher PM, Sutherland HW, and Bewsher PD: Insulin response to glucose infusion in normal human pregnancy, Diabetologia 19:15, 1980.

37. Freeman RK, Anderson G, and Dorchester W: A prospective multi-institutional study of antepartum fetal heart rate monitoring. I. Risk of perinatal mortality and morbidity according to antepartum fetal heart rate test results, Am J Obstet Gynecol 143:771, 1982.

38. Freeman RK, Anderson G, and Dorchester W: A prospective multi-institutional study of antepartum fetal heart rate monitoring. II. Contraction stress test versus nonstress test for primary surveillance, Am J Obstet Gynecol 143:778, 1982.

39. Freinkel N: Of pregnancy and progeny, Diabetes 29:1023, 1980.

40. Freinkel N, and others: Gestational diabetes mellitus: heterogeneity of maternal age, weight, insulin secretion, HLA antigens and islet cell antibodies and the impact of maternal metabolism on pancreatic beta-cell and somatic development in the offspring, Diabetes 34(suppl 2):1, 1985.

41. Gabbe SG and others: Management and outcome of class A diabetes mellitus, Am J Obstet Gynecol 127:465, 1977.

42. Gabbe SG and others: Management and outcome of pregnancy in diabetes mellitus, classes B to R, Am J Obstet Gynecol 129:723, 1977.

43. Gabbe SG: Medical complications of pregnancy. Management of diabetes in pregnancy: six decades of experience. In Pitkin RM and Zlatnik FJ, eds: Yearbook of obstetrics and gynecology. Part I: Obstetrics, Chicago, 1980, Yearbook Medical Publishers.

44. Gabbe S, Mestman J, and Hibbord L: Maternal mortality in diabetes mellitus: an 18-year survey, Obstet Gynecol 48:549, 1986.

45. Gant NF and others: The metabolic clearance rate of dehydroisoandrosterone sulfate. III. The effect of thiazide diuretics in normal and future preeclamptic pregnancies, Am J Obstet Gynecol 123:159, 1975.

46. Gillis S and Hisa D: The infant of the diabetic mother, J Doctor Child 97:1, 1959.

47. Ginsberg-Fellner F and others: Islet cell antibodies in gestational diabetes, Lancet 2:362, 1980.

48. Ginsberg-Fellner F and others: HLA antigens, cytoplasmic islet cell antibodies, and carbohydrate tolerance in families of children with insulin-dependent diabetes mellitus, Diabetes 31:292, 1982.

49. Golde SH and others: Insulin requirements during labor: a reappraisal, 144:556, 1982.

50. Golde SH and others: The role of nonstress tests, fetal biophysical profile and contraction stress tests in the outpatient management of insulin-requiring diabetic pregnancies, Am J Obstet Gynecol 148:269, 1984.

51. Gyves MT and others: A modern approach to management of pregnant diabetics: a 2-year analysis of perinatal outcome, Am J Obstet Gynecol 128:606, 1977.

52. Hadden DR and others: Physical and psychological health of children of type I (insulin-dependent) diabetic mothers, Diabetologia 26:250, 1984.

53. Hanson U, Persson B, and Thowell S: Relationship between haemoglobin A_{1C} in early type 1 (insulin-dependent) diabetic pregnancy and the occurrence of spontaneous abortion and fetal malformation in Sweden, Diabetologia 33:94, 1990.

54. Haworth JC, McRae KN, and Dilling LA: Prognosis of infants of diabetic mothers in relation to neonatal hypoglycaemia, Dev Med Child Neurol 18:471, 1976.

55. Hollander P and others: Optimal therapy for improved outcome in gestational diabetes, Diabetologia 30:224A(suppl 1), 1987.

56. Hollander P and others: Insulin therapy and improved outcome in gestational diabetes, Diabetes 37(suppl 1):261A, 1988.

57. Jackson WV: Studies in prediabetes, Brit Med J 2:690, 1952.

58. Javier Z, Gershberg H, and Hulse M: Ovulatory suppressants, estrogens, and carbohydrate metabolism, Metabolism 17:443, 1968.

59. Jervell J and others: Diabetes mellitus and pregnancy: management and results at Rikshopitalet Oslo 1970-1977, Diabetologia 16:151, 1979.

60. Joslin EP and others: The treatment of diabetes mellitus, ed 8, Philadelphia, 1948, Lea & Febiger.

61. Jovanovic L and Peterson CM: Management of the pregnant, insulin-dependent diabetic woman, Diabetes Care 3:63, 1980.

62. Jovanovic L, Douzin M, and Peterson C: Effect of euglycemia on the outcome of pregnancy in insulin dependent diabetic women as compared to normal control subjects, Am J Med 71:921, 1981.

63. Jovanovic L and Peterson CM: Optimal insulin delivery for the pregnant diabetic patient, Diabetes Care 5:24, 1982.

64. Jovanovic L and Peterson CM: Insulin and glucose requirements during the first stage of labor in insulin-dependent diabetic women, Am J Med 75:607, 1983.

65. Jovanovic-Peterson L and Peterson CM: Screening for gestational diabetes with solid-phase reagent strips, Diabetes Professional pp 5, 20, 1988.

66. Kalkhoff RK, Jacobson M, and Lemper D: Progesterone, pregnancy and the augmented plasma insulin response, J Clin Endocrinol 31:24, 1970.

67. Karlsson K and Kjellmer I: The outcome of diabetic pregnancies in relation to the mother's blood sugar level, Am J Obstet Gynecol 112:213, 1972.

68. Kitzmiller J and others: Diabetic pregnancy and perinatal morbidity, Am J Obstet Gynecol 131:560, 1978.

69. Kitzmiller JL and others: Diabetic nephropathy and perinatal outcome, Am J Obstet Gynecol 141:741, 1981.

70. Kitzmiller J and others: Preconception care of diabetes, glycemia control prevents congenital anomalies, JAMA 265:731-736, 1991.

71. Klein B and Klein R: Gravidity and diabetic retinopathy, Am J Epidemiol 119:564, 1984.

72. Klein B, Moss S, and Klein R: Effect of pregnancy on progression of diabetic retinopathy, Diabetes Care 13:17-22, 1990.

73. Landon MB and Gabbe SG: Antepartum fetal surveillance in gestational diabetes mellitus, Diabetes 34 (suppl 2): 50, 1985.

74. Landon MR and Cembrowski GS: Capillary blood glucose screening for gestational diabetes: a preliminary investigation, Am J Obstet Gynecol 155:717, 1986.

75. Langer O and Mazze RS: Diabetes in pregnancy: evaluation self-monitoring performance and glycemic control with memory-based reflectance meters, Am J Obstet Gynecol 155:635, 1986.

76. Langer O and others: Gestational diabetes: insulin requirements in pregnancy, Am J Obstet Gynecol 157:669, 1987.

77. Langer O and others: The significance of one abnormal glucose tolerance test value on adverse outcome in pregnancy, Am J Obstet Gynecol 157:758, 1987.

78. Like A and Orci L: Embryogenesis of the human pancreatic islets: a light and electron microscopic study, Diabetes 21:511, 1972.

79. Lufkin G and others: An analysis of diabetic pregnancies at Mayo Clinic 1950-79, Diabetes Care 7:539, 1984.

80. Malins JM and others: Sulphonylurea drugs in pregnancy, Br Med J 3:187, 1964.

81. Martin T, Allen A, and Stinson D: Overt diabetes in pregnancy, Am J Obstet Gynecol 133:275, 1979.

82. Mazze R and others: Reliability of blood glucose monitoring by patients with diabetes mellitus, Am J Med 77:212, 1984.

83. Menon RK and others: Transplacental passage of insulin in pregnant women with insulin-dependent diabetes mellitus; its role in fetal macrosomia, N Engl J Med 321:15, 1990.

84. Metzger B and others: Gestational diabetes mellitus: correlations between the phenotypic and genotypic characteristics of the mother and abnormal glucose tolerance during the first year postpartum, Diabetes 34(suppl 2);111, 1985.

85. Meuller-Beubach E and others: Lecithin/sphingomyelin ratio in amniotic fluid and its value for the prediction of neonatal respiratory distress syndrome in pregnant diabetic women, Am J Obstet Gynecol 130:25, 1978.

86. Miller E and others: Elevated maternal hemoglobin A in early pregnancy and major congenital anomalies in infants of diabetic mothers, N Engl J Med 304:1331, 1981.

87. Mills J and others: Lack of relation of increased malformation rates in infants of diabetic mothers to glycemic control during organogenesis. National Institute of Child Health and Human Development Diabetes in Early Pregnancy Study, N Engl J Med 318:671, 1988. 88

88. National Diabetes Data Group. Diabetes 28:1039, 1979.

89. National Research Council: Recommended dietary allowances, Washington, DC, 1989, National Academy Press.

90. O'Sullivan JB and Mahan CM: Criteria for the oral glucose tolerance test in pregnancy, Diabetes 13:278, 1964.

91. O'Sullivan JB and others: Gestational diabetes and perinatal mortality role, Am J Obstet Gynecol 116 901, 1973.

92. O'Sullivan JB: Long-term follow-up of gestational diabetes. In Camerini-Davolos RA and Cole HS eds: Early diabetes in early life, Orlando, FL, 1975, Academic Press.

93. O'Sullivan JB: Gestational diabetes: factors influencing rates of subsequent diabetes. In Sutherland HW and Stowers JM eds: Carbohydrate metabolism in pregnancy and the newborn, New York, 1978, Springer-Verlag.

94. O'Sullivan JB: Body weight and subsequent diabetes mellitus, JAMA 248:949, 1982.

95. O'Sullivan JB: Subsequent morbidity among gestational diabetic women. In Sutherland HW and Stowers JM eds: Carbohydrate metabolism in pregnancy and the newborn, Edinburgh, 1984, Churchill Livingstone.

96. Papaspyros NS: The history of diabetes mellitus, ed 1, Stuttgart, 1952, Thieme.

97. Pederson J: The pregnant diabetic and her newborn, Baltimore, 1977, Williams & Wilkins.

98. Personal communication.

99. Persson B and Gentz J: Follow-up of children of insulin-dependent and gestational diabetic mothers, Acta Paediatr Scand 73:349, 1984.

100. Pettitt D and others: Excessive obesity in offspring of Pima Indian women with diabetes during pregnancy, N Engl J Med 308:242, 1983.

101. Pettitt D and others: Congenital susceptibility for development of NIDDM, Diabetes 37:622, 1988

102. Proceedings of the Second International Workshop-Conference on Gestational Diabetes Mellitus, 1984, Chicago, Diabetes 34(suppl 2):1-30, 1985.

103. Rednon C: Treatment of hypertension in pregnancy, Kidney Int 18:267, 1980.

104. Reece EA and Robbins JC: Diabetic embryopathy pathogensis prenatal diagnosis and prevention, Obstet Gynecol Surv, 41:325, 1986.

105. Reece EA and others: Diabetic nephropathy: pregnancy performance and fetomaternal outcome, Am J Obstet Gynecol 159:66, 1988.

106. Rigg L and Petrie R: Fetal biochemical and biophysical assessment. In Reece E and Coustan D eds: Diabetes mellitus in pregnancy: principles and practices, New York, 1988, Churchill Livingstone.

107. Roberts AB and others: Fructosamine estimation, a possible screening test for diabetes mellitus, Br Med J 287:863, 1983.

108. Rovergi GD and others: A new approach to the treatment of diabetic pregnant women, Am J Obstet Gynecol 135:567, 1979.

109. Sabata V, Wolf H, and Lausmann S: The role of fatty acids, glycerol, ketone bodies and glucose in the energy metabolism of the mother and fetus during delivery, Biol Neonate 13:7, 1968.

110. Sadler TS: Effects of maternal diabetes on early embryogenesis. I. The teratogenic potential of diabetic serum, Teratology 21:339, 1980.

111. Silfen SL, Wapner RJ, and Gabbe SG: Maternal outcome in class H diabetes mellitus, Obstet Gynecol 55:749, 1980.

112. Soler NG, Nicholson HO, and Malins JM: Serial determinations of human placental lactogen in the last half of normal and complicated pregnancies, Am J Obstet Gynecol 120:214, 1974.

113. Soler N, Soler S, and Malins J: Neonatal morbidity among infants of diabetic mothers, Diabetes Care 1:340, 1978.

114. Soubrane G, Conivet S, and Coscas G: Influence of pregnancy on the evolution of background retinopathy, Int Ophthalmol Clin 8:249, 1985.

115. Spellacy WN and Goetz FC: Plasma insulin in normal late pregnancy, N Engl J Med 268:988, 1963.

116. Steel SM and others: Can pregnancy care of diabetic women reduce the risk of abnormal babies, Br Med J 301:1070-1074, 1990.

117. Stephens JW, Page OC, and Hare RL: Diabetes and pregnancy: a report of experiences in 119 pregnancies over a period of ten years, Diabetes 12:213, 1963.

118. Stowers JM, Sutherland HW, and Kerridege DF: Long-range implications for the mother: the Aberdeen experience, Diabetes 34(suppl 2):106, 1985.

119. Subcommittee on Nutritional Status and Weight Gain During Pregnancy, Food and Nutrition Board, National Academy of Sciences: Nutrition during pregnancy, Washington, DC, 1990, National Academy Press.

120. Susa J and others: Chronic hyperinsulinemia in the fetal rhesus monkey, Diabetes 28:1058, 1979.

121. Tallarigo L and others: Relation of glucose tolerance to complications of pregnancy in nondiabetic women, N Engl J Med 315:989-992, 1986.

122. Tattersal R and Pyke D: Diabetes in identical twins, Lancet 2:1120, 1972.

123. Taylor P and others: Hyperbilirubinemia in infants of diabetic mothers, Biol Neonate 5:289, 1963.

124. The DCCT research: Diabetes control and complications trial. Results of the feasibility study, Diabetes Care 10:1, 1987.
125. The Kroc collaborative study: Blood glucose control and the evolution of diabetic retinopathy and albuminuria, N Engl J Med 311:372, 1984.
126. Troug AI and others: Pregnancy and diabetes: the improving progress, Ulster Med J 52:118, 1983.
127. Tyron F: Medical aspects of diabetes in pregnancy and the diabetogenic effects of oral contraceptives, Med Clin North Am 55:947, 1971.
128. Ulmsten U: Treatment of normotensive and hypertensive patients with labor using oral nifedipine, a calcium antagonist, Arch Gynecol 236:69, 1984.
129. Walker J and others: Antihypertensive therapy in pregnancy, Lancet 1:932, 1983.
130. Warran JH and others: Differences in risk of insulin-dependent diabetes in offspring of diabetic mothers and diabetic fathers, N Engl J Med 311:149, 1984.
131. Widness JA and others: Neonatal morbidities in infants of mothers with glucose intolerance in pregnancy, Diabetes 34(suppl 2):61, 1985.
132. White P: Childhood diabetes: its course and influence on the second and third generations, Diabetes 9:345, 1960.
133. White P: Pregnancy and diabetes. In Marble A and others, eds: Joslin diabetes mellitus, ed 12, Philadelphia, 1988, Lea & Febiger.

PART TWO

DIABETES MANAGEMENT ACROSS THE LIFE SPAN

CHAPTER **10**

Social Contexts of Management: Family and Community Environments

WENDY AUSLANDER

Consideration of the social context of the individual is critical for successful coping and management of diabetes. In the next five chapters, the impact of diabetes will be described as it interacts with the unique developmental and psychosocial milestones of each stage of the life cycle. Yet, it is important to view these developmental influences within a *social-environmental context*. This chapter provides an overview of several theoretic frameworks that have been used to examine the social context of diabetes management. Diabetes management and regimen-related behaviors are influenced not only by intra-individual factors but also by the system that surrounds the individual. The biopsychosocial model has emerged as a paradigm that has replaced the traditional biomedical model, and maintains that disease and behavior is a function of the interaction of biological, psychosocial, developmental, sociocultural, and ecologic factors.[14] The model is broadly based on the general systems approach that proposes that there are bidirectional influences between a person and his environment, and multiple factors that interact to influence health and disease. The biopsychosocial or systems model has provided several theoretic perspectives that have been used to study the interaction among disease, family, and community environments of individuals with diabetes.

THE FAMILY CONTEXT

The family is the most frequently mentioned social context in the psychosocial literature in diabetes. While many studies have examined the associations between family and disease factors, it is generally accepted that there are bidirectional influences among family, disease, and regimen-related factors.[1] One of the first theoretic perspectives to link family interactional patterns with the health status of diabetic children was Minuchin's structural family systems perspective in his work with "psychosomatic families." Specifically, Minuchin and colleagues[30] formulated the view that four family characteristics—enmeshment, overprotectiveness, extreme rigidity, and lack of conflict resolution—are necessary for the development of "psychosomatic diabetes" in children. Although it is important to note that less than 5% of diabetic children are considered "psychosomatic" (i.e., containing all of the above-mentioned characteristics accompanied by metabolic instability),[31] the work of Minuchin and colleagues triggered a wealth of research that examined the associations between family system variables and metabolic control.

Several consistent findings across studies have emerged relating to family interactions and metabolic control in children and adolescents with insulin-dependent diabetes mellitus (IDDM). Anderson and associates [3] found that high levels of cohesion and independence and low levels of conflict were significantly associated with better metabolic control. Evidence of the association between family cohesion and children's metabolic control was provided by other studies.[5,19,24] Family conflict has also been shown to relate to the children's metabolic control, with higher levels associated with poorer control.[5,24,35] Other studies have focused on family behaviors or factors that support adherence to the treatment regimen. For example, nonsupportive family behaviors were associated with poorer adherence to glucose testing, diet, and insulin injections among diabetic adults.[34] Among children with diabetes, patterns of sharing diabetes-related responsibilities between mothers and children were related to metabolic control. Disagreements between mothers and children about who is assuming responsibility for regimen tasks were significantly associated with poorer metabolic control.[2] These findings provide evidence for the strong linkage among the family context of the diabetic individual, adherence behaviors, and metabolic control.

A second theoretic perspective that has guided research of family factors and diabetes is the Family Adaptation and Adjustment Response or Double ABCX Model formulated by McCubbin and colleagues.[29] Briefly, this is a supply-demand model that examines the interaction of family stressors (demands) and resources (coping skills, extended family support, finances, and family strengths) to determine the degree to which a family adapts to the crisis of diagnosis.

In recent research,[7] this perspective was utilized to study family coping with the crisis of diagnosis of diabetes. Assessments were performed one year after diagnosis. Family stressors were found to be the strongest predictor of the children's control, when controlling for C peptide levels and family resources.[7] These data indicate that family variables such as stress are more strongly associated with metabolic control than the child's level of endogenous insulin after the first year following diagnosis. This is an important finding given other research (e.g., Kovacs and colleagues[26]) that challenges the influence of family variables as influences to the health status of diabetic children. Results from other investigations that include measures of family stress, coping, and levels of metabolic control have been contradictory. Several studies of diabetic children have found stressful family life events to be significantly associated with poor metabolic control.[8,11,18] In contrast, others have found no significant relationship between frequency or severity of stress and metabolic control.[10,13] Inconsistent findings across studies are probably a result of differences in the patient populations, in instruments used to measure stress and coping, and whether a family or individual perspective is examined. In addition, as McCubbin's model points out, the impact of chronic stress on individuals and families with diabetes varies according to the resources available to buffer the impact and the definition or perception that the individual or family attributes to the stressor.[28] Certainly family stress, family resources, and the family's perception of these two factors are potential areas for intervention with diabetic individuals.

Although it is acknowledged that the developmental stage of the individual with diabetes is an important variable in the education and medical management of the disease, less attention has been given to the different phases of an illness (i.e., crisis phase, chronic phase, and terminal phase[32]) and how this affects the educational and psychosocial needs of diabetic patients and their families. This is related in part to the difficulty that researchers experience in conducting longitudinal studies, in addition to the fact that health professionals rarely follow a chronically ill patient throughout the "illness life cycle." Yet, the time phase of an illness is an important dimension in diagnosing the educational and psychosocial needs of the patient with diabetes and the family.

Several family-based studies of children with IDDM have acknowledged that the phase following diagnosis may be unique in terms of the needs of diabetic families and thus have focused on recently or newly diagnosed children and adolescents with diabetes and their families. One study examined the predictors of the acquisition of diabetes knowledge within the year following diagnosis in children and adolescents with diabetes and their parents.[6] Problem-solving knowledge relating to disease management was poorer than general knowledge in both parents and children. Both demographic (age, family, socioeconomic status [SES]) and family variables (family communication skills, financial resources) were predictive of general information and problem-solving knowledge, suggesting that family factors should be considered in the education of newly diagnosed children and families.

Another investigation of newly or recently diagnosed children and families found that coping with the diagnosis and early impact of diabetes lasts up to 9 months for most children and that psychiatrically diagnosable reactions were more likely among children of lower SES families, and from families with marital distress.[25] Other studies of recently diagnosed children and families examined predictors of compliance[23] and family environmental characteristics of diabetic versus acutely ill adolescents.[20]

Research that has taken into account the illness phase has primarily focused on newly or recently diagnosed individuals and their families. The interest in newly diagnosed families is based on the premise that if health care professionals intervene immediately following diagnosis, new patterns of cooperation and interaction can be learned that would facilitate the successful integration of the treatment regimen into daily routines. In doing so, the prevention of psychosocial and management problems could be attained.

Because most health professionals rarely work with only newly diagnosed patients and their families, more information is needed regarding the family reactions, needs, and types of coping with diabetes at other phases of the illness. Diabetes is a disease that is characterized by "predictable crises" or predictable complications in the course of the disease.[16] Health professionals with their expertise in knowing this course can prepare families how to anticipate, prepare, and cope with diabetes-related complications at each phase of the disease.

THE COMMUNITY CONTEXT

Health education and promotion has primarily focused on facilitating behavior change through interventions that target the individual rather than the environment. However, within the biopsychosocial framework, health behaviors are a function of the interaction of both intraindividual and environmental factors. The community is the environmental context of individuals who share similar values and institutions. Community components include ethnocultural and socioeconomic characteristics of groups of people.

The African American and Native American communities recently have received considerable attention in epidemiologic reports because of the increased prevalence of diabetes in these populations. Subsequently, health professionals have increased their attention to racial, ethnic, and cultural factors in the education and disease management of individuals with diabetes. According to the National Diabetes Data Group,[33] the rate of non–insulin-dependent diabetes mellitus (NIDDM) in African Americans is 50% to 60% higher than that in Caucasians. The rate of diabetes among African American women is alarming—1 in 4 black women over 55 years has diabetes.[33] Among Native Americans the diabetes-related mortality rates are 2.3 times higher those in the general population. The prevalence rate of NIDDM for the Pima Indians is the highest in the world—10 to 15 times the rate for the general U.S. population.[21] African Americans and Native Americans incur higher rates of three complications of diabetes: end-stage renal disease, blindness, and amputation.[21]

The disparity in the health status between minority and nonminority populations has also been noted in pediatric populations with IDDM. In one study of recently diagnosed children and adolescents,[5] youths from African and/or single-parent families were in significantly poorer metabolic control than were children from Caucasian and two-parent families when controlling for family factors and socioeconomic levels. Moreover, this pattern persisted 2 and 3 years after diagnosis. Likewise, a study comparing African American and Caucasian children with IDDM revealed that African American children were in poorer metabolic control, were hospitalized more frequently for diabetic ketoacidosis, and missed more clinic visits than did their Caucasian counterparts.[12] A third study by Hanson, Henggeler, and Burghen[17] found that adolescent African American females were in poorer metabolic control than were their white male adolescent counterparts.

What are the factors that contribute to the poorer health status of minority populations? Lower SES levels among minority families explain part of the effects of race on the diabetic individual's metabolic control, since fewer financial and educational resources are associated with lower quality of medical services and less emphasis on preventive care.[4,15] However, in many of the above-mentioned studies, the difference in metabolic control between African Americans and whites was not explained only by SES levels. Physiologic factors such as increased frequency of hyperlipidemia among African Americans may be related to poor metabolic control.[17] Likewise, there is reason to believe that minority populations experience more stress than nonminorities through interactions with a racist climate that denies personal values, identity, and economic opportunities.[27] Moreover, cultural barriers to effective communication and treatment planning between minority patients and health care providers may also contribute to the disparity in health status between minority and nonminority populations. For example, in a study of low income, predominantly African American older adults with NIDDM, diet was reported as the most problematic aspect of the regimen.[22] The authors suggest that this may in part be related to the lack of sensitivity to social and cultural factors in the assessment and prescription of the dietary component of the treatment regimen.

Although the reduction of risk factors (e.g., obesity, smoking) among minorities continues to be a priority as recommended by the Secretary's Task Force on Black and Minority Health,[21] there is an increased awareness that an effective strategy to accomplish this goal is through already established minority community networks. Community organization is a strategy that is being utilized to promote health through citizen participation and ownership in the defining, planning, and implementing of disease prevention programs.[9] Several community-based programs have been implemented in African American communities to reduce smoking as a rick factor to cardiovascular disease, such as *Richmond Quits* in the San Francisco Bay area and *Neighbors for a Smoke-Free Northside,* located in North St. Louis. Key principles previously outlined by Bracht and Kingbury[9] were critical in the *Neighbors* program: facilitating community ownership of the program by integrating community values and norms into educational messages and materials, and integrating the intervention activities into already existing networks. Implicit in this approach is the strategy of "empowerment"—to provide the neighbors with opportunities for increased mastery and control over their circumstances. Community organization as a strategy to prevent diabetes and its complications is an approach that has not been utilized in a systematic or comprehensive manner but may prove to be an effective strategy in minority and low-income communities in which more traditional methods have failed.

The biopsychosocial approach to diabetes management involved the interaction of persons with their environment. Health professionals are traditionally trained in the biomedical model that emphasizes individual influences to diabetes management: physiologic, physical, and developmental factors. Of equal importance are the social contexts in which diabetic individuals live, primarily because of the influence that environment has on human behavior, particularly health preventive and management behaviors. Two social contexts—the family, and the community—have considerable impact on individuals with diabetes throughout their lives. Consideration of the social context is critical in the design and implementation of interventions with these individuals. Ideally, interventions should also be focused to change the environment or the system in which health care behaviors occur so that individual change is supported and reinforced by the norms of the social context.

REFERENCES

1. Anderson BJ and Auslander WF: Research on diabetes management and the family: a critique, Diabetes Care 3:696-702, 1990.
2. Anderson BJ and others: Assessing family sharing of diabetes responsibilities, Pediatr Psychol 15:477-492, 1990.
3. Anderson BJ and others: Family characteristics of diabetic adolescents: relationship to metabolic control Diabetes Care 4:586-594, 1981.
4. Angel R and Worobey JL: Single motherhood and children's health, J Health Social Behav 29:38-52, 1988.
5. Auslander WF and others: Risk factors to health in diabetic children: a prospective study from diagnosis, Health Social Work 15:133-142, 1990.
6. Auslander WF and others: Predictors of diabetes knowledge in newly diagnosed children and parents, J Pediatr Psychol 16:213-228, 1991.
7. Auslander WF, Rogge M, and Jung K: Family resources and stress: areas of intervention to improve management in IDDM, Diabetes 37(suppl 1):19A, 1988.
8. Barglow P and others: Diabetic control in children and adolescents: psychosocial factors and therapeutic efficacy, J Youth Adolesc 12:77-94, 1983.
9. Bracht N and Kingsbury L: Community organization principles in health promotion. In Bracht N, ed: Health promotion at the community level, Newbury Park, CA, 1990, Sage.
10. Brand AH, Johnson JH, and Johnson SB: Life stress and diabetic control in children and adolescents with insulin-dependent diabetes, J Pediatr Psychol 11:481-495, 1986.
11. Chase HP and Jackson GG: Stress and sugar control in children with insulin dependent diabetes mellitus, J Pediatr 98:1011-1013, 1981.
12. Delamater AM and others: Racial differences in metabolic control of children and adolescents with Type I diabetes mellitus, Diabetes Care 14:20-25, 1991.
13. Delamater AM and others: Stress and coping in relation to metabolic control of adolescents with type I diabetes, Development Behav Pediatr 8:136-140, 1987.
14. Engel GH: The need for a new medical model: a challenge for biomedicine, Science 196:129-136, 1977.
15. Guendelman S: At risk: health needs of Hispanic children, Health Social Work 10:183-190, 1985.
16. Hamburg BA and Inoff GE: Coping with predictable crises of diabetes, Diabetes Care 6:409-416, 1979.
17. Hanson CL, Henggeler SW, and Burgen GA: Race and sex differences in metabolic control of adolescents with IDDM: a function of psychosocial variables, Diabetes Care 10:313-318, 1987.
18. Hanson CL, Henggeler SW, and Burghen GA: Social competence and parental support as mediators of the link between stress and metabolic control in adolescents with insulin dependent diabetes mellitus, J Consult Clin Psychol 55:529-633, 1987.
19. Hanson CL and others: Family system variables and the health status of adolescents with insulin-dependent diabetes mellitus, Health Psychol 8:239-254, 1989.
20. Hauser ST and others: The contribution of family environment to perceived competence and illness adjustment in diabetic and acutely ill adolescents, Fam Relations 34:99-108, 1985.
21. Heckler MM: Report of the Secretary's Task Force on Black and Minority Health, 1985, Executive Summary, Washington DC, 1985, US Government Printing Office.
22. Hopper SV and Schechtman KB: Factors associated with diabetic control and utilization patterns in a low-income, older adult population, Patient Educ Counsel 7:275-288, 1985.
23. Jacobson AM and others: Psychologic predictors of compliance in children with recent onset of diabetes mellitus, J Pediatr 110:805-811, 1987.
24. Klemp SB: Adolescents with IDDM: the role of family cohesion and conflict, Diabetes 36(suppl 1):18A, 1987.
25. Kovacs M and others: Initial coping responses and psychosocial characteristics of children with insulin-dependent diabetes mellitus, J Pediatr 106:827-834, 1985.
26. Kovacs M and others: Family functioning and metabolic control of school-aged children with insulin-dependent diabetes mellitus, Diabetes Care 12:409-414, 1989.
27. McAdoo HP: Societal stress: the black family. In McCubbin HI and Figley CR, eds: Coping with normative transitions, New York, 1983, Brunner/Mazel.
28. McCubbin HI and Patterson JM: Family adaptation to crisis. In McCubbin HI, Cauble E, and Patterson JM, eds: Family stress, coping, and social support, Springfield, IL, 1982, Charles C Thomas.

29. McCubbin HI and Patterson JM: The family stress process: The double ABCX model of adjustment and adaption, Marriage Fam Rev 6:7-37, 1982.
30. Minuchin S and others: A conceptual model of psychosomatic illness in children, Arch Gen Psychiatr 32:1031-1038, 1975.
31. Minuchin S, Rosman BL, and Baker L: Psychosomatic families, Cambridge, MA, 1978, Harvard University Press.
32. Rolland JS: Toward a psychosocial typology of chronic and life threatening illness, Fam Sys Med 2:245-263, 1984.
33. Roseman JM: Diabetes in Black Americans. In: Diabetes in America, NIH publ no 85-1468, Washington, DC, 1985, US Government Printing Office.
34. Schaefer LC, McCaul KD, and Glasgow RE: Supportive and nonsupportive family behaviors: relationships to adherence and metabolic control in persons with Type I diabetes, Diabetes Care 9:179-185, 1986.
35. White K and others: Unstable diabetes and unstable families: a psychosocial evaluation of diabetic children with recurrent ketoacidosis, Pediatrics 73:749-755, 1984.

CHAPTER 11

Diabetes Mellitus and the Preschool Child

BARBARA SCHREINER AND SHARON PONTIOUS

Diabetes occurring in childhood can be devastating to the child and to the parent. When that child is an infant or toddler, the impact can be even more pronounced. Yet diabetes in the very young can be managed effectively, both from a metabolic/physiologic standpoint and an emotional focus. The guiding principle seems to be a balance of "ideal" care and metabolic control with what is "realistic" or practical for this particularly vulnerable age group.

The diabetes health care team must work closely with the child and his or her family to develop optimal management strategies. In assessing and planning for the care of the infant or preschooler with diabetes, a knowledge of normal physical, cognitive, and social development is important. A necessary overall goal will be to nurture the "normal" developmental needs of the child less than 5 years old, while maintaining near normoglycemia.

By convention, and for our purposes, infants are children aged 2 to 12 months, toddlers are 1 to 3 years old, and preschool children are 3 to 5 years old.

This chapter, then, will address how these aspects of normal growth and development are affected by diabetes mellitus and its required care; common concerns that parents and siblings have in living with a young child with diabetes; practical applications of the diabetes meal plan for infants and toddlers; typical health concerns for the infant, toddler, and preschooler in terms of diabetes management; the role of blood glucose monitoring as a tool in making daily decisions about diabetes management; considerations in selecting and preparing a babysitter to safely care for the infant with diabetes; approaches to giving injections to young children; techniques helpful in approaching and communicating with a young child in the clinical setting; guidelines for managing hypoglycemia and sick days in the infant, toddler, or preschool child.

Normal Physical Development

Physical growth and development occur in several dimensions. Cephalocaudal development progresses from head to toe. For example, in neuromuscular development, the child gains head control (cephalo) before gaining the ability to walk (caudal). Another dimension of growth occurs from near to far, or proximodistal. The child develops, for instance, gross motor skills (large muscle) prior to fine motor control (small, distal muscles). Finally, growth and development moves from simple to more complex operations. The infant is able to crawl, but the older child is able to synchronize the complex actions of running.

In general, growth is predictable and orderly but it progresses at varying rates within the individual. New behaviors and growth patterns arise from existing ones, given a suitable environment and the proper timing. Such critical periods are dependent on the careful interplay of environment and biology. Brain development is dependent on a continuous supply of glucose, for example. While such critical periods are important for physiologic development, it appears that emotional or psychologic growth also requires an ideal or opportune time. Learning, for instance, occurs during optimal periods of development.

Skeletal growth

Growth rate in children is characterized by periods of acceleration, "spurts," occurring at different times but in similar sequences for healthy children.[43] By age 2, the child has achieved 50% of his or her adult height.[74] By age 3 years, the child is expected to be 3 feet tall. Linear growth is rapid in the first year of life, then slowly decelerates until puberty.[43] From 1 to 6 years, there is an average annual increase in height of 7.6 cm.[62]

Despite growth delays caused by disease or nutritional deprivation, catch-up growth is possible. Once an adequate diet or recovery from illness occurs, the child may experience a rapid acceleration in growth.[37] How much of lost linear growth can be recovered is determined by the timing, severity, and duration of the interruption.

Standardized growth charts provide a means of evaluating the progression of normal growth or the detection of changes in linear growth.[31] Clearly, sequential measurements are necessary in any evaluation of growth. Not only the rate of growth but also the pattern is assessed from a growth chart. Those children whose height falls under the fifth percentile or over the ninety-fifth percentile for age, or who demonstrate a loss of several percentiles on the growth chart, should have a growth assessment conducted. Such an evaluation should include physical assessment, previous history of illness, nutrition history, and family patterns of growth. Specialized growth charts allow for the parents' heights to be considered in assessing the child's growth potential.[70]

Physical growth is measured also by monitoring head circumference. At birth, the neonate's head circumference measures 34 to 35 cm. The infant's head may increase by 10 cm in the first year. By the end of infancy, growth in head circumference has slowed to 2 to 5 cm per year. By age 5 years, the child's head circumference is expected to increase less than 1.25 cm per year. Head circumference equals chest circumference by ages 1 to 2 years.

Neuromuscular development

In the infant, neuromuscular growth occurs rapidly and in a predictable sequence. The central nervous system develops rapidly, resulting in the infant's increasing ability to perform gross motor and fine motor tasks. From kicking and waving arms to reaching, rolling over and, finally, walking, the developing infant achieves milestones swiftly.

At birth, the human brain is 25% of its adult size. By the end of the first year of life, the brain has grown to two thirds its final size, and by the end of age 5, 90% of brain mass is present. Although brain growth is nearly complete by school age, there are critical times of especially rapid brain cell replication: at 15 to 20 weeks' gestation and from 30 weeks' gestation to the end of the first year of life. A growth spurt occurs first and fastest in the cerebellum, the site of coordination and balance. Later, growth predominates in the forebrain and stem. This nervous system development is dependent on a constant, unfailing supply of glucose as nerve cell replication and myelination progresses.[64,74]

Nerve cell myelination sheaths and protects neurons and allows impulses to travel more rapidly and accurately. Myelination follows a cephalocaudal direction, with the pathways for sensory nerves myelinating before motor pathways. Myelination in the spinal cord is nearly complete by age two years, allowing for the gross motor development in the toddler.

While the infant concentrates on large muscle development in rolling over and reaching, the toddler refines gross motor tasks and performs increasingly more sophisticated fine motor tasks. Toddlerhood is characterized by the child's ability to walk and run. Toddlers can hold writing tools and scribble.

The preschooler has even more refined large muscle control. This child is able to ride a bike and catch a ball. Fine motor skill is evident in the child's ability to button and unbutton clothing.[64]

Even vision is affected by the progression of muscular development. Binocular vision is established in the infant by 4 months old, with mature functioning of the ocular muscles by age 1 year. As the eye achieves a more adult shape, the child is able to focus both for near vision and for far vision.

Other system development

The child's gastrointestinal system is also in a state of rapid growth and change from infancy through young childhood. At birth, the infant's stomach is very small and empties relatively quickly (from 2 to 6 hours). In infancy, regurgitation is common because of an immature cardiac sphincter. Because of these anatomic characteristics, the young child requires small, frequent feedings.

Voluntary control of elimination occurs around ages 18 to 24 months, following central nervous system maturation. Children at these ages not only can detect a full bladder but can often control its emptying. Bowel control precedes bladder control, and daytime toilet training precedes nighttime control.

In addition to central nervous system (CNS) development, the infant is developing a more mature immune system. By birth, the neonate has received passive immunity to many viral and bacterial organisms through the transplacental transfer of maternal immunoglobulin G (IgG).[74] This maternal IgG is virtually the neonate's only protection against infection. By three months of age, maternal IgG is waning and the infant is actively producing his or her own immunoglobulin. By age 1 year, the child is producing about 40% of the adult levels of IgG.[75] Other immunoglobulins (A, D, and E) are produced more gradually, with maximum levels reached in early childhood. During this process, however, the infant and young child are prone to upper respiratory illnesses and common childhood diseases.

Dentition

The calcification of deciduous teeth begins in the seventh month of gestation. At term, calcification begins to occur in the permanent teeth. By 5 to 9 months of age, the first deciduous teeth erupt, beginning with the lower central incisors. Most 1-year-olds have 6 to 8 teeth, and by age 2 years most children have a full set of 20 deciduous teeth. By 6 to 7 years old, these primary teeth begin to fall out, initially with the lower central incisors.

Sleep and rest patterns

Sleep and rest in the young child progressively changes both in quantity and quality. Sleep occupies as much as 15 hours per day in the infant. The newborn infant is beginning to establish his or her biologic rhythms and by age 3 months demonstrates diurnal patterns of waking and sleeping. By 4 to 6 months, the child is often sleeping through the night. The 1- to 2-year-old child may be taking one to two naps per day, decreasing to one nap per day by age 3. Most 5-year-olds have virtually eliminated the daily nap.

Not only does the quantity of sleep change, but the quality or duration of REM sleep changes. REM sleep is characterized by rapid eye movements and increased brain activity as evidenced by brain wave patterns that are low in voltage and relatively fast.[2] In the neonate, 50% of sleep occurs in the REM state, while only 20% of sleep is REM for the older child.[69] REM sleep for the infant is a source of internal stimulation to higher brain centers. As the child increasingly interacts with the environment, less endogenous stimulation is necessary.

HEALTH CONCERNS FOR THE YOUNG CHILD
Physical Injuries and Accidents

Injuries and accidents are the leading cause of death in the young child. In the infant, falls, aspiration of small objects, poisoning, burns, and drowning contribute to mortality and morbidity. Many accidents in this age group result from the parent's lack of knowledge of normal child development. Knowing the general age when a child will roll over, reach for objects, and begin crawling are important to making his or her environment safe. For the infant, a safe environment includes an infant car seat, medications and household chemicals locked away, small objects and toys out of reach, and pacifiers, toys, and clothing that are well made, fire resistant, and appropriate for age.

The toddler's natural curiosity and unsteady gait make him or her a candidate for se-

Table 11-1   Recommended Schedule for Active Immunization of Normal Infants and Children*

Recommended age	Immunization(s)†	Comments
2 mos.	DTP, OPV	Can be initiated as early as age 2 wks. in areas of high endemicity or during epidemics
4 mos.	DTP, OPV	2-mo. Interval desired for OPV to avoid interference from previous dose
6 mos.	DTP	A third dose of OPV is not indicated in the U.S. but is desirable in geographic areas where polio is endemic
15 mos.	Measles, mumps, rubella (MMR)	MMR preferred to individual vaccines; tuberculin testing may be done at the same visit
18 mos.	DTP, ‡§OPV, II PRP-D	See footnotes
4-6 yrs.	DTP,¶ OPV	At or before school entry
14-16 yrs.	Td	Repeat every 10 yrs. throughout life

From American Academy of Pediatrics: Report of the Committee on Control of Infectious Diseases, ed 21, Elk Grove Village, IL, 1988, American Academy of Pediatrics.

*For all products used, consult manufacturer's package insert for instructions for storage, handling, dosage,and administration. Biologics prepared by different manufacturers may vary, and package inserts of the same manufacturer may change from time to time. Therefore the physician should be aware of the contents of the current package insert.

†DTP = diphtheria and tetanus toxoids with pertussis vaccine; OPV = oral poliovirus vaccine containing attenuated poliovirus types 1, 2, and 3; MMR = live measles, mumps, and rubella viruses in a combined vaccine (see text for discussion of single vaccines versus combination); PRP-D = *Haemophilus* b diphtheria toxoid conjugate vaccine; Td = adult tetanus toxoid (full dose) and diphtheria toxoid (reduced dose) for adult use.

‡Should be given 6 to 12 months after the third dose.

§May be given simultaneously with MMR at age 15 months.

‖May be given simultaneously with MMR at 15 months of age or at any time between 12 and 24 months of age.

¶Up to the seventh birthday.

rious accidents in the home. Reaching for boiling pots, putting small fingers in electrical outlets, and tumbling down stairs are all activities typical for the inquisitive, "omnipotent" toddler or preschool child. Injury prevention for the toddler and preschooler include use of approved car seats, close supervision at playgrounds, ponds, swimming pools, lakes, and locking away medicines, firearms, and house and garden chemicals. In addition, because the toddler and preschool child can begin to understand safety precautions, teaching the young child about general safety precautions is possible.

Immunizations

Immunizations against childhood diseases is a necessary aspect of child health care for this age group (Tables 11-1 and 11-2).

Table 11-2   Recommended Immunization Schedules for Children Not Immunized in First Year of Life

Recommended time	Immunization(s)	Comments
Less than 7 years old		
First visit	DTP, OPV, MMR	MMR if child $\geq$ 15 mos. old; tuberculin testing may be done at same visit
Interval after first visit: 1 mo.	PRP-D	For children aged 18-60 mos.; can be given concurrently with DTP (at separate sites) and other vaccines*
2 mos.	DTP, OPV	
4 mos.	DTP	A third dose of OPV is not indicated in the U.S. but is desirable in geographic areas where polio is endemic
10-16 mos.	DTP, OPV	OPV is not given if third dose was given earlier
4-6 yrs. (at or before school entry)	DTP, OPV	DTP is not necessary if the fourth dose was given after the fourth birthday; OPV is not necessary if recommended OPV dose at 10-16 mos. following first visit was given after the fourth birthday
10 yrs. later	Td	Repeat every 10 yrs. throughout life
7 years old and older		
First visit	TD, OPV, MMR	
Interval after first visit:		
2 mos.	Td, OPV	
8-14 mos.	Td, OPV	
10 yrs. later	Td	Repeat every 10 yrs. throughout life

From American Academy of Pediatrics: Report of the Committee on Control of Infectious Diseases, ed 21, Elk Grove Village, IL, 1988, American Academy of Pediatrics.

*The initial three doses of DTP can be given at 1- to 2-month intervals; so, for the child in whom immunization is initiated at age 24 months or older, one visit could be eliminated by giving DTP, OPV, and MMR at the first visit; DTP and PRP-D at the second visit (1 month later); and DTP and OPV at the third visit (2 months after the first visit). Subsequent DTP and OPV 10 to 16 months after the first visit are still indicated. PRP-D, MMR, DTP, and OPV can be given simultaneously at separate sites if return of vaccine recipient for future immunizations is doubtful.

The infant and toddler require a series of immunizations against measles, mumps, and rubella (MMR), polio, diphtheria, and tetanus. The recommended age to begin immunizations is age 2 months, with repeat inoculations at scheduled intervals throughout childhood. MMR inoculations are given at 15 months. Normal consequences from immunizations include fever, malaise, and pain or swelling at the injection site. Some youngsters will have malaise or feeding irregularities following their immunizations. Elevated temperature (>39.5° C) for more than 48 hours should be further evaluated.[64,74]

Dental

Once teeth begin to erupt, oral hygiene should be implemented. Removing plaque and food particles will need to be the parent's job for several years, until the child's dexterity allows self-care. Visits to the dentist should begin no later than 2 to 2½ years old, with initial appointments simply to meet the dentist and his or her staff. Routine check-ups allow the dentist to establish a relationship with the child and parents and to begin preventive measures for healthy dentition.[64,74]

Nutrition

The demand for adequate nutrition and calories is greatest during infancy and childhood. The infant requires 110 to 120 kcal per kilogram per day, while the toddler requires around 100 kcal/kg/day. Providing a suitable diet for the growing young child demands a combination of creativity, patience, and perseverance in the parent. Eating behaviors are closely linked to other aspects of cognitive and social development. Consequently, the young child is apt to provide challenging situations for the busy parent. From food jags to mealtime rituals to dawdling at the dinner table, the young child is a study in the growth of independence and fine motor skills.[4,42]

Between 3 to 4 months, the infant must change from sucking and swallowing skills to the ability to eat solid foods. This is really no small task, as the infant learns to control his or her tongue to take in food rather than to spit it out. During the first year, the child is introduced to new flavors and new textures in food. Foods should be offered in small amounts, simple in preparation but with variety.[42] Typically, infants prefer individual foods rather than mixtures of foods. As the youngster gains dexterity and fine motor skills, self-feeding should be allowed.

A typical food plan is included in Table 11-3.

Children require a combination of foods from all the food groups. Yet, variety is important not just in the type of food but in its texture. A balance of dry and moist foods should be offered to the toddler. One recommendation is to serve one soft food, one chewy food, and one crisp food at each meal. The child may prefer meals served at room temperature, as very hot foods are sometimes frightening.

Factors that help to shape food patterns in the young child include parents' food preferences, the sweetness and familiarity of foods, the food's preparation, the nutrition knowledge of the caregivers, and other influences such as television.[42] Overcooking, for

Table 11-3 Suggested Serving Portions for Toddlers and Preschoolers

Type of food	Suggested portion					Number per day
	1 year	2 years	3 years	4 years	5 years	
Milk	4 oz.	5 oz.	6 oz.	6 oz.	6 oz.	Total intake of 16-24 oz.
Meats and alternatives	1 tbsp.	2 tbsp.	3 tbsp.	4 tbsp.	4 tbsp.	3-4
Egg	1	1	1	1	1	0-1
Cooked legumes	1 tbsp.	2 tbsp.	3 tbsp.	4 tbsp.	4 tbsp.	0-2
Fruits and vegetables						At least 4
Citrus juice or other vitamin C source	¼ c.	¼ c.	⅓ c.	½ c.	½ c.	1
Dark green, leafy, or yellow vegetable	1 tbsp.	2 tbsp.	3 tbsp.	4 tbsp.	5 tbsp.	1 on alternate days
Other fruits and vegetables	1 tbsp.	2 tbsp.	3 tbsp.	4 tbsp.	5 tbsp.	
Breads (enriched or whole grain)	¼ sl.	⅓ sl.	⅓ sl.	½ sl.	½ sl.	4 or more
Cooked cereal	1 tbsp.	2 tbsp.	3 tbsp.	4 tbsp.	4 tbsp.	0-2
Ready-to-eat dry cereal	2 tbsp.	¼ c.	⅓ c.	½ c.	½ c.	0-2

From McWilliams, M: Nutrition for the growing years, ed 4, New York, 1986, John Wiley & Sons, Inc.

instance, has been cited as the most common offender in the child's dislike for vegetables and other foods.[45] A relaxed mealtime, with simply prepared foods of balanced nutrients, will permit the child an appropriate food intake.

Parents worry about their child's food intake, especially between 2 and 4 years of age. During this time, the child's appetite may in fact be erratic and unpredictable. Play and other distractions make the child a picky eater. Parents should remove the plate at the end of the meal regardless of the amount eaten.[20] No foods should be offered until the next planned eating/snack time. Some parents will worry that the child's nutrient intake will suffer with this approach. Keeping a food diary for several days and consulting the pediatrician or dietitian should assure parents that nutritional needs are being met.

Food jags and rituals are normal developmental stages for the child that may persist for several days or even weeks. Sometimes, food jags are related to the child's physical development. For example, many youngsters prefer carbohydrate-rich foods over protein foods because they are easier to masticate. Chewing is a challenging activity for the 1- to 4-year-old. Finger foods, such as carrot sticks, green beans, small sandwiches, or hard cooked eggs cut in quarters, are ideal snack and meal items. Serving small portions of food on large plates encourages a child's perception that there is less food.

Food rituals too have a place in the child's development. Children may prefer a certain food preparation or utensil. Some, for example, always want the crust cut from the sandwich, or will drink milk only from a special cup.

Regular meal and snack times are important for the picky eater. Snacks should be offered more than 1 hour from the next meal. Snacks are important adjuncts to the typical

American plan of three large meals per day and hold particular importance for the child with diabetes, which will be discussed in a later section. In the young child, glycogen stores in the liver are limited and easily depleted between meals. Snacks provide a more constant source of glucose for energy and storage.

Self-feeding is a developmentally based activity that should be promoted by parents. As the child gains dexterity, his or her use of fine motor skills are tested during mealtime. Handedness is generally not well-established in the first year, but increasingly the toddler and preschool child will demonstrate a preference. By 16 to 17 months, the child has more dexterity in using a spoon because of better wrist control. By 2 years of age, the child demonstrates a preference for right- or left-handedness.

Role of Play Activities of Childhood

Play has been termed the "work of childhood,"[5,16] for it is during play that the child learns about self and others. Only animals high on the evolutionary scale play, and the more advanced they are, the more they play. Humans have a long infancy to allow the extensive time for play necessary for development of sophisticated cognitive skills. Development progresses in several dimensions during play, from socialization to communication, from stress relief to problem-solving. Play is "extraordinary and supremely serious."[16] It is the child's mechanism for investigating the world, for learning adult roles, and for mastering physical challenges.

There are several primary types of play. *Practice* (or *sensorimotor*) play is the infant's and toddler's mechanism for investigating self and the world by using his or her body, motion, and senses to explore and manipulate objects. Young infants (0 to 6 months) enjoy *exercise play*—repetition of actions and sounds for pleasure (e.g., getting their feet into their mouths, kicking at toys hung above their crib, rolling over, and babbling).[49]

Infants who are 6 to 12 months old enjoy *exploratory play*—attain pleasure by causing effects and reconfirming skills. For example, they play "pat-a-cake" and throw mashed potatoes on the floor to see what will happen.

Babies 12 to 24 months old have increased mobility and are developmentally driven to explore and manipulate their involvement. Play is used to practice their newly developed physical skills of walking, running, and climbing. They also need to test and reexamine objects from all angles for shape, size, weight, texture, color, function, spatial relationship, and interaction with themselves.

Toddlers 18 to 36 months old enjoy *deferred imitation*—imitating previously observed actions (not the reasons for or purposes of actions) from memory.[49] For example, they pretend to be "daddy" and shave, walk outside to "go to work," then come back inside and snore to "take a nap." At this age, play is parallel and personal, rather than reciprocal or interactive. Conflicts are common as the youngster claims his or her "property rights."

By the preschool years, child's play is more interactive and more cooperative. They engage in *symbolic play*—play in which children represent or reenact experiences and reflect on people, things, and events they have experienced.[49] Symbolic play enables children to turn reality into what they wish reality was; for example, imaginary friends are common. Preschoolers also engage in social play. They play games in which rules are collectively made up so everyone wins and has fun. Hopscotch, jump rope, and tag are examples of social play.

Research suggests that parental expectations and resources for play vary across cultures and socioeconomic backgrounds. Parents in lower socioeconomic brackets, for example, play less often with their children and speak less often to them during play.[74]

Impact of Television

More than 98% of households in the United States have at least one television. Children between 2 and 11 years average 4 hours per day in front of the "electronic babysitter."[20] As a solitary activity, television viewing promotes increased passivity, and decreased physical activity and social interaction.[14,75] Heavy viewing is not conducive to the development of imaginative capacities.[68] In at least one study, exposure to television violence increased children's subsequent aggressive behaviors in a laboratory setting.[20] It has been estimated that by high school graduation, the average American child has seen 18,000 televised murders.

The average child is exposed to 20,000 television commercials each year. Typically the ads concern toys or sugary treats or fast foods, influences of special concern to the child with diabetes. Watching hours of television at a time increases the consumption of snack foods and indirectly, may have a role in promoting obesity in some children. Gender-stereotyped programs deliver a message of values not necessarily held by the parents.

Parents have a decided role in promoting constructive television viewing.[68] Developing viewing habits and setting limits must be started early in the child's development. Viewing should be planned rather than random. More importantly, the parent should interact with the child, clarifying what is being seen, discussing sensitive issues, sharing personal values, and analyzing commercials. The parent's important job is to help the child to see cause and effect, not just the action.[20,68]

IMPACT OF DIABETES MELLITUS ON NORMAL PHYSICAL DEVELOPMENT
Physical Examination

The young child with diabetes needs a physical examination at least quarterly, with special attention paid to the following aspects:

- Height and weight (plus head and chest circumference until 2 years) measurement and comparison with standardized norms.
- Evaluation of pulses and blood pressure.
- Cardiac, neurologic, dental, and ophthalmoscopic examinations.
- Thyroid palpation.
- Skin examination (including inspection of injection sites for lipodystrophies, infec-

tion, or redness of fingertips to determine frequency of blood glucose testing and identify errors in technique).
- Laboratory test for glycated hemoglobin, urine ketones, and protein.[41,64]

If findings indicate a fasting lipid profile, urine culture or thyroid function tests are added. The child who has ketones and/or is not gaining weight, growing, or appears wasted or dehydrated may have had hyperglycemia for days or weeks and may need hospitalization for determination of causes and major insulin dose adjustment.

Growth Retardation

On a more long-term basis, diabetes mellitus can affect the young child's linear growth.[39,71] The complex interaction of insulin, growth hormone, and somatostatin result in a normal growth pattern. When this balance is altered, as in diabetes, growth may suffer. Golden and associates[28] found that intensified management with frequent glucose monitoring and multiple injections resulted in a more normal growth pattern when compared with a group of children managed less optimally. Jackson[37] reported that catch-up growth is possible in children formerly in poor metabolic control. Once glycemic balance was achieved, these children reestablished and maintained normal growth. Other authors, too, have noted, with intensification of insulin treatment, that growth velocity markedly improves.[48]

CNS Growth and Hypoglycemia

Without an available source of glucose, the central nervous system will not develop normally. Animal studies suggest that prolonged hypoglycemia results in diminished brain weight, cellularity, and protein content. Myelinization is also decreased.[17] Complex motor functions require an intact nervous system. Thus, probably the single most serious impact of diabetes in the infant or toddler is the potential for severe or prolonged hypoglycemia. Goals for diabetes control must account for the child's inability to accurately communicate hypoglycemic symptoms. Therefore, most diabetes specialists recommend maintaining blood glucose levels between 100 and 200 mg/dL as a precaution against undetected hypoglycemia during the years before school age.

Dental Care

Because the oral mucosa and gums are also bathed in glucose during periods of hyperglycemia, the child with diabetes is prone to gum infections and dental problems. Strict oral hygiene and, of course, controlling glucose levels are necessary. Children with diabetes are generally not exposed to as many cariogenic snacks as other children. However, selecting snack foods that limit plaque formation is wise. Popcorn and raw fruits and vegetables provide a mechanical cleaning of the teeth while the child is enjoying the snack. Sweet foods are less damaging to the teeth when eaten immediately after a meal than when eaten alone. This practice actually is better in blunting a postprandial glucose rise as well.[44,64]

Schedules and the Sleep Cycle

Diabetes requires a fairly rigid schedule of meals, snacks, blood glucose testing, insulin injections, and exercise. Yet the young child is often not consistent in his or her activity or appetite. Adjusting diabetes care to a young child's routine is demanding.

Parents often worry about how their child will fare during the night or during nap time. What will happen to the blood glucose? Will the child awaken if hypoglycemic? Before nap time and sleeptime, parents should check the child's blood glucose. Naps should follow either a meal or a snack, particularly if there will be an insulin peaking during the sleep period. Parents should be reassured that most children will awaken when hypoglycemic and that the child's normal counterregulatory hormones will provide some safety in buffering low blood glucose.[10]

Bedtime blood glucose values and snacks are especially important for young children with insulin-dependent diabetes mellitus (IDDM) because they can prevent the relatively common occurrences (approximately once a week) of silent nocturnal hypoglycemia. This is a problem partly because nocturnal insulin requirements are lower between 1 to 2 AM.[19,65] Nocturnal hypoglycemia is manifested by nightmares, sleep walking or sleep talking, and restlessness, as well as the common daytime symptoms such as sweating, feeling shaky, and/or starving. The best predictor of 1 to 3 AM hypoglycemia is the blood glucose level at bedtime.[65,76] A child who has a bedtime glucose below 120 mg/dL has a 25% chance of a subsequent episode of hypoglycemia at 2 AM. The bedtime snack can be used to reduce the risks of a 1 to 3 AM hypoglycemia by doubling its protein content.

Illnesses and Diabetes

Young children with IDDM are not more likely to be ill than children without diabetes. However, infections in children with IDDM stimulate wide fluctuations in blood glucose levels; some infections cause hypoglycemia whereas others, or chronic infections, tend to cause hyperglycemia and insulin resistance. Infections frequently stimulate the development of the stress response and ketoacidosis. Thus insulin requirements are variable during illness episodes. In general, during illness children with IDDM need frequent blood glucose and urine ketone testing along with variable amounts of insulin based on the glucose and ketone levels during illness. Young children will often exhibit *low* blood glucose because of smaller glycogen reserves and loss of appetite during illness. Both reasons contribute to the hypoglycemia often seen in the young child.

Immunizations can affect the blood glucose levels, again as a result of the child's lack of desire to eat. Some youngsters, however, will demonstrate hyperglycemia for up to 24 hours following immunizations. In either case, extra blood glucose tests and adjustment of insulin doses may be necessary.[63,64,72]

Children with IDDM are especially susceptible to dehydration. Thus, during illness, especially when diarrhea occurs, these children should be encouraged to drink 4 to 8 ounces of fluid every hour. If they are unable or unwilling to ingest fluids, they need to be taken to the physician's office or emergency room for intravenous (IV) fluid therapy.

Whenever children with IDDM are sick for any reason, "sick day" management rules should be followed.

Insulin requirements can be quite variable during illness episodes. Generally the parent should continue to administer the routine insulin doses, with amounts based on fluctuations in the blood glucose. For example, the ill child with hyperglycemia and ketones will require additional regular insulin as often as every 2 to 3 hours. If, however, the ill child's blood glucose falls below normal, a reduction in the usual dose will be necessary. Parents should be in close contact with their diabetes team or pediatrician during their child's illness.

NORMAL COGNITIVE AND LANGUAGE DEVELOPMENT
Cognitive Development

Just as physical development follows predictable patterns, cognitive development has established milestones. The infant learns about the world through his or her developing senses. Sucking and grasping are early means for experiencing the environment. The young infant has relatively no sense of time. Gradually the infant begins to appreciate object permanence. Play becomes more goal directed. By the first birthday, the youngster can understand some cause and effect and can remember events.

The toddler uses symbols, can recall past events, and has an initial understanding of the future. By the fourth year, the child can begin to understand the perspective of others and uses classification, although nonsystematically. The 3- to 5-year-old has an active imagination and explains much of the world in terms of fantasy. These children are particularly vulnerable to medically invasive procedures. Body integrity and regeneration of lost body fluids are foreign concepts to the preschooler.

Piaget[26,51] contributed to our understanding of how infants and children form their impressions of reality. Piaget recognized that there is a regular sequence to this development and that each step is a necessary predecessor to the next phase. He described the processes of internal structuring and organizing of reality as using "schemas," primitive mental structures that evolve from both assimilation or accommodation. Assimilation involves the incorporation of a stimulus into an existing schema, while accommodation involves the reshaping of an existing schema to adapt the new information. The repetition of play, for example, is a form of assimilation, as the child repeats patterns of experiences.

Piaget described two developmental stages for children from birth to 7 years of age: (1) sensorimotor (0 to 2 years) and (2) preoperational (2 to 7 years). Each of these stages has characteristic attributes that affect how children perceive, comprehend, problem-solve, and reason about themselves and their environment.[50,52]

Sensorimotor stage

Infants and young toddlers (birth to 2 years) are in Piaget's sensorimotor stage of cognitive development. Their senses and motor skills are actively used to define and interpret objects and events.[53] The infant learns about the environment through reflex activity, simple repetitive behaviors, imitation, and, ultimately, trial-and-error problem-solving. Between 1 and 4 months of age, the child enters a stage of primary circular reaction, a time of repetition and imitation. The infant discovers that moving is pleasurable and thus kicks his or her legs or waves his or her hands repeatedly. The child in this stage will love to shake a rattle, but, if he or she drops it, the rattle no longer exists.

During secondary circular reaction, the 4- to 6-month-old has a growing interest in the results or consequences of his or her actions. The child can now recognize his or her ball from seeing only a portion of it hidden under a blanket. The child is able to use combinations of reflexes and senses purposely.[53] From 6 to 12 months of age, the infant progresses through the stage of "coordination of secondary schemas," demonstrating purposeful actions and understanding object permanence. For example, an infant will begin crying as soon as an alcohol pad is wiped on the skin, anticipating the stick to follow.[53] An appreciation for cause and effect is also developing.

Around 12 months of age, toddlers begin to reason by using familiar actions to achieve results. They reason by perceiving only the whole, not parts, which results in connecting a series of separate actions or ideas into one confused whole.[50] For example, if a toddler wants the squeaky toy to make noise, he or she "reasons" that the toy squeaks when Dad touches it, so the toy is taken to Dad and the child cries if Dad fails to make it squeak.

The 12- to 18-month-old experiments with new means of achieving familiar results. Unlike the earlier stages of repetition and anticipating results from usual actions, the child in the tertiary circular reaction substage prefers to try different approaches toward a goal. For example, the child will slowly pour out supper on the floor to watch the effect.

By the last stage in the sensorimotor phase, the 18-to 24-month-old is now making mental combinations to solve problems. "Out of sight, out of mind" no longer works with this age group. If Daddy goes into another room and closes the door, the toddler now knows that he still exists behind that door.

Preoperational stage

The child in Piaget's preoperational phase has an increasingly sophisticated use of language. The child interprets the world in quite egocentric ways. Objects and events occur only in relationship to the child and there is no seeing another person's point of view.

By ages 4 to 7 years, the child enters Piaget's stage of intuitive thought, a time of concrete, tangible thinking. Thought is dominated by what is seen, heard, and experienced. The child can make simple associations and begins to understand weight, length, size, and time. Children in this stage love to classify objects, to separate them into groups, to sort them into categories.

Another aspect of cognitive development for the 4-to 7-year-old concerns conservation of length, quantity, mass, weight, and volume. Conservation occurs when the child understands that changing the outward appearance of an object does not change its permanent characteristics.

Fantasy and play are predominant in the preschool child's life, and inanimate objects take on rich and sometimes frightening lives of their own. Inanimate objects not only are viewed as living entities but have feelings, thoughts, and intentions.

Preschool and school-age children differ in how they think.[20] As previously noted, toddlers and young preschoolers exhibit egocentrism, which means they perceive situations only in terms of immediate personal outcomes (things they enjoy are good, things that hurt or frustrate them are bad). *Absolutism,* exhibited by 2- to 5-year-olds, is the belief that things are right or wrong, good or bad, hurt or don't hurt. For example, a finger-stick or injection either hurts or does not hurt. *Artificialism,* the belief that natural events are created by humans, influences the 2- to 5-year-old to believe someone made him or her get sick. *Animism* is the belief that all things have intention, feelings, and thoughts. Children of this age often ask "When do the stars go to bed?" and "Where does the sun play when it rains?" *Irreversibility,* the belief that actions or thought cannot be reversed or compensated for, causes children who receive fingersticks or injections to think all their blood will leak out of this hole and they will die, or that a cast placed on their leg is now their leg.[53]

Preoperational children exhibit magical thinking, the belief that their own thoughts or actions influence events outside of their control. For example, an angry child who wishes a sibling would no longer be there to pester him or her feels guilt when the sibling becomes ill, believing his or her wish came true. The type of thinking exhibited by the child has implications for diabetes management that are discussed in depth later in this chapter.

Speech and Language

The infant is particularly responsive to high-pitched voices, and reacts to the cadence and melody of voice. By 3 months old, the child is cooing and reciprocating certain sounds with the caregiver. By 4 months, the infant laughs, and by 6 months, babbles in monosyllables. It is during this phase of development that the infant begins experimenting with sound production and virtually makes all human speech sounds. By the end of the first year, the child is attentive to his or her own name and knowingly uses ma-ma or da-da.

The toddler begins using short sentences and has a vocabulary developing from 50 to 200 words. Clearly, the toddler understands more than he or she can verbalize.

The child from 3 to 5 years old has a much larger vocabulary, ranging from 850 to 2000 words. This child begins to use plurals and past tense. By 3 years old, the child can verbalize two to three sentences together. By age 4, he or she is making grammatically complete sentences. As the child's social world expands to include peers, repetition and songs become tools for language development.

It must be emphasized that preschoolers do not necessarily understand the meaning of the words used unless they have had direct contact in learning to apply them.[8,53] Words used in relation to time, causality, and left and right are incorrectly employed because a child of this age does not understand these concepts.

It is imperative that health care providers know the cognitive development of the specific child they are working with to understand what the child is thinking. In addition, it is essential they explain any special medical treatments or tests before their occurrence using words and phrases that the child can understand. When there is no explanation, toddlers and preschoolers will conjure up their own reasons that contain elements of self-reproach and punishment.[8,53] For example, telling children you will take their temperature connotes taking something from them; it is better to say you are "checking" it. Testing often implies determining if they are good or bad; while, "checking" is less challenging.

Developing Concepts of Health and Illness

The preschooler's understanding of health and illness is very much linked to cognitive development and holds special pertinence to understanding the child with diabetes. Fantasy thinking and past experiences all contribute to the child's developing understanding of health. Health is viewed as a positive state, associated with the ability to play.

Robinson[55] studied preschool children in an effort to determine how children explain illness causality. In general, the youngsters understood illness better than health. One could be sick and healthy at the same time, and the relative degree of health or illness was determined by the kind of activity permitted. For example, one with a cold could still play inside and was healthier than one who had to stay in bed. The cause of illness was viewed as multifactorial and externally located. Often, children interpreted ill health as the result of some misdeed or as punishment. The transfer of illness was often accomplished magically.[9,53]

Other patterns became clear to Robinson. First, there was a relative lack of self-blame in any of the explanations by the children. Second, verbal explanations contributed only a small part to the child's understanding. Rather, sensory experiences were more important. And, finally, in explaining illness to preschool children, it was important for there to be congruency between the verbal explanation and the child's sensory experiences. Preparing children for health care encounters should therefore include the sights, sounds, and sensations to be expected.

IMPACT OF DIABETES ON COGNITIVE AND LANGUAGE DEVELOPMENT
Perceptions and Feelings

The onset of diabetes is harrowing to the parent, and necessitates an abrupt life-style change for the family. The sensitive child will soon learn mother's or father's reactions to testing, injections, and meal plans. By school-age, a child with very early onset of diabetes may have experienced the rigors of diabetes care for several years.

According to Brewster,[12] children at this age believe illness is the outcome of wrongdoing. Frequent fingersticks (testing blood glucose levels) and insulin injections validate these beliefs. Parents and children need to be frequently reassured there was nothing they thought or did to cause the diabetes and nothing they could have done to prevent it.

Effect of Early Onset of Diabetes

Infants, toddlers, and preschool children with IDDM are subject to the same cognitive development as are children without IDDM. Some studies have found preschool children with chronic illnesses (e.g., IDDM) may develop delays in cognition as compared with those without chronic illness.[25] Researchers have shown that even mild hypoglycemia (45 to 60 mg/dL blood glucose) causes visual-spatial, visual-motor, cognitive speed, and global cognitive skills to deteriorate in adults.[60,66,77] Ryan and associates[61] found that after 21 minutes of induced mild hypoglycemia, there was a significant compromise of mental efficiency, especially on measures of attention and sustained concentration, for 12- to 17-year-old children. Another study found children with early onset of IDDM had lower scores on the Wechsler Intelligence Scale for Children–Revised (WISC-R).[34] Rovet found children with earlier onset and longer duration of IDDM and more frequent hypoglycemic seizures scored lower on visuospatial tests.[56-59] Thus even mild hypoglycemia impairs mental functioning to some degree.[33] At this time, we do not know if or how many hypoglycemic events or what magnitude or duration, will cause permanent impaired mental functioning.

NORMAL PSYCHOSOCIAL DEVELOPMENT
Erikson's Theory of Personality Development

Erikson[23] theorized several stages of development leading to a psychologically healthy adulthood.

Infants, through the use of their senses, are in a stage of developing trusting relationships. Successful movement through this stage results in an individual who is able to maintain hope, optimism, and faith in his or her environment and abilities. A caring, consistent parent is necessary to this development of trust. Lack of such care results in the child's inability to trust the caretaker and presumably, later, to lack a sense of faith and confidence. Thus the development of "fear of strangers" is positive in that infants demonstrate bonding to their primary caretakers and learn to be wary of those they do not know yet.

Toddlers are in Erickson's stage of "autonomy versus shame and doubt." The toddler must establish autonomy by gaining control of his or her body, its functions, and its mobility. If repeatedly thwarted in attempts at self-control, toddlers begin to question their abilities with a sense of shame and self-doubt. Central to this stage are the parents and the child's desire to imitate their actions.

Preschoolers are in Erickson's "initiative versus guilt" stages. The child is vigorous, intrusive, and enterprising. Imagination guides the child into new adventures, and his or her inner voice or early conscience warns of limits in the environment. Successfully starting and completing tasks results in a long-term sense of direction and purpose. Conflicts during this stage, with frequent severe criticisms of efforts, leaves the child feeling guilty and worthless.

Erikson's concepts continue through several additional stages, including adulthood and aging, which are addressed in other chapters of this text.

Family Systems

The social domain for the infant, toddler, and preschool child is the family. For the infant, parents (and especially the mother) are the borders of the social world. As the child matures and is exposed to other social systems (day care, babysitters), siblings, peers, and extended family members become increasingly important to social development.

Families as units have developmental tasks and responsibilities. From providing physical needs to allocating resources, to socializing its members, the family system is responsible for ultimately incorporating its members into the society at large. The family provides the growing child with the "rules" for its society. Families develop a system of communication and interaction, with unwritten rules for expressing affection and aggression. The family must interface with society, through interaction with work, church, school, day care, or extended family members. They, too, must maintain motivation and morale in its members by rewarding achievements, confronting personal and family crises, setting goals, and developing family values.[15] Interactions within and outside the family in a variety of contexts, a sense of coping and mastery in the members, and a flexible internal organization characterize the "energized" family.[54]

Role of Siblings

Siblings are the child's first peer group. They are important participants in the preschool child's social development. As much as one third of the interactions between a toddler and an older sibling, for example, consist of imitation.[20] This imitation is important as the child learns social, cognitive, and moral lessons. Often older siblings share in parenting responsibilities and provide security and language enhancement.[6] Sibling relationships may have increasing relevance because of shrinking family size, blended families as a result of divorce and remarriage, geographic mobility, maternal employment, and day care.[6]

Day Care

As increasingly more mothers work outside the home, issues of child care surface. About 50% of infants and approximately ⅔ of preschool children have mothers in the workplace.[74] Most mothers feel some guilt over leaving their infants or toddlers in another's care, feelings that may be intensified in mothers of children with diabetes. Brazelton[11] encourages families to wait until the infant is at least 4 months old before entering day care. The American Academy of Pediatrics has a reference manual to assist parents in selecting appropriate child care.[1]

Parenting Styles

Children seem to cycle in their behavioral patterns of equilibrium and disequilibrium. The smooth, consolidated behaviors of the 2-year-old become the disturbed, erratic behaviors of the 2½-year-old, become the rounded, balanced and happy patterns of the 3-year-old, and so on.[36] Such flux in behavior typically marks surges of growth toward new developmental challenges. Parents, however, often find that while one approach to parenting was effective for the toddler, that same technique no longer works with the preschooler.

Parenting styles seem to fit one of three patterns: authoritarian, permissive, or authoritative.[74] The authoritarian style sets absolute standards for behavior. The permissive style is tolerant, allowing for considerable self-regulation by the child. Few demands are made for mature behavior. The authoritative style sets standards, expects developmentally appropriate behavior, encourages independence, and allows for open communication between parents and children in decision making.

Setting limits and maintaining consistency in reinforcing those limits are concerns for most parents. Structuring the child's interpersonal and physical environment to minimize misbehavior and applying behavior management techniques when misbehavior has occurred are skills parents often learn by doing. Minimizing the opportunity for misconduct includes setting clear and simple rules, modeling appropriate actions, and frequently reminding the youngsters about the established rules.

Despite a parent's best efforts, misbehavior will occur. Common strategies for discipline include spanking, time out, reasoning or scolding, or ignoring.[46,47]

Regardless of the disciplining approach, parents should initiate it immediately. Young children have short attention spans, and immediate feedback is necessary for the child to attach the discipline to the precise action. In selecting a disciplining approach, parents must consider the temperament of their child and the severity of the misbehavior. Furthermore, once the behavior is disciplined, the parents should express concern for the child's feelings and should consider the issue closed.

Temperament

Temperament has been defined as that manner of thinking, behaving, or reacting that characterizes an individual and is an important component to consider in terms of the planning of the diabetic regimen.[75] Chess and Thomas[18] identified nine qualities contributing to differentiations in temperament: (1) motor activity, (2) rhythmicity, (3) approach-withdrawal, (4) adaptability, (5) threshold of responsiveness, (6) intensity of reaction, (7) quality of mood, (8) distractibility, and (9) attention span and persistence. The child's response to new stimuli is assessed in terms of the amount of mobility the child displays, how quickly the child approaches a new stimulus, the energy level of the response, and how easily the child is distracted from the stimulus. Taken together, the researchers were able to classify children into three broad descriptive groupings. The "easy" child was one of even temper, who approached new stimuli in open and positive ways. These children seemed to adapt to changing situations, demonstrated mild to moderately intense moods, and accounted for 40% of the children.

The "difficult" child (10% of the sample) was highly active, irritable, irregular in feeding schedules and other habits, and adapted more slowly to new routines, people, or situations. These children fared better in an environment with structure, low stimulation, and gradual introductions to new experiences.

The "slow-to-warm-up" child, accounting for 15% of the study group, reacted to new situations slowly and preferred repeated contact. They showed mild resistance to change or novelty and were inactive and somewhat moody.

Vaughan[74] has warned that labeling infants and children in this way may promote a self-fulfilling prophecy. Rather, the classifications should be considered in terms of how well the infant's temperament fits with the environment and specifically with the parent's personality. Behavior problems are likely when the child's approach to the world differs markedly from the parent's expectations or child-rearing practices.

Fears and Stresses of Young Childhood

The nature and impact of childhood fears and stressors relate to the child's level of cognitive development, temperament, and overall vulnerability to stress (Table 11-4). Children that are active, energetic, resourceful, and willing to take risks are more resilient to the effects of stress than are children who are more withdrawn, timid, stubborn, impulsive, or dependent.[75]

Infants are frightened by loud noises or by loss of physical support. The older infant (6 months to 1 year) shows fear of strangers, heights, things looming over them, or of separation from the caregiver. By ages 2 to 4 years, the child's knowledge of the world is still fragmented, and fantasy is used to invent explanations. These children are particularly frightened by animals, scary masks, and the darkness. For the toddler, bedtime, visits to the pediatrician, or loss of a security toy may be sources of stress. Because the sense of personal boundaries is poorly defined, the toddler fears the loss of body parts.

For the preschooler, additional fears include fantasies about ghosts and concerns about bodily harm or castration. Invasive procedures, such as needle sticks, are a real threat to body integrity and are viewed with fear. Stressors for these children center around changes in their routines. Nightmares are also common at this age.

Helping the child to master a problem encourages cognitive and psychosocial development.[69,75] Dealing with children's fears in general could include giving the child who is fearful of the dark a flashlight. Some youngsters may draw a picture of the scary creature and then tear it up in a ritualized banishing.

IMPACT OF DIABETES ON PSYCHOSOCIAL DEVELOPMENT
Parental Coping

The effect of diabetes on the very young child's psychosocial development relates indirectly to the reactions of parents and family members to the illness.

Table 11-4 Children's Fears by Age and Behaviors Indicative of Fears

Age	Major fears	Behaviors
Infants (0-3 mos)	Sudden movements Loud noises Loss of physical support	Generalized total body reaction, crying Clinging to adult

Infants (4-12 mos)	Strange objects and people
	Heights
	Anticipation of previous uncomfortable situations
	Change in routines
	Separation from loved ones
		Crying
		Clinging to adult
		Pulling away, crying
		
		Difficulty eating and sleeping
		Separation anxiety
		  Protest
		  Despair
		  Denial, detachment

Toddlers (1-3 yrs)	The unknown, the dark Being alone and separation Large or scary animals Loss of control Body injury/pain	Delay bedtime Separation anxiety Crying, clinging to adult Regression, negativism, temper tantrums, resistance Physical aggression, verbal uncooperativeness
Preschool (3-5)	The unknown; supernatural Monsters and ghosts Body mutilation Separation and abandonment Loss of control Change in routine Body injury and pain Fear of body mutilation	Refusing to sleep Aggressive behavior Separation anxiety Aggression: physical and verbal Regression, withdrawal, guilt, anxiety Aggression, withdrawal anxiety

Parents (and other caretakers) experience the full range of emotional reactions when a young child is diagnosed with diabetes, including anger, guilt, resentment, and blaming. As the demands of daily care become more clear, parents can become apprehensive, over-protective, and depressed.[32]

Parents of chronically ill children often view them as vulnerable or endangered.[44] For example, the child with diabetes may have activities restricted because of parental fear of hypoglycemia. Choices in foods may be severely limited because of uncertainty of the glycemic effect. At a time when the child is struggling to gain independence, the parent may feel obligated to maintain a rigid schedule of meals and activities.

How parents, particularly mothers, adjust to diabetes in their preschool children has been the focus of a few recent studies. Wysocki and associates[78] surveyed 20 mothers of preschool children using various behavioral scales and stress indices. In this sample, mothers of children with IDDM reported more sleep problems, social withdrawal, and somatic complaints in their children, although *overall* the mothers did not score their children as abnormal. The mother's also identified more overall family stress with the child with diabetes seen as the source of that stress.

Parental stress and negative feelings are communicated and responded to by young children.[41] The more attention parents place on diabetes activities, the more children are reminded of being different, and the more they resist.

The stress of managing diabetes can certainly stretch a parent's coping abilities. Horan and associates[35] have speculated that children with IDDM may be at risk for child abuse and neglect. Abuse incidence data are higher in chronically ill children, although there are no good data about cases involving children with IDDM specifically. Marital strife, parental hopelessness, unrealistic or exaggerated parental expectations, and inconsistent parenting may all be indicators of poor adaptation to the child's diagnosis and care needs.

Well-meaning friends may also offer a variety of how-to approaches or share stories of what can happen when the management plan is not compulsively followed. Thus, underlying the day-to-day anxieties associated with diabetes self-management are the parents' worst fears of long-term complications and poor health. Such fears may manifest as overprotective limitations on the child's life.

Parents may benefit from contact with other families with young children with IDDM within the parameters of a diabetes education program.[67] Diabetes education provides the opportunity for parents of young children to share other concerns, fears, and anxieties as well as ideas on how to handle problem times like fingersticks, injections, and meals or snacks. Parents learn their "worst fears" may be positively handled when others describe their crises, what they did, and the outcome to the child[41] (see accompanying box).

___ PARENTAL CONCERNS AND THE YOUNG CHILD WITH DIABETES ___

Fear of hypoglycemia, especially undetected hypoglycemia
Fear of hyperglycemia and long-term complications
Accepting their child has diabetes
Dealing with the opinions of relatives and friends
Lack of support or help from spouse
Adapting to a rigid schedule
Feeling alone
Dealing with siblings' reactions and behaviors
Fear of making a mistake in the management
Finding and trusting other caregivers
Developing a working relationship with the medical community
Guilty feelings about all the invasive procedures

Behavior Management

Knowing when and how to discipline the very young child with diabetes can be quite a dilemma for parents. For example, the child who is irritable or combative may be having a low blood glucose or may be having normal difficulty with impulse control. The physical sensations of blood glucose fluctuations are often not recognized by the child and can be misdiagnosed by the parent. Parents need to be taught how to differentiate these symptoms from behaviors caused by poor impulse control. Hypoglycemic symptoms in young children include feeling shaky, sweaty (but cool to touch), starving (will happily eat their least favorite foods), stubborn, having an abrupt change in activity level, and becoming pale and irritable, whiney, or clinging without provocation.[10,13] Nocturnal hypoglycemia is evidenced by any of the above plus nightmares, restless or noisy sleep, and sleep walking, or sleep talking.

Hypoglycemia often occurs when children are late for meals, eat part of their meal, are more active than usual (excess exercise can cause hypoglycemia up to 12 hours afterwards), take long naps (especially when they are then late for a meal or snack), or if appetite is decreased during illness. Parents should test the blood glucose or, if not possible, treat a possible "low" by giving the child ½ glass of juice or 1 to 2 teaspoons of sugar or pancake syrup. If this doesn't help, discipline should be instituted. Candy and extra attention should *not* be given for hypoglycemia because children will use these symptoms for secondary gain.

Hyperglycemia causes children to look for something to drink, urinate frequently, feel "lazy" and tired, and become irritable, frustrated, and less able to follow directions. Many infants and toddlers become flushed, cry, or fuss and rub their eyes for no apparent reason. Hyperglycemia occurs when children are not as active as usual, eat more than planned, have an infection, or develop relative insulin deficiency as a result of a growth spurt or inadequate insulin adjustment during growth.

Children with hyperglycemia should be given extra non–glucose-containing fluids and should be encouraged to remain active unless they have ketones, blood glucose over 350 mg/dL, or fever. Children with ketones may require additional insulin, according to the recommendation of the physician. In addition, 4 to 8 ounces of fluid per hour for 2 to 3 hours and frequent testing are recommended. If the ketones and blood glucose are not diminishing, or if the child cannot drink and retain fluids one hour without vomiting, the parents should call the diabetes nurse clinician or physician regardless of the time of day. Careful discussions with the parent as to strategies for differentiating diabetes symptomatology from behavioral changes is needed.

Siblings

The impact of diabetes in the family on a well sibling can be profound. Older siblings may feel guilty that their brother or sister developed diabetes. They may assume management anxieties and worries of their parent. In a study of 30 well siblings, Ferrari[24] found lower self-concept scores when compared with control subjects. Siblings of diabetic children were more concerned about their school status, their personal happiness, and their popularity.

Baby Sitters

Finding adequate and knowledgeable child care is an additional demand for parents of the child with diabetes.[22] The babysitter must know how to handle hypoglycemia. Emergency protocols, including ready access to juice or glucose gels must be stressed. Meal times, snack foods and what to do if the child will not eat must be shared with the sitter. Access to the parent or a capable family friend by phone, as well as a physician's phone number, should be available.

Some diabetes centers and hospitals offer training courses for babysitters.[27] The American Diabetes Association or Juvenile Diabetes Foundations in the area are good resources for such classes.

TEACHING/LEARNING IMPLICATIONS

An underlying philosophy for teaching the young child and parent includes an appreciation that knowledge and skill acquisition can be gradual and that children will eventually attain self-management behaviors.[64] Young children require a gradual introduction of concepts and skills. This introduction should not necessarily be in the logical order that adults learn. For instance, it may seem more reasonable to teach drawing the dose first, followed by injection procedures. However, the young child (5 to 6 years old) will have the fine motor skill to inject *first*. It will not be until perhaps 8 to 10 years old that the child will have the fine motor and the cognitive skills required to accurately draw and mix insulin doses.[63] Together, parents and professionals should plan for the gradual introduction of self-care skills consistent with the child's developmental level (Table 11-5).

Strategies

Teaching/learning strategies for the young child with diabetes and the family are dictated by several aspects of learner readiness. Clearly, most of the training will be directed toward the parents or significant caregivers. These individuals must be assessed for their desire and ability to learn the information necessary for safe management of the child. Strategies that enhance learning include early introduction and direct application of necessary diabetes skills, such as injections, fingerstick procedures, and record keeping. By becoming actively involved from the beginning, the parent is better able to regain a sense of control. For the child, having a parent perform the necessary procedures can be much less threatening. Consequently, if hospitalization is necessary at diagnosis, the parents should be encouraged to stay with their child and participate actively in his or her care. Often, parents are so overwhelmed at the time of diagnosis that they are unable to fully

Table 11-5   Effect of Diabetes on the Child and Parent

Developmental tasks	Effect of diabetes on child's development	Effect of diabetes on parents	Suggested approaches
Infancy (0-1 year)			
Trust vs mistrust Sensorimotor stage	Confused by parents inflicting pain Frequent feedings are required to maintain blood glucose levels Frequent, severe or prolonged hypoglycemia is dangerous to developing CNS Immunizations may elevate glucoses	Grief over loss of perfect child Selection of day care and babysitters is affected Anxiety over fear of hypoglycemia	Parents should reassure, cuddle, hold child after injections and fingersticks Use fingerstick BG tests to monitor and alter care Use external clues with bedtime and midnight blood glucose levels to detect hypoglycemia during night
Todder (1-3 years)			
Autonomy vs shame and doubt Sensorimotor and preoperational	Depends on parents for BG tests, diet, and insulin Food jags lead to diet inconsistencies Childhood illnesses and growth spurts affect BG levels Older toddler begins to know if "low" Older toddler can begin assisting with fingersticks	Difficulty distinguishing misbehavior from blood glucose levels Difficulty in allowing child some autonomy	Offer the child choices in food selection, injection, and BG testing sites Matter-of-fact and quick with procedures Use BG tests to help identify symptoms Provide consistency in discipline, setting limits, and routines Use a flexible insulin program Prevent mealtime battles

Preschool (3-6 years)
Initiative vs guilt
Preoperational stage

Begins to feel different from peers
Views any aspects of diabetes management as punishment
Fantasizes that fingersticks and injections may result in bleeding to death
Needs to control own environment; wants to cooperate
Fears body mutilation

Overprotective behaviors as child becomes increasingly independent
Working with preschool teachers

Have a plan for managing sick days
Child needs to be told didn't cause IDDM, and not punishment
Avoid giving candy/extra attention for hypoglycemia
2- to 3-year-old child can identify "low" and tell adult.

Use play and drawings to express feelings
Encourage child's participation in simple diabetes tasks
Basic diabetes education includes choosing proper foods, identifying symptoms, and knowing what to do for "lows"
Knowing if BG high - needs to wait to eat
Can do own fingerstick, may try to give own injection
Plan for parties and holidays to minimize child's feelings of "differentness"
Encourage child's participation in sports, swimming, dancing, gymnastics

attend to all the new information. Modeling diabetes skills for these parents permits them to gradually assume the care in a less threatening manner.

Techniques directed at adult learning are used for the parents (see Chapter 16). Thus, understanding how the parent approaches new information will be important. Some parents learn best through self study, others need more direction from the educator.

In any teaching plan for the very young child, a component of behavior management and parenting skills must be included. How to assess the need for discipline and when to begin the child's self-care training must be addressed. Parents need to be given information about what to expect as the child grows, both in terms of predictable changes in diabetes management and in normal child development. Parents should be introduced to the use of positive reinforcement and praise for acceptable behavior and time out for unacceptable behavior.[46,47]

Teaching toddlers and preschoolers about diabetes is difficult since no educational materials are currently available for young children. Diabetes educators and parents need to use play, older children's drawings, cartoons, and story telling to teach about diabetes.[29,53] For example, telling a story about another child who has the same symptoms, fears, and behaviors as does the toddler or preschooler is very helpful. Emphasizing the child did nothing to cause the diabetes and restating that fingersticks and injections are *not punishment* is essential. The story can be repeated often, adding new behaviors and feelings of the child. Also, having preschool children tell the health care professional a story helps reveal their thoughts, feelings, and misperceptions.

Approaching the young child must be done with caution and caring. Young children are fearful of strangers, particularly those dressed in white lab coats. The child should be allowed time to observe and inspect the professional from a safe distance, often while securely in mother's arms. Toddlers and preschool children are also frightened by prolonged eye contact or staring. The professional should avert his or her gaze, talk with the child's toy animal first, and approach the child slowly, unhurriedly, and quietly. Preschool children need to handle equipment to assure themselves that the stethoscope or reflex hammer is not alive. Analogies escape these children. "Taking your blood pressure" or "giving a little stick on your arm" are taken quite literally.

Children should be encouraged to give their doll/stuffed animal injections and fingersticks just before and just after they receive their own. This helps them express their thoughts and feelings and attain mastery and a feeling of control over these situations. It also allows adults to correct any misperceptions or fantasized fears present.

Assessment and Planning

Diabetes in the child less than 2 years old is reported to be increasing in most diabetes centers in the United States and Great Britain. The child may present with gastrointestinal symptoms, dehydration, or some precipitating viral or bacterial infection.[38] Frequently, a random blood glucose result directs the physician to the diagnosis of diabetes. The young child has the potential for rapid dehydration and acidosis.

Management of DKA in the very young child focuses primarily on correcting fluid, electrolyte, and acid-base balance along with insulin replacement. (Management of DICA is addressed in Chapter 8.) Once past the crisis of acidosis, the health team's plans are directed at long-term management centered on the goals of adequate blood glucose control and promotion of normal growth and development. To this end, blood glucose and urine ketone testing, a meal plan, insulin therapy, and an activity plan are established with the parents.

Nutrition

The chief aim of dietary management in this age group is providing sufficient calories and nutrients for normal growth, while limiting the amount of simple sugars. Unlike the adult with diabetes, these children *need* extra calories for impending growth demands.[72,73]

In the case of an infant, demand feeding is allowed with adjustments made to the insulin program. Mothers who are breastfeeding can be assured that, with blood glucose monitoring and use of a short-acting insulin, their babies' blood glucose can be adequately controlled. Once the switch is made to baby foods, a more standard exchange system can be used.[7]

Toddlers are notoriously picky about their foods. Food jags and faddisms are common. At times, they will be ravenous and other times will refuse food altogether. Such behaviors play havoc on diabetes control but can be managed with insulin adjustments. Often a parent will need to give the insulin *after* the child's meal, and in amounts based on food intake. Obviously this is not the ideal approach to good control, but such adaptations are necessary to avoid battles and manipulation by the youngster at meal times.

The preschool child is increasingly able to accommodate to a diabetes exchange plan. It is important that any child less than 6 years old has small frequent meals throughout the day (i.e., three meals and three snacks).[40] Because of limited storage of glycogen, the child cannot safely delay meals or snacks. Snacks such as finger foods (breadsticks and cheese) provide not only needed nutrition but opportunity for fine motor development and independence. Parents may try some creativity in appealing to the young child's appetite. Mixing fruit juice with seltzer and freezing the combination makes a nice alternative to soda pop. Raw vegetables in yogurt dip is an ideal choice for the extra hungry child.

Mealtime battles may be avoided or managed with a reward system of stars or smiley faces.[30] Children should be given no more than 25 minutes to eat a meal and 15 minutes to eat snacks, after which time leftover food is removed. No additional food is given until the next meal, or hypoglycemic symptoms begin. If hypoglycemic symptoms begin, blood glucose is tested and treatment initiated. Five minutes following treatment the child should be reminded that hypoglycemia occurs when he or she doesn't eat most of the food planned for meals or snacks. Since children do not like to feel hungry or "low," these experiences are their best teachers. In contrast, children who become hypoglycemic following excessive activity should be given an extra bread, fruit, or meat. If hypoglycemia occurs 2 to 3 days in a row, parents should call the diabetes professional for a meal plan/insulin adjustment.

Monitoring Blood Glucose Levels

Self-monitoring of blood glucose has afforded the parents of infants and very young children a practical and expedient means of evaluating effects of the management plan.[13] Typical sites for testing include fingertips, earlobes, toes, and outer aspect of the heel. With such small surface areas available, the parents will need to rotate puncture sites and carefully observe the areas for any skin breakdown or infection. Parents should be cautioned about using the central portion of the heel because repeated punctures in that site may be associated with osteomyelitis. The formation of callouses following continual use may decrease discomfort.

As with injections, parents must be quick, reassuring, and calm to gain the child's confidence. As the child becomes old enough to actively participate, the parent can begin to offer choices (e.g., which finger, do you want to push the button, help hold the strip). Fingersticks can be completed at the kitchen table or in the living room while the child is distracted (e.g., sitting on the couch watching cartoons). Even 2-year-olds like to wash their hands, unwrap and hold the bandage, and select the finger to be used this time. Most 3- and 4-year-olds like to do the fingerstick by themselves (with parents right there). It seems to hurt less and provides them a sense of accomplishment and control.

Blood glucose methods should be chosen that operate with accuracy using small amounts of blood.

Exercise

While there is no question that exercise is an important component of the diabetes care plan, it is probably the most inconsistent parameter in the young child. Exercise in the young child is not easy to schedule, nor does the child participate in the same degree each day. For example, once the child begins walking, parents may notice more hypoglycemia and a subsequent need to adjust insulin doses. Because of this, blood glucose monitoring and diet adjustment are essential to assist in adjusting insulin doses. If prolonged or excess activity is anticipated, a decrease in the insulin dose or additional complex carbohydrates (e.g., peanut butter or cheese and crackers) may be required.

Insulin Management

Infants and young children require correspondingly lower doses of insulin than older children or adolescents. This presents unique management challenges. Insulin syringe manufacturers now market syringes measured by 1/2 unit increments with a total of 25 units (Terumo), and Becton-Dickinson produces a 30 unit U-100 syringe. Both are ideal for small doses.

Infants may require very small portions of an insulin unit. In such cases, diluting the insulin to either U-10 or U-25 concentration may be required.[64] Diluting insulin is not ideal because of the extra manipulation in preparing the dose and the potential error in drawing up insulin in a U-100 syringe. Thus, other alternatives should be employed before diluting is selected. If dilution is required, the parent must clearly understand how the conversions are made.

Current insulin therapy suggests that frequent doses will provide a more smooth pattern of glycemic control across the day. Often two mixed doses a day will provide adequate glucose control in the young child. More intensive insulin therapy regimens are available. They use doses of regular insulin before meals and an intermediate insulin at bedtime or with the evening meal and allow the parent or physician to make rapid adjustments as appetite and activity levels change. However, the parent and diabetes team members must consider the ideal management against the most practical and reasonable protocol for the young child.

Because the child is smaller, insulin injection sites are, of course, limited. Thighs, arms, and upper buttocks are generally acceptable. The abdomen is acceptable when sufficient subcutaneous tissue is present. Parents must be taught ways to hold the child comfortably while giving the injection.

The child's attitude about injections closely approximates the parents' responses.[22] Parents should be encouraged to approach the procedure in a matter-of-fact manner, quickly preparing and giving the injection, with plenty of hugs and reassurances afterward. Parents often find it helps to give preschoolers stickers for holding still and then going to the park or playing a favorite game when five stickers are earned. Pleading and negotiating with the struggling toddler or preschooler is futile and accelerates both the child's and the parent's stress levels.

Unless the parent has personally experienced an injection, he or she may believe that there is a great deal of pain inflicted on the child. Simulated injections (with an empty insulin syringe or with saline) are potent teaching aids for frightened parents. Many parents will appreciate the opportunity to practice on themselves and each other, gaining confidence and skill before giving the child an injection.

For the child who continues to be anxious about injections, therapeutic play with syringes and dolls is beneficial. Extreme behavioral responses may require the expertise of a behavioral specialist.

Several "jet" injector devices are on the market. These needleless injectors operate under high-pressure air blasts that propel the insulin under the skin. Although seemingly a wonderful idea for small children, pressure settings that are not properly adjusted result in bruising or painful "injections." In addition, the cost of these devices ($500 to $700) are prohibitive for many.

Schedules

Despite careful planning, the parent will often find that the child will not always eat or sleep on schedule and will not always be cooperative with testing and injections. Parents need guidance in knowing which aspects of care cannot be changed and which areas of care can be more flexible. For example, there is no question that the child must have insulin several times each day. It may be possible, however, to establish a standard routine for weekdays with a more flexible schedule for weekends. Any alterations in the treatment plan must be carefully monitored with blood glucose checks to determine the effect.

Naps should be preceded by a snack. Parents will feel more confident and safe if they observe the sleeping child once or twice during the sleep hours, checking for external symptoms of hypoglycemia such as sweating or restless sleep. Silent nocturnal hypoglycemia occurs between 1 and 3 AM rather frequently, especially if the blood glucose is less than 120 mg/dL at bedtime.[65] If the bedtime blood glucose is less than 120 or if the child has had excess vigorous exercise during the late afternoon or early evening, parents may need to double the amount of protein in the bedtime snack and check the blood glucose again at 2 AM.[65] The evening intermediate insulin may need to be decreased if blood glucose is consistently low over three to five nights.

Nighttime hyperglycemia is often detected because of extra wet diapers, enuresis, or frequent trips to the bathroom during the night. If nighttime hyperglycemia occurs more than three of five nights, the evening intermediate insulin (NPH or Lente) may need to be increased.

Children who awake with ketones may be "running out of insulin" overnight and may require dosage adjustments. This most commonly occurs in children after the honeymoon period, in those with frequent nocturnal hyperglycemia, and during rapid growth spurts.

Management of Acute Problems

Hypoglycemia

As noted earlier, hypoglycemia is often difficult to detect in the preverbal child. Subtle symptoms such as sleepiness, change in personality, fussiness, sweating, pallor, and dilated pupils are typically all that clues a parent to problems.[4]

Hypoglycemia is most likely to occur around the peak action of insulin or following excessive activity. In the case of infants who receive a morning dose of intermediate insulin, for example, peak action may occur at nap time. Parents should be made aware of the subtle changes that indicate hypoglycemia in a sleeping infant, and taught to establish a pattern of blood glucose monitoring that will help to avoid such problems.

Managing hypoglycemia in an infant or small child is no different, in concept, than handling hypoglycemia in an older child or adult. The object is to provide an adequate glucose source to raise blood glucose. Two teaspoons of most table syrups, molasses, corn syrup, or jelly are effective treatments. Infants can be fed regular cola or sugar water from the bottle. Honey should generally be avoided in infants because of recent reports of associated infant botulism.

Parents may carry a tube of cake-decorating frosting (in the child's favorite color or flavor) and a can of apple juice in the glove compartment of the car at all times in case of traffic delays. Parents may need to use the same word ("low," "funny," "need sugar") each time hypoglycemia occurs so the child learns to associate the feelings with the term.

All parents should be taught how and when to administer glucagon. Glucagon is used whenever the child passes out or has a seizure or in situations in which oral treatment would be dangerous. For preschool children, 1/3 to 1/2 vial (0.3 mg to 0.5 mg) is recommended, with dilution required immediately before intramuscular administration. If blood glucose does not improve in 15 minutes, more aggressive treatment may be required by emergency medical personnel. All such episodes should also be reported immediately to the diabetes team.

Illnesses and infection

The effect of illness on diabetes control in the infant or toddler can be variable. Some children will experience a drop in blood glucose level, especially during the initial illness onset. Others will exhibit a rise in blood glucose associated with the release of counter-regulatory hormones during illness. As previously noted, routine immunizations may also result in variations of blood glucose.

Guidelines for sick day management are addressed in Chapter 2. For children, these guidelines include the following: (1) Monitor blood glucose and urine ketones every 2 to 3 hours. Placing cotton balls in the infant's diaper to absorb urine is one method of monitoring ketones. Using urine collection bags may be discouraged because of possible damage to the child's skin with repeated use. (2) Ill children with IDDM need insulin, and usually will require more than the usual dose. Parents should call the diabetes team whenever the child is ill for adjustment of insulin doses. (3) If hyperglycemia or ketones are present, give the child 4 to 8 ounces of fluid hourly (depending on the child's age and size) for 2 to 3 hours and retest. If blood glucose and ketones remain the same or increase, call the diabetes team for insulin dose adjustment. (4) If the child has diarrhea or vomits, omit solid foods and give only clear liquids for the next 4 to 8 hours. (5) Call the diabetes physician immediately if the child vomits more than once in a 4- to 6-hour period or if he or she refuses fluids.[7,30,64]

IMPLEMENTATION AND EVALUATION
Self-Management

Choices are important for the developing child's growing independence and sense of self. Parents can foster this developmental need even in the arena of diabetes care. As previously discussed, the young child can gather the supplies for testing, pick a finger for sticking, press the button on the meter, or compare the color on the strip with the chart. Even before recognizing numbers, preschool children could color in a block on a record sheet to match the color of the glucose strip.

Offering choices at meal time is equally important. Allowing the child to choose between two starch groups or to select which sugar-free drink he or she would like all contribute to the child's need to master his or her environment.

While there may not seem to be many choices in the area of injections, some options can be offered. The preschool child can select which of two sites to use, can wipe the site with alcohol, and can even push the plunger in after the parent injects. Each small step in this process moves the child closer to self-care.

The very young child will not be able to formulate words to describe symptoms. Parents can foster this language development by identifying symptoms and using simple words to describe the sensations. For example, "You look shaky—shaky means you need sugar." Explaining other aspects of care are also useful. For instance: "It's time for your insulin. Insulin keeps you healthy." Such an explanation reminds the child that this is a part of daily life.

Role of the Diabetes Health Care Team

The health care team serves the family in various ways. From initial diagnosis and training to long-term follow-up and support, the physician, nurse, and dietitian provide a core group of professionals. Reaching a team member quickly at any time of the day provides immense support and reassurance. Parents need diabetes professionals versed in well-child needs and who are willing to collaborate with the pediatrician or family physician as needed. In addition, parents may benefit most from a single, continuously available team member who can provide ongoing support and expertise.[3]

The diabetes professional working with children must keep current with resources available to families and provide case management and referral services.

The diabetes team is also responsible for offering follow-up assessments. Infants, toddlers, and preschoolers should be evaluated at least every 3 months (Table 11-6). A typical visit should include height and weight assessments, blood glucose and glycated hemoglobin levels, and review of current management, symptoms, and blood glucose levels. Additionally, adjustments to the meal plan are warranted during periods of rapid growth.

Many families are unable to access an interdisciplinary team and must rely on diabetes care and supervision from their pediatrician or family practice physician. Because of the complexity of the disorder, involvement with a team is preferred and often necessary. However, the pediatrician can establish a "quasiteam" within his or her community. Working with public health department nurses, dietitians, and social workers is one avenue.[21] In addition, many communities now provide diabetes classes and diabetes educators in the local hospitals and clinics. Networking with these individuals provides a valuable source of information and support to families followed by a primary care physician.

Role of the Family

Because diabetes is a disease requiring daily and, sometimes, hourly adjustment and management, the family becomes the ongoing provider of care. Parents are expected to assume this task and participate in this decision-making.

Outcome Evaluation

If the diabetes team and the parents have accomplished their goals, several factors will be apparent. First, the child and parents will have established a comfortable system of managing diabetes. This is not to say that all anxieties and misbehavior will abate. Rather, the

Table 11-6 Suggested Diabetes Care and Follow-Up for Children

	First year of diabetes						Routine diabetes care after first year				Comments
	Diagnosis	6 weeks	3 months	6 months	9 months	1 year	3 months	6 months	9 months	12 months	
Primary physician	X					X				X	More often as needed
Core diabetes team											
Diabetes physician		X	X	X		X	X	X		X	
Diabetes nurse		X	X	X		X	X	X	X	X	
Diabetes dietitian		X	X	X	X	X		X	X	X	
Diabetes consultant team											
Ophthalmologist						X				X	Every 5 years until puberty, then yearly
Dentist						X				X	
Podiatrist		As needed or referred									
Diabetes counselor		As needed or referred									
Laboratory studies											
Glycated hemoglobin (Hgb A$_{1c}$)	X		X	X	X	X	X	X	X	X	Every 3 months
Urine for microalbumin	X					X				X	Yearly
Urine for culture (females)	X					X				X	Yearly
Thyroid studies	X					X					Optional: yearly
Lipid studies	X					X				X	Yearly (cholesterol, triglycerides)
Serum creatinine										X	Yearly starting at 5 years' duration at puberty

Developed by Children's Diabetes Management Center, Galveston 1991, University of Texas Medical Branch.
Home testing: blood glucose testing—2 to 8 times per day. Minimum: 14 tests per week.
urine ketone testing—whenever blood glucose is 240 mg/dL or more, and during illness.

family will find a schedule and a routine that is no longer disruptive to the overall needs of the family.

Second, the child will be developing normally, both physically and emotionally. Growth will occur as expected and typical infant, toddler, or preschool behaviors will be apparent. The child will achieve normal developmental milestones.

Another outcome is related to metabolic control. Blood glucose and glycosylated hemoglobin levels should reach acceptable ranges, with few extremes of severe hypoglycemia or ketosis.

Finally, parents will have developed a realistic plan for encouraging the child's growing involvement in self-care. Parental expectations for the child participating in care should be consistent with normal maturation patterns.

In summary, the infant, toddler, and preschool child with diabetes present several management challenges. The ideal approach to diabetes management in the young child must often be balanced against the practical and realistic. Managed with sensitivity by knowledgeable caregivers, the young child with diabetes has every opportunity to grow physically and emotionally healthy.

REFERENCES

1. American Academy of Pediatrics Committee on Early Childhood, Adoption and Dependent Care: Health in day care: a manual for health professionals, Elk Grove Village, IL, 1987, American Academy of Pediatricians.
2. Anders TF, Carskadon MA, and Dement WC: Sleep and sleepiness in children and adolescents, Pediatr Clin North Am 27:29-43, 1980.
3. Anderson B: The impact of diabetes on the developmental tasks of childhood and adolescence: a research perspective. In Natrass M and Santiago J, eds: Recent advances in diabetes, London, 1984, Churchill and Livingston.
4. Arky R: Nutrition therapy for the child and adolescent with type I diabetes mellitus, Pediatr Clin North Am 31:711-719, 1984.
5. Axline V: Play Therapy, Boston, 1947, Houghton-Mifflin.
6. Bank S and Kahn M: The sibling bond, New York, 1982, Basic Books, Inc.
7. Benz M and Kohler E: Baby food exchanges and feeding the diabetic infant, Diabetes Care 3:554, 1982.
8. Betz C and Poster E: Communicating with children: more than just words, Paedovita 1:11-16, 1984.
9. Bibace R and Walsh M: Development of children's concepts of their illness, Pediatrics 69:355-362, 1980.
10. Brambilla P, and others: Glucose counterregulation in pre–school-age diabeteic children with recurrent hypoglycemia during conventional treatment, Diabetes 36:300-304, 1987.
11. Brazelton T: Stress for families today, Infant Ment Health J 9:65-71, 1988.
12. Brewster A: Chronically ill hospitalized children's concepts of their illness, Pediatrics 69:355-362, 1982.
13. Brouhard B: Management of the very young diabetic, Am J Dis Child 139:446-447, 1985.
14. Bryant J and Anderson D: Children's understanding of television, New York, 1983, Academic Press.
15. Burr C: Impact on the family of a chronically ill child. In Hobbs N and Perrin J, eds: Issues in the care of children with chronic illness, San Francisco, 1985, Jossey-Bass.
16. Caplan F and Caplan T: The power of play, Garden City, NY, 1974, Anchor Press.
17. Chase HP and others: Hypoglycemia and brain development, Pediatrics 52:513-520, 1973.
18. Chess S and Thomas A: Temperamental differences: a critical concept in child health care, Pediatr Nurs 11:167-171, 1985.
19. Clarke W, Haymond M, and Santiago J: Overnight basal insulin requirements in fasting insulin-dependent diabetics, Diabetes 29:78-80, 1980.
20. Clarke-Stewart A and Friedman S: Child development: infancy through adolescence, New York, 1987, Wiley & Sons, Inc.

21. Drash A and Berlin N: Juvenile diabetes. In Hobbs N and Perrin J, eds: Issues in the care of children with chronic illness, San Francisco, 1985, Jossey-Bass.
22. Ducat L and Cohen S: Diabetes, New York, 1983, Harper & Row.
23. Erikson E: Childhood and society, ed 2, New York, 1959, WW Norton & Co.
24. Ferrari M: The diabetic child and well sibling: risks to the well child's self-concept, J Child Health Care 15:141-148, 1987.
25. Garrison M and McQueston A: Chronic illness during childhood and adolescence, Newbury Park, CA, 1989, Sage Publications.
26. Ginsberg H and Opper S: Piaget's theory of intellectual development: an introduction, Englewood Cliffs, NJ, 1969, Prentice-Hall.
27. Giordano B and Edwards L: Meeting the needs of parents of children with diabetes: a babysitter's course, Diabetes Educ 6:26, 1980.
28. Golden M and others: Management of diabetes mellitus in children younger than 5 years of age, Am J Dis Child 139:448-452, 1985.
29. Hahn K: Therapeutic storytelling: He]ping children learn and cope, Pediatr Nurs 13:175-178, 1987.
30. Hall J and Keltz J: What to do when your child won't eat, Diabet Forecast May-June, 27-29, 1980.
31. Hamill PV and others: Physical growth: Nationa] Center for Health Statistics percentiles, Am J Clin Nutr 32:607-629, 1979.
32. Hauenstein E and others: Stress in parents of children with diabetes mellitus, Diabetes Care 12:18-23, 1989.
33. Holmes C and others: Verbal fluency and naming performance in type I diabetes at different blood glucose concentrations, Diabetes Care 7:454-459, 1984.
34. Holmes C and Richman L: Cognitive profiles of children with insulin-dependent diabetes, Dev Behav Pediatr 6:323-326, 1985.
35. Horan P, Gwynn C, and Renzi D: Insulin-dependent diabetes mellitus and child abuse: is there a relationship? Diabetes Care 9:302-207, 1986.
36. Ilg F and Ames L: Child behavior, New York, 1955, Harper & Row.
37. Jackson R: Growth and maturation of children with insulin-dependent diabetes mellitus, Pediatr Clin North Am 31:545-567, 1984.
38. Jefferson I, and others: Insulin-dependent diabetes in under 5 year olds, Arch Dis Child 60:1144-1148, 1985.
39. Jivani S and Rayner P: Does control influence the growth of diabetic children? Arch Dis Child 48:109-115, 1973.
40. Kinmonth A, Magrath G, and Reckless J: National Subcommittee of the Professional Advisory Committee of the British Diabetic Association, Dietary recommendations for children and adolescents with diabetes, Diabetic Med 6:537-547, 1989.
41. Kushion W, and others: Issues in the care of infants and toddlers with insulin-dependent diabetes mellitus, Diabetes Educ 17:107-110, 1991.
42. Lowenberg M: The development of food patterns in young children. In Pipes PL, ed: Nutrition in infancy and childhood, ed 3, St. Louis, 1985, CV Mosby.
43. Lowrey G: Growth and development of children, Chicago, 1986, Year-Book Medical Publishers.
44. McCollum A: The chronically ill child: a guide for parents and professionals, New Haven, 1975, Yale University Press.
45. McWilliams M: Nutrition for the growing years, ed 4, New York, 1986, Wiley & Sons, Inc.
46. Patterson GR: Families, Champaign, IL, 1979, Research Press.
47. Patterson GR: Living with children, Champaign, IL, 1980, Research Press.
48. Petersen H, and others: Growth, body weight and insulin requirement in diabetic children, Acta Pediatr Scand 67:453-457, 1978.
49. Piaget J: Play, dreams and imitation in childhood, New York, 1962, WW Norton & Co.
50. Piaget J: The construction of reality in the child, New York, 1971, Ballantine.
51. Piaget J: The child's conception of the world, Totowa, NJ, 1976, Littlefield, Adams & Co.
52. Piaget J and Inhelder B: Memory and intelligence, New York, 1973, Basic Books.
53. Pontious S: Communicating with children. In Servowsky J and Opus S, editors: Nursing management of children, Boston, 1987, Jones & Bartlett Publishing Co.
54. Pratt L: Family structure and effective health behavior: the energized family, Boston, 1976, Houghton-Mifflin.

55. Robinson CA: Preschool children's conceptualizations of health and illness, J Child Health Care 16:89-96, 1987.
56. Rovet J and Ehrlich R: Effect of temperament on metabolic control in children with diabetes mellitus, Diabetes Care 11:77-82, 1988.
57. Rovet J, Ehrlich R, and Hoppe M: Behaviour problems in children with diabetes as a function of sex and age of onset of disease, J Child Psychol Psychiatr 28:477-491, 1987.
58. Rovet J, Ehrlich R, and Hoppe M: Intellectual deficits associated with early onset of insulin-dependent diabetes mellitus in children, Diabetes Care 10:510-515, 1987.
59. Rovet J, Ehrlich R, and Hoppe M: Specific intellectual deficits in children with early onset diabetes mellitus, Child Dev 59:226-234, 1988.
60. Ryan C, Vega A, and Drash A: Cognitive deficits in adolescents who developed diabetes early in life, Pediatrics 75:921-927, 1985.
61. Ryan C and others: Deterioration of mental efficiency associated with experimentally induced mild hypoglycemia in children with IDDM, Diabetes 38(suppl 2):8A, 1989.
62. Sahler 0 and McAnarnwy E: The child from three to eighteen, St Louis, 1981, Mosby–Year Book, Inc.
63. Schreiner B and Travis L: When your child has diabetes: the preteen years, Diabet Forecast 40:37-41, 1987.
64. Schreiner B and Travis L: The child less than 3 years old. In Travis L, Brouhard B, and Schreiner B, eds: Diabetes mellitus in children and adolescents, Philadelphia, 1987, WB Saunders Co.
65. Shalwitz R and others: Prevalence and consequences of nocturnal hypoglycemia among conventionally treated children with diabetes mellitus, J Pediatr 116:685-689, 1990.
66. Schroeder DB and others: Cognitive and motor effects during hypoglycemia and recovery, J Am Diabetes Assoc 38(suppl 2):108a, 1989.
67. Simpson 0 and Smith M: Lightening the load for parents of children with diabetes, Matern Child Nurs J 4:293-296, 1979.
68. Singer J and Singer D: Television, imagination and aggression, Hillsdale, NJ, 1981, Erlbaum Associates.
69. Smart M and Smart R: Children: development and relationships, ed 3, New York, 1977, Macmillan Publishing Co.
70. Tanner J, Goldstein H, and Whitehouse R: Standards for children's height at 2-9 years allowing for height of parents, Arch Dis Child 45:755-762, 1970.
71. Tattersall R and Pyke D: Growth in diabetic children, Lancet 2:1105, 1973.
72. Thorp F: Infants and children. In Powers M: Handbook of diabetes nutritional management, Rockville, MD, 1987, Aspen.
73. Travis L, Brouhard B, and Schreiner B: Diabetes mellitus in children and adolescents, Philadelphia, 1987, WB Saunders Co.
74. Vaughan VC and Litt IF: Child and adolescent development: clinical implications, Philadelphia, 1990, WB Saunders Co.
75. Whaley L and Wong D: Nursing care of infants and children, ed 3, St. Louis, 1987, Mosby–Year Book.
76. White N, and others: Identification of type 1 diabetic patients at increased risk for hypoglycemia druing intensive therapy, N Engl J Med 308:485-491, 1983.
77. Wedin B, Topliffe L, and Simonson D: The effect of glycemic control on hypoglycemia-induced neuropsychologic dysfunction in IDDM, Diabetes 38(suppl 2):4A, 1989.
78. Wysocki T and others: Adjustment to diabetes mellitus in preschoolers and their mothers, Diabetes Care 89:524-529, 1989.

CHAPTER 12

Diabetes Mellitus and the School-Age Child

SHARON PONTIOUS AND BARBARA TESNO

Over 1 million, or 1 in every 500 children, have type I or insulin-dependent diabetes mellitus (IDDM). For school-age children with IDDM between the ages of 6 and 11 years, this means they must master the diabetes care regimen while they also master the common developmental tasks of latency, industry, and concrete cognitive operations. This developmental period is characterized by freedom, expansion, and, sometimes, inexhaustible energy that enables children of this age to explore the world beyond the home. They have enough self-confidence to begin new activities and to independently explore ideas and the environment without the need for excessive parental supervision or approval. Throughout this developmental period, the parent's roles diminish while the role of other important adults commonly increases.[116] The school introduces these children to their culture and teaches them how to get along with other people while following societal rules. Significant adults help children learn the various roles and technical skills essential to function as a competent adult.

The purpose of this chapter, then, is to describe how diabetes mellitus influences the normal physical development of the school-age child; describe the impact of diabetes mellitus on the cognitive and language capacity of the school-age child; summarize cognitive problems associated with school-age children; assess normal psychosocial development of the school-age child; identify factors associated with diabetes mellitus that impact psychosocial development; describe the family and child adaptation process associated with a diagnosis of diabetes mellitus; discuss the importance of individualizing treatment goals for the school-age child with diabetes; summarize the content associated with an individualized, developmentally based program; assess issues related to regimen adherence; address the role of the diabetes health care team.

NORMAL PHYSICAL DEVELOPMENT

A description of the general characteristics of children throughout the school-age years is now presented. These characteristics should not be taken as absolute and are meant only to suggest common growth and behavior trends that occur at different ages within the school-age period.

Growth

Children enter the school-age period with a body type and a linear rate of growth of 5 to 7 cm/year that they maintain until the changes of puberty begin—10 to 12 years for girls and 12 to 14 years for boys. Children grow approximately 6 to 7 cm (2.5 to 3 inches) in height and gain 2 to 3.5 kg (5 to 7 pounds) in weight each year until puberty. It is important for parents, teachers, and physicians to accept that, in general, short children remain short and thin ones thin. Over the last 3 decades, it has become apparent that the secular trend of constantly increasing size of successive generations of American children has ended. Black and white children have been found to be of essentially the same height.[77] Thus, the parent's height and weight is a major predictor of their children's ultimate height and weight.

Disproportionate growth of the lower extremities during early and middle childhood gives them a taller and thinner appearance. However, boney epiphyses are largely cartilaginous and soft in early childhood. Thus, physical activities for the school-age child should be supervised to avoid bone or joint injuries. Rapidly growing children often complain of knee pains that can be increased by overexertion or injury.[10] These pains are usually not significant if they occur late in the day or night and disappear in the morning, but children with persistent leg pains should be referred to a physician.[116] Facial bones grow faster than the skull because over 90% of brain growth occurs by age 6.[10]

Overall, school-age children look slimmer, more graceful, and better coordinated than the pre-schooler. Their posture improves and their legs are longer. Movements are more skilled and precise.

Eighty percent of the height and weight measurements of children at a given age are expected to fall between the tenth and ninetieth percentiles of the National Center for Health Statistics' anthropometric charts. Children with height and weight measurements that fall in markedly different percentile groups, as well as those who shift by more than 25 percentiles or fall near to or outside the fifth and ninety-fifth percentiles, need to be referred for potential growth abnormalities.

Motor Coordination

During the school-age period, fine motor coordination improves greatly, as do writing and printing skills. Children now enjoy writing plays and stories and developing artistic talents such as drawing, ceramics, and macrame.

Children learn to refine their gross motor skills by practicing sports and games. Exercise is required for muscle development and tone, refinement of balance and coordination, gaining strength and endurance, and maintaining normal weight.[113] Exercise is especially important for children with IDDM. It increases insulin sensitivity and decreases insulin requirements and has beneficial effects on blood pressure, blood lipids, and emotional status.[47] During this period children's muscular strength doubles so they can play increasingly strenuous games for longer time periods. It is essential that all school-age children adhere to the following guidelines for sports: proper physical conditioning, proper grouping according to body size, skill, and maturation, good protective equipment, periodic health appraisals, and availability of an experienced health professional during games and practice sessions. Noncontact sports such as swimming, gymnastics, track and field, martial arts, tennis, and skating are recommended for 6- to 7-year olds. Later, they can add basketball, volleyball, soccer, and wrestling. Some authorities recommend that collision sports such as football, rugby, and hockey be delayed until age 11.[84]

IMPACT OF DIABETES ON PHYSICAL DEVELOPMENT

IDDM has the highest incidence of all serious, life-threatening diseases of children in the United States.[71] Approximately 120,000 young people in the United States, [70] or 1 in every 500 children, will develop IDDM by the end of high school. The non–age-adjusted mortality rate associated with IDDM is at least four times greater than that for non–insulin-dependent diabetes mellitus (NIDDM). Patients with IDDM also develop retinopathy, neuropathy, and renal disease earlier and in more severe forms than those with NIDDM. Thus, IDDM is likely the most important and costly chronic illness affecting children in the U.S.[88]

IDDM can affect the normal physical development of school-age children in three ways: (1) stunted growth in those very poorly controlled, (2) delayed puberty, and (3) enhanced risk for development of early retinopathy, nephropathy, or neuropathy, particularly during adolescence.[1,77,105]

Growth Rate and Height at Diagnosis

Drayer,[37] in a study of 62 children with diabetes, found 4- to 9-year-old boys with IDDM, but not girls, were significantly taller than control subjects. The mid-parent height or parental age of the children with IDDM was not significantly different from that of the controls. A more recent study of a population of 200 newly diagnosed children, 187 nondiabetic siblings and 169 parents at the University of Pittsburgh confirmed and extended these findings. They found 5- to 9-year-old children with IDDM were consistently taller than the national average, as were their nondiabetic siblings. Children positive for islet cell antibodies were taller than those without these antibodies.[77] The cause of this increased height is not known and is difficult to reconcile with other studies indicating that monozygotic twins with diabetes are shorter at diagnosis than their unaffected twins at diagnosis.

Growth Failure

Diabetic dwarfs were common when insulin treatment of IDDM was first begun. The growth failure was clearly related to an inadequate amount of insulin and a negative nitrogen and carbohydrate balance. It was frequently associated with Mauriac syndrome, which also includes truncal obesity, round facies, delayed puberty, and an enlarged fatty liver. Growth failure, alone or with other associated physical findings of Mauriac syndrome, is still seen sporadically today, primarily in those children who consistently fail to administer all their prescribed insulin or who falsify their blood glucose records for various reasons and are in poor metabolic control.[2,75]

More recently, a number of studies have found children with IDDM are statistically likely to be shorter than their initial genetic make-up would have suggested.[77,108] To date, there is no evidence to suggest that children with IDDM are more likely to be obese nor, if they are, that obesity leads to the development of IDDM.[1] It is currently unclear whether or not children in good metabolic control, as measured by glycated hemoglobin, attain their full growth potential.[77,93] Conflicting data also exist regarding whether delayed puberty or an abnormal growth spurt exists today for children who are in moderate or good-to-average metabolic control.[23,27,102,107] It does seem that girls with average or good metabolic control no longer have pubertal or menarcheal delay. It is now clear that children with IDDM who are in poor metabolic control with glycated hemoglobin values indicating average blood glucose values greater than 240, have inadequate weight gain, poor growth, delayed pubertal onset and menarche, and decreased peak pubertal height velocity.[77,86]

Children with IDDM who are in poor metabolic control most often have insulin deficiency. This prevents the appropriate maintenance of a positive nitrogen balance that may be responsible for some of the growth failure observed. In addition, glycosuria leads to urinary loss of minerals and loss of normal vitamin homeostasis. Specifically, a zinc deficiency has been associated with poor growth and delayed puberty.[20] Hypercalcuria and hyperphosphaturia was noted in children with IDDM and correlated closely with reduced height.[83] Two other autoimmune disorders that are found more frequently in IDDM, chronic lymphocytic thyroiditis and Addison's disease, may also be associated with growth failure or poor weight gain, respectively. Hashimotos thyroiditis may occur in as many as 20% of the white and 5% of the black children with IDDM.[86] The most common findings are an elevated thyroid-stimulating hormone (TSH) value in serum and a modest goiter.

Physiologic growth hormone peaks have been found to be more pronounced in children with IDDM. Normal stimuli of growth hormone release (i.e., exercise, glucagon, arginine, and falling blood glucose levels) also lead to an exaggerated release of growth hormone. However, all of these abnormal responses of growth hormone release can be normalized by good control of the blood glucose. On the other hand, the somatomedin C (also known as insulin-like growth factor or IGF-l) levels tend to be lower than normal and negatively correlate with glycohemoglobin.[77] The lower somatomedin C levels may be responsible for poor growth in poorly controlled IDDM.

Diabetes-Related Health Complications

Consistently higher levels of plasma glucose place affected children at a higher risk for the development of specific diabetes-related health complications.[22,55,65,105] As a result, health care providers emphasize the importance of maintaining a glycated hemoglobin of 9% or less and mean blood glucoses below 200 mg/dL, to lessen children's risk of developing dangerous health problems such as retinopathy, neuropathy, and renal disease. The presence of limited joint mobility of the metacarpophalangeal and interphalangeal joints is common, is associated with children's level of glycemic control, and increases the risk of microvascular complications.[86]

Maintaining adequate glycemic levels is a very difficult task for most school-age children and their families. It requires frequent insulin dose adjustments, because insulin replacement regimens rarely duplicate normal patterns and are hard to replicate because of erratic patterns of absorption of injected insulin. Some degree of individual differences in insulin sensitivity/resistance and the degree to which catecholamines (epinephrine and norepinephrine), glucagon, cortisol, and growth hormone are secreted contribute to problems with glycemic control among young persons.[15,26,92,121] Thus, frequent and substantial adjustment in the insulin requirements of prepubertal, and especially of pubertal youth, are essential to maintain acceptable levels of glycemia.[14,83] School-age children typically receive 0.5 to 1 unit of insulin per kilogram of body weight per day with two thirds of their total insulin dose given before breakfast and one third before supper. However, during illness and growth spurts, especially the pubertal growth spurt, these same children often require as much as 1.5 units or more of insulin per kilogram.[2] It is essential that children and their parents learn when and how to change the insulin doses and that insulin requirements change with amount of food, growth, activity, illness, and stress as well as other factors such as erratic absorption. Insulin doses are generally adjusted by 0.5 to 2 units per type of insulin or by no more than 10% of the total insulin per day.

Physical Examination

The physical examination of children with IDDM must include an evaluation of growth and screening for early development of micro- and macrovascular complications. Evaluation of growth includes recording accurate measurements of the height and weight of children every 3 to 4 months and plotting on the standardized weight and height charts. Blood pressure should be plotted on age- and sex-standardized curves. Determining the specific Tanner stage is important because the pubertal growth spurt routinely requires an increase of 20% to 50% in insulin doses as well as an increase in food.[15,107] Children with poor growth or abnormal weight should be evaluated for meal plan adherence, insulin deficiency, or autoimmune diseases such as celiac syndrome and Addison's disease. If children have a goiter, they should be evaluated for hypothyroldism. Finally, children should be screened for the presence of limited joint mobility by having them place their hands in the prayer position. If limited joint mobility is present, children should be carefully examined for the presence of retinopathy, nephropathy, and neuropathy.[77,93]

Nutrition

Caloric, protein, vitamin A, carbohydrate, and calcium needs increase slowly and steadily during the school-age years. A rule of thumb is that children need 1000 plus 100 calories for each year of age up to puberty; thus, they require between 1600 to 3000 calories, depending on their activity levels. Maintenance of the basal metabolism of the school-age child uses approximately 50% of the caloric intake.[116]

The school-age child usually eats well and has fewer food fads. Children 9 years of age or less need to eat every 2½ to 3 hours; children between 9 to 12 years need to eat every 3 to 3½ hours.[106] Midmorning snacks are thus often discontinued in children after age 9. Meals and snacks should be spaced appropriately to counterbalance peaks of insulin actions.

Breakfast is an especially important meal for the 6- to 11-year old. Children who eat a well-balanced breakfast may perform better academically than those who do not.[110] Because of their desire not to be viewed as different from peers, lunch preferences are often based on whether friends take lunch to school or eat in the school cafeteria. In addition, children often eat as fast as possible to be able to go outside and be with their friends. Thus, variable amounts of well-planned lunches are often not eaten, posing potential problems for children with IDDM.

School-age children want and need snacks. The 6- to 8-year old benefits from a midmorning snack of milk and or juice. Most children want after-school snacks. These snacks can help make up for the lack of food consumed at lunch. Snacks eaten more than an hour before meals do not usually decrease the child's food intake at mealtimes. Acceptable nutritious snacks include milk, cheese, fresh fruits and vegetables, raisins, peanut butter, unsugared nuts, yogurt, and fruit juices.

Dietary adherence is the most difficult part of the diabetes regimen.* The overall nutritional requirements for a child with well controlled IDDM are essentially the same as those for the same age child without diabetes. The main difference is that meals should be consumed at similar times and should have similar protein, carbohydrate, and fat distributions from one day to another so that the insulin needs are more predictable. The goals for nutritional management of IDDM in childhood include: promoting normal growth, enabling and encouraging normal physical activity for age, and maintenance of acceptable blood glucose levels.[66]

Children weighing 20 to 70 kilograms need 1500 calories plus 20 calories per kilogram of body weight; the distribution of these calories varies slightly. The American Diabetes Association recommends between 50% and 65% of the calories be from carbohydrates (of which 70% are from complex carbohydrates), 12% to 20% from protein, and less than 30% from fat.[18] The recommended daily intake of protein is 0.8 g per kilogram of body weight and of fiber is 35 to 40 g per day. Intake of highly refined sugars or simple carbohydrates should be minimized because they tend to exaggerate glucose incre-

---

*References 3, 4, 18, 32, 42, 81.

ments after meals. In general, 20% of the total calorie intake is at breakfast, 20% at lunch, and 30% at supper, leaving 10% each for morning, midafternoon, and bedtime snack. In older school-age children (9 years and older), the midmorning snack is omitted and the calories at lunch increased to 30%.

Meal plans are designed to take into account the consistency, timing, composition, and caloric content of foods ingested and physical activity, age, sex, and pubertal status.[18] The keys to successful adherence to meal plans are to allow flexibility and to require as few major changes as reasonable. However, meal plans must take into consideration the pharmacokinetics of previously injected insulin and the need to consume adequate food to prevent hypoglycemia with exercise.[42] The experienced dietitian commonly evaluates the current eating patterns, preferences, and nutritional needs of children before negotiating an acceptable meal plan with them and their families.

Maintaining a consistent eating pattern is the most difficult behavioral task for families of children with IDDM.[18] Children who lack predictable daily eating and activity patterns have the greatest difficulty maintaining adequate blood glucose control. Younger children do not possess the cognitive knowledge and skills required for good dietary adherence. [32,82,95]

Both children and their parents have common and substantial dietary knowledge and skills deficits. Research found that on the average, only 54% of the meal plan was accurately recalled, with particularly poor recall of afternoon (40%) and bedtime snacks (42%).[32,66,67] Even more impressive was the poor performance (50% or less) of both children and mothers when asked to estimate amounts and identify their exchange groups for 20 food models of common foods. Younger children and mothers of older children were the worst at estimating amounts of foods. Underestimation errors were found for meats and fruits, while overestimation errors were found for fats.

Over one third of the children in one study reported problems with adhering to their meal plan.[32] These problems occurred most often for the afternoon snack, while at school or in restaurants, and when with their friends. Children with poor adherence at school and while with their friends were more likely to have worse metabolic control. Thus, health care providers' expectation that children and their parents adhere strictly to any prescribed meal plan is not only incorrect but unrealistic.

Dietary knowledge and skills can be enhanced through the use of behavioral rehearsal, problem-solving, role playing, and supervised practice. Demonstrating how to substitute some of the popular "teenage," "snack," or "junk" foods for appropriate bread and fruit exchanges is extremely helpful. Teaching children self-management strategies for coping with urges while alone at home, especially for the afternoon and bedtime snacks, and for coping with temptation and peer pressure while with friends at school or in restaurants is also very helpful.

Self-monitoring of blood glucose (SMBG) values can be used to demonstrate the effects of various foods on the blood glucose after eating. This is a superb way of demonstrating to children the effects foods have on blood glucose. This also may assist children to feel that controlling what they eat really does affect their blood glucose control.[18]

Parents should avoid getting into power struggles with their child over food. Maintaining an open attitude in which "dietary indiscretions" are openly acknowledged and conditionally accepted by all parties concerned is crucial. Children who can discuss situations in an honest dialogue with family and health care team members can be helped to problem solve preplanned eating deviations by increasing activity or insulin.[118] The family that allows some members to consume forbidden foods in front of children probably contributes to the child's dietary indiscretions.[18] It is not surprising that children with IDDM who feel different from, or not adequately supported by their family and peers "act out" through dietary or insulin administration noncompliance.

Exercise

Regular strenuous exercise by children with IDDM increases insulin sensitivity and lowers insulin requirements. However, hypoglycemia may occur immediately after strenuous activity (up to 24 hours after) if moderately severe exercise is prolonged for several hours.[47] Snacks eaten just before, during, or just after strenuous activity are helpful in preventing hypoglycemia. Foods such as fruit, crackers with cheese or peanut butter, and/or milk are often recommended for prevention or treatment of hypoglycemic episodes. In addition, some foods like ice cream may be more acceptable at these times because, despite the high carbohydrate content, they contain sufficient protein, fat, and guar gum (used in processing ice cream) that blunts the rapid absorption of the carbohydrate. Therefore, ice cream is a good choice to counterbalance the immediate carbohydrate need after exercise.

Bedtime snacks

Bedtime snacks are an important part of the meal plan of children with IDDM because they can help prevent the relatively common occurrences (approximately once a week) of often silent early morning hypoglycemia. Nighttime hypoglycemia is sometimes manifested by nightmares, sleep-walking, or sleep-talking and restlessness as well as the common daytime symptoms such as sweating, feeling shaky, sleepy, and/or starving.

During the early morning hours (1 to 3 AM) insulin requirements are lower than at any other time of the day. Since most episodes of hypoglycemia during sleep go undetected, it is not surprising that in some studies over 50% of all episodes of severe hypoglycemia occur during sleep. The best predictor of 1 to 3 AM hypoglycemia is the blood glucose level at bedtime.[104,114] A child who has a bedtime glucose below 120 mg/dL has a 25% chance of a subsequent episode of hypoglycemia at 2 AM. Thus, the bedtime snack can be used to reduce the risks of a 1 to 3 AM hypoglycemia by increasing calorie and protein content.

Children whose bedtime glucose value is less than 120 mg/dl should eat double the usual amount of protein for their bedtime snack to avoid silent nocturnal hypoglycemia between 2 and 4 AM. In addition, if the blood glucose is over 300 mg/dL at bedtime, the carbohydrate portion may be omitted for that bedtime snack, but the protein portion should still be consumed.

Sweeteners

A common concern of most parents is the safety of available nonsugar sweeteners. Recent evidence suggests that the use of alternative sweeteners such as aspartame and saccharin is safe. The Diabetes Task Force Report for the Committee on Nutrition of the American Academy of Pediatrics in 1985 suggested combining alternative sweeteners as a means of limiting their potential toxicity. Aspartame has been found to cause headaches, stomach upsets, and dizziness in a few susceptible people. Its use should be limited in those with phenylketonuria (PKU) since aspartamine is a derivative of phenaylalanine. The total consumption of nutritive sweeteners should be limited to 10% of the total calories.[18,46]

In summary, the nonnutritive alternative sweeteners aspartame and saccharin can be safely used; fructose and sugar alcohols may also be used in limited amounts. However, more expensive food sweetened with fructose or sorbitol have no proven ability to help promote weight loss or improve overall blood glucose control in children with diabetes.[46,47]

OTHER HEALTH CONSIDERATIONS
Physical Injury

School-age children are at high risk for physical injuries. Developmental characteristics that place them at risk include independence, growth in height exceeding muscular growth and coordination, daring and adventurous activities, frequently playing in hazardous places, attempting dangerous feats, confidence often exceeding physical capacity, overdoing, and having a strong need for activity.[113] Children who have an attention deficit disorder and the immature child are at higher risk for injuries. They often attempt dangerous acts to prove themselves worthy of acceptance and improve their status in their peer group.[78,79]

Motor vehicle accidents are the most common cause of accidental injury and death among 6- to 12-year olds. Ninety percent of fatal bicycle injuries are the result of collision with motor vehicles. The rate of bicycle injuries not involving motor vehicles is twice that of teenagers and four times that of preschool children.[43,51] Bicycle injuries are often related to violations of traffic laws or the result of "dashing out." In addition, the peak incidence of child pedestrian fatalities is between the ages of 5 and 9 years.[99]

Teaching and modeling accident prevention activities such as correct pedestrian behavior, use of restraint systems, door lock mechanisms, appropriate passenger seating and behavior, and the use of protective equipment for the more dangerous sports is essential. Children should also be taught to refuse to accept things from, speak to, or ride with strangers.

Children with IDDM must be taught that episodes of hypoglycemia may be increased with strenuous exercise. Most experienced pediatric diabetologists encourage, rather than discourage, normal sports and physical activity. This requires extensive training regarding the causes, recognition, and prompt treatment of exercise-related hypoglycemia. SMBG as well as diet and insulin adjustments before, during, and after sports or strenuous exercise greatly reduces the risks of hypoglycemia.

Infections

School-age children with IDDM who are well controlled are not more likely to become ill than children of this age without IDDM. Chronic hyperglycemia may, however, increase risks of common bacterial and viral infections for children with IDDM because of impaired granulocytic and immune function in debilitated children.

Parents of children with IDDM must check their children's urine for ketones whenever an illness related to a viral or bacterial infection is suspected or they complain of nausea, stomachache, have acetone-smelling breath, have trouble breathing, or develop vomiting or abdominal pain. Regardless of the blood glucose level, the presence of large amounts of ketones in the blood or urine indicates the need for increased insulin.

Children with IDDM who have gastrointestinal upsets or diarrhea are prone to become dehydrated more quickly. When they are vomiting or have abdominal pain, they should be taken off solid foods and given ample fluids to avoid dehydration—8 to 12 ounces every hour until the ketones are negative and the vomiting or diarrhea is resolved. Those who cannot keep liquids down need to be taken to the emergency room or clinic for rehydration until the vomiting resolves. Although hydration with sugar-free fluids is sometimes done for short periods (4 to 8 hours), carbohydrate-containing fluids and insulin are often required to clear the ketones. A common error that sometimes has disastrous consequences is to attempt to correct hyperglycemia with sugar-free fluids and to simultaneously withhold insulin from children who cannot eat or who are vomiting.

Dental Health

Dental health is of particular importance to school-age children because all of the permanent teeth, except wisdom teeth, erupt during this period. Prolonged undernutrition, such as might occur with undiagnosed or poorly controlled IDDM, may delay the eruption of permanent teeth. All children should receive regular preventive dental care and supervision in daily hygienic care. Inadequate dental care results in the most prevalent childhood health problems, dental caries, malocclusion, and peridontal disease.[113]

Children with IDDM have been shown to develop early, severe periodontal disease more often than those without IDDM. Poor removal of food debris allows for the development of caries and periodontal disease from proliferation of acid-forming bacteria and dental plaque. Frequent oral hygiene and dental checkups every 6 months are highly recommended for all school-age children. Note that children with IDDM with extensive dental and periodontal disease often have a worsening of glycemic control as a result of these chronic infections.

Obesity

Obesity commonly begins during middle childhood. A combination of factors contribute to obesity: inactive life-styles with too much time spent watching television, frequent snacking to treat hypoglycemia, physical or emotional stress, lower socioeconomic status, and having obese parents. Overweight children are often teased, ridiculed, and left out of activities, which results in feelings of inferiority, rejection, and isolation. The child then tends to withdraw or act out, which may continue a cycle of rejection and overeating. Overeating becomes the main source of emotional gratification.

The goal for obese children is to allow them to "grow into their weight" by stabilizing their weight rather than encouraging them to lose large amounts of weight over a short time. Parents can help by removing junk foods from the home and having low-calorie snacks and foods instead. Having at least 30 to 60 minutes of strenuous activity every day is essential. Overweight children should be encouraged to take part in group activities such as the Scouts, YMCA or YWCA, and after-school programs.[90] Children with IDDM are taught these same dietary goals as a component of their regimen. Adherence to these goals and scheduled physical activity prove to be of benefit in maintaining appropriate body weight.

Enuresis

Enuresis (bedwetting) is usually nocturnal and occurs in 17% of the children over 5 years of age. Primary enuresis occurs in a child who has never attained a dry period and is usually caused by delayed or incomplete neuromuscular maturation of the bladder. Secondary enuresis, which occurs after a child has been dry for over a year, may be caused by bladder infections, urinary tract infections or structural disorders, major neurologic deficits, nocturnal epilepsy, chronic renal failure, sickle cell disease, diabetes insipidus, or diabetes mellitus. These organic causes must first be ruled out.[113] Parents need reassurance that bedwetting is not willful misbehavior.[35,36] They should know that punishing, shaming, or scolding are useless and harmful.

Children with IDDM can be taught to avoid IDDM-triggered nocturnal enuresis by keeping blood glucose values less than 200 during the night. Children's self-esteem and self-confidence must also be enhanced. They must believe they can help themselves and achieve independent self-control.

YOUNGER SCHOOL-AGE CHILDREN'S NORMAL COGNITIVE AND LANGUAGE DEVELOPMENT
Cognitive Development

During the school-years, intense intellectual and conceptual growth occurs and reasoning becomes more logical. Cognitively, younger school-age children (6- to 8-year olds), are in transition between Piaget's "preoperational" and "concrete" stages (see Table 12-1). These children have learned to (1) seriate, (2) classify by one primary characteristic, (3) realize that numbers and words stand for objects, events, and feelings, (4) perceive common objects and events from others' perspectives, (5) use systematic trial-and-error problem-solving, (6) make judgments based on outcomes to themselves but verbalize the intent behind the actions, and (7) play alone or socially with others.[94,95,97]

Table 12-1 Characteristics of School-age Childrens' Thinking: Transitional and Concrete Stages

Transitional stage (6 to 8-year-olds)	Concrete state (9 to 11-year-olds)
Major task	
Conquest of symbol	*Mastery of classes, quantities, and relations*
Thought is influenced almost completely by the child's own perceptions, personal actions, and experiences. Thinking moves from perceptual illusion and egocentricity (from the child's own viewpoint and in the child's own way) toward the beginning of sociocentricity (socially validated ideas from others' perspectives) and manipulating symbols.	Thought processes are not internalized so that overt actions on objects or experiences are not essential; thought is limited by dependence on reality and past experiences, therefore it is of limited complexity; observation is now accurate (not perceptually bound) and objective.
Perception	**Perception**
Less egocentric, begins to appreciate other person's point of view and feelings although does not comprehend other's viewpoints when there is conflict with own perspective.	View of world is concrete but objective and can encompass a variety of perspectives of others.
Thought	**Thought**
Views world in terms of a combination of own and beginning awareness of others' perspectives. World exists independent of self, but all events still have a purpose.	Animism is now confined to natural phenomena, but loss of animism causes need to cope with concept of death.
Decentering begins: can focus on two or more aspects of an event at the same time; begins to seriate and classify by dominant feature.	The following concepts are mastered. Reversibility: can perform opposite or compensating act to undo first one.
Animism: believes only things that move have consciousness. Words and numbers: begins understanding concepts of number and spatial relations.	Measurement: and use of various measuring devices. Association, combination, negation.
The concept of length, number, amount and distance is attained at the approximate age of 6 to 7 years.	Causality: as different from association or combination.
	Classification and seriation.
	Conservation: mass of an object remains the same even if the form and shape change.
	The following concepts are attained at the approximate ages indicated:
	7 to 8 years
	substance, area, space, mass
	9 to 10 years
	weight, time
	11+ years
	volume, speed (time plus distance), velocity, density

Table 12-1   Characteristics of School-age Childrens' Thinking: Transitional and Concrete Stages—cont'd.

Transitional stage (6 to 8-year-olds)	Concrete state (9 to 11-year-olds)
Reasoning	**Reasoning**
Systematic trial-and-error problem solving and reasoning begins. Judgements still made based on outcomes for self but now verbalizes intent behind actions.	Is concrete: mental experiements are done on things that were actually sensed previously or currently by directly organizing immediately given or remembered data Lacks ability to transfer learnings immediately because the learning is still tied to particular objects and situations. Progresses from inductive reasoning (8 to 11 years) to deductive reasoning (11 years and over) and uses elementary logic. Judges actions by logical effect; separates cause and intent from outcome.
Language	**Language**
Words: represent one or more common names or uses of things; still understands words more generally and less completely than adults; has learned the power of words (words more effective in creating reactions than are actions). Questions: asked now to learn about the "how" of things and to express frustration.	Symbols now truly represent real objects and events as well as those concepts attained so far; structure of language now more important; progresses toward increasingly more sociocentric verbal exchanges, sharing ideas among people.
Play	**Play**
Symbolic: satisfies self needs and means of coping with conscious or unconscious conflicts by transforming what is real into what is wished was real (e.g., via painting, drawing, puppets, plays). Social: plays games where rules are collectively made up so everyone wins and has fun (e.g., hopscotch, jumprope, tag).	Symbolic play continues Collaborative play in groups (detailed rules to maintain equality and mutual respect) progresses toward competition (object is to win after "fair" play).

Perception

Younger school-age children view the world primarily in terms of how they perceive it or how it appears on the outside; thus they are extremely susceptible to perceptual illusion. For example, 10 cars spread out are "more" than 20 cars bunched together. Because of the perceptual illusions, they can easily be tricked into eating or drinking even when they do not want to. For example, bunching foods together on a large plate and giving an ounce of fluid in a round, fat glass looks like a lot less, so the child may eat or drink it.[98]

Thought

Since children are more sociocentric, they can begin to compare their own thoughts and feelings with those of another person. However, if the person's viewpoints conflict with their own, they still cannot comprehend the other's thoughts or feelings. Their thinking is still based on their own past experiences—literal interpretations of words or parts of things they have centered on. Although they are no longer bound by rigid centering, artificialism, or irreversibility, thinking is still colored by their beliefs in animism, absolutism, irreversibility, and magical thinking.[95,98]

Animism

Children of this age think animistically and believe nonliving, moving things have their own consciousness and intention. Cars, computers, machines, and even bicycles are believed to have childlike characteristics. They are heard to say things such as, "The candy machine ate my quarters, it didn't want me to have any."[98]

Absolutism

Absolutism, the belief that things are good or bad, work or don't work, hurt or don't hurt, is still present but now modified. These children say, "the shot hurt but not that long" or, "The nurse hurt me when doing my fingerstick but she didn't mean to." However, they still cannot see the gray areas between right and wrong or good and bad, nor perceive pain or punishment in degrees. Children at this age still believe that if an adult is wrong or has lied about one thing, they are wrong or lie about everything.[39] Thus, it is essential that all health care providers honest with children.

Irreversibility

Irreversibility, the belief that actions or thoughts cannot be undone or compensated for, is present only for those things children have not actually seen changing. For example, they know that an IV is not going to be a permanent part of their arm. However, many still believe that a fingerstick or cut not covered by a bandage may kill a person because losing blood equals death.[98]

Magical Thinking

Children believe their own thoughts or actions influence events outside of their control. For example, a brother, when angry at his sister, wished she would become ill. When he was told she had IDDM, he was certain he had caused it. Many 6- to 8-year-old children newly diagnosed with IDDM are sure they caused it by going outside without their hats or coats or by eating too many sweets. In addition, thinking about their internal body parts or functions, which they cannot touch or see, is primitive, fear-provoking, influenced by fantasy, magical thinking, and absolutism.[97] It is not surprising, therefore, that children under 9 become panicky when the well-meaning physician says their "islet cells don't make insulin and they now need insulin injections," since the children reason they will be getting "shots ιn their eyelids."

Reasoning

Younger school-age children reason inductively, from a particular action or event to a whole group of similar actions or events. For example, children may state, "A nurse sticks me with a needle to help my 'diabetes' so any needle (e.g., straight or safety pin) poking me will help me feel better." Health care providers must show 6- to 8-year-olds how water comes out of the syringe needle so they can reason: "When I push on the syringe, water comes out of the needle, so when I get an injection, medicine goes into my body."[98]

Language

The 6-year-old understands 2500 to 3000 words, carries out commands involving three to four actions, and, to a large extent, comprehends "if," "because," and "why." They receive and give information, take turns in conversation, but still make grammatic errors.[49] From the time children enter school, the extent and precision of their speaking vocabulary and reading skills attained will be the predominant factors that determine their success or failure.[12]

It is essential to remember that younger children (6 to 8 years old) still use many words without understanding their meaning because they are simply imitating what they have heard others say.[39,97] Elkind revealed children's imitation and use of words conceal many limitations of their understanding and thinking. One reason is that they assume words convey their own particular meaning to others because of the egocentrism they still have. Thus, if they make a word up, they think others know its meaning. Another reason is that they have no concept of relativeness, and words are taken extremely literally.[137]

Many terms commonly used to help children understand are actually very fear-provoking. For example, using *bug* for germ when discussing infections conveys the idea of insects crawling around inside their bodies. *Shot* implies a violent, punishing, or aggressive act and instills fears of being severely hurt or killed. *Take* or *test* implies removal of something from the children.[98] The term *diabetes* implies "die-of-betes"; they become very afraid they are going to die of something called "betes" or "beets." Even *glucagon,* the hormone used for low blood glucose emergencies, stimulates the fear that they will be "shot with gluc from a gun."

Moral Development

Younger school-age children are extremely egocentric and behave to avoid punishment and parental disapproval. They are just beginning to use self-control to resist temptation.

Children begin to incorporate the same-sex parent's moral values into their behavior by thinking of these values as precepts, "I must" or "I must not." Thus, their conscience initially is tyrannical and rigid; they apply the rules of right and wrong in a rigid, strict, and absolute manner with no allowances made for extenuating circumstances.[63] This unyielding standard of right and wrong causes children to be very critical or other's behavior and the "unfairness" of uncontrollable events.[116]

Kohlberg found most 6- to 9-year olds were in stage 1, punishment and obedience, or moral reasoning.[63] In this stage, children decide whether or not to break a rule based on the type of physical punishment they anticipate. Parents are viewed as all powerful and rules as being rigid and unbreakable.[41] In essence, they feel no guilt for doing things forbidden; they only wish to avoid punishment. Discipline for children of this age needs to include clear limits, with consistent rewards for good behavior and punishment for bad behavior.

OLDER SCHOOL-AGE CHILDREN'S COGNITIVE AND LANGUAGE DEVELOPMENT
Cognitive Development

Older school-age children, 9 to 11 years old, are in Piaget's concrete stage of cognitive development. The major task for this age is to master concepts of classes, quantities, and relationships. Although the thought processes of these children are now internalized (concrete objects or experiences are not absolutely necessary), their thinking is still limited because of their dependence on reality and the limited number and quality of their past experiences.[94,95]

Thought

Older school-age children can use symbols to organize their ideas and manipulate the world around them. They can experience an event without touching or seeing it.[116] The 9- to 11-year-old now can think about the present, the past, and to some extent, the future. Because they can perceive objects and events more objectively, they can correct some perceptual distortions and illusions. However, their thought is still less complex and flexible than that of adults (see Table 12-1). The most important concepts needed to understand children of this age are described below.

Animism

The 9- to 11-year-old believes in animism only for natural events like tornadoes, hurricanes, and earthquakes. When they lose their animistic belief that objects have intention, they now must deal with what death is. They begin asking many questions about death, such as; "Where do people who die go?" "What happens to your body when you die?" and "Will I die of diabetes?"[98]

Reversibility

Older children now comprehend the concept of reversibility—that an act can be undone by performing an opposite act or compensated for by other behaviors. They understand a person who feels ill today can feel good tomorrow. In addition, they perceive thoughts, actions, and events from another's point of view.[98]

Conservation

Older school-age children understand conservation—things are the same even when their form and shape change. They now know that the amount of water in a tall, thin glass is the same when poured into a short, fat glass and that the amount of clay in two equal balls is the same even when the shape of the balls is changed.

Relationships

Older children seriate and classify things by many characteristics simultaneously (e.g., color, size, weight, and number). This, along with reversibility, measurement, and conservation, allows them to comprehend relations and degrees of things such as "hurting a little bit."

Reasoning

Older school-age children can do experiments in their minds instead of requiring the concrete manipulation of objects. But they cannot transfer what they learned from one situation to another because they still need actual data to organize and manipulate. They begin to reason deductively, from groups of experiences to a particular experience.[94] For example, "The nurse says injections hurt less if muscles are relaxed, so if I relax the muscles in my leg, this insulin shot will not hurt as much." They can also separate consequences to them from the causes and intentions, "Mom hurt me when she gave my insulin shot but I need the insulin and she didn't want to hurt me."

Health care providers should determine whether school-age children are in the transition phase or concrete cognitive development stages to know what words and terms are appropriate to use in teaching them.[98] For learning to occur, those in the transitional phase need multisensory teaching techniques and careful use of words and avoiding homonyms and synonyms that may cause misinterpretation of information.[111] Those in the concrete stage develop fearful misperceptions less often when only pictures or concrete teaching materials are used.

Coping Mechanisms

School-age children use a variety of defense mechanisms to cope with feelings of anxiety or inadequacy. Extreme independence is usually expressed in relation to denial of fears. They display the greatest amount of bravado when they are feeling the most helpless. They use compulsive rituals or "magic incantations" to defend themselves from anxiety related to aggression. They believe these expressions of their new awareness of death prevents something happening to them or to their loved ones.[98]

Language

Words and other symbols now represent real objects, actual actions, and experiences. Jokes that play on words are especially appreciated. Because the structure of language is becoming important, children enjoy arguing and trying to stump adults with jokes that have multiple meanings, depending on the way one structures the sentence.[98] For example, "What animals can jump as high as a tree? Answer: All animals because trees can't jump." Language is now used to truly share ideas, communicate thoughts, and to learn others' perspectives.[48]

Moral Development

The majority of children aged 10 to 12 recognize the intent of laws and consequences of disobeying them, but typically obey only to avoid personal discomfort. In essence, they believe rules should be followed and will try to bargain with others to get those rules and laws to meet their own needs. Children of this age have no true understanding of abstract concepts such as fairness, loyalty, or laws.[115,116]

Discipline

Adults must establish consistent rules and discuss the issues involved in setting each of the rules. Punishment must be consistent, immediate, and appropriate to the nature of the misdeed. Experiencing the natural or logical consequences for actions is helpful. Children must understand what distinguishes right from wrong and the rationale for any punishment. They must understand that they are punished for the misdeeds done, not because they are not liked as a person.

Lying and Cheating

Kohberg[63] found that all school-age children cheat and that the amount of cheating varies with the amount of pressure they feel to succeed. Children will cheat to blame others for their misdeeds, appear more knowledgeable or skilled in activities, and to avoid punishment or a "lecture" from significant adults. Children 9 to 12 have a strong need for peer group membership and for approval from authority figures, which lessens the frequency and degree of lying and cheating behaviors.

Play

Play is a natural for children, follows a developmental sequence, and is dependent on cognitive and language development as well as on environmental, cultural, and familial factors. Play is the most significant way in which children learn. Play is also the child's chief medium of communicating their ideational and fantasy preoccupations. Because it is self-revealing, it should be used to better understand children's concerns and feelings. It must be remembered that children communicate their unconscious conflicts or wishes through play and create new situations or put real and imagined experiences together in new combinations.

School-age children participate in various types of play including pretend or dramatic, quiet, aggressive, and cooperative play. Play gives them renewed energy to tackle their problems at a later time.[46] At this age, pretending becomes less overt and more covert. This is the age of "games with rules." Play becomes more realistic while fantasy play gradually goes underground.

Cognitive Problems: Learning Problems With and Without Hyperactivity

Approximately 4,000,000, or 12%, of school-age children have some form of learning problem. Three-fourths are actually diagnosed with a learning disability. Of these, two-thirds are boys. The number of children with learning problems is currently growing at an alarming rate, which suggests this is a problem that potentially has an impact on more children with diabetes. Learning disability is now diagnosed as either an undifferentiated attention deficit disorder (ADD: DSM-III-R, 3.400) or as attention deficit hyperactivity disorder (ADHD: DSM-III-R, 314.014). The primary difference between these two is that children with ADHD are also hyperactive. While the etiology is unknown, a strong familial tendency exists. In 1987, the Interagency Committee on Learning Disability defined them as follows:

Learning disability is a generic term that refers to a heterogeneous group of disorders manifested by significant difficulties in the acquisition and use of listening, speaking, reading, writing, reasoning, or mathematical abilities, or of social skills.[49]

There are four types of learning disabilities: receptive, integrative, expressive, and diffuse, which is a combination of the three previous categories. Children with a receptive type of learning disability have trouble getting information into their brains. Those with the expressive type have difficulty getting the information out, in speaking, spelling, writing, calculating, or drawing. Those with the integrative type can get the information in but have difficulty in organizing their thoughts, as is noted in trouble with sequencing, understanding cliches, and in analyzing or synthesizing information.[49,76] Although each child is unique, children with ADD or ADHD exhibit most of the specific behaviors identified in the box on p. 418.

Learning-disabled children function best when they have clear guidelines, structure, routine, and consistency. They should be given directions one at a time and not be overwhelmed with having to make a number of decisions at any one time, especially pertinent considerations in teaching the child with IDDM.

Learning occurs best when 5- to 10-minute teaching sessions are given in a quiet room away from any extraneous stimuli. Careful structuring of diabetes content is essential. These children need to feel successful at understanding the previous content before

___ BEHAVIORS COMMON TO CHILDREN WHO HAVE ADD AND ADHD ___

Behaviors common for children with ADD

Hear only the beginning or end of set of directions.
Start work before getting the directions.
Often lose things necessary for tasks or activities.
Ignore and impatient with details because they feel have the general idea.
Do not recognize relationships of parts to whole task.
Resist going back over new material.
Resist correcting work.
Want black-and-white, simple, uncomplicated answers.
Do not consider all variations of problems, arrive at quick, simple answers and decisions.

Behaviors common for children with ADHD

All behaviors listed for children with ADD plus:
Difficulty sustaining attention in tasks or play.
Talk excessively.
Interrupt or intrude on others.
Blurt out answers before question is completed.
Rush into potentially dangerous situations.
Quick to anger in unpredictable and explosive ways.
Very short attention spans.
Easily distracted by extraneous stimuli.
Constantly moving; great difficulty in sitting or staying still.
Difficulty in waiting turns.
Lack of concern for rules and the rights of others.

moving onto new ideas. For example, present *only* five ways they will feel if they have low blood glucose on a chart with each symptom written and pictures illustrating each one. Have the children look at the chart, read it aloud, act out each symptom and then write each one down. When they can state these symptoms, teach them to take 5 to 6 sugar cubes or 4 ounces of juice whenever they feel this way. Then help them transfer this information to various situations they will be in. For example, ask, "What should you do if you feel shaky and starving in math class?"

IMPACT OF DIABETES ON NORMAL COGNITIVE/LANGUAGE DEVELOPMENT

School-age children with IDDM are subject to the same cognitive development as children who do not have IDDM. However, it is possible that children who experience multiple, severe episodes of low blood glucose may develop learning disabilities or delayed or impaired cognition. It is now recognized that all school-age children with chronic illnesses (e.g., IDDM), may have either regressed or delayed cognitive development when compared with those without illnesses.[38,48] In one study 25% of 7- to 10-year-old children with IDDM were still preoperational, while none of those without illnesses were preoperational at these ages.

Perceptions of Diabetes

Children's understanding of illness is primarily determined by their level of cognitive maturation. Preoperational children have numerous misperceptions about what diabetes is. For example, a 7-year-old said IDDM is "something where you have to take blood out. Getting holes in you." Even children in the concrete stage of cognitive development have misperceptions about IDDM. For example, "The insulin in your body isn't traveling right. I'm eating too much sugar and it goes into my blood system and blocks the insulin passage."

Preoperational children also tend to think the cause of any disease results from human action or the outcome of wrongdoing—such as, God gave it to them, they caught it, or they ate too much sugar. Children in the transitional stage perceive germs as the physical cause for all illness. During the concrete stage, they perceive that illness can have multiple causes.[13,17,38,48]

After 1 year, school-age children perceive their diabetes as caused by several reasons: (1) a mechanical breakdown (i.e., "insulin producing cells are sick"), (2) simplified cause and effect, (i.e., "ate too much candy"), (3) being punished, (i.e., got diabetes because I fought with my brother), (4) it just happened, or (5) for a *specific* reason to *help* that child in some way[34,74] (e.g., Jeff felt he got IDDM as a message to give up alcohol, smoking, and hanging around a bad group of kids[17,23,99]).

Feelings About Having Diabetes

Children clearly remember how they felt and what they thought when they first heard they had diabetes. Most of the children say they were confused, sad, mad, and frightened of needles.[74] Other feelings about having diabetes included fear of death and feelings of acceptance and rejection toward having IDDM.[19] Feelings of acceptance include statements about the perceived good aspects of having IDDM, such as not getting many cavities, getting to eat snacks at school when others do not, never getting fat, feeling special, and being spoiled. Major negative feelings about having IDDM focus on being "different," the inconvenience and extra time caring for it takes every day, having to eat when you're not hungry, and not being able to eat sweet treats whenever friends do.[34,74] It is important to note that having to take "shots" is not usually identified as the worst thing about having IDDM.

Many children are unable to verbalize their feelings. Drawing and painting are extremely useful communication techniques to help children express their thoughts, feelings, and misperceptions in a very nonthreatening and revealing manner.[60] Art is less subject to control by defense mechanisms and allows children to reveal unconscious tensions, feelings, and perceptions of deeper reactions to events.[39,98] Drawings are projections of children's concerns, fears, and thoughts because they represent their inner reality.[12] Children draw what is important to them and what they think and feel, not necessarily reality. This enables them to express taboos and release hostility and other socially nonacceptable feelings through artwork.[98] Drawings also provide children with the opportunity to master feelings they have. They can alert health care providers to the misperceptions and fantasies children have about IDDM that then can facilitate the development of more positive feelings and correct knowledge.[11,47]

The verbalized feelings cited previously have been validated by analyzing drawings completed by children with IDDM. In one study, Italian children with IDDM drew healthy and ill children smaller than did their nondiabetic peers, indicating these children may not be as well adjusted to their environment. In addition, they seemed to have less clear-cut images or stereotypes of sick and healthy persons.[91] In another study, drawings completed in response to "What is it like to have diabetes?" yielded emotional themes such as insecurity, anxiety, ambivalence, rigidity, isolation, anger, sadness, and fear. Parental drawings had similar themes but more frequently included anxiety, insecurity, and powerlessness.

School-age children have varied feelings about each component of the required daily diabetes care regimen including the diet, insulin, insulin reactions, exercise, and testing. In general, they feel a sense of achievement and pride when they can test their own blood glucose and give themselves insulin injections,[19,34,74] but some complain blood testing takes too much time and that it hurts. Others have misperceptions of these skills. For example, a 9-year-old used only one finger for blood tests because she thought it was "the only one with blood in it."[74]

PSYCHOSOCIAL DEVELOPMENT

School-age children are now in Freud's "latency" period and Erickson's "industry" versus "inferiority" stage. They become immersed in learning vast amounts of knowledge and developing a variety of new skills to master the environment, affirm their sexual identity, and find their place in a peer group. A sense of industry and self-esteem is acquired from frequent successes, significant others encouragement of and recognition for achievement. They rely on their peers and develop close relationships. With help and guidance, inferiority is conquered and self-worth, cooperation, and competition emerge.

Self-Esteem

Children gain self-esteem and appreciation of their own worth by being accepted by parents and peers and by having clear, consistent limits flexible enough to permit individual actions.[103] Those with high self-esteem can accept criticism, state their beliefs even if they challenge authority, and confidently enter new situations. They respect other's thoughts and opinions, and begin to feel empathy for others.[116]

Behavior Style

Six- to 11-year-old children have a very rigid behavior style; they follow rules closely and use lots of rituals. They complete tasks in a specific order, continuously practice skills, and precisely carry out new roles. Rules reduce anxiety, give specific guidelines, and provide an external standard against which to measure themselves. Older children try to control their fear of death by being good.[98,116]

Peers

Peers provide children with feedback, which encourages self-evaluation, teaches how to compromise individual needs for the group's benefit, encourages sharing of information and feelings, and provides an environment in which the child can safely practice sex role behavior. In addition, an older friend of the same sex often is a "worshipped" hero who provides support as the parental ties become loosened, and who helps soften the child's previous dependence on parents.

Significance of Family

For school-age children, mastery of each developmental task is dependent upon the family's ability to create a positive, nurturing environment in which they can thrive. The tasks of the family include meeting the basic physical needs of the family, providing emotional support, and opening communication. Mastering these tasks helps each member develop to their fullest potential. Parental responsibilities include supporting children in forming academic and social skills needed for achievement, adjusting to rules and laws, and developing values of justice while respecting others' differences.[57]

Significance of Community

Establishing some independence from the family is important to develop relationships in the community. Children need to participate in sports events, community clubs, and overnights at peers' homes. As their world expands beyond that of the family's home, parents must maintain effective communication with their children. Although much of children's time is now spent outside the home, the family remains the most important emotional refuge.[57]

IMPACT OF DIABETES ON PSYCHOSOCIAL DEVELOPMENT

The management of diabetes in children requires a complicated treatment regimen that includes: one to four daily insulin injections, two to four daily blood glucose tests, dietary regulation, consistent timing of meals and snacks, and careful monitoring of physical activities.[44,68] In addition, both children and their parents must know which behaviors can cause or correct high blood glucose, ketones, and low blood glucose.

They must know what to do when any of these occur. These management tasks must be carried out on a daily basis, with no vacations.[22] Thus, diabetes care is time-consuming, difficult, complex, requires a high degree of self-discipline and regulation, and often a change in life-style for children with IDDM and their families.[3,44,58]

Children's Reactions to Diabetes

In general, most children adequately cope with diabetes, although some do have considerable difficulty.[68] To adequately care for their diabetes, school-age children must comprehend the disease, have positive attitudes toward themselves and their diabetes, plus have social and environmental support.[62] To avoid emotional difficulties, they also need confidence that they can follow the diabetes regimen.

While most families receive extensive instruction regarding the diabetes care regimen, many studies suggest that school-age children have much lower levels of essential skills and knowledge about their regimen than health care professionals expect.[44] In fact, a number of studies have demonstrated that children made numerous errors in insulin injections and urine and blood testing.[23,28,40,61,117] While most had some understanding of the need for insulin, many did not comprehend the route insulin takes in the body or the reason for rotating injection sites. Most children know that eating candy is forbidden and eating too much contributes to high blood glucoses, but do not really understand how choices or the timing of food affects them. Many admitted to sneaking a candy bar[34] and then feeling guilty, but did not know *why* they should not eat it. Although some children understand that exercise brings their blood glucose down, many use diabetes as a reason for not participating in activities.[74] Thus, children must be provided with extensive cognitively appropriate information and hands-on practice sessions to learn how food, exercise, and insulin influence blood glucose levels.[44] They must be frequently helped to apply this information to their daily activities.[7,61,74]

Children's cognitive developmental level should be the determinant of what they are taught and how they are taught.[59] Diabetes educators can use the numbers, water, and clay Piagetian tasks to identify their current cognitive level. Children must be retaught this content each time they reach a new cognitive level and re-evaluated on their skills abilities at least twice a year.

Personality Development

No specific pattern of personality traits have been found to characterize children with diabetes. In addition, the levels of emotional disturbance are no higher among these children than for children with any other chronic illness or even in the general population.[33,89] Several studies have found no difference between the levels of behavioral problems or self-esteem of school-aged children with and without diabetes.[19,72,73]

Children who do exhibit emotional problems need to be referred for psychologic of psychiatric assistance. Since stress may negatively influence metabolic control of diabetes, children with IDDM need to be taught stress reduction techniques to modulate their stress reactions and be encouraged to participate in activities and exercise that will help to disperse their anxious feelings.[16]

Children's Adaptation to Diabetes

School-age children often adapt quite well to the diagnosis of diabetes, at least initially.[45] One study of children newly diagnosed with IDDM illustrated this phenomena and demonstrated two general modes of coping to the initial strain of living with IDDM. The majority of the school-age children were found to be emotionally resilient and psychologically adapted with comparative ease to the new life demands. In fact, 64% had a rather subdued reaction to the diagnosis throughout the first year after. Their reaction consisted of mild sadness, anxiety, feelings of friendlessness, and social withdrawal. The rest of the children exhibited a depressive syndrome that included an anxious, apprehensive, and depressed mood, anger, irritability, suicidal ideation, and excessive somatic complaints. However, recovery from these symptoms occurred over the 9-month period after diagnosis.

Healthy attitudes toward having diabetes are best developed by an environment that is relatively stress-free and by parents, teachers, and other significant adults who acknowledge the presence of diabetes but who treat it in a matter-of-fact and supportive manner. Disturbed family environments are often associated with poor diabetic control.[4,6,7,85] Children from low socioeconomic, single parent homes are at higher risk for poor diabetes management.[6] Children are also at risk for poor diabetes control if they are from homes in which the family patterns are overprotective and overanxious, overindulgent and overpermissive, perfectionistic and controlling, or indifferent and rejecting. In the school setting, teachers who treat the child with IDDM the same as others and who assist other children in the classroom to understand diabetes promote positive adaptation.

Family's Reaction to Diabetes

Three major factors have an impact on the family's ability to achieve each developmental task and meet the needs of all members: family's perception of the task, the availability or resources to achieve each task, and the family's ability to cope with problems. Incorporating the management of children's diabetes into the family can dramatically affect the family's healthy development.

The initial goal in the treatment of children with diabetes is to empower the family with the knowledge required to participate in and gain independence with self-care management. Formal educational programs are designed to assist the family in learning and integrating two levels of knowledge regarding diabetes. Basic knowledge includes an understanding of the physiologic processes of IDDM and the ability to perform the psychomotor skills, which include insulin administration, blood glucose monitoring, urine ketone testing, and diet management. A higher level of knowledge requires applying the basic information to everyday problems.[44] This level of understanding allows the family to actively problem-solve and negotiate independent decisions about the child's everyday management, such as handling hyperglycemia with or without the presence of ketones before a sport's event and when and how to permit sweets in children's diets.

Diabetes education is best viewed as an ongoing process that must be continually reevaluated and reinstituted as the developmental needs of the children and family change. Parents of younger school-age children have been found to have higher levels of knowledge, especially in the problem-solving area, than parents of older school-age children.[7] Recent research found that mothers are more knowledgeable about children's diabetic management than either fathers or children. In the preadolescent population, it is the knowledge level of the mother, not of the children, that is closely associated with treatment adherence and metabolic control.[61]

Family's Adaptation to Diabetes

Healthy family adaptation and rearing children with a chronic illness such as IDDM requires collaboration and sharing or responsibilities among all family members. However, the primary responsibility for diabetes care tasks often falls upon mothers. Hauenstein and colleagues [54] studied 52 mothers who had children with IDDM and found over 50% reported excessive maternal stress caused by negative characteristics of their children. These negative characteristics included poor adaptability, demanding behaviors, and distractability resulting in children's stress. In another study, school-age males with IDDM were found to have more behaviors associated with neurotic tendencies and personality disturbances than females with IDDM of the same sage. Such behaviors included withdrawal, anxiety, hyperactivity, and aggression.[24,59,73]

A significant association between parental stress, age of the child, and glycemic control has been found. Low levels of parental stress in mothers of younger school-age children were associated with good glycemic control, but the same levels in mothers of older children were associated with poor metabolic control.[54] Future research needs to more definitively describe the relationship between children's personality, parental stress, family adaptation, and glycemic control.

Adaptation and coping behaviors of parents of children with IDDM have not been extensively investigated. One study found parental coping methods included expressions of anger, trying again, talking with friends and hospital staff, and learning more.[11] Such coping behaviors may assist parents in becoming more aware of their added responsibilities associated with the care of their children's diabetes.[96]

The complex array of daily tasks that must be followed to manage children with IDDM required families to adjust and rearrange their established routines. Family organization and control are necessary for successful management of children with IDDM.[112]

Participation of *all* family members in the diabetes care regimen is essential for healthy adaptation and good glycemic control.[21,50] Research on sharing of diabetes responsibilities among family members found 72% of the sample families reported areas of disagreement between the child and mother about who took ultimate responsibility for 22 diabetes-related tasks. The mother-child dyads that reported multiple areas of disagreement and whose mothers admitted low levels of adherence to the care regimen had children at risk for poor glycemic control.[4] These results emphasize the need for clearly defined expectations within the family and the need for each family member to have agreed on responsibility for specific diabetes-related tasks.

Adaptation to School

School entry brings about a new set of hurdles for parents and children with IDDM. Normal childhood activities, such as swapping of food between friends and spontaneous exercise sessions, place these children at risk for diabetes problems.[64] Parents worry most about their children's diabetes management while they are at school. They often lack confidence in teachers' abilities to recognize insulin reactions and to understand their children's special dietary needs.[56] These concerns are legitimized by recent research that found that schoolteachers often have an inadequate understanding of IDDM and its management. In one study of over 400 teachers, 55% could not identify symptoms of hypoglycemia and only 26% could identify when a hypoglycemic reaction is most likely to occur.[80]

Throughout the elementary school years, peer relationships become increasingly important and are essential for the healthy socialization of the child. Perceived restrictions imposed by the diabetes regimen may hinder some children's active participation in normal childhood activities. Parents agonize over whether or not to allow their child to attend slumber parties, go on outings with friends, and attend birthday parties without parental supervision. It is the uncertainty over whether their children may stray from the diabetes regimen or will become ill and not be properly treated that causes much of this parental anxiety and fear.

Information and support from national organizations, current publications, and community resources are of assistance to families with children who have IDDM. Such organizations and publications offer ideas on living with diabetes and current information regarding new trends in diabetes management.

Assessment of the Family

The success of the health care team in caring for school-aged children with IDDM begins with a complete and thorough family assessment (see box on pp. 426-427). The initial assessment is critical in planning children's education and care and the ongoing assessment of the family's development and reveals current and new information.

The socioeconomic status (SES) of the family affects the child's compliance with the diabetes regimen and with their glycemic control. Children with IDDM, living in a family with relatively high SES, tend to have parents who possess higher education levels, more financial resources, and greater problem-solving skill. These children are able to achieve better metabolic control than those from families with relatively low SES[4,6,7] who continually struggle to meet their basic needs.

—————————— **FAMILY ASSESSMENT TOOL** ——————————

Child's name_____Age_____School grade_____

Race_____Nationality_____Religion_____

Household members

Name	Relationship to patient	Age	Pertinent information

Family/healthcare/community support

Name	Address	Phone	Comments

Socioeconomic status

Variable	Adequate	Inadequate	Excellent
Income			
Housing			
Neighborhood			
Telephone			
Transportation			
Resources for dietary needs			
Resouces for medical equipment			
Resources for health care needs			

Communication patterns/family functioning

Family stability_____

Family flexability_____

Support from extended family_____

Decision-making process_____

Communication patterns_____

Family's feeling of closeness_____

Satisfaction with relationships_____

Sharing of IDDM responsibilities_____

Understanding child development_____

Impact of IDDM on family members_____

————————————— **FAMILY ASSESSMENT TOOL**—cont'd. ——————————————

Functioning in community

Variable	Adequate	Inadequate	Excellent
Knowledge of community resources			
Utilization of community resouces			
Social activities of family			
Social activities of child			
Adequate babysitting resources			
Support from school system			

Treatment knowledge/management skills

Ability to learn psychomotor skills

Ability to problem-solve

Knowledge of healthcare management

Over the past 30 years changes in the structure of the American family have resulted in a dramatic increase in single parent homes. According to the U.S. 1984 Bureau of Census, over 25% of all children in the United States are now living with only one parent. The majority of these families are headed by women and are more likely to live in poverty than two-parent households.[5] Children with IDDM who live in such families are at risk for poor compliance and poor metabolic control. Auslander and colleagues[7] found the glycated hemoglobin levels were 30% higher in children from African American families and single-parent homes than those in children from white or two-parent families. This may be true in part because cohesion and emotional expressiveness between members within the African-American and single-parent families is significantly lower than those for the white and two-parent households.[6] Another study found children with IDDM living with their mothers and a stepfather or with adoptive parents have even worse glycemic control than those living in single-parent homes, regardless of SES.

Families that have open communication patterns and frequent sharing of ideas create a nurturing atmosphere that encourages learning about diabetes. Marteau and associates[85] concluded that ". . . happy families may produce happy children who carry out a diabetic regimen compatible with good control and consequently have good diabetic control."

TEACHING/LEARNING IMPLICATIONS

It is clear from many studies that school-age children need a developmentally based education program that not only presents knowledge at an understandable cognitive level but also emphasizes the application of that knowledge in their daily activities.[6,7] Since studies also identified variability in the levels of knowledge about diabetes within specific age groups,[19] educators need to be conscious not only of individual differences but also of the cognitive development level on which children are currently operating.

Frequent reassessment of children's skills and knowledge is essential. Educators can employ children's drawings to assist them to communicate their fears, misperceptions, and current understanding of the various components of the diabetes care regimen.[19,25,98] When fears and anxieties are revealed, parents and health care providers need to let the children know they are recognized and assist them in coping with these feelings.

Individualizing Treatment Goals for the School-Age Child

A common assumption among health care providers is that children with diabetes should assume as much responsibility for self-care as possible. A recent summary of over 200 diabetes professionals found the average expectation of mastery for 14 to 20 selected skills was below the age ranges recommended by the American Diabetes Association in 1983.[120] Therefore, numerous diabetes providers have inappropriate age-related expectations for school-age children. In fact, recent research demonstrated that children given more responsibility for their diabetes care make more errors, are less adherent, and are in poorer metabolic control than children whose parents are more involved.[44,45,68] Therefore, the determination of the amount of self-management responsibility for diabetes care must not be based on age alone.

The responsibility for diabetes management must be shared between parents and children with more gradual responsibility being assumed by children as determined by their demonstrating correct skills and wanting more independence. A recent study found that of 400 children, 50% of the 10- to 11-year olds wanted more help with recording their blood glucose values and thought they should be at least 9.5 years old before giving their own insulin injections, and 150 wanted their families to keep sweets out of the house.[49a] Another study found children who were more prone to worry and apprehension had better blood glucose control than those without emotional or adjustment problems. It is likely these children are more diligent in monitoring the subjective signs of poor blood glucose control and, thus, counteract them more effectively. It may also be that these children do not take responsibility for their diabetes care and their dependence on their parents protects them from the adverse effects of precocious self-care.[45]

Currently, empirical information, is needed to define appropriate developmental expectations for acquisition of self-care independence by children with IDDM.[44] What is clear is that any guidelines about age-related expectations of children' learning knowledge or assumption of diabetes care skills must be individualized for that specific child.

Goals of an Individualized Developmentally Based Education Program

There are three major goals of a developmentally based diabetes education program: (1) to facilitate parents' and children's positive knowledge of and adjustment to diabetes; (2) to help the parents and children attain and maintain shared interdependence and responsibility for assuming diabetes management skills that enhance good metabolic control; and (3) to enhance parents' and children's self-esteem and independence as part of their normal development. To attain these goals, the diabetes health care providers must provide the family with cognitively appropriate knowledge, guidelines for age-related expectations, information on how to apply the diabetes care knowledge and skills in a flexible way to meet everyday activities, and encourage the learning of appropriate behavioral management strategies.

Several research studies found that to assume responsibility for IDDM self-care, children must be provided with the knowledge base needed via multiple senses, active participation, and behavioral demonstration, not just through verbal information.[29,111] Second, it is important to assess the current knowledge and perceptions of both parents and children before beginning an education program. In addition, parental involvement is critical for school-aged children since parental knowledge, especially the mother's knowledge, has been found to be significantly related to both adherence and control for 7- to 11-year olds. Knowledge of diabetes care is a necessary, but not sufficient, prerequisite to good self-management, adherence, and metabolic control. Behavioral strategies aimed at improving various skills children need to use in diabetes-related situations (e.g., social skills) should be included. As previously noted, many studies have shown that even children with good information about diabetes skills make numerous and serious errors in estimating amounts of foods, in drawing up insulin doses, and in testing and recording urine ketone and blood glucose values.[32,40] These errors are serious enough to have a negative impact on metabolic control. It is also clear that skill or adherence in one area of care does not predict adherence in other(s).[100]

School-age children are at an ideal age to *begin* taking some responsibility for their own insulin injections, glucose testing, and diet control. However, it is important to implement changes gradually, frequently assessing both specific areas of knowledge and specific skills to determine children's readiness to perform self-care tasks.[44]

Assessing children's current cognitive level via Piagetian Tasks along with their ability to manage complex information in areas other than diabetes provide important clues about their ability to manage the multiple and complex aspects of their diabetes.[44] Children who demonstrate deductive reasoning abilities in school or in the types of questions they ask educators are most likely to understand more advanced principles of diabetes care and to assume an increased role in diabetes care skills. In these cases, the educator should encourage implementation of a gradual transfer of appropriate responsibilites from parents to children.

Optimal metabolic control is encouraged in families that value and affirm structure and organization and who also maintain good communication with their children. Parents who provide consistent guidance to the child with diabetes, in a cooperative, shared way without nagging or being perfectionistic, promote behaviors that contribute to better metabolic control.[4,7] In contrast, overprotectiveness and indifference are associated with poor metabolic control and should be discouraged.

The overall goal for diabetes education of school-age children and their parents is to

---

DIABETES CONTENT

For younger school-age children

    I. What is diabetes?

Explain by using an analogy like blood sugar is like gasoline. Gasoline must get into the car's engine to make it run and blood sugar must get in so you can run and play.

Diabetes is not caused by thoughts or misdeed.

Diabetes is not a punishment.

Diabetes will not go away.

    II. How to check blood for amount of sugar.

    III. How to check urine for ketones.

    IV. What it feels like to have low blood sugar (shaky, sweaty, sleepy, and starving).

    V. What to do if you have low blood sugar. Tell your mom, dad, teacher, coach, or friend. Always carry cubes of sugar or packs of honey in pocket and keep these in desk at school. Treat low blood sugar by eating one tsp. sugar, honey, jelly, or syrup, or drink 3 oz unsweetened juice.

    VI. When low blood sugars are likely to occur.

When not all food at a meal is eaten.

When a snack is skipped.

When playing sports longer and harder than on other days.

When too much insulin is accidently given.

    VII. What it feels like to have high blood sugar (thirsty, have to pee alot, pee is sticky; feel very tired and crabby).

    VIII. What to do if you have high blood sugar. Tell your mom, dad, teacher, coach, or friend. Drink a large glass of water, ice tea, sugar-free Koolaid, or diet soda.

    IX. When likely to have high blood sugar.

When snacks and food are eaten that mom does not know about.

When an apple is traded for a candy bar with a friend.

Forgot to take insulin injection.

    X. What it feels like to have ketones (sick to stomach, throw-up, stomach hurts, breathe funny, and bad breath that does not brush away).

---

provide both with complete diabetes education and to facilitate the child's ability to become active and knowledgeable participants in diabetes care. Diabetes instruction needs to be geared toward the conceptual/developmental level of the child, with very strong messages for both parents and children to work as a team. Education programs must teach by using multiple senses, behavioral demonstrations, and unannounced, frequent "spot checks" of parents' and children's performances.

Content of Educational Program

The content for an individualized developmentally based diabetes education program is similar for both newly and previously diagnosed children with IDDM and their families.

———————————— **DIABETES CONTENT—cont'd.** ————————————

For older school-age children

I. What is diabetes?

Explain using three-dimensional doll.

Explain location of pancreas and define insulin.

Explain "cells" to child and how insulin is their best friend because it gets sugar into the cells so the body can grow and work well.

Diabetes was not caused by them. It is not a punishment for being bad or lying. They did not catch diabetes from someone.

II. How to check blood sugars.

III. How to check urine for ketones.

IV. How to give self insulin injections (not until 10 to 11 years to draw dose up).

Wash hands.

Clean top on insulin bottles.

Place air into NPH insulin bottle.

Place air into regular insulin bottle.

Draw up regular insulin.

Draw up NPH insulin.

Clean off injection site.

Bunch up skin with free hand.

Break skin with needle using a 90-degree angle.

Inject insulin.

Rotate needle before removing.

Remember to rotate site (arms and abdomen 1 week and legs and abdomen the next).

Use abdomen when blood sugars are high (insulin is absorbed more quickly).

V. Symptoms of high and low blood sugar.

VI. Treatment of high and low blood sugar.

VII. Causes of high and low blood sugar.

VIII. Problem-solving skills.

What would you do if:

You were locked out of your house and your blood sugar was low?

It was a schoolmate's birthday and the class was having cake?

You are in the middle of a science test and you suddenly realize you forgot to eat lunch?

(See Appendix C for a list of content provided children with IDDM and their families by an interdisciplinary team at St. Louis Children's Hospital.) After an extensive initial in-hospital education, all families and children with IDDM need frequent reeducation and retraining. Topics frequently reevaluated are presented in the box above.

Self-monitoring of blood glucose

Children should be taught to select three fingers that are to be used for blood testing so that in 3 to 4 weeks, callouses will develop and the fingersticks will not be so painful.

Be sure children stick the sides of their fingers to minimize pain and to prevent pads from losing their sense of touch over the next few years.

As these SMBG skills are mastered, the educator should teach the child to try to keep most blood glucoses between 80 to 180 mg/dL. This is a more realistic target for school-age children than is the normal range of 60 to 140 mg/dL. Keeping most glucoses in this target range usually results in adequate glycemia without markedly increasing the number of frequent, severe hypoglycemia episodes. Maintaining most blood glucoses between 80 and 180 mg/dL is often easier during the first few months when a child's ability to produce insulin temporarily increases. This period, called the honeymoon, commonly lasts for several months during the first year after diagnosis and may result in excellent glucose control even when the diabetes regimen is not followed closely. Subsequently, as maintaining good control becomes more difficult, higher and more erratic blood glucose readings become more common.

Hypoglycemia and hyperglycemia

As early as possible, children must be taught to recognize when a "low" blood glucose occurs and to immediately either tell someone or treat it. A "low" is defined as having less than 60 mg/dL blood glucose. The child often can be taught to remember the 6 Ss of low blood glucose; shaky, sweaty (but cool to touch), sleepy (not tired), starving, stubborn, and spacey. Parents should also watch for children to become pale, quiet, whiny, or irritable. Emphasize to parents that candy is not to be used to treat a "low" because some kinds of candy may not have enough sugar, it must be eaten too quickly to enjoy, and many children cannot resist eating the candy even when they know they are not "low." Whenever a "low" occurs more than 1 hour before the next scheduled snack or meal, the child should ingest at least one-half glass of milk or six saltine crackers with cheese, meat, or peanut butter. This avoids hypoglycemia every 20 to 30 minutes.

Children with markedly elevated glucoses over 240 mg/dL for several hours or more have to urinate often, feel thirsty or exhausted, are crabby, and may develop refractive errors. When blood glucoses are over 240 mg/dL or whenever children with IDDM become ill, someone should check the urine for ketones. Children should avoid strenuous exercise when large amounts of ketones are present in the urine.[52]

If hyperglycemia occurs before a scheduled insulin injection, children should learn when and how to adjust the insulin dose. When ketones are present, children should drink at least 8 ounces of sugar-free liquid per hour for 2 to 3 hours and then retest. If the blood glucose or ketones have not gone down after taking appropriate fluids and/or extra insulin, they should call the diabetes health professional who may then order a supplemental amount of regular insulin.

Sick day management

Parents must know that children with IDDM who are ill are very susceptible to dehydration that can increase the concentration of both glucose and ketones. Children can develop diabetic ketacidosis within a few hours when dehydrated or febrile. Thus, sick day management requires that children drink large amounts of fluids. A rule of thumb is to take children off solid food and have them alternate 6 to 8 ounces of sugared with sugar-free fluids every hour. Children should be seen by their physician or brought to an emergency room for IV therapy if they cannot keep liquids down or vomit more than once within 4 to 6 hours.

Giving injections

Giving insulin injections can be frightening for parents and children alike. Diabetes educators can reduce this anxiety by demonstrating and then expecting the parents to give each other saline injections. School-age children who want to can give the educator saline injections early in the education program. Parents are usually surprised at how little the injections hurt and children are very proud of themselves afterward. Both must be taught to quickly insert the needle through the skin to minimize pain. Using insulin syringes calibrated to the smallest amount of units possible makes it easier for all to accurately see the unit markings. For example, Terumo makes a 25 unit syringe that is marked in ½ units and Becton-Dickenson makes a 30-unit syringe for U100 insulin. However, neither should be used unless the total number of insulin units per dose is 5 units less than the amount held by the syringe. Younger children, during the honeymoon period, may require half-unit insulin doses, e.g. ½ regular and 3½ NPH. One-half units can be fairly accurately measured on either of the new small insulin syringes just described.

Parents and children must know that both glucagon and insulin need to be kept between 32° and 86° Fahrenheit; keeping them in the refrigerator is best during warm months. Once opened, insulin should be used within 45 days. Otherwise, unexplained high blood glucoses are sometimes caused by insulin that has "gone bad." This can be noted when older NPH or Lente insulin looks thready or crystallized or if the bottle appears frosted.

Rotation of injections is extremely important. Injections should be given 1 inch apart. Some studies found insulin is absorbed faster and more completely from the abdomen (than from arms, buttocks, and legs).[8] This suggests rotation should not be taught clockwise around the body as previously thought. Instead, all sites on the arms should be used 1 week, then all leg sites should be used on alternate weeks (buttocks used only in children who do not mind). The abdominal sites should probably be used whenever hyperglycemia is present prior to injections. In addition, injections should be avoided in the legs or arms if the child is about to participate in strenuous activities, using these limbs within the next 2 hours.

Behavioral strategies

Parents help children become active participants in their care by not expecting perfection, making is easy for children to remember care activities by leaving written reminders in visible places, or by using simple, matter-of-fact verbal reminders.[101] Parents who encourage their children to be progressively more involved in their self-care, while providing structure and working together with them, send their children the message that they trust them and see them as competent and worthwhile persons who can do increasingly complex skills. Successful parents list clearly what each family member's responsibilities are. In addition, they set up natural or logical consequences for predictable outcomes related to diabetes. For example, natural consequences for being late for a meal is having a "low" reaction and for eating too many snacks at bedtime at a friend's house may be to wet the bed. A logical consequence for choosing not to measure blood glucoses is the need for a parent to come to a friend's house, with whom the child is sleeping overnight, to test blood at bedtime and before breakfast.

Diabetes health care providers need to help parents set up natural or logical consequences for children's actions. This is a much more instructive way for children to learn the consequences of their various actions and may reduce parental guilt or anger.

Health care providers should emphasize to school-age children, in front of their parents, that adults will not become angry with them, like them less, or punish them if their blood glucose values are not within the target range or if they honestly say they ate a candy bar or other food that raised their blood glucose. Encouraging children to be honest and to eat sweet foods, within clearly established limits, prevents the need to sneak foods or lie about blood glucose values.

On the other hand, parents should know the various ways and reasons children "cheat" on their diet and should be encouraged to closely supervise their children. For example, some children place ketchup on their glucose test strips to make the blood test come out within range, whereas others may spit on the blood test strips or run diluted koolaid or milk over them in order to obtain low readings.

Parents need to be reminded that younger school-age children think differently from adults and cannot comprehend the wisdom of doing something difficult today to prevent something bad from occurring in 5, 10, or more years. Furthermore, causing fear of some dreadful consequence like loss of a leg or vision is likely to cause them to feel depressed or hopeless.

Parents must also be cautioned not to feel that children need to eat all their food or have blood glucose values between 80 to 180 all of the time; these are unreal expectations. Behavioral management strategies such as the use of sticker charts, earning tokens to be traded in for activities they like to do, and the use of practical positive and negative reinforcers to make diabetes activities easier is helpful. For example, completing 3 or 4 "good" behaviors earns a reward. Allow the child to negotiate the reward, such as extra TV time or a walk in the park with parents. It is necessary to change the tasks and rewards biweekly to keep the child interested and motivated.

Parents must also be taught to avoid power struggles with their children over food. It is better to let children experience the "low" as a consequence of not eating all their food or exercising too much without eating extra food than for parents and children to argue about it. Experiencing low blood glucoses under parental supervision provides a safe and effective learning experience.

Parents must remember the primary goal is to encourage children to become independent, develop normally, and feel as similar as possible to their peers. Parents must openly be in agreement, as a couple, on the goals they wish to establish for their children.[59] Then they must *consistently* encourage their children to attain these goals or discipline them for misbehavior or misdeeds.

DIABETES REGIMEN ADHERENCE ISSUES

The overall level of metabolic control is related to the following categories of variables: regimen adequacy; knowledge/management skills; psychosocial adjustment/dysfunction of children, family, and peers; stress; and adherence or self-care management of the diabetic regimen.[70] Regimen adequacy, self-care/adherence to the diabetes regimen and stress are directly related to metabolic control. Psychologic adjustment/dysfunction and knowledge/ correct management skills are directly related to each other and self-care/adherence and, thus, indirectly related to metabolic control.

Regimen Adequacy

Encouraging children with IDDM to maintain good metabolic control may reduce the risks of future development of diabetes-related health problems such as retinopathy.[105] School age is a time of rapid physical, cognitive, and social change. Thus, children undergo difficult development changes while having to follow a complex diabetes regimen. Studies report 10- to 15-year olds are at very high risk for poor metabolic control because of rapid growth, less parental supervision, inadequate problem-solving ability, and difficulty in adhering to the diabetic regimen.[14,26,69]

Knowledge and Management Skills

Recent research studies have found the following to be associated with good metabolic control. (1) General and problem-solving levels of knowledge. Higher levels are related to better control for older adolescents and for parents of younger children.[69] In contrast, the levels of knowledge attained by children were not related to their knowledge of diabetes management. (2) Age of the child. Children between 6 and 11 have better control, whereas midadolescents have the worst.[4,6] These data suggest it is not the information per se that is important, but the child's and/or family's ability to understand and use the information to solve daily problems and correctly adjust the diabetes regimen.[7]

Psychosocial Adjustment, Dysfunction, and Stress

Research findings regarding the effects of children's stress on metabolic control are conflicting. Studies have found stressful life events of children were associated with poor glycemic control,[16,53] while others found the frequency and intensity of daily stressors or of laboratory-induced stress did not differentiate between levels of glycemic control.[30,31]

Anxiety, depression, and interpersonal conflict among children with IDDM has been found to have an impact on glycemic control.[70] These findings indicate that children who are depressed or whose families are in stress (e.g., family conflict, decreased cohesion, financial problems) are more likely to have worse glycemic control.

Positive family factors, family cohesion, and organization are associated with the child's improved self-care management and improved glycemic control.

Adherence and Self-Care

Treatment adherence refers to how closely children or their parents follow the prescribed diabetes management regimen. In general, self-monitoring of blood glucose alone is not sufficient to achieve good metabolic control.[9,28,119] Knowledge about diabetes management is higher in youth who are responsible for their own self-care and is related to better control.[4] In contrast, children who report more depression and anxiety display less problem-solving knowledge and worse control. Those who identify barriers to adherence also exhibit poorer control[69] (i.e., meal plan barriers included social interference, planning and problem-solving difficulties, and appetite problems).

Overall, these and other data suggest that adherence-control relationships must take into account the individual child's knowledge and management skills, the adequacy of the treatment regimen, and the presence of stress factors that together contribute to disruptions in metabolic functioning, since even children who adhere to the diabetes regimen may not have improved metabolic control.

ROLE OF THE DIABETES HEALTH CARE TEAM

The diabetes health care team needs to consist of a physician, nurse, dietitian, social worker, and/or psychologist. Team members need to frequently reassess parents and children's levels of knowledge, care and coping skills, and to confer with each other to devise effective management plans. Team members should be available to both parents and children by phone to answer the myriad of questions that arise on a day-to-day basis. However, the team's goal must be to assist parents and children to become independent in diabetes management, not dependent on team members.

RESEARCH IMPLICATIONS

Research is needed to determine the factors that influence the development of positive and negative emotional and psychosocial behaviors in children who have chronic illnesses such as diabetes.[89] In addition, research is needed to define the interrelationships of these behaviors with children's adherence to illness management and ultimately to a good or poor metabolic control outcome.

The critical periods when children are most receptive to basic and advanced knowledge and implementation of diabetes management skills have not been clearly identified.

Future research needs to determine when children with IDDM are best able to assume responsibility for specific components of diabetes management. Guidelines for self-care management skills need to be identified for specific developmental stages, especially for cognitive levels of children.

REFERENCES

1. Abusrewil S and Savage D: Obesity and diabetic control, Arch Dis Child 64:1313-1315, 1989.
2. Ainslie M and Spencer M: New approaches to diabetes in the young, Compr Ther 14:65-70, 1988.
3. Anderson B: The impact of diabetes on the developmental tasks of childhood and adolescence: a research perspective. In Nattrass M and Santiago J, eds: Recent advances in diabetes, London, 1984, Churchill and Livingston.
4. Anderson B and others: Assessing family sharing of diabetes responsibilities, J Pediatr Psychol 15:477-492, 1991.
5. Angel R and Worobey J: Single motherhood and children's health, J Health Soc Behav 29:38-52, 1988.
6. Auslander W and others: Risk factors to health in diabetic children: a prospective study from diagnosis, Health Soc Work 15:133-142, 1990.
7. Auslander W and others: Predictors of diabetes knowledge in newly diagnosed children and parents, J Pediatr Psychol 16:213-228, 1991.
8. Bantle JT: Injection site rotation: the downside, Pract Diabet 9:1-3, 1990.
9. Belmonte M and others: Impact of SMBG on control of diabetes as measured by HBA1: a three year survey, Diabetes Care 11:484-488, 1988.
10. Behrman R and Vaughn V, eds: Nelson's textbook of pediatrics, ed 12, Philadelphia, 1983, Saunders.
11. Betschart J: Parent's understanding of and guilt over children's blood glucose control, Diabetes Educ 13:393-401, 1987.
12. Betz G and Poster E: Communicating with children: more than just words, Paedovita 1:11-16, 1984.
13. Bibace R and Walsh M: Development of children's concepts of illness, Pediatrics 66:912-916, 1980.
14. Blethen S and others: Effect of pubertal stage and recent blood glucose control on plasma somatomedin C in children with insulin-dependent diabetes mellitus, Diabetes 30:868-872, 1981.
15. Bloch C and others: Puberty decreases insulin sensitivity, J Pediatr 110:481-487, 1987.
16. Brand A, Johnson J, and Johnson S: Life stress and diabetic control in children and adolescents with insulin-dependent diabetes, J Pediatr Psychol 11:481-495, 1986.
17. Brewster A: Chronically ill hospitalized children's concepts of their illness, Pediatrics 69:355-362, 1982.
18. Brink S: Pediatric adolescent, and young-adult nutrition issues in IDDM, Diabetes Care 11:192-200, 1988.
19. Brown A: School-Age children with diabetes: knowledge and management of the disease, and adequacy of self-concept, Matern Child Nurs J 14:47-61, 1985.
20. Canfield W, Hambidge K, and Johnson L: Zinc nutriture in type I diabetes mellitus: relationship to growth measures and metabolic control, J Pediatr Gastrolenteral Nutr 3:577-584, 1984.
21. Cerreto M and Travis L: Implications of psychological and family factors in the treatment of diabetes, Pediatri Clin North Am 31:689-707, 1984.
22. Cerutti F and others: Course of retinopathy in children and adolescents with insulin-dependent diabetes mellitus: a ten-year study, Ophthalmologica 198:116-123, 1989.
23. Clarson C and others: Residual beta-cell function in children with IDDM: reproducibility of testing and factors influencing insulin secretory reserve, Diabetes Care 10:33-38, 1987.
24. Court S and others: Children with diabetes mellitus: perception of their behavioral problems by parents and teachers, Early Hum Dev 16:245-252, 1988.
25. Cross B and others: Metabolic and endocrine function and alterations. In Servonsky J and Opas S, eds: Nursing management of children, Boston, 1987, Jones and Bartlett.
26. Cryer P and Gerich J: Relevance of counter regulatory system to patients with diabetes: critical roles of glucagon and epinephrine, Diabetes Care 6:95-99, 1983.
27. Daneman D and Ehrlich R: Management of insulin-dependent diabetes mellitus in childhood, Med North Am 15:1852-1859, 1984.
28. Daneman D and others: The role of self-monitoring of blood glucose in the routine management of children with insulin-dependent diabetes mellitus, Diabetes Care 8:1-4, 1985.
29. Delamater A and others: Randomized prospective study of self-management training with newly diagnosed diabetic children, Diabetes Care 13:492-498, 1990.

30. Delameter A and others: Stress and coping in relation to metabolic control of adolescents with Type I diabetes, Dev Behav Pediatr 8:136-140, 1987.

31. Delamater A and others: Physiologic responses to acute psychological stress in adolescents with type I diabetes, J Pediatr Psychol 13:69-86, 1988.

32. Delamater A and others: Dietary skills and adherence in children with type I diabetes mellitus, Diabetes Educ 14:33-36, 1988.

33. Delamater A and others: Diabetes management in the school setting: the role of the school psychologist, School Psychol Rev 13:192-203.

34. Delp R: Kids speak up: a special article for the young set, Diabetes Forecast 36:38-40, 1983.

35. Dische S and others: Childhood nocturnal enuresis: factors associated with outcome of treatment with an enuresis alarm, Dev Med Child Neurol 25:67-80, 1983.

36. Doleys D: Behavioral treatments for nocturnal enuresis in children: a review of the recent literature, Psychol Bull 84:30-54, 1977.

37. Drayer N: Height of diabetic children at onset of symptoms, Arch Dis Child 49:616-620, 1974.

38. Eisner C: The psychology of childhood illness, New York, 1985, Springer-Verlag.

39. Elkind D: Children and adolescents: interpretive essays on Jean Piaget, ed 3, New York, 1981, Oxford University Press.

40. Epstein I and others: Measurement and modification of the accuracy of determinations of urine glucose concentration, Diabetes Care 3:535-536, 1980.

41. Esslinger P: The preschooler. In Smith M, Goodman J, and Ramsey N, eds: Child and family: concepts of nursing practice, New York, 1987, McGraw-Hill Publishing Co.

42. Faro B: Maintaining good control in children with diabetes, Pediatr Nurs 9:368-373, 1983.

43. Feldman K: Prevention of childhood accidents: Recent progress, Pediatr Rev 2:75-82, 1980.

44. Follansbee D: Assuming responsibility for diabetes management: What age? What price? Diabetes Educ 15:347-352, 1989.

45. Fonagy P and others: Psychological adjustment and diabetic control, Arch Dis Child 62:1009-1013, 1987.

46. Franz M: Use of nonnutritive and nutritive sweeteners, Diabetes Educ 14:357-359, 1988.

47. Franz M and Norstrom J: Diabetes actively staying healthy: your game plan for diabetes and exercise, Wayzata, MN, 1990, DCI Publishing.

48. Garrison M and McQueston A: Chronic illness during childhood and adolescence, Newbury Park, CA, 1989, Sage Publication.

49. Gearheart BR: Learning disabilities: educational strategies, ed 4, St. Louis, 1989, Mosby–Times Mirror.

49a. Giordano B, Neuenkirchen G, Banion C: Diabetes management responsibilities: assessment for readiness, Presented at American Association of Diabetes Educators, Cincinnati, OH, 1990.

50. Gray D and others: Chronic poor metabolic control in the pediatric population: a stepwise intervention program, Diabetes Educ 14:516-520, 1988.

51. Guyer B and Gallagher S: An approach to the epidemiology of childhood injuries, Pediatr Clin North Am 32:5-15, 1985.

52. Hamburg B and Inoff G: Coping with predictable crises of diabetes, Diabetes Care 6:409-415, 1983.

53. Hanson S and Pichert J: Perceived stress and diabetes control in adolescents, Health Psychol 5:439-452, 1986.

54. Hauenstein E and others: Stress in parents of children with diabetes mellitus, Diabetes Care 12:18-23, 1989.

55. Hausdorf G, Rieger U, and Koepp P: Cardiomyopathy in childhood diabetes mellitus: incidence, time of onset, and relation to metabolic control, Intern J Cardiol 19:225-236, 1988.

56. Hodges L and Parker J: Concerns of parents with diabetic children, Pediatr Nurs 13:22-24, 1987.

57. Hymovich D and Chamberlin R: Child and family development, New York, 1980, McGraw-Hill.

58. Ingersoll G and others: Cognitive maturity and self-management among adolescents with insulin-dependent diabetes mellitus, J Pediatr 108:620-623, 1986.

59. Jacobson A and others: Psychologic predictors of compliance in children with recent onset of diabetes mellitus, J Pediatr 110:805-811, 1987.

60. Johnson BH: Children's drawings as a projective technique, Pediatr Nurs 16:11-17, 1990.

61. Johnson S and others: Cognitive and behavioral knowledge about insulin-dependent diabetes among children and parents, Pediatrics 69:708-713, 1982.

62. Johnson S and Rosenbloom A: Behavioral aspects of diabetes mellitus in childhood and adolescence, Psychiatr Clin North Am 5:357-369, 1982.

63. Kohlberg L: The child as a moral philosopher, Psychol Today 2:25-30, 1968.
64. Krauser K and Madden P: The child with diabetes mellitus, Nurs Clin North Am 18:749-762, 1983.
65. Krolewski A and others: Risk of proliferative diabetic retinopathy in juvenile-onset type 1 diabetes: a 40-year follow-up study, Diabetes Care 9:443-452, 1986.
66. Kupper N, Foster M, and MacMillan D: Treating children with type 1 diabetes mellitus: choosing an appropriate nutritional treatment strategy, Diabetes Educ 14:238-242, 1988.
67. Kurtz S: Adherence to diabetes regimens: empirical status and clinical applications, Diabetes Educ 16:50-56, 1990.
68. LaGreca A: Children with diabetes and their families: Coping and disease management, In Field T, McCabe P and Schneiderman N, eds: Stress and coping across development, Newark, NJ, 1988, Erlbaum.
69. La Greca A, Follansbee D, and Skyler J: Developmental and behavioral aspects of diabetes management among children and adolescents, Child Health Care (in press).
70. La Greca A and Skyler J: Psychosocial issues in IDDM: A multivariate framework. In McCabe P and others, eds: Stress, coping and disease (in press).
71. LaPorte R and Cruickshanks K: Incidence and risk factors for insulin-dependent diabetes. In: Diabetes in America, National Diabetes Data Group, NIH Publication 85-1468, DHHS, Washington, DC, 1985.
72. Lask B: Psychosocial factors in childhood diabetes and seizure disorders: the family approach, Pediatrician 15:95-101, 1988.
73. Lavigne J and others: Parental perceptions of the psychological adjustment of children with diabetes and their siblings, Diabetes Care 5:420-426, 1982.
74. Leach D and Erickson G: Children's perspectives on diabetes, J School Health 58:159-161, 1977.
75. Lee R and Bode H: Stunted growth and hepatomegaly in diabetes mellitus, J Pediatr 91:82-84, 1977.
76. Lerner J: Learning disabilities: theories, diagnosis, and teaching strategies, Boston, 1981, Houghton Mifflin.
77. Levitsky L: Growth and pubertal pattern in insulin dependent diabetes mellitus, Sem Adolesc Med 3:233-239, 1987.
78. Levine M: Middle childhood. In Levine M and others: developmental-behavioral pediatrics, Philadelphia, 1983, WB Saunders.
79. Lewis C and Lewis M: Peer pressure and risk-taking behaviors in children, Am J Public Health 74:580-584, 1984.
80. Lindsay R, Jarrett L, and Hillman K: Elementary Schoolteachers' understanding of diabetes, Diabetes Care 13:312-314, 1987.
81. Lockwood D and others: The biggest problem in diabetes, Diabetes Educ 12:30-33, 1986.
82. Lorenz R, Christensen N, and Pichert J: Diet-related knowledge, skill, and adherence among children with insulin-dependent diabetes mellitus, Pediatrics 75:872-876, 1985.
83. Mann N and Johnson D: Improvement in metabolic control in diabetic adolescents by the use of increased insulin dose, Diabetes Care 7:460-464, 1984.
84. Martens R and Seefeldt V: Guidelines for children's sports, 1979, The American Alliance for Health, Physical Education, Recreation, and Dance.
85. Marteau T, Bloch S, and Baum J: Family life and diabetic control, Child Psychol Psychiatr 28:823-833, 1987.
86. Menon R and Spearling M: Childhood diabetes, Med Clin North Am 72:1565-1576, 1988.
87. Minuchin S and others: A conceptual model of psychosomatic illness in children, Arch Gen Psychiatr 32:1031-1039, 1975.
88. Moy CS and LaPorte RE: Why do so many children in U.S. develop diabetes? Pract Diabetol 8:1-8, 1989.
89. Nelms B: Emotional behaviors in chronically ill children, J Abnormal Child Psychol 17:657-668, 1989.
90. Neumann C: Obesity in pediatric practice: obesity in the preschool and school-age child, Pediatr Clin North Am 21:117-122, 1977.
91. Nuvoli G and others: Diabetes and illness image: an analysis of diabetic early-adolescents' self-perception through the draw-a-person test, Psychol Rep 65:83-93, 1989.
92. Pedersen O and Beck-Nielsen H: Insulin resistance and insulin-dependent diabetes mellitus, Diabetes Care 10:516-523, 1987.
93. Peterson H and others: Growth body weight and insulin requirement in diabetic children, Acta Pediatr Scand 67:453-457, 1978.
94. Piaget J: The construction of reality in the child, New York, 1971, Ballantine.
95. Piaget J and Inhelder B: Memory and intelligence, New York, 1973, Basic Books.

96. Pond H: Parental attitudes towards children with a chronic medical disorder: special reference to diabetes mellitus, Diabetes Care 2:425-431, 1979.

97. Pontious S: Practical Piaget: helping children understand, Am J Nurs 82:112-114, 1982.

98. Pontious S: Communication with children. In Servonsky J and Opas S, eds: Nursing management of children, Boston, 1987, Jones and Bartlett Publishing Co.

99. Rivara F and Barber M: Demographic analysis of childhood pedestrian injuries, Pediatrics 76:375-381, 1985.

100. Schafer L and others: Adherence to IDDM regimens: relationship to psychosocial variables and metabolic control, Diabetes Care 6:493-498, 1983.

101. Schreiner B and Travis L: When your child has diabetes: the preteen years, Diabetes Forecast 40:37-41, 1987.

102. Schriock E, Winter R, and Traisman H: Diabetes mellitus and its effects on menarche, J Adolesc Health Care 5:101-104, 1984.

103. Sieman M: Mental health in school-age children, Am J Mater Child Nurs 3:215, 1978.

104. Shalwitz R and others: Prevalence and consequences of nocturnal hypoglycemia among conventionally treated children with diabetes mellitus, J Pediatr 116:685-689, May, 1990.

105. Skyler JS: Why control diabetes? Influence on chronic complications of diabetes, Pediatr Annu 16:713-724, 1987.

106. Steranchak I: When the lunch bell rings, Diabetes Forecast 39:32-37, 1986.

107. Stewart-Brown S, Lee T, and Savage D: Pubertal growth of diabetes, Arch Dis Child 60:768-769, 1985.

108. Tattersal R and Pyke D: Growth in diabetic children, studies in identical twins, Lancet 2:1105-1109, 1973.

109. Templeton C and others: A group approach to nutritional problem solving using self-monitoring of blood glucose with diabetic adolescents, Diabetes Educ 14:189-191, 1988.

110. Tuttle WW and others: Effect on school boys of omitting breakfast, J Am Diet Assoc 30:674-678, 1974.

111. Vessey J, Braithwaite K, and Wiedmann M: Teaching children about their internal bodies, Pediatr Nurs 16:29-33, 1990.

112. Wertlieb D, Hauser S, and Jacobson A: Adaptation of diabetes: behavior symptoms and family context, J Pediatr Psychol 11:463-479, 1986.

113. Whaley L and Wong D: Nursing care of infants and children, ed 3, St. Louis, 1987, Mosby–Year Book.

114. White N and others: Identification of type I diabetic patients at increased risk for hypoglycemia during intensive therapy, N Engl J Med 308:485-491, 1983.

115. Wilcox M: Developmental journey—a guide to the development of logical and moral reasoning and social perspective, Nashville, 1980, Abingdon.

116. Wilde J: The school-age child. In Smith M, Goodman J, and Ramsey N: Child and family: concepts of nursing practice, New York, 1987, McGraw-Hill.

117. Wing R and others: Behavioral skills in self-monitoring of blood glucose: relationship to accuracy, Diabetes Care 9:330-333, 1986.

118. Winter R: Special problems of the child with diabetes. Comp Ther 8:7-13, 1982.

119. Wysocki T, Green L, and Huxtable K: Blood glucose monitoring by diabetic adolescents: compliance and metabolic control, Health Psychol 8:267-284, 1989.

120. Wysocki T and others: Survey of diabetes professionals regarding developmental changes in diabetes self-care, Diabetes Care 13:65-68, 1990.

121. Yki-Jarvinen H and Kovisto V: Natural course of insulin resistance in Type I diabetes, N Engl J Med 315:224-227, 1986.

CHAPTER 13

The Adolescent With Diabetes

DENIS DANEMAN AND **MARCIA FRANK**

Anna Freud characterized the period between childhood and young adulthood thus: "Adolescence is by its nature an interruption of peaceful growth, and . . . the upholding of a steady equilibrium during the adolescent period is in itself abnormal. . . . Adolescence resembles in appearance a variety of other emotional upsets and structural upheavals. The adolescent manifestations come close to symptom formation of the neurotic, psychotic, or dissocial order and merge almost imperceptibly into . . . almost all the mental illnesses."[37] This view of adolescence, which has been supported by many of the earlier commentators, however, has been based more on "confident assertion than by the presence of well-based knowledge."[99] Even today debate rages as to whether the view of adolescence as a time of turmoil and significant emotional upheaval is fact or fiction. More recent studies have concluded that while adolescent turmoil may be a fairly frequent finding, its psychiatric importance has been greatly overestimated.[58,99]

Similarly, early research on the relationship between both the cause and course of diabetes on the one hand and psychosocial factors on the other was most influenced by psychoanalytic theory and sought to find a "diabetic personality" that predisposed the individual to this disease. Research and clinical experience have failed to support this concept; nevertheless, interest in the interaction between diabetes and behavioral, social, and emotional factors has flourished.[57,58,72] Thus, while early research on psychosocial aspects of diabetes in adolescence focused primarily on personality issues, current models are much more complex and presume psychosocial adjustment and health status to be the result of multiple patient and environmental variables.

Adolescence is clearly a time of rapid biologic change accompanied by increasing physical, cognitive, and emotional maturity. It is a time of increasing independence from family and the start of peer conformity, experimentation, and limit testing. The presence of a chronic disease such as insulin-dependent diabetes mellitus (IDDM) may have an impact on both biologic and psychologic aspects of adolescent development.

In this chapter the focus will be on normal adolescent development, both physical and emotional, and the impact of IDDM on this development. We will highlight how these interactions may have an impact on both the short- and long-term outcome of diabetes. Since the adolescent with diabetes is often characterized as being in poor metabolic control, we will also explore the reasons for such metabolic deterioration. Following this we outline a treatment approach to adolescents with IDDM, stress the importance of anticipatory guidance with respect to the long-term micro- and macrovascular complications, and suggest directions for future research in this population.

The objectives of this chapter then, are to develop an understanding of teens with diabetes as normal adolescents in an abnormal situation; describe the normal biology of adolescence; discuss the psychology of adolescence; describe the impact of diabetes on the normal processes of adolescence; summarize factors contributing to poor health outcomes (poor metabolic control); explain the effects of exercise, alcohol, drugs, and smoking on diabetes; describe the epidemiology of diabetes-related complications in teenagers; summarize the goals of diabetes management in this age group; evaluate the impact of diabetes on career planning; and assess strategies to improve metabolic control and general well-being.

PHYSICAL DEVELOPMENT
Growth and Development

The onset of adolescence is heralded biochemically by activation of the "gonadostat," the hypothalamic-pituitary-gonadal axis, by mechanisms that remain largely unknown.[105] This change from tonic suppression of gonadotrophin secretion to its pulsatile release begins a period of the most rapid hormonal and physical changes since early infancy. The pulsatile nature of secretion of a number of hormones, including gonadotrophins, sex steroids, and growth hormone, are important in both the initiation and maintenance of sexual maturation. The period ends with the achievement of full sexual and physical development. There are very good correlations during adolescence between sex hormone concentrations found in the plasma (either in the basal state or in response to dynamic testing) and the stage of physical development achieved.

The onset of puberty in the female (noted by the onset of breast development between 9 and 13 years of age) occurs slightly earlier than that in the male (testicular enlargement starting between 10 and 14 years).[112] Furthermore, pubertal progression in the female is much more rapid with achievement of peak height velocity soon after the onset of puberty (Tanner stages 2 to 4) and virtual completion of maturation with the onset of menstruation (menarche occurs on average 2 years after the onset of puberty, i.e. 11 to 15 years). In males, peak height velocity is reached later in puberty (Tanner stages 3 to 5). The later onset of puberty and the later achievement of peak height velocity in the male account for the final adult height differential between the sexes, adult men being on average 12.5 cm taller than women. Females appear more sensitive to small changes in gonadotrophin-releasing hormone concentrations than males. This explains why puberty begins slightly earlier in girls. The reason for the difference in timing of peak height velocity is uncertain but may relate to differences in sex steroid–growth hormone relationships between the sexes. In females, low levels of estradiol may stimulate growth hormone secretion, while high levels block insulin-like growth factor 1 (IGF-1) production. In males, relatively higher levels of testosterone are required to accentuate the effects of growth hormone.[105]

Impact of Diabetes on Physical Development

The relationship between diabetes and adolescence may be viewed from a number of different directions: first, do factors during adolescence trigger the onset of the disease and its complications; second, what is the impact of diabetes on normal adolescent development; and, third, what are the effects of the hormonal changes of adolescence on metabolic control?

IDDM affects both sexes equally; it can occur at any age but it has its peak incidence in late childhood/early adolescence, this peak being somewhat earlier in females than males.[31] However, IDDM can occur at any age. It remains largely speculative as to the reasons why the peak incidence of IDDM occurs at this age. Whether the changing hormonal milieu is responsible in any way remains unknown. It seems possible that in those with declining B-cell mass, a rapid increase in counterregulatory hormones, accompanied by the metabolic needs for growth, may tip the balance leading to exhaustion of the remaining functional B-cells and presentation of the disease. By the end of adolescence, the prevalence of IDDM will be one in 500 to 600, making it one of the most common chronic disorders of childhood.[31]

The severity of the presenting metabolic derangement tends to be greater in younger children, particularly infants and toddlers, and less so in adolescents. Clinical remission (the "honeymoon period") occurs shortly after diagnosis and is associated with metabolic stability, declining insulin dose requirement, and usually, partial recovery of B-cell function.[102] This remission period tends to last longer and be of greater magnitude clinically in the adolescent than in the younger child.

The impact of IDDM on adolescent physical and sexual development has been studied ever since the availability of insulin therapy in the 1920s.[8,53,74] At onset of diabetes, children have been reported to be of average to slightly above average height, suggesting that there is no impact of the "preclinical phase of IDDM" (marked by the presence of immunologic abnormalities and also by abnormalities in insulin secretion, but with normal glucose homeostasis) on physical development. After initiation of insulin therapy, normal growth and sexual development depend more on the presence of adequate insulinization than on the achievement of near normoglycemia.[19]

Early reports suggested that children with IDDM grew more poorly than their nondiabetic peers, entered puberty at a later stage, and achieved a significantly decreased final adult height.[8,53,74] The most striking illustration of the impact of underinsulinization on adolescent growth and development was described in 1934 by Mauriac and others.[79] The Mauriac syndrome, fortunately now quite rare, comprises hepatomegaly, growth failure, and pubertal delay, all resulting from prolonged and profound underinsulinization. Several authors in the 1950s and 1960s reported a significant decrease in height, caused by a reduced growth velocity in children studied from 6 months to 3 years after diagnosis.[8,53,74] Some also found a decrease in final adult height in those with IDDM, particularly boys.[8,68] More recent studies have reported that children with diabetes display normal growth patterns and normal onset and progression of pubertal development.[19,54]

We recently evaluated growth and pubertal development and their relationship to metabolic control in a representative subgroup of 122 children in our Diabetes Clinic.[19] These children were found to have growth characteristics similar to those of children without diabetes, not only in terms of distribution of height and weight percentiles, but also of height and weight velocity percentiles. Specifically, we were unable to find any relationship between metabolic control, as reflected by hemoglobin A_{1c} levels, and growth parameters. We concluded that conventional management of IDDM children should be associated with normal growth and puberty and that normal development did not necessarily indicate optimal, but rather only "average" control.

There are many factors influencing growth in children, some of which, such as genetic background and nutrition, are major determinants of growth velocity, onset of puberty, and final adult height achieved. It may be that any contribution of diabetic control to growth is very small and only apparent at the very extreme of poor metabolic control. These data indicate that the presence of normal growth and physical development in IDDM children should not lull health care providers into a false sense of security that this reflects good metabolic control. Conversely, although extremely poor metabolic control may contribute to poor growth and delayed adolescence, the latter finding in an adolescent with IDDM warrants thorough investigation.

Early data also suggested a delay in the onset of menstruation in IDDM girls compared with their nondiabetic counterparts.[55,106,114] In 1948, Beal[8] reported that diabetic girls continued to increase in height until age 17.5 years, indicating a delay in either the onset or progression of puberty. Sterky[106] found menarche to occur 4 months later than normal in 27 girls with IDDM onset before 12 years of age, and Jackson[54] reported that delayed menarche occurred in girls with poor metabolic control. The most striking evidence for delayed menarche occurring in association with diabetes was found in the report by Tattersall and Pyke:[114] menarche occurred 4 and 5 years later in the diabetic than in the nondiabetic identical twins. Unlike the older reports, more recent research has revealed a normal distribution of the onset of menarche.[19]

Taken together, the older data revealed poorer growth in adolescents with IDDM, while more recent evidence has suggested that in adequately treated IDDM, growth is normal. This change is likely a result of more comprehensive treatment strategies that include appropriate insulinization and provision of calories.[24] This allows for normal growth and development within a wide spectrum of metabolic control. An extension of this is the finding of excessive weight gain in those IDDM individuals treated more intensively with either continuous subcutaneous insulin infusion systems or with multiple daily injections (3) of insulin and in whom normoglycemia has been targeted.[29]

Finally, what is the impact of the changing hormonal milieu during adolescence on the ability to achieve and maintain adequate metabolic control in these children? There is convincing evidence that metabolic control, as noted by increasing glycated hemoglobin (HbA$_{1c}$) levels, deteriorates during adolescence despite significantly higher insulin doses.[11,26] Research has demonstrated that glycated hemoglobin levels increase with age, the highest levels being found in the age group 12 to 16 years[26] (see Fig. 13-1).

This deterioration in glycated hemoglobin levels was more marked in females than males with IDDM. Furthermore, this increase with age was independent of disease duration. Blethen and others[11] reported a similar finding in relation to pubertal staging. This deterioration in control is all the more striking when the relative increased insulin dose requirements during adolescence are noted.[11,31] In Blethen's study, for example, HbA$_{1c}$ levels increased in pubertal boys from 11.6% to 14.1% despite an increase in insulin dose (expressed as u/kg per day) of 36% to 44%.

The report of the initial feasibility phase of the Diabetes Control and Complications Trial (DCCT) highlights differences between adolescents and adults with IDDM both at initiation and during the first year of therapy in the study: first, at randomization into the trial, HbA$_{1c}$ levels and insulin dosages were significantly higher in the adolescents than in adults.[28] For example, in those randomized to conventional (standard) insulin treatment, adult volunteers had a mean HbA$_{1c}$ and insulin dose of 9.0% and 0.65 u/kg respectively; in the adolescents these were both significantly higher, 9.8% and 0.94 u/kg. In the intensive (experimental) treatment group, adult HbA$_{1c}$ of 9.2% and insulin dose of 0.62 u/kg were similarly less than the adolescent, 10.1% and 0.95 u/kg respectively. Second, throughout the first year of study, HbA$_{1c}$ levels in adolescents remained about 1% higher whether they were assigned to the standard or experimental group. Nevertheless, the reduction in mean HbAlc and blood glucose levels in the "experimental" adolescents was of the same order of magnitude as that seen in the "experimental" adults when compared with their respective standard groups.

These data suggest that there are substantial impediments to the achievement of good

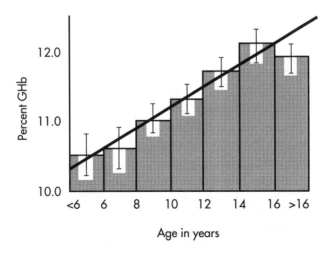

Fig. 13-1 Relationship of age of the patient to glycosylated hemoglobin (GHb) (r = 0.24, p < 0.001). (Modified from Daneman D and others: Factors affecting glycosylated hemoglobin values in children with insulin-dependent diabetes, J Pediatr 99:847-853, 1981.)

metabolic control in adolescents with IDDM. The deterioration in metabolic control during adolescence has long been attributed to problems with compliance in these youngsters.[18,51,57,61] However, recently compelling data have emerged that suggest that biological factors may also be operative, namely declining peripheral insulin action and changing counterregulatory hormonal responses.[4,12,91,111]

While IDDM is a disease of B-cell destruction, what is also becoming increasingly clear is that peripheral insulin action ("sensitivity") is impaired in all hyperglycemic states and more particularly at certain times, specifically during adolescence and times of poorer metabolic control.[4,12,17] Using the euglycemic, hyperinsulinemic clamp technique, several groups have been able to demonstrate convincingly that peripheral insulin sensitivity is decreased during adolescence in nondiabetics when compared with that in younger children and adults.[4] At each stage (Fig. 13-2) of development, insulin action is more impaired in those individuals with IDDM, such that the most impaired insulin action is seen in adolescents with IDDM.[4,12,91] Although as yet not conclusive, the data also suggest that this "resistance" may be most marked in the female adolescent. The reasons for declining insulin action remain speculative, but are likely related to at least some of the attendant hormonal changes. Since sex hormones in adolescents are lower than those in adults, it seems unlikely that these would be the prime suspects. More probably, changes in growth factors, specifically changes in the growth hormone–IGF-1 axis, will be found to be the cause.[4,12,91] In fact, in the study of Bloch and others,[12] a correlation was noted between insulin resistance and IGF-1 concentrations.

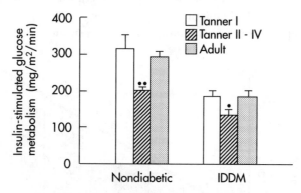

Fig. 13-2 Effect of puberty on insulin-stimulated glucose metabolism in nondiabetic and diabetic subjects. Value (means ±SE) in prepubertal children (Tanner stage I) are shown by open bars, those in pubertal (Tanner stages II to IV) by hatched bars, and those in adults by the shaded bars. The double asterick denotes p < 0.01 for nondiabetic children in Tanner stages II to IV versus nondiabetic children in Tanner Stage I and adults; the single asterisk denotes p < 0.05 for children with IDDM in Tanner stages II to IV versus children with IDDM in Tanner stage I. Insulin-stimulated glucose metabolism was also significantly lower in patients with IDDM than in nondiabetics at each stage of development (p < 0.01). (From Amiel D and others: Impaired insulin action in puberty: a contributing factor or poor glycemic control in adolescents with diabetes, New Engl J Med 315:215-219, 1986.)

Furthermore, it appears that counterregulatory hormone responses, and specifically those of epinephrine, may be more brisk in children with diabetes than in those without, and also more so than in diabetic or nondiabetic adults.[111] In at least one study, epinephrine responses were shown to occur at higher blood glucose concentrations and to reach a greater magnitude in children with diabetes than in adults.[111] These rapid changes in epinephrine may contribute, at least in part, to the metabolic instability that characterizes some, but not all, adolescents with IDDM.

PSYCHOLOGIC DEVELOPMENT
Normal Development

In attempting to understand the psychosocial impact of diabetes on adolescents and their families, it may be helpful for the health care provider to view these young people as normal teens in an abnormal situation. Such an approach casts adolescents with diabetes in a normalizing framework and permits the use of developmental theories to conceptualize and predict the difficulties that they and their families may encounter.[17,90] This section will begin with a review of normal psychosocial and cognitive growth during adolescence and then focus on the interrelationship between normal development and diabetes.

Adolescence is a phase quite distinct from both childhood and adulthood in terms of emotional focus and psychologic needs. Furthermore, within adolescence three distinct stages of development are recognized, specifically early, middle, and late adolescence.[27,89] Briefly, early adolescence is characterized by rapid physical growth and maturation. These changes are accompanied by intense self-examination; body image is of paramount importance. Young teens need to know that they are normal; reassurance is sought by comparison with peers.[89] Emotional normalcy is tested by acceptance into the peer group. To be excluded is the worst possible scenario.[27] As teens move into midadolescence, the struggle for autonomy and control of personal destiny become more prominent. This period is often associated with varying degrees of parental conflict as the peer group replaces parental influence and sets behavior standards.[17,27,89] With late adolescence comes increasing stability. Successful conclusion of adolescent development is accompanied by the establishment of clear vocational goals and a global sense of personal identity.[33]

In a comprehensive review of normal adolescence, Orr and Ingersoll emphasize the wide variability in adolescent development.[89] They stress that differences do not occur only across age groups but also within age groups and within individuals. Taken as a whole however, the teen's central developmental task is to establish a new sense of personal identity that involves adjusting to a new physical self, a new cognitive self, and a new social self. For many people this level of maturation does not occur until their mid-twenties.

Cognitive development

Included in the many transitions that occur during adolescence are a number of important changes in cognitive abilities. Cognitive development is more than an accumulation of new knowledge: it also involves a new way of thinking and speculating about one-self and the environment.[44,89] Piaget and Inhelder[52] have provided the most useful model for the understanding of development. During preadolescence, children operate on a cognitive level that has been termed "concrete operational thought." During this early stage young people require concrete references to solve problems. Clearly, this way of thinking is limiting, and one's ability to adapt to the environment depends on moving beyond this stage. As teens progress through adolescence, it is expected that they will become more capable of abstract thinking and shift into what has been termed "formal operational thought." Along with increasing cognitive maturity comes more latitude in the adolescent's ability to consider hypothetical situations and to speculate about various possibilities for future consequences based on current actions. Furthermore, as young people progress toward social cognitive maturity, egocentrism diminishes permitting the adolescent to understand the perspectives of others, to better tolerate ambiguity and differences, and to recognize the interdependence of oneself with others. Orr and Ingersoll[89] point out that all of these attributes can be related to positive health care.

Included in the adolescents' cognitive structure and of particular relevance to the health practitioner are the teen's concepts of health and illness. Theoretically these views will have an impact on his or her willingness and ability to deal with health-related behaviors. In general, researchers have found that such concepts develop parallel with other aspects of cognitive maturation.[10,81,86] In their study of normal adolescents, Millstein and associates[81] found a shift from magical and mystical thinking in identifying causes of illness in younger children to a more conceptually sophisticated understanding of the disease process in older adolescents. However, they also reported a persistence of concrete explanations for illness in some older adolescents. This variation that is also described by others who study cognitive development underlines the fact that qualitative shifts in concepts are age-related rather than age-dependent.[17,44,90] Consequently, health professionals are wise to avoid assumptions regarding a teen's level of maturity simply on the basis of age and/or physical maturity.

Social development

Critical to adolescent psychosocial development is the emergence of a new sense of self.[33] Adolescents who successfully complete this task will enter the adult years with a feeling of competence. Preparation for adulthood, though, is a gradual and somewhat painful process. In the context of self-exploration and uncertainty, teens must make some sense out of the world, set realistic goals and limits, learn that rules are not the same for everyone everywhere, and learn to balance their own individual rights with the rights of others. It is not surprising, then, that many young people experience a considerable degree of inner turmoil at this time. Epidemiologic studies of normal adolescents summarized by Rutter and co-workers indicate that 14- and 15-year-old children commonly experience feelings of misery and self-deprecation. Many reported ideas of reference; that is, feeling that people were looking at them or talking and laughing about them. Only a small percentage had suicidal ideation. The results of these same studies also suggested that adults do not seem to appreciate how miserable these teens may feel.[99]

As teens progress through normal adolescence, their questions about who they are become multifaceted and their self-concept more complex. Self-concept is an accumulation of personal perceptions of one's own physical, social, educational, intellectual, and psychologic characteristics. In their review, Orr and others found evidence to support the smooth continuous development of self-concept over the teen years. They also suggest that significant social and psychologic crises, such as a move or a change in schools, may temporarily or permanently alter one's self-concept. The occurrence of major life events and the ability of the teen to manage them contributes to adolescents' feelings of self-worth.[89]

Within the context of the social milieu, other important transitions are occurring for the adolescent. Relationships with family members, especially parents, are changing; the peer group is increasingly influential. Teens beg and bargain for more freedom and responsibility; rules and limitations are frequently challenged. Conflict develops when the new values of the adolescent clash with the existing family values. How common and how serious are these conflicts? The epidemiologic studies summarized by Rutter and associates showed parent/adolescent conflict to be very common. Conflict issues, however, were generally trivial; that is, related to clothes, hair, and going out. Major parent/adolescent alienation however appeared to be unusual; physical and emotional withdrawal was uncommon; most teens were not especially critical of their parents; very few rejected them. This and other studies indicate that parents continue to have substantial influence on their children right through adolescence and into early adulthood. As expected, peer influence increased during the teen years sometimes to the point of rivaling parental influence but rarely replacing it.[99] Health professionals can use such data to reassure parents of normal adolescents and to indicate earlier evaluation and treatment for the troubled adolescent and his or her family.

Sexuality

Puberty is accompanied by the development of secondary sex characteristics and a change in the teen's self-concept. Young teens often feel frightened and overwhelmed by their lack of control over the rapid changes occurring in their bodies and self-conscious about differences between themselves and their peers. Body image is influenced not only by these rapid changes but also by perceived cultural norms. Adolescents who view their bodies as being less ideal than their peers may have less favorable feelings about themselves.[46]

Teenagers learn about body changes and develop sexual and social behavior through their peer relationships. In early adolescence, a same sex best friend is very important; intimate ideas and concerns are shared. Best friends experience a closeness that will develop into the capacity to form intimate heterosexual relationships.[46]

Adolescents become sexually active for a variety of reasons that tend to change as they mature. Younger teens may use sexual experimentation as a way of being accepted into a specific peer group or as a means of bolstering their self-esteem. These youngsters are less likely to consider the long-term outcomes of their sexual activity.[32] Conversely, older adolescents who have had opportunities to work through their sexual role are likely to be more comfortable with who they are and more capable of establishing intimacy in their relationships. Furthermore, these youngsters are more inclined to be thoughtful about the reasons for having intercourse, to plan for safe sex, and to use effective contraception.[32]

Impact of Diabetes on Psychologic Development

Since diabetes and its management are unavoidably intertwined with the complexities of growing up, an understanding of the normal process of adolescent development is essential for the health professional caring for teens with IDDM. In general, adolescents are highly concerned about their physical development, appearance, and emotions and are worried about being considered "normal." Teens with IDDM are faced with constant reminders that they are different each and every time that they inject insulin, monitor their blood sugar, or even eat a mouthful of food. The degree to which they and their families are able to meet the daily demands of self-management and still participate in life is a function of their coping.

Coping with diabetes

Diabetes management requires a degree of responsibility and behavioral control uncharacteristic of adolescents.[78] The daily demands of diabetes has an impact on the personal and public lives of adolescents, interacting with vital developmental tasks: independence, body image, identity, sexuality, responsibility, and self-esteem.[17] How well do young people and their families cope with the combination of diabetes and adolescence?

Psychosocial adjustment to diabetes has been the focus of considerable research. A number of earlier investigators reported that children and adolescents with diabetes, when compared with their healthy peers, were more commonly maladjusted and neurotic and had an inadequate self-image and weaker personalities.[69,110] More recently, however, a growing body of research suggests that diabetes in children and adolescence does not typically lead to psychologic disruption and that these young people are in fact quite well adjusted.[*]

The level of adjustment to diabetes is a reflection of the child and family's ability to cope with the additional tasks imposed by the disorder. According to Wexler, families are required to master both cognitive/practical (e.g., develop a satisfactory understanding of diabetes and demonstrate an ability to apply the necessary skills) as well as certain psychosocial tasks.[119] The latter include coping with the impact of the diagnosis, and experiencing a sense of mastery over diabetes thereby maintaining good self-esteem, and finally striving for and attaining a balanced acceptance of diabetes with positive expectations for the immediate and long-term future.

Coping with the demands of diabetes is probably most difficult immediately after diagnosis but also continues to require considerable effort over time. Coping is influenced

---

*References 1, 14, 56, 65, 72, 108.

by past experience and life-style and is affected by strengths in the adolescent, the family, and the environment.

Initial coping. Kovacs and associates[71-73] investigated the course of adjustment of children and families to diabetes from the time of onset. The coping responses and well-being of 74 children and their parents were assessed both retrospectively to and following diagnosis. They found that the majority of children were no different from those in the nondiabetic population before diagnosis in terms of psychosocial functioning. Furthermore, most children weathered the diagnosis and initial treatment quite well, although they commonly exhibited some psychologic upset in the beginning. During the adaptation phase, they typically experienced at least one of the following symptoms: periods of depression, feelings of friendlessness, irritability, anxiety, and some social withdrawal. These complaints declined within the first year of IDDM.

The study of Kovacs and others showed that emotional and behavioral disturbances that met criteria for psychiatric disturbance were not the norm but were nonetheless quite prevalent (36%). Adjustment disorders with anxiety and depression were most common; there was a 50% recovery rate within 3 months. Abnormal coping responses occurred more often in families from lower socioeconomic classes and in families who were experiencing severe marital difficulties. These children may have fewer coping resources available to them and lack in environmental and social assets or parental support.

Kovacs[73] also studied the coping responses of parents of children with diabetes. When compared with a control group, mild-to-moderate depression was two to three times more common in mothers of children with diabetes. Mothers were also more preoccupied with diabetes than were fathers and they "worried" all the time. Even when psychologic tests indicated that the parents were functioning well, they frequently became tearful, upset, and anxious and expressed feelings of hopelessness when asked about the child's diabetes. As with the children, the symptoms of depression and anxiety lessened over time.

The findings of this study demonstrate the emotional resilience of youngsters with diabetes and their families. Clinical experience and the reports of other investigators concur with Kovacs' conclusions. For example, Jacobson and associates assessed the psychosocial adjustment of children with recently diagnosed diabetes and found their levels of self-esteem, locus of control, and psychologic symptoms to be comparable to those of children with a recent, acute medical problem.[56] In another study, Hauenstein and co-workers evaluated stress in parents of children with diabetes and demonstrated that most mothers of children with diabetes have coping skills that are adequate to deal with the added stress posed by diabetes.[47]

Although healthy adaptation is the usual outcome for most children with diabetes, all of these studies, and that of Kovacs in particular, indicate that initially a negative emotional reaction should be expected. Health care professionals aware of these patterns of adjustment are better prepared to (1) help the child and family to anticipate the initial psychosocial effect of diabetes; (2) intervene with short-term supportive counseling knowing that most reactions are self-limited; and (3) identify those in need of more intensive psychosocial intervention.

Long-term coping.   Current evidence also supports a picture of psychologic health for those adolescents with diabetes of longer duration. Sullivan[108] found no differences in the self-esteem of adolescent girls with and without diabetes. Kellerman and associates[65] reported a similar finding when they assessed the relationship between chronic illness and psychologic functioning in adolescents. The results of this study further suggest that, even though chronically ill adolescents report high levels of situational stress, they generally do not become chronically anxious or react with inordinate distress to the problems of daily living.

In examining a number of studies on the psychologic adjustment of adolescents to diabetes, Cerreto and Travis[17] found evidence to show that, on the whole, teens with diabetes view themselves as being similar to their peers in the areas of personal freedom and responsibility in their daily lives. The studies reviewed also indicate that most adolescents reported telling their friends about diabetes, developing occupational goals sooner than their nondiabetic peers, and planning to marry and have children.

Thus, it would appear that for most adolescents, diabetes neither prevents nor seriously disrupts accomplishment of the developmental tasks viewed as essential for entry into psychologically healthy adulthood. Their sense of identity, self-esteem, autonomy, and future goal orientation seems to remain intact.

The documented evidence of healthy attitudes and lack of psychopathology in adolescents with diabetes is encouraging. Several authors postulate that this positive response is related to adolescents' denial of some of the hard realities of their illness.[113] This denial, however, is not necessarily inappropriate; rather, it can be viewed as part of the adaptation process.

Compliance and adherence

Haynes and colleagues[49] defined compliance as "the extent to which a person's behavior (in terms of taking medication, following a diet, or executing life-style changes) coincides with medical advice." For simplicity we have chosen to abandon the semantic arguments for and against use of the term "compliance" versus "adherence"; rather, we have used them interchangeably.

Poor adherence to health recommendations, particularly those that involve a life-style change, is widespread, perhaps more so in adolescents, including those with IDDM.[49,50,72] The factors that account for nonadherence are best understood within the context of normal adolescent development. Attitudes of experimentation, rebellion, and risk taking are commonly associated with the teen's struggle for control of his or her own destiny. It has been suggested that among adolescents with IDDM, management issues may become the battleground upon which the struggle for independence is fought.[60]

Disregard for the diet, infrequent monitoring, and insulin dose manipulation are behaviors observed in many of these young people. Blood glucose monitoring is especially difficult for the nonadherent adolescent; tests are often missed and/or the results fabricated. From the adolescents' perspective, this behavior is understandable since test results may provide evidence of poor performance and reinforce lack of control. As one 15-year-old girl said, "I can't make myself test because if I do I'll see how bad I am and I'll have to do something about it and I'm not ready yet." This girl and other poorly adherent adolescents are at risk for deteriorating metabolic control that may jeopardize their future health. Few of them, however, will experience any immediate health consequences as a result of paying minimal attention to their diabetes regimen, and many of them will perceive an immediate reward; that is, acceptance into the peer group. Thus, for teenagers, the reasons NOT to follow good diabetes management practices may far outweigh those that promote compliance.

Parents and health care providers also play a role in adolescent noncompliance. As teens mature, there is often a mismatch between what is expected of them in terms of independent self-care and their own interest and capabilities in this regard.[44] Establishment of unrealistic goals for the adolescent frequently results in premature withdrawal of active parental involvement in daily diabetes management, contributing to poor adherence and poor metabolic control. Sometimes, noncompliance may represent a deliberate disruption in order to get other needs met, such as attention from parents and health care providers. It may also result from denial of the reality or implications of the disease, or it may be the result of genuine lack of knowledge or self-management mistakes.[58]

To a large extent, the health care providers rely on the information provided to them by teens and their families in order to make suggestions regarding changes in the management regimen. Ability to offer safe, sensible advice depends on the teen's level of compliance and the reliability of his or her reporting to the team. Thus, health care providers must be able to assess compliance accurately. Most adolescents respond to a direct, nonjudgemental approach. For example, to assess adherence to self monitoring blood glucose, one may ask "How many times a week do you *manage* to check your blood sugar?" Or, when insulin omission is suspected, teens often find it easier to admit to *forgetting* their insulin rather than deliberately not taking it. In assessing dietary adherence we have most success when we begin by acknowledging how difficult it must be to follow a meal plan, by alluding to the problems that other teens have, especially when they are out with friends, and then by giving the teen an opportunity to discuss his or her own feelings, experiences, and concerns about food.

Extracting an admission from adolescents about noncompliant behavior rarely solves the problem. It is more important to find out what is interfering with their ability to care for their diabetes and to work with them and their families to develop strategies to deal with these issues.

FACTORS ASSOCIATED WITH POOR HEALTH OUTCOME

Most adolescents with diabetes are healthy and well adjusted. A few teens, however, encounter serious problems characterized by persistently poor metabolic control and/or impaired psychologic functioning. (See the box on p. 454 for a listing of factors associated with poor metabolic control.) This minority has been the focus of considerable attention both in the clinical setting and in the research literature, thus clouding the view of just how well most teens do.

FACTORS ASSOCIATED WITH POOR METABOLIC CONTROL IN ADOLESCENTS WITH IDDM

A. Biologic
   1. Impaired insulin action ("insulin resistance") during adolescence
   2. Counterregulatory hormone responses
B. Medical
   1. Acute intercurrent disease (e.g., dental abscess, influenza)
   2. Chronic intercurrent disease
      a. Diabetes-related (e.g., hypothyroidism, celiac disease)
      b. Unrelated to diabetes (e.g., chronic infection, malignancy)
C. Psychologic
   1. Lack of knowledge of diabetes and its management
   2. Poor social support—including unrealistic expectations for self-care
   3. Psychosocial issues
      a. Psychophysiologic response to stress
      b. Psychiatric disease
      c. Adolescent noncompliance
      d. Poor self-esteem and self-efficacy
      e. Family dysfunction
      f. Parental "collusion"
      g. Eating disorders—anorexia and bulimia nervosa and their subclinical variants

---

What factors account for this difference in outcome? The role of specific biologic and psychosocial variables in mediating health outcomes of teens with diabetes warrant further discussion.

Biologic

As stated earlier, the adolescent with IDDM is less sensitive to the action of insulin than either children or adults with the disease.[4,12] In addition, epinephrine responses to moderate drops in blood glucose concentration occur earlier and to a greater extent than in adults.[111] These two factors may contribute not only to the higher insulin dose requirement but also to some of the lability in metabolic control noted in some adolescents. Biologic factors are probably not central to the poorest level of metabolic control that characterizes a small group of adolescents with IDDM.

Medical

Occasionally, intercurrent illnesses may interfere with the ability to achieve good blood glucose control (e.g., chronic pyelonephritis, malabsorption). These are relatively rare occurrences, but they do warrant a thorough evaluation before problems with blood glucose regulation are ascribed to the other causes listed.

Knowledge and Level of Cognitive Maturity

The daily demands of diabetes are complex, requiring technical competence with routines, comprehension of complicated concepts related to blood glucose balance, and an appreciation of future implications and complications. Knowledge about diabetes and the self-management routines is a prerequisite for self-care. Thus, inadequate knowledge will potentially have an impact on metabolic control. Knowledge alone, however, is not sufficient to predict good diabetes control.

Many children develop diabetes at a time when their cognitive or emotional maturity is insufficiently well-developed to allow a thorough understanding of IDDM and its therapy.[69] It is essential to continuously upgrade the understanding and self-care skills of these youngsters in order to ensure that a simple "knowledge deficit" is not at the root of their inability to achieve adequate metabolic homeostasis. We believe that such a pure knowledge deficit is only occasionally the cause of metabolic deterioration. However, in these few individuals, correction of the deficit or misconception (e.g., timing of insulin injections and blood glucose testing) can greatly improve their control. Educational efforts must be tailored to the specific cognitive capabilities of each teen and his or her family. Occasionally, specific learning disabilities hamper understanding of diabetes care. Such situations may warrant changes in the basic approach to self-care, for example, more frequent contact with the health care team to discuss insulin dose adjustment.

Supportive

Two of the major causes leading to deterioration in adolescent diabetes control are: (1) the setting of unrealistic expectations for treatment outcome (blood glucose and glycated hemoglobin levels) by parents and health care providers, and (2) too early and too rapid transfer from parent- to adolescent-oriented diabetes care.

Many health care providers target unrealistic and unachievable goals such as euglycemia and normal HbA_{1c} levels in all children with IDDM. A number of studies have suggested just how unreasonable these goals are for the majority of adolescents.[9,11,26,43] Rather, the diabetes regimen should be tailored to suit each individual adolescent and his/her family taking into account their intellectual, economic, and social abilities. Health care providers should avoid being excessively judgmental in the way they deal with these youngsters and their families: often the behavior of the health care provider leads directly to fabricated test results and implicit parental support for their noncompliant behaviors in an effort to satisfy the health care team.

The issue of when to encourage transfer of responsibility from parent- to self-oriented diabetes care has been dealt with in a number of studies.[1,69] For example, Ingersoll and colleagues[51] asked their adolescent patients to indicate who was making the adjustments in their insulin dosage: in children <15 years of age, parents made some or all adjustments in 15 of 18 subjects, in those >15 years, parents adjusted insulin in only 2 of 23 subjects. Nevertheless, increased self-management did not necessarily translate into "good" care. On the contrary, in some it led to deterioration in metabolic control.

It becomes clear that age is not the only criterion for transfer of responsibility: cognitive and emotional maturity are more important. The process is not—and should not be—sudden; that is, one day the parent gives the insulin injection and the next day the teen does it alone behind a closed door. Rather, a gradual evolution should take place with direct parental involvement in the daily routines and decision-making receding slowly as the adolescent demonstrates willingness *and* ability to take over. During times of stress; for example intercurrent illness—parental supervision once again becomes mandatory. By making responsibility contingent on performance, we hope to reinforce appropriate self-care.

Psychosocial issues

Since individuals with IDDM live their lives under the constant threat of both acute (hypoglycemia and ketoacidosis) and chronic (macro- and microvascular) complications, it is not surprising that attention would be focused on the psychosocial impact of this disease. The recent studies by Kovacs and Jacobson and their colleagues[56,57,71-73] are most reassuring in that they show that, after significant emotional trauma at the onset of their disease, most children with IDDM and their families learn to cope quite admirably. It is obvious however that the presence of one or more psychosocial stresses may play havoc with metabolic stability. Among the stresses that have been identified are those discussed below.

Psychophysiologic response to stress

Poor metabolic control has sometimes been blamed on a heightened physiologic response to stress. Indeed laboratory studies have shown an increase in blood glucose levels and a release of free fatty acids in the blood during psychologic stress.[82] The clinical importance of this hormonal response as a direct cause of serious metabolic disturbances leading to diabetic ketoacidosis, however, has been overestimated. More recent studies link diabetes stability and control to the level of adherence with the treatment regimen.[38,42,62,100,120]

Psychiatric disease

Although overt psychopathology has not been shown to be more common in teenagers with IDDM or other chronic diseases, it is clear that the chance association of IDDM with a psychiatric disorder may lead to enormous difficulties with glycoregulation.[73]

Adolescent noncompliance

See the section on Compliance and Adherence on p. 452.

Self-efficacy and self-esteem

Issues of personal control are important to adolescents with and without diabetes. Recent studies have shown that teens who are confident in their ability to control their diabetes are, in fact, able to achieve better metabolic control than teens who feel overwhelmed and helpless in this regard.[45,76] The notion that self-perceived confidence in performing a task is a strong predictor of performance is termed self-efficacy. Adolescents with weaker levels of self-efficacy also report less personal control and lower self-esteem. Poor self-efficacy and poor self-esteem may put youngsters at risk for depression.[45] Indeed Sullivan has reported an association between depression, low self-esteem, and poor adjustment in adolescent girls with diabetes.[107] All these factors may interfere with motivation to adhere to self-care routines and have a negative impact on metabolic control. Since self-reliance and instrumentality are critical issues during adolescent years, health care professionals should consider the teen's current estimation of his or her abilities and needs in planning treatment and education.

Family functioning

In her review of the psychologic aspects of diabetes in children and adolescents, Johnson[59] states that high levels of conflict, disorganization, and poor supervision within the family appear to be linked to poor health and adjustment to diabetes. Teens who do well generally report that their families are supportive, make them feel good about taking care of their diabetes, listen to their problems about having diabetes, and engage in efficient negotiation and problem-solving. Conversely, adolescents who do poorly experience less effective communication within their families[14,108]; these adolescents frequently put on a facade of ignoring their parents, especially their mothers, or responding to them with arguments, heckling, or needling. In turn, mothers of poorly adherent adolescents often challenge their teens with examples of their misdemeanors, an approach that frequently leads to an escalation of conflict and increased alienation.[108] This pattern of interaction does not allow for discussion of deeper concerns, problem-solving, or modification of behavior; hence adherence problems and resulting poor metabolic control persist.

Minuchin and colleagues[82] have done much to highlight pathologic family patterns in causing poor metabolic control. Some family characteristics of adolescents with unstable diabetes include (1) enmeshment to the extent that there is no clear distinction between the role of the child and the role of the parents; (2) overprotectiveness; (3) rigidity for maintaining the status quo leaving no room for decision making by the teen, and (4) lack of conflict resolution. In disturbed families the adolescent with diabetes sometimes assumes an important role in the family's attempt to avoid conflict; he or she becomes the scapegoat or the symptom bearer of the family. As long as the adolescent with diabetes remains unstable, the family can focus on the diabetes and avoid dealing with more threatening issues such as marital difficulties, alcoholism, or abuse.

Parental collusion

In certain families, parents can either implicitly or explicitly support the noncompliant behaviors of their children. The reasons for this are uncertain, but likely relate to their unwillingness to admit that either their children or they themselves may be less than "perfect." This is an exceptionally difficult situation to deal with, since attempts to increase parental supervision of routines are unlikely to be of any real benefit.

Eating disorders

Recent data suggest that eating disorders (anorexia nervosa, bulimia, and their subclinical variants) may be somewhat more common in teenage girls with IDDM than in the general population.[96,98] The reasons for this association may be multiple: the alterations in body image, the sense of autonomy and identity, self-esteem, mood regulation, and family interactions described in IDDM are all common in individuals with eating and weight pathology.[96] Thus it is possible that IDDM could potentiate this psychopathology in the individual, almost invariably a teenage girl, predisposed to the development of anorexia or bulimia.

Metabolic control in those girls with overt and subclinical eating disorders is likely to be poorer than in those without. Mechanisms for the deterioration in metabolic control include the direct metabolic effects of binge eating, self-induced vomiting or laxative abuse, and noncompliance with specific aspects of the diabetes treatment regimen. A high incidence of insulin omission with the specific intent of producing glycosuria and weight loss in these girls has been documented.[95] Thus in young women with IDDM poor metabolic control may be the result of eating pathology with binge eating and insulin omission as common features.

Recurrent Diabetic Ketoacidosis

During a 5-year period in the mid-1970s a group of 4 teenage girls with IDDM provided our house staff with 130 opportunities to manage diabetic ketoacidosis (DKA). Careful attention to educational deficiencies and to the complex psychosocial situations of these four failed to break the pattern of recurrent DKA. This experience is certainly not unique.[34,38,42,120] More recently, however, health care professionals involved with IDDM in young people have become increasingly aware that intentional omission of insulin is overwhelmingly the most common immediate cause of recurrent DKA.[42,62] Schade and colleagues[100] developed a useful algorithm to determine the cause of life-threatening brittle diabetes: over 90% of their subjects responded normally to insulin, administered subcutaneously or intravenously, effectively ruling out insulin resistance as a cause of this problem.

Golden and associates[42] pointed out that recurrent DKA is a problem of insulin omission: elaborate tests to diagnose its cause are unnecessary. When asked directly, most of these adolescents admit to either omitting or reducing their insulin dose. Weight loss by self-induced glycosuria, attempted suicide and desire to get out of a dysfunctional family situation have been associated with this behavior. Episodes of DKA cease when responsibility for insulin administration is assumed by a reliable family member, while attempts are made to define and to deal with the underlying reasons. This approach to management of recurrent DKA is simple, logical, and effective. Nevertheless, it was overlooked until recently with more emphasis placed on the physiologic response to stress as the cause of recurrent DKA, rather than nonadherence to the insulin regimen.[42] This way of thinking precluded any expectation that recurrent DKA would cease without long-term psychosocial intervention. While individual or family therapy is a crucial part of management, this step alone rarely, if ever, eliminates the immediate risk of DKA. To reduce the risk requires guaranteed insulin administration.

Among health care providers, there is a certain unwillingness to acknowledge or deal with the possibility of intentional insulin omission. They are often concerned about the risk of breaking the patient's or family's trust in the care giver and/or interfering with normal adolescent development by asking parents to assume or resume responsibility for the diabetes routines. Yet it is apparent from these youngsters' behavior that they need and want additional parental involvement.

Surreptitious Insulin Administration

Most studies of youth with IDDM have focused on defining characteristics of those with poor compliance, including those who omit treatment (see recurrent DKA above). The opposite, repeated administration of extra insulin, secretly or surreptitiously, has received considerable less attention despite a number of reports in the literature.[6,88,100,117] The prevalence of this syndrome is unknown but likely much higher than suspected.

The reasons for surreptitious insulin administration may be varied, but most would agree that this behavior invariably indicates serious underlying psychologic disturbance.[88,100] This behavior may represent a suicidal attempt or gesture. It may also be a misguided attempt to manipulate family members and health care providers.

Suspicion of this syndrome should be triggered when hypoglycemia persists despite an unusually large decrease in perceived insulin dose requirement, particularly in adolescents with IDDM noted to have psychosocial difficulties. Direct confrontation of the adolescent and his or her family is essential to diagnose the problem. Psychiatric evaluation and therapy are mandatory.

Hypoglycemia

Hypoglycemia is the most common acute complication of IDDM and, therefore, represents a significant and constant risk for all adolescents with the disease.[25] This subject is more fully dealt with elsewhere, but a few comments are pertinent here.

Virtually every individual with IDDM experiences some of the symptoms of hypoglycemia on a regular basis.[28] Many clinicians believe that the absence of any hypoglycemia may indicate metabolic control that is less than optimal[116]; mild occasional hypoglycemia that can be recognized and treated is, therefore, one of the prices to be paid in the achievement of acceptable levels of glycemic control. Teens, however, are often unwilling to pay this price. Their concern is not for the future; rather, they are more interested in avoiding any situation where they feel out of control, singled out, or inconvenienced. Thus, overeating and insulin manipulation may represent their attempt to prevent even the mildest hypoglycemic reactions.

As much as teens want to avoid hypoglycemia, however, a number of important lifestyle factors put them at increased risk for reactions, including erratic physical activity, sleeping in, dieting, and experimenting with alcohol. Many teens refuse to wear their diabetes identification bracelet or necklace. When adolescents are secretive about their diabetes, the risk is compounded. In this situation there is more potential for missed snacks and delayed or inadequate meals. For example, one youngster became hypoglycemic during a sleepover at a friend's home because his friend's family was unaware of his diabetes. At dinner he failed to eat all his food choices because he did not want to "look like a pig." The embarrassing hypoglycemic episode might have been avoided had he discussed his diabetes and its requirements with his friend before the visit.

Severe hypoglycemia (defined by an episode of coma, convulsion, or confusion) is to be avoided at all costs, both because of its potential for morbidity and because of the anxiety that it creates in the teens and their families. For youngsters who have experienced severe insulin reactions, fear of hypoglycemia may be a source of more anxiety for them and their families than the fear of long-term diabetes-related complications. As a result, metabolic control may be compromised.

The frequency of episodes of severe hypoglycemia is unevenly distributed throughout the diabetic population.[39] Studies suggest that up to a third of those with IDDM will have an episode of severe hypoglycemia during their lifetime with the disease.[25,39] Many studies attest to tighter metabolic control as a risk factor for severe hypoglycemia.[25,28] For example, in the DCCT, those in the experimental treatment group were 2.5 to 3 times more likely to experience an episode of severe hypoglycemia than were those receiving standard treatment.[28] Data also suggest that between 4% and 20% of those with IDDM will suffer such an episode in any one year.[25] In our review of 311 children attending our clinic, we found that 31% had experienced a severe episode in the past, and that in 16% at least one episode had occurred in a particular year. Younger age, longer duration of IDDM, and lower HbA_{1c} levels were risk factors associated with the occurrence of severe hypoglycemia.

The majority of hypoglycemic reactions, whether mild or severe, are related to the known predisposing factors: decreased or missed meal or snack, extra exercise without additional caloric intake, or inadvertent (or occasionally, intentional) insulin overdosage. However, there will always be a number of episodes that cannot be explained on the basis of these factors but likely relate to the variations in insulin dosage and absorption, food intake, and daily activity that are common in these children.

Although the potential exists for significant morbidity (and even mortality) from severe hypoglycemic episodes, virtually all such episodes have an uneventful outcome in adolescents with IDDM. Nevertheless, these adolescents must be taught about the factors predisposing to hypoglycemia, how to recognize early warning symptoms, and what measures to take to prevent an episode from becoming more severe. Equally important, health professionals must explore the adolescent's concern about reactions and identify life-style factors that increase their risk of such events. Teens need to be engaged in active problem-solving around these issues. For example, they can be encouraged to take an extra late-night snack in anticipation of sleeping in on the weekend. They need to understand the effect of alcohol on blood glucose so that they will eat when they consume alcoholic beverages. Whenever possible, meals and snacks should be planned to fit in with the school schedule: if a snack must be eaten in class then the use of "low noise" foods such as dried fruit can be suggested.

Teens need encouragement to carry some form of sugar with them at all times. Prepackaged dextrose either in tablet or gel form is convenient to carry and less likely to be consumed than candies, chocolate bars, etc. Should a severe episode of hypoglycemia occur, parents need to be taught how to use glucagon. Unfortunately research has shown that glucagon is used in only about one third of severe episodes.[25] Reasons for failure to use this hormone included inability to locate the glucagon at the time of the event, panic or fear during the event, absence of glucagon in the home and forgetfulness about its availability, or denial of the severity of the episode. Similar findings have been reported in adults with diabetes.[20] This finding underlines the need to regularly update the adolescent's and his or her parents' understanding of hypoglycemia and checking that glucagon is available and accessible. Glucagon can only help, not harm. When a glucagon vial expires, the adolescent or parent should "practice preparing it" prior to discarding.

Somogyi Phenomenon

Poor metabolic control in adolescents with diabetes is often ascribed to overinsulinization with the Somogyi phenomenon (i.e., posthypoglycemic hyperglycemia and ketonuria). A number of recent studies have shown this phenomenon to occur infrequently. A more likely explanation for fasting hyperglycemia (with or without ketonuria) is underinsulinization, or the waning of the effect of insulin in the early morning hours.[48,75]

CHRONIC COMPLICATIONS OF DIABETES

Based on the absence of either retinal microvascular changes or incipient nephropathy (defined by the presence of microalbuminuria) in the prepubertal child with IDDM, researchers have speculated that the years of diabetes prior to the onset of puberty contribute little, if at all, to the risk of the long-term complications related to diabetes.[35,66,70,85] Recent epidemiologic data support this notion, indicating that postpubertal diabetes duration is a more accurate determinant of the development of microvascular disease and diabetes-related mortality than total duration.[70] For example, Kostraba and associates[70] examined the relationship between diabetic complications and duration, both before and after puberty, in three large cohorts of subjects with IDDM: retinopathy, overt nephropathy, and mortality were all more prevalent in subjects diagnosed during or after puberty than in those diagnosed before puberty. Subtraction of the prepubertal years from the total duration led to disappearance of these differences. Similarly, Klein and associates[66] reported on the relationship between the time of menarche and diabetic retinopathy. The duration of diabetes after menarche conferred about 1.3 times the risk of retinopathy compared with duration before menarche. Murphy and others[85] found this risk to be even greater, of the order of 4.8-fold.

The available data suggest that certain events occurring at the time of puberty contribute or are related to the development of microvascular complications. While glycemic control often deteriorates during adolescence, other factors would appear to be involved. Recent work suggests that IGF-1, similar to other growth factors, may contribute to angiogenesis and atheromatous lesions. Merimee and associates[80] have postulated a direct association between IGF-1 and retinopathy. Whatever the reason, hyperglycemia and puberty are a potentially sinister combination. Correction of the hyperglycemia may require significant hyperinsulinemia, which is itself a further risk factor to hypertension and macrovascular disease.[93]

It is reassuring that the prepubertal years contribute so little to the development of complications. The fact that the clock starts ticking with puberty, however, highlights the need for health care professionals to be aware of the known and presumed/potential risk factors for the development of diabetes-related macro- and microvascular complications. These include: (1) obesity, (2) hypertension, (3) lipid abnormalities, (4) smoking, and (5) metabolic control.[2,64]

The nature and risk of diabetes-related complications are very sensitive topics for adolescents, their families, and health care providers. Yet, it is essential that the realities of potential problems be discussed openly and honestly. Teens and their parents need to understand the importance of metabolic control and other factors that may contribute to the development of the complications so that they will have the opportunity to choose behaviors that may reduce their risk.

When adolescents do not adhere to the treatment regimen, parents and health professionals are often tempted to threaten them with blindness, kidney failure, and loss of limbs. In our experience, threats have no impact on metabolic control and may lead to feelings of hopelessness and helplessness. Alternate and more successful strategies for enhancing compliance in these less mature teens include focusing on the immediate rewards for adherence (e.g., maintaining a high-energy level, avoiding parents' nagging) and ensuring adequate parental support in daily diabetes management.

Advanced diabetes-related complications are rare during adolescence; thus, it is essential that anticipatory steps be taken in the care of their diabetes. These include routine blood pressure measurements and eye examinations, appropriate counseling that stresses avoidance of excess weight gain and cholesterol intake, avoidance of smoking, regular urine checks for protein, and measurement of glycated hemoglobin and serum lipid levels.

Dietary counseling must include information regarding the relationship between hyperlipidemia and macrovascular disease. It is clear that improving metabolic control (by lowering HbA_{1c} levels) will decrease serum cholesterol and triglyceride levels. However, in the adequately "controlled" teen, lowering or maintaining lipid levels will depend on attention to a diet low in total cholesterol intake, specifically decreasing saturated and increasing polyunsaturated fat intake. Snack foods are a major source of excess fat intake. Annual or more frequent measurement of serum cholesterol and triglyceride concentrations will help facilitate dietary adjustments. Frequent dietary review in a nonthreatening manner may also help to forestall excess weight gain and the onset or worsening of obesity.

With respect to retinopathy, the American Diabetes Association has issued a position statement called "Eye Care Guidelines for Patients with Diabetes Mellitus."[3] See the box below for guidelines of importance to the care of the adolescent with IDDM.

Experience with teens with IDDM suggests that very few reach the stage of proliferative retinopathy requiring intervention with laser therapy. In teens who exhibit the poorest metabolic control, as evidenced by the presence of Mauriac's syndrome, sudden improvement in glucose homeostasis may lead to a rapid deterioration in diabetic retinopathy.[23] This suggests that extra vigilance is required in such teenagers to diagnose and treat proliferative changes before sight is threatened. The reason for the deterioration has not been elucidated, but may be related to changes in hormones, specifically growth hormone and IGF-1, that occur during catch-up growth.

Just as the early detection and management of retinopathy may decrease visual loss by over 80%, so may the detection and management of hypertension decrease the progression of diabetic nephropathy.[83] Whether reduction of blood pressure in normotensive adolescents with IDDM who have incipient nephropathy (microalbuminuria) will be equally effective remains under investigation.[22] The outcome of the latter investigations will dictate whether screening for microalbuminuria is indicated in the normotensive adolescent population with IDDM.[21] A number of studies have revealed that about 5% to 20% of all teens with IDDM have significant microalbuminuria (defined by albumin excretion rates >20 µg/min) suggesting that they are at greatest risk for progression to overt nephropathy.

Reduction of the major risk factors for macrovascular disease (e.g., obesity, lipid abnormalities, hypertension, and smoking) during adolescence may have a major positive effect in the long term. The importance of these risk factors in those adolescents with diabetes compared with that in the nondiabetic population is still being examined.

**EYE CARE GUIDELINES FOR THE ADOLESCENT WITH
DIABETES MELLITUS**

1. All patients should be informed that
   a. sight-threatening eye disease is a common complication of diabetes mellitus and is often present even with good vision.
   b. early detection and appropriate treatment of diabetic eye disease greatly reduces the risk of visual loss.
2. People between 12 and 30 years of age with a diagnosis of diabetes mellitus of at least 5 years' duration should have a baseline ophthalmic examination, including
   a. history of visual symptoms.
   b. measurement of visual acuity and intraocular pressure.
   c. ophthlamoscopic examination through dilated pupils.
3. After the initial eye examination, it is suggested that people with diabetes mellitus should receive the above ophthalmic examinations annually unless more frequent exams are indicated by the presence of abnormalities.

Source: Position Statement of the American Diabetes Association: Eye care guidelines for patients with diabetes mellitus, Diabetes Care 11:745, 1988.

The role of health care providers of adolescents with IDDM is to be aware of the risk factors, provide anticipatory guidance, and detect complications as early as possible. Results of long-term trials will determine whether intensified insulin therapy or the use of specific agents such as neuronal sorbitol levels (aldose reducase inhibitors) or intraglomular pressure (angiotensin conversing enzyme inhibitors) will have a major impact on the development and/or progression of IDDM complications.

SPECIAL CONSIDERATIONS
Risk-Taking Behaviors

Risk taking is part of the natural expression of independence that all teenagers go through to some extent. Crucial to the psychologic maturation of adolescence is the pursuit of new activities and taking of initiative. Teens do a lot of exploring at a time when their cognitive skills are insufficiently well honed to allow them to make decisions that will keep them out of trouble (e.g., sex without contraception, driving too fast or while drinking, or illicit use of drugs and alcohol). They tend to have the idea that they are invulnerable; for example, if a teen drives a car while under the influence of alcohol and does not have an accident, he or she may begin to believe that they can safely take this risk again. Conversely, for many teens taking a drink, smoking cigarettes or marijuana, having sex is, in fact, risk-avoidant. It is sometimes easier for these teens to go along with their peers, rather than running the risk of being shunned or ridiculed for not "indulging."

Teens with diabetes are no different from their nondiabetic peers in respect to the usual risk-taking behaviors of adolescence. However, the diabetes regimen itself may become a focus for risk taking (e.g., insulin omission, dietary and testing nonadherence). Furthermore, certain risks may be greater in those with diabetes (e.g., alcohol ingestion as a risk factor for acute hypoglycemia, marijuana use as a stimulus to increased food intake, smoking and unplanned pregnancies as risk factors for long-term complications).

Alcohol

Metabolic consequences of alcohol ingestion include inhibition of hepatic gluconeogenesis, enhanced fatty acid and triglyceride synthesis, impaired hepatic fatty acid oxidation leading to fatty liver, diversion of fatty acids into ketone bodies producing ketosis, and enhanced conversion of pyruvate to lactic acid (producing lactic acidosis).[40] The impact of these metabolic changes on the individual with diabetes may include: hypoglycemia (direct effect of alcohol on the liver), hyperglycemia and weight gain (if alcohol ingestion is accompanied by increased caloric intake), hyperlipidemia, gastrointestinal upset, and, in the longer term, neurotoxocity and sexual dysfunction.

Adolescents with IDDM should be made aware of all these implications of alcohol use in a nonjudgemental manner. However, the dangers of alcohol use listed above do not imply that those with diabetes must all abstain. As a general rule, it is better to educate appropriately about responsible alcohol use rather than to forbid it. Adolescents should be encouraged to wear identification that states that they have diabetes, to drink in moderation, and not to drive when drinking. To avoid the alcohol-induced hypoglycemia, it is advisable never to drink on an empty stomach or after vigorous exercise. Also, although it may be important to "count" alcohol-derived calories when counseling teens, it is essential not to cut down on food intake during alcohol use.

Only Glasgow and associates[41] have commented on the frequency of alcohol use in teens with IDDM: of 101 adolescents surveyed, 49 denied any alcohol use, 26 admitted to having tried it, 19 to occasional use, and only 7 to alcohol use once or twice a week. Alcohol use was more common among older patients and among white as compared with black youngsters.

Smoking and drug abuse

Most teens try smoking cigarettes at some stage. Only some will become regular users. The same is likely also true for the use of street drugs. Educational programs are required that stress the risks of smoking and drugs in general, and to the diabetic teen in particular (namely the relationship of smoking to the macro- and microvascular complications of the disease). Adolescents experiment with and continue to use these substances for a variety of reasons, including peer pressure, risk taking and experimentation, feeling "grown-up," pleasurable relief from anxiety, and imitation of family members.

Primary prevention should start during the early school years and continue through adolescence. Education programs should focus on providing information to help young people make responsible decisions regarding the use of drugs and tobacco. If they are to be successful, such programs must take into account the teen's social context. Programs that utilize teen role models and peers are more likely to be successful than those that appear to the teen to be yet another example of the "establishment" preaching at them. Health care providers are obliged to ensure that their young patients are aware of the special hazards and risks in using these agents: smoking may accelerate the development of micro- and macrovascular disease.

The impact of other "recreational" drugs" in diabetes has been less extensively investigated. Nevertheless, certain drugs cause a change in appetite and alter level of awareness and concentration, effects which may interfere with safe diabetes management.[30] Because use of these agents is so common among adolescents, we should routinely ask about their use. Establishing open dialogue with these teens may allow them to seek sound answers to their questions and discuss their concerns. Indications of drug use such as deterioration in school performance, personality change, mood swings, sleeplessness, or fatigue should be assessed. When drug abuse is suspected, the issue needs to be addressed in a sensitive, nonjudgmental manner. The teen's motivation for drug use and extent of use must be explored. This information will help guide the health care provider in making appropriate decisions about the need for referral for further assessment and/or treatment.

There is little information about the prevalence or incidence of concurrent diabetes and drug use or dependency.[102] In two studies of adult IV drug users, 1.4% of 2911 and 3.2% of 1780 individuals in Baltimore and New York, respectively, volunteered a history of diabetes.[15,87] In the report of Glasgow and colleagues,[41] only 1 of 97 consecutive urine specimens from adolescents with diabetes was positive for marijuana. This compares with a 24% positive rate among teens attending the adolescent clinic at the same hospital.[101] About 20% of teens in Glasgow's study reported having tried drugs with none admitting to frequent use. The reported use of drugs in these studies is lower than might be expected from studies in the nondiabetic population.[15]

Contraception and avoidance of sexually transmitted diseases (STDs)

Those involved in the continuing care of adolescents with diabetes have an excellent opportunity and an obligation also to provide teens with accurate information and a forum for discussion of sexuality and sexual activity. There is no evidence that youth with IDDM are more susceptible to STDs. However, like their peers, they need to be informed about the risks of STDs and how they can be prevented by safe sex practices, including avoidance of sexual contact with an infected person and routine use of condoms.

Information and counseling regarding sexuality and contraception should not be limited to adolescent girls. Young men also need to understand methods of birth control and where to obtain advice and help. For example, one misguided adolescent male was responsible for his girlfriend's unplanned pregnancy because he believed himself to be sterile because of his diabetes. Furthermore, many teenage boys with diabetes fear the possibility of impotence. They should be reassured that this problem rarely affects the teenage population; however, the possibility that it may occur at a later stage in their lives should be addressed as questions arise.

In sexually active girls with IDDM, contraception is essential to avoid unwanted pregnancies. Again anticipatory guidance is required. Although use of oral contraceptives may occasionally be associated with such complications as deterioration in metabolic control, hypertension, and hyperlipidemia, these agents constitute the preferred method of contraception for the adolescent with diabetes. In fact, recent data from Klein and associates failed to reveal an association between either current or past use of oral contraceptives and severity of retinopathy, hypertension, or current metabolic control.[67] Thus, the risks of unwanted pregnancies and abortions likely far outweigh those from use of birth control pills.

Driving

Most countries have laws that limit to some degree the rights of individuals with diabetes to operate motor vehicles in an unrestricted fashion. These restrictions have been based on the acute threat of hypoglycemia in insulin-requiring individuals, and the chronic complications such as retinopathy, coronary disease, and hypertension in those with longer standing disease. Unfortunately the laws are not based on appropriate data, and studies are underway to establish whether individuals with IDDM do in fact constitute an increased risk on the roads. A recent case control study by Songer and associates attempted to examine accident rates for a cohort of individuals with IDDM and their relationship to hypoglycemia.[104] In brief, the overall accident risk rate did not differ between persons with diabetes and controls; however, female drivers with diabetes did show a marked increased risk for accidents. Furthermore, in nine of eleven individuals who admitted that a health-related problem was the cause of the accident, hypoglycemia was the recorded reason. In the other two limited vision was the cause noted. Clearly, more data are required to assess the association between diabetes and accident risk.

Based on the available data, most countries require physician notification of the condition of the disease and the occurrence of any episodes of severe hypoglycemia particularly while driving. In addition, many countries forbid insulin-requiring persons with diabetes from driving commercial vehicles.[92]

The implications of these rules and regulations for adolescents with IDDM are as follows:

1. Teens about to obtain their driver's permits should be fully informed once again about the hazards of hypoglycemia and its prevention.
2. They should be instructed to keep a source of concentrated carbohydrate readily available at all times (e.g., packet of glucose tablets in the glove compartment) as well as identification that they have diabetes.
3. They should avoid driving at a time when hypoglycemia is most likely, such as immediately following vigorous exercise. Rather, they should take some food to prevent possible hypoglycemia, and monitor their blood glucose before getting back in the driver's seat to ensure that it is in a "safe" range.
4. They should monitor blood glucose concentrations regularly as a method of preventing hypoglycemia.
5. They should submit to regular medical check-ups and report immediately the occurrence of any episodes of severe hypoglycemia or any visual problems.

Employment

Most health care providers are likely to be asked by their adolescents with IDDM about educational and employment opportunities. Even if not asked, these subjects should be broached as part of ongoing care. The questions that require attention are (1) Are there any jobs not available to individuals with IDDM? (2) Do employers tend to be discriminatory in their hiring practice when it comes to employing these individuals? The answer to both questions is "yes."

A number of industries do not employ people with diabetes for specific jobs, and, in fact, will remove employees from such positions should they acquire diabetes. Since there are blanket rules preventing operation of commercial vehicles, trains, and aircraft by individuals with IDDM, employment in these positions is impossible in most places. Similarly, the military in many countries has traditionally denied employment to those with diabetes; recently, in some countries military employment in noncombat positions has been allowed. The same is true in many police forces. Before applying for a particular educational or employment opportunity, individuals with IDDM should inquire as to their employability in these areas. For example, it would be unwise for an adolescent to enter training in criminology at a college, only to find out years later that he or she is not eligible for employment by the local police force. It is in situations such as this that the health care team can provide important counseling and support.

Employer discrimination has been documented in some recent reports both from the United States and United Kingdom.[94,103] Songer and others[103] report that individuals who told job interviewers about their diabetes were more likely to experience job refusal than were their nondiabetic siblings, whereas if they did not mention their diabetes, employment rates were similar.

Furthermore, Robinson[94] found that people with diabetes had to change their jobs more frequently because of their illness and (particularly in shift workers) experienced more problems with their jobs than did controls. Absenteeism from work was similar in both persons with diabetes and controls in both of these studies.

In the report of Tebbi and associates[115] young adults with IDDM appeared about as successful in obtaining and maintaining employment as a control group, despite an apparent deficit in their perceived general well-being. Those with diabetes seemed more likely to experience job-related problems; the results, however, did not suggest a pervasive deficit in overall job adjustment and performance.

The young person with IDDM seeking employment should be encouraged to stress personal qualifications, abilities, and ambitions to prospective employers. They should not withhold information about their diabetes from these employers, and should not expect particular concessions, such as "better" shift rotations or more frequent sick leave. Satisfactory employment will depend on an enlightened attitude of both the employer and employee. Diabetes should not be allowed to prevent productive employment. Young adults with diabetes, 18 years of age and older, who are experiencing difficulty acquiring and maintaining employment may be eligible for vocational rehabilitation services. These services vary from country to country and state to state, but generally help with job training and placement. Individuals who feel they have suffered job discrimination should be encouraged to seek counsel from Human Rights Commissions or other employee advocate groups.

ROLE OF DIABETES HEALTH CARE TEAM

Adolescents with IDDM should have the opportunity for health care delivery by a multidisciplinary health care team experienced in their care. Members of such a team should include physicians, nurse educators, dietitians, behavioral specialists (e.g., social workers, psychologists, psychiatrists), public health nurses, and support groups (e.g., national diabetes associations, local teen support groups). Clearly, not all teens live in centers large enough to warrant such a team. However, referral to such a center may be most beneficial at the onset of the disease and/or in those experiencing difficulty with one or more aspects of their diabetes care. Furthermore, as outlined above, the problems of these adolescents are sufficiently different from those of adults with the disorder, that they should not be lumped together with adults for education and care unless attention is paid to their specific needs. For example, information regarding foot care will be of much less relevance to a new-onset diabetic teen than will information about activities such as vigorous exercise, eating out, and partying.

The three components of health care that should be offered to teens with diabetes and their families include education, support, and care. Each part of this package must be sensitive to the teen's increasing needs for self-responsibility, integrity of body image, and self-esteem.

Education

Initial education requires that the teens and their families acquire an understanding of diabetes and the components of care essential to function adequately at home, e.g., insulin injection, blood glucose monitoring, urine ketone testing, hypoglycemia recognition and treatment, and nutritional planning. In the early weeks it is essential that they learn about and experience the various facets of diabetes management. Wexler[119] has referred to this period as the time for acquisition of "cognitive-practical tasks." Diabetes education for children and adolescents with IDDM starts at diagnosis and continues for the rest of their lives. For those who develop diabetes at a younger age, the onset of puberty signals an ideal time to update diabetes knowledge and to integrate developmental concepts into the discussion. Anticipatory guidance concerning psychosocial issues such as alcohol and drug use, smoking, sexuality, and normal parent-child conflict should be offered to all young teens and their families and reinforced on a regular basis.

For adolescents, the approach to diabetes education needs to be informal and interactional; both facts and feelings should be addressed. For example, it is natural for teens to have some difficulty with rules, yet these are unavoidable with diabetes management. Diabetes educators should encourage teens to question these rules: this affords the opportunity to provide a solid rationale for each aspect of therapy and to discuss various options with them. Teens should also be encouraged to use a problem-solving approach to develop solutions to their diabetes-related dilemmas and to add flexibility to their routines.

Education and treatment goals must be practical and achievable and should take into account the teen's estimates of his or her own needs and abilities. Regardless of the adolescent's age, parents must be included in the learning process so that they can offer the appropriate level of support and guidance. Initially, some teens may resist parental involvement in the diabetes education program. They want privacy and autonomy: it is important to respect these needs and spend at least some time in discussion with the teen alone. It is also essential that the youngster understand that inclusion of the parents in the education program is required to ensure consistency of understanding of diabetes in the teens and their parents and to promote self-efficacy. An often successful strategy is to encourage the teen to actively participate in teaching his or her parents about the diabetes. Hopefully such an approach will lessen family conflict around the diabetes and increase the parent's respect for and confidence in their teen's self-care abilities.

Clearly, some teens welcome the chance to learn more about diabetes: it makes them feel one step closer to independence. Others, however, refuse all offers of diabetes education: for these teens, it is essential that parents remain responsible for daily diabetes management. At the same time, health professionals should maintain a nonjudgmental attitude when dealing with these youngsters and keep the door open for future opportunities to learn.

An excellent source of additional information for health professionals regarding specific educational strategies with a developmental focus is the *Diabetes Youth Curriculum: A Tool for Educators.*[113]

Support

Adolescents and their families must assume ultimate responsibility for daily diabetes management. The health care team, however, has an important role in enabling these families to cope with this onerous task. Some supportive and motivational strategies recommended and/or employed by health professionals include the use of the therapeutic relationship, contracting, social learning interventions, camps, counseling, and support groups.

The importance of a satisfying relationship between adolescents with diabetes and health care providers in promoting positive coping and enhancing compliance is well described.[13,16,97,109,115] Key to this therapeutic alliance is the health care provider's interest in and respect for the teen and his or her point of view. When social and psychologic issues are considered as carefully as physical concerns, caregivers are much more likely to arrive at an interpretation of facts that is congruent with that of the teen and his or her family and thereby earn their trust. Once this has been established, teens and health care providers may be better able to negotiate realistic management goals and plan appropriate strategies to achieve them.

For many teens, "contracting" can be used to encourage good self-care behaviors. Contracting, which is addressed in detail in Chapter 16 of this text, involves an agreement that details specific rewards for specific behaviors. Contracts provide youths with an opportunity to become increasingly involved in planning for their own care as they become more independent. They also provide a mechanism for clear communication and help all parties understand the division of responsibilities.[118]

Peer acceptance is extremely important during adolescence; thus peer group interventions may be effective in mediating health care goals. Social learning strategies are designed to provide groups of teens with opportunities to identify difficult situations, develop and practice creative solutions, and learn to counter argue. According to Kaplan,[63] such interventions have been used successfully to discourage smoking, truancy, and antisocial behavior in the adolescent population. Anderson and others[5] used an activity-based peer group intervention with teens with diabetes to prevent the expected deterioration in metabolic control during adolescence. Their strategy provided teens with the problem-solving skills and support needed for adjusting the insulin dose, exercise, and meal plan.

Camps for youth with diabetes allow these youngsters to participate in a variety of new activities (e.g., marathon swimming, overnight canoe trips) and at the same time to consider their diabetes-related needs. The new learning that occurs during camp not only boosts their self-confidence but can also be applied to situations that youngsters encounter outside the camp environment.

It is critical that health professionals not limit their supportive efforts to the teens themselves. Families should be assessed for their adjustment and adaptive capabilities early in the course of the diabetes and periodically thereafter.[31,119] Most parents need help in finding the balance between the youngster's need to feel in charge and their need not to be abandoned. Once teens have assumed responsibility for their own routines, there is the risk that parents (and health providers) will pay only negative attention to the diabetes regimen; that is, nag when a task is not completed.[17] Families should be encouraged to maintain a system of positive reinforcement throughout the youngsters' diabetes career. Youths and adults have a need to be recognized for their efforts. When adolescents and parents find themselves in a pattern of negative interaction to the extent that diabetes control suffers, family counselling may be indicated.[17]

Finally, parents and other family members may benefit from participation in therapeutic and/or self help groups. Self-help groups for people with diabetes are frequently affiliated with organizations such as the American/ Canadian Diabetes Associations or the Juvenile Diabetes Foundation. Such groups provide families with peer support, modeling, a sense of not being alone with diabetes as well as an opportunity for sharing different attitudes and catharsis. Therapeutic groups refer to those organized and facilitated by experienced health professionals. Goals of the group are quite specific (e.g., to promote an understanding of emotional reactions to diabetes or to develop an awareness of the impact of diabetes on normal developmental tasks and to learn ways of coping).

Care

Since diabetes is a life-long disorder, continuity and consistency of care are important. This is particularly so during the adolescent years when noncompliance, mistrust, and rebellion are most likely to be at a peak. In the ideal situation some members of the health care team (physician, nurse educator, social worker/psychologist, and dietitian) develop a relaxed, trusting, and caring relationship with the teen and his or her parents. This is unlikely to occur at the first meeting, but may take months or even years to develop. The clinic visits should be unhurried and focus on understanding the teen as an individual: what does he or she know about diabetes and its management, and what are his or her major fears and dislikes about the disorder?

It is necessary for the teen to begin to assume membership in his or her health care team. Decisions made by members of the team without consulting the teen will often be seen as arbitrary and intrusive and will likely be disregarded. When the teen's view is respected and incorporated into the treatment regimen he or she is much more likely to comply. Noncompliance is virtually ensured when unrealistic goals and punitive action or judgmental attitudes are foisted on these youngsters.

The tools of therapy (namely the balance between insulin administration and food intake) are imprecise at best. Subcutaneous injection of insulin is unphysiologic; for most teens, then, euglycemia is an unrealistic goal. The overzealous demand for tight control in the teen will frequently lead to noncompliance with many or all aspects of diabetes care. Often it will lead to poor clinic attendance, fabricated test results, sneaking food, etc. See the box on p. 472 for goals of therapy for adolescents.

No guidelines are available as to what constitutes good and safe glycemic control in adolescents with IDDM: "good" control implies levels that may prevent the onset and/or

---

_____ **GOALS OF THERAPY** _____

(1) To maintain normal growth and physical development.
(2) To encourage normal psychosocial development leading to acquisition of the cognitive and emotional skills necessary to carry out all aspects of self-care.
(3) To control symptoms of hyperglycemia, such as polydipsia, polyuria, nocturia.
(4) To maintain normal blood lipid profiles.
(5) To achieve acceptable metabolic control as evidenced by the majority of self-monitored blood glucose concentrations in the 4 to 10 mmol/L (70 to 180 mg/dL) range preprandially and "good" HbAlc levels.
(6) To avoid severe hypoglycemia (mild, occasional hypoglycemia that can be easily recognized and treated is virtually ubiquitous) and ketoacidosis.

---

progression of long- term complications, while "safe" control refers to prevention of severe hypoglycemia. The line between "good" and "safe" has not been established, but studies such as the DCCT underline the increased frequency of severe hypoglycemia associated with intensification of the treatment regimen in an attempt to achieve near normoglycemia.[28] Whether the risk of hypoglycemia will be offset by a decrease in long-term complications remains uncertain.

Complete normalization of blood glucose levels for adolescents with IDDM seems at this time to be both an unrealistic and potentially dangerous goal. Efforts (or demands) to keep preprandial glycemia in the 3.3 to 6.7 mmol/L (60 to 120 mg/dL) range will ensure frequent levels below 3.3 mmol/L (60 mg/dL), whether asymptomatic or symptomatic. Attention should focus not only on blood glucose targets, but also on the prevention of severe hypoglycemia (and diminution of episodes of asymptomatic or mild hypoglycemia as harbingers of more severe episodes), avoidance of repeat hospitalization whether for hypoglycemia, ketoacidosis, or generally poor overall control, and encouraging normal adjustment and optimal self-care practices as adolescence ends and young adulthood begins.

Insulin

Children and adolescents with new-onset IDDM typically begin on twice-daily injections of mixtures of a short- and intermediate-acting insulin, the first injection before breakfast and the second before the evening meal.

In nonadherent teens in poor metabolic control, there is often the temptation to intensify treatment to improve the situation, for example, by adding more insulin injections, demanding more frequent blood glucose testing, or tightening up the nutritional plan. Such strategies are probably doomed to failure; increasing demands of the treatment regimen may lead to a vicious cycle of fabricated tests, insulin omission, worse control, more demands, and on and on.

Instead of a more complex treatment regimen, such situations often call for a back-to-basics approach in which a simpler regimen may actually lead to improvements. Increased parental support may be needed at this time as well. This approach requires two components: (I) What is the teen willing to do (as opposed to being told to do)? (2) Support of the health care team to help the teen meet the mutually agreed-on (and often, at least initially, meager) goals.

Nutrition and exercise planning

Although the approaches to nutritional planning and exercise in individuals with diabetes are dealt with in Chapters 2 and 3, it is warranted to highlight some issues relating to these that have an impact specifically on the adolescent with diabetes.

As described before, adolescence is a time of increasing independence from family, peer conformity, and experimentation. All of these factors may significantly affect compliance with the treatment regimen and perhaps most importantly with the nutritional plan.[18,61] It becomes essential to keep adolescents with diabetes well informed about their diet and the reasons for consistency in timing of meals and snacks, amount, and types of food eaten. More important, however, is the need to provide a meal plan that provides sufficient calories to the rapidly growing adolescent and to provide these on an individual basis by tailoring each youngster's meal plan to his or her own needs. Similarly the plan must be flexible enough to accommodate "nonbasal" conditions, such as extra exercise, eating out, partying, etc. One thing that will ensure dietary noncompliance is provision of a meal plan that is inflexible and provides insufficient calories.

At the end of the growth spurt, adolescents in general and the females in particular may need a reduction in caloric intake to forestall excessive weight gain. The teen should be prepared for this in advance so that adjustment in his or her nutritional plan is not seen as punitive and can be carried out, wherever possible, before unwanted weight gain occurs.

Some adolescents, more commonly girls than boys, become concerned about their weight and wish to lose a few pounds. At this time, the health care professional must work along with the teen to establish realistic goals in terms of weight loss and to make rational adjustments in the meal plan to accommodate this change. Failure to support the adolescent's efforts in this way may result in the utilization of fad diets or cycles of insulin omission, intentional glycosuria, binging, etc. Whenever the diet is decreased, insulin dosage must be adjusted appropriately to avoid hypoglycemia and/or excessive hunger that will jeopardize adherence. The role of self monitoring of blood glucose to facilitate the changes in insulin dosage cannot be overemphasized.

Similarly adolescents must be instructed in dealing with the metabolic impact of extra exercise.[121] Whereas during earlier childhood most compensation is made by parents and other caretakers, during adolescence this task falls increasingly on the shoulders of the youngsters themselves. Not only do they need to know about extra caloric intake before and during exercise, but also about the possibility of late postexercise hypoglycemia.[77,121] This latter condition most commonly occurs late at night or in the early morning hours after a bout of strenuous exercise after the evening meal. What is needed in this situation is not necessarily extra calories during the exercise, but rather afterwards to prevent the later drop in blood glucose. Nevertheless, these requirements may differ greatly from one individual to another and it is only with the help of increased glucose monitoring that the specific needs of each adolescent can be addressed adequately.

Crisis Intervention

All teens with IDDM are susceptible to the acute complications of the disease, namely hypoglycemia and ketoacidosis, as well as to the impact of intercurrent illness on glucose homeostasis. Availability of medical personnel on an around-the-clock basis to help cope with such emergencies is, therefore, essential.

Transition From Pediatric to Adult Diabetes Care

Most children and adolescents with IDDM receive ongoing care from health professionals experienced in pediatric diabetes. This system, though ideal in many respects, ultimately leads to a disruption in the continuity of medical care. There comes a time when the teen must leave the nurturing environment of the pediatric center and establish himself or herself with an adult center. When the shift in care is abrupt and the adolescent and his or her family are ill-prepared to deal with transition, regular follow-up may cease. Recent data show that 25% of adolescents graduating from our diabetes clinic at age 18 years dropped out of medical care for months to years, resurfacing when they experienced a diabetes-related crisis that otherwise may have been averted.[36]

An extended transition period and anticipatory guidance may ease the teenager's transfer to adult diabetes care. Teens who are approaching "graduation" from the clinic should understand the reasons for ongoing regular medical care, specifically to maintain good metabolic control and screen for or treat the complications of IDDM. In addition, they should have the opportunity to discuss various options for ongoing care and be prepared for a health care approach that may differ from that used in the pediatric center. They may need coaching on how to be a "good" consumer of health services. Finally, the pediatric diabetes team can facilitate the teen's transition by making the first appointment at the adult center and contacting the teen after the visit to discuss the success of the transfer.

Perhaps the ideal method of providing comprehensive care to adolescents and young adults with IDDM is through a transition clinic where pediatric and adult specialists join forces to provide developmentally appropriate care. Baum and Kinmonth have used and described that such an approach reduced the dropout rate from 20% to 3%.[7]

RESEARCH DIRECTIONS

Several directions of research should be encouraged in order to better understand and manage the adolescent with IDDM:

(1) Studies of IDDM pathogenesis and immune modulation must of necessity include the late childhhood and adolescent population since this is the group at greatest risk for

developing the disease. Studies that employ only adults with new-onset IDDM may provide some confusing data because there may be contamination of the study group with non–insulin-dependent diabetic patients and also because IDDM has been noted to have a less severe course when it begins later in life.

(2) Research must be directed at improving our understanding of the reasons for deteriorating metabolic control in the adolescent population. These studies must focus on the interaction between biologic and psychosocial factors.

(3) The earliest lesions of diabetic microvascular disease must be sought in these youngsters and methods for halting or slowing their progression developed.

It is incumbent on those dealing with large numbers of teenagers with IDDM to involve them in studies aimed at helping both health care providers and the teens themselves to better understand their disease.

SUMMARY

In this chapter both physical and psychologic factors having an impact on adolescents with diabetes have been reviewed. Hopefully, we have painted a picture of hope: most teens with diabetes achieve adequate to good degrees of metabolic control and make a satisfactory transition to self-care and young adulthood. For those in whom adolescence is a stormy period, every effort must be made to define the cause(s) of their problems and construct therapeutic interventions that can best help them achieve mastery over their condition.

REFERENCES

1. Ahlfield JE, Soler NG, Marcus SD: The young adult with diabetes: Impact of the disease on marriage and having children, Diabetes Care 8:52-56, 1985.
2. American Diabetes Association Consensus Statement: Role of cardiovascular risk factors in prevention and treatment of macrovascular disease in diabetes, Diabetes Care 12:573-579, 1989.
3. American Diabetes Association Position Statement: Eye care guidelines for patients with diabetes mellitus, Diabetes Care 11:745-746, 1988.
4. Amiel S and others: Impaired insulin action in puberty: a contributing factor to poor glycemic control in adolescents with diabetes, New Engl J Med 315:215-219, 1986.
5. Anderson B and others: Effects of peer-group intervention on metabolic control of adolescents with IDDM. Randomized outpatient study, Diabetes Care 12: 179-183, 1985.
6. Arem R and Zogbhi W: Insulin overdose in eight patients: Insulin pharmacokinetics and review of the literature, Medicine 64:323-332, 1985.
7. Baum JD and Kinmonth AL: Care of the child with diabetes, New York, 1985, Churchill Livingstone.
8. Beal C: Body size and growth rate of children with diabetes mellitus, J Pediatr 32:170-179, 1948.
9. Belmonte M and others: Impact of SMBG on control of diabetes as measured by HbA1: 3-year survey of a juvenile IDDM clinic, Diabetes Care 11:484-488, 1988.
10. Bibace R and Walsh ME: Development of children's concept of illness, Pediatrics 66:912-917, 1980.
11. Blethen S and others: Effect of pubertal stage and recent blood glucose control on plasma somatomedin C in children with insulin-dependent diabetes mellitus, Diabetes 30:868-872, 1981.
12. Bloch C, Clemons P, and Sperling M: Puberty decreases insulin sensitivity, J Pediatr 110:481-487, 1987.
13. Blum R: Compliance with therapeutic regimens among children and youth. In Blum RW, ed: Chronic illness and disabilities in childhood and adolescence, Orlando, 1984, Grune and Stratton.
14. Bobrow ES, AvRuskin TW, and Siller J: Mother-daughter interaction and adherence to diabetes regimen, Diabetes Care 8:146-151, 1985.

15. Brown LS: Clinical aspects of drug abuse in diabetes, Diabetes Spect 4:45-47, 1991.

16. Bynam L and Vickery C: Compliance and health promotion, Health Values 12:5-12, 1988.

17. Cerreto MC and Travis LB: Implications of psychological and family factors in the treatment of diabetes, Pediatr Clin North Am 31:689-710, 1984.

18. Christensen N and others: Quantitative assessment of dietary adherence in patients with insulin-dependent diabetes mellitus, Diabetes Care 6:245-250, 1983.

19. Clarson C and others: The relationship of metabolic control to growth and pubertal development in children with insulin-dependent diabetes, Diabetes Res 2:237-341, 1985.

20. Collier A and others: Comparison of intravenous glucagon and dextrose in treatment of severe hypoglycemia in an accident and emergency department, Diabetes Care 10:712-715, 1987.

21. Cook J and Daneman D: Microalbuminuria in adolescents with insulin dependent diabetes mellitus, Am J Dis Child 144:234-237, 1990.

22. Cook J and others: Angiotensin converting enzyme inhibitor therapy to decrease microalbuminuria in normotensive children with insulin-dependent diabetes mellitus, J Pediatr 117:39-45, 1990.

23. Daneman D and others: Progressive retinopathy with improved control in diabetic dwarfism (Mauriac syndrome), Diabetes Care 4:360-365, 1981.

24. Daneman D and Ehrlich R: Children with insulin-dependent diabetes mellitus, Medicine North Am 15:2926-2934, 1987.

25. Daneman D and others: Severe hypoglycemia in children with insulin-dependent diabetes mellitus: frequency and predisposing factors, J Pediatr 115:681-685, 1989.

26. Daneman D and others: Factors affecting glycosylated hemoglobin values in children with insulin-dependent diabetes, J Pediatr 99:847-853, 1981.

27. Daniel WA: Impact of diabetes on adolescents, Texas Med 71:56-60, 1975.

28. The DCCT Research Group: Diabetes Control and Complications Trial: results of feasibility study, Diabetes Care 10:1-19, 1987.

29. The DCCT Research Group: Weight gain associated with intensive therapy in the Diabetes Control and Complications Trial, Diabetes Care 11:567-573, 1988.

30. Dinwiddie S: Psychiatric aspects of drug abuse in diabetes, Diabetes Spect 3:353-356, 1990.

31. Drash A: Clinical care of the diabetic child, St. Louis, 1987, Mosby–Year Book.

32. Emans SJ: The sexually active teenager, Dev Behav Pediatr 4:37, 1983.

33. Erikson E: Identity, youth and crisis, New York, 1968, WW Norton.

34. Flexner C and others: Repeated hospitalization for diabetic ketoacidosis, Am J Med 76:691-695, 1984.

35. Frank R and others: Retinopathy in juvenile-onset type 1 diabetes of short duration, Diabetes 31:874-882, 1982.

36. Frank M, Perlman K, and Ehrlich R: Factors contributing to non-compliance with medical follow-up after discharge from a pediatric diabetes clinic, Diabetes 39:55A, 1990.

37. Freud A: Adolescence, Psychoanal Stud Child 13:255-278, 1958.

38. Fulop M: Recurrent diabetic ketoacidosis, Am J Med 78:54-60, 1985.

39. Gale E: The frequency of hypoglycernia in insulin-treated diabetic patients, In Serrano-Rios M, and Lefebvre P, eds: Diabetes, Amsterdam, 1985, Elsevier.

40. Gaudiani L and Feingold K: Alcohol and diabetes: mix with caution, Clin Diabetes 2:121-132, 1984.

41. Glasgow AM and others: Alcohol and drug use in teenagers with diabetes, Adolesc Health 12:11-14, 1991.

42. Golden M, Herold A, and Orr D: An approach to prevention of recurrent diabetic ketoacidosis in the pediatric population, J Pediatr 107:195-200, 1985.

43. Goldstein D: Is glycosylated hemoglobin clinically useful? New Engl J Med 310:384-385, 1984.

44. Grossman HY: The adolescent with insulin-dependent diabetes mellitus: psychological considerations. In Brink SJ: Pediatric and adolescent diabetes mellitus, Chicago, 1987, Yearbook Medical Publishers.

45. Grossman HY, Brink S, and Hauser ST: Self-efficacy in adolescent girls and boys with insulin-dependent diabetes mellitus, Diabetes Care 10:324-329, 1987.

46. Hancock LA, and Fast GP: Adolescence. In Edelman C and Mandel C, eds: Health promotion throughout the lifespan, St. Louis, 1986, Mosby–Year Book.

47. Hauenstein E and others: Stress in parents of children with diabetes mellitus, Diabetes Care 12:18-22, 1989.

48. Havlin C and Cryer P: Nocturnal hypoglycemia does not commonly result in major morning hyperglycemia in patients with diabetes mellitus, Diabetes Care 10:141-147, 1987.

49. Haynes RB, Taylor DW, and Sackett DL: Compliance in health care, Baltimore, Md, 1979, Johns Hopkins University Press.
50. Hays RD and DiMatteo MR: Patient compliance assessment, J Compliance Health Care 2:27-53, 1981.
51. Ingersoll G and others: Cognitive maturity and self-management among adolescents with insulin-dependent diabetes mellitus, J Pediatr 108:620-623, 1986.
52. Inhelder B and Piaget J: The growth of logical thinking from childhood to adolescence, New York, 1958, New York Basic Books.
53. Jackson R: Growth and development of children with diabetes mellitus, Diabetes 2:90-92, 1953.
54. Jackson R and others: Growth and maturation of children with insulin-dependent diabetes mellitus, Diabetes Care 1:96-107, 1978.
55. Jackson R and others: Growth and maturation of children with insulin-dependent diabetes mellitis, Diabetes Care 1:96-107, 1978.
56. Jacobson A and others: Psychological adjustment of children with recently diagnosed diabetes mellitus, Diabetes Care 9:323-329, 1986.
57. Jacobson A and others: Psychologic prediction of compliance in children with recent onset of diabetes mellitus, J Pediatr 110:805-811, 1987.
58. Johnson S: Psychological aspects of childhood diabetes, J Child Psychol Psychiatr 29:729-738, 1988.
59. Johnson SB: Annotation: psychological aspects of childhood diabetes, J Child Psychol Psychiatr 6:729-738, 1988.
60. Johnson S and Rosenbloom A: Behavioral aspects of diabetes mellitus in childhood and adolescence, Psychiatric Clin North Am 5:357-369, 1982.
61. Johnson S and others: Assessing daily management in childhood diabetes, Health Psychol 5:545-564, 1986.
62. Kanimer Y and Robbins D: Insulin misuse: a review of an overlooked psychiatric problem, Psychosomatics 30:19-24, 1989.
63. Kaplan R, Chadwick M, and Schimmel L: Social learning intervention to promote control in type 1 diabetes mellitus: pilot experiment results, Diabetes Care 8:152-155, 1985.
64. Keen H: Chronic complications of diabetes mellitus. In Galloway J, Potvin J, and Shuman C, eds: Diabetes mellitus, ed 9, Indianapolis, 1988, Eli Lilly, Inc.
65. Kellerman J and others: Psychological effects of illness in adolescence. 1. Anxiety, self-esteem, and perception of control, J Pediatr 97:126-131, 1990.
66. Klein B, Moss S, and Klein R: Is menarche associated with diabetic retinopathy? Diabetes Care 13:1034-1038, 1990.
67. Klein B, Moss S, and Klein R: Oral contraceptives in women with diabetes, Diabetes Care 13:895-898, 1990.
68. Knowles H and others: The course of juvenile diabetes treated with unmeasured diet, Diabetes 14:239-273, 1965.
69. Koski ML: The coping processes in childhood diabetes, Acta Pediatr Scand 188(suppl):7-56, 1969.
70. Kostraba J and others: Contribution of diabetes duration before puberty to development of microvascular complications in IDDM subjects, Diabetes Care 12:686-693, 1989.
71. Kovacs M and others: Children's self-reports of psychologic adjustment and coping strategies during first year of insulin-dependent diabetes mellitus, Diabetes Care 9:472-479, 1986.
72. Kovacs M and others: Initial coping responses and psychosocial characteristics of children with insulin-dependent diabetes mellitus, J Pediatr 106:827-834, 1985.
73. Kovacs M and others: Initial psychologic responses of parents to the diagnosis of insulin-dependent diabetes mellitus in their children, Diabetes Care 8:568-575, 1985.
74. Larsson Y and Sterky G: Long-term prognosis in juvenile diabetes mellitus, Acta Pediatr Scand 130(suppl S1):20-21, 1962.
75. Lerman I and Wolfsdorf J: Relationship of nocturnal hypoglycemia to daytime glycemia in IDDM, Diabetes Care 11:636-642, 1988.
76. Littlefield C and others: The relationship of self-efficacy and bingeing to adherence to diabetes regimen among adolescents, Diabetes Care (in press).
77. MacDonald M: Postexercise late-onset hypoglycemia in insulin-dependent diabetic patients, Diabetes Care 10:584-588, 1987.
78. Marrero DG and others: Problem-focused versus emotion-focused coping styles in adolescent diabetes, Pediatr Adolesc Endocrinol 10:141-146, 1982.

79. Mauriac P: Hepatomegalies de l'enfants avecs troubles de la croissance et due metabolisme des glucide, Paris Med 2:525-528, 1934.

80. Merimee T: A follow-up study of vascular disease in growth-hormone deficient dwarfs with diabetes, N Engl J Med 298:1217-1222, 1978.

81. Millstein SG, Adler NE, and Irwin CE: Conceptions of illness in young adolescents, Pediatrics 68:834-839, 1981.

82. Minuchin S, Rosman B, and Baker L: Psychosomatic families, Cambridge, Mass, 1978, Harvard University Press.

83. Mogenson C and Christensen C: Predicting diabetic nephropathy in insulin dependent patients, N Engl J Med 311:89-93, 1984.

84. Moynihan P and others: Diabetes youth curriculum: a textbook for educators, Waysata, Minnesota, 1988, Diabetes Center Inc.

85. Murphy R and others: The relationship of puberty to the onset of diabetic retinopathy, Arch Ophthalmol 108:215-218, 1990.

86. Natapoff JN: A developmental analysis of children's ideas of health, Health Education Quart 9:34-45, 1982.

87. Nelson KE and others: Diabetes is protective against HIV infections in IV drug users. In Proc Sixth Int Conf on AIDS, San Francisco, 1990, Abstract FC 109.

88. Orr D and others: Surreptitious insulin administration in adolescents with insulin-dependent diabetes mellitus, JAMA 256:3227-3230, 1986.

89. Orr DP and Ingersoll GM: Adolescent development: a biopsychosocial review, Curr Probl Pediatr 18:441-499, 1988.

90. Perrin JM and MacLean WE: Children with chronic illness: the prevention of dysfunction, Pediatr Clin North Am 35:1325-1337, 1988.

91. Press M, Tamborlane W, and Sherwin R: Importance of raised growth hormone levels in mediating the metabolic derangements of diabetes, N Engl J Med 310:810-815, 1984.

92. Ratner R and Whitehouse F: Motor vehicles, hypoglycemia, and diabetic drivers, Diabetes Care 12:217-222, 1989.

93. Reaven G: Role of insulin resistance in human disease, Diabetes 37:1595-1607, 1988.

94. Robinson N: Employment of people with diabetes in the United Kingdom, Diabetes Care 13:538-539, 1990.

95. Rodin G and others: Eating disorders and intentional insulin undertreatment in adolescent females with diabetes, Psychosomatics 32:171-176, 1991.

96. Rodin G and others: Eating disorders in female adolescents with insulin-dependent diabetes mellitus, Int J Psychiatr Med 16:49-57, 1986.

97. Rosenstock I: Understanding and enhancing patient compliance with diabetic regimens, Diabetes Care 8:610-616, 1985.

98. Rosmark B and others: Eating disorders in patients with insulin-dependent diabetes mellitus, J Clin Psychol 47:547-550, 1988.

99. Rutter M and others: Adolescent turmoil: fact or fiction? J Child Psychol Psychiatr 17:35-56, 1976.

100. Schade D and others: The etiology of incapacitating, brittle diabetes, Diabetes Care 8:12-20, 1985.

101. Silber TJ and others: Adolescent marijuana use: concordance between questionnaire and immunoassay for Cannabinoid metabolites, J Pediatr 111:299-303, 1987.

102. Sochett E and others: Factors affecting and patterns of residual insulin secretion during the first year of Type 1 diabetes mellitus in children, Diabetol 30:453-459, 1987.

103. Songer T and others: Employment spectrum of IDDM, Diabetes Care 12:615-622, 1989.

104. Songer T and others: Motor vehicle accidents and IDDM, Diabetes Care 11:701-707, 1988.

105. Stanhope R and Brook C: An evaluation of hormonal changes at puberty in man, J Endocr 116:301-305, 1988.

106. Sterky G: Diabetic school children, Acta Pediatr Scand 144(suppl 1):1-36.

107. Sullivan B: Adjustment in diabetic adolescent girls. 1. Development of the diabetic adjustment scale, Psychosomat Med 41:119-126, 1979.

108. Sullivan B: Adjustment in diabetic adolescent girls. 11. Adjustment, self-esteem, and depression in diabetic adolescent girls, Psychosomat Med 41:127-138, 1979.

109. Surwit R, Scovern A, and Feinglos M: The role of behavior in diabetes care, Diabetes Care 5: 337-342, 1982.

110. Swift CR, Seidman F, and Stein H: Adjustment problems in juvenile diabetes, Psychosomat Med 29:555-571, 1967.
111. Tamborlane W: Personal communication, 1991.
112. Tanner J: Growth at adolescence, ed 2, Oxford, 1962, Blackwell.
113. Tattersall RB and Lowe J: Diabetes in adolescence, Diabetol 20:517-523, 1981.
114. Tattersal R and Pyke D: Growth in diabetic children: studies in identical twins, Lancet 1:1105-1109, 1973.
115. Tebbi C and others: Vocational adjustment and general well-being in young adults with IDDM, Diabetes Care 13:98-103, 1990.
116. Travis L: Hypoglycemia in insulin-dependent diabetes mellitus, J Pediatr 115:740-741, 1989.
117. Weintrob N and others: Severe hypoglycemia and hepatic dysfunction due to surreptitious insulin overdose, J Pediatr Endocrinol 3:277-280, 1989.
118. Wesolowski C: Self-contracts for chronically ill children, Maternal Child Nursing 13:20-23, 1988.
119. Wexler P: The social worker and the child with juvenile diabetes mellitus, In Traisman HJS, ed: Management of juvenile diabetes mellitus, St Louis, 1980, Mosby–Year Book.
120. White K and others: Unstable diabetes and unstable families: a psychosocial evaluation of diabetic children with recurrent ketoacidosis, Pediatrics 73:749-755, 1984.
121. Zinman B: Exercise in diabetes treatment, Clin Diabetes 1:18-22, 1983.

CHAPTER 14

Diabetes Mellitus in Young and Middle Adulthood

JAMES A. FAIN AND GAIL D'ERAMO-MELKUS

Diabetes mellitus is a chronic illness that can occur at any age throughout the life span. The period of young adulthood (20's and 30's) is often thought to begin with separation from parents, ideas of seeking education, a career, and finding a partner with whom to share one's life. It is conceptualized as a time when individuals are willing to unite their identity with others. In general, by young adulthood, individuals reach the highest level of intellectual efficiency and cognitive development. Middle adulthood (40's and 50's) represents a stage of self-review—a time of questioning accomplishments, successes, and value to society. During both periods, the impact of diabetes mellitus affects physical, cognitive, and psychosocial aspects of development.

In this chapter, the physical, cognitive, and psychosocial tasks of young and middle adulthood are discussed. It is important, however, that as members of the health care team we consider all changes as interrelated processes that affect and are affected by each other.

The objectives of this chapter are to identify physical changes associated with young and middle adulthood; contrast the cognitive abilities of the young adult with those of middle adulthood; differentiate normal psychosocial tasks of development in young and middle adulthood; discuss specific health needs of the young adult with diabetes; describe the impact of drug/alcohol abuse in young adulthood; discuss unique health problems associated with diabetes and middle adulthood; outline sociocultural and economic factors that can affect young and middle adults with diabetes; and describe the role of the health care team in providing care to individuals in young and middle adulthood.

NORMAL PHYSICAL TASKS OF DEVELOPMENT IN YOUNG ADULTHOOD
Physical Changes

Young adulthood is thought to be the healthiest time of life. During a 15-year span (20 to 35), the young adult's physical abilities are at a peak with body systems compensating optimally during illness.[15] Physical growth is usually completed by age 20, while muscular strength is at peak efficiency by age 25 to 30. The young adult can expect to have strong muscles and bones free from serious infections or degenerative disease. Physical stamina is usually sufficient to keep up with all the social, economic, and emotional tasks of this period.

Ninety percent of the adult height and weight are attained during young adulthood.[41] Body shape and proportions finally reach their finished state, with the exception of weight and muscle mass. Fat accumulation and muscle mass are under more environmental influence (diet and exercise) and may fluctuate throughout a person's life. Skeletal development is completed as the long bones of the upper legs and arms finish their ossification process. Attainment of final adult height coincides with epiphyseal fusion. A few millimeters may be added to the width of some bones later by surface deposition. Head length and breadth, facial diameters, and the width of bones in the legs and hands may increase slightly by this process throughout life.

Muscles continue to gain strength throughout the twenties and reach peak strength at about age 30, depending on exercise and genetic endowment. Men have larger muscles that can produce more force than the muscle tissue of women. They also have a greater capacity for carrying oxygen in the blood to the muscles and a greater capacity for neutralizing the chemical products of exercising muscle. Dental maturity is finally achieved in the twenties with the emergence of the last four molars or wisdom teeth.

During young adulthood the senses are functioning appropriately. Ocular functioning is completely developed by age 20 and starts to decline during middle adulthood. Hearing is best at age 20 with higher tone sounds tending to be gradually lost. The other senses of touch, smell, and taste remain intact until 45 to 50.[43]

The peak efficiency of cardiac output, which was achieved during adolescence, continues throughout the adult years to accommodate typical activity.[7] Changes in heart size and cardiac function occur with age and have a direct relationship to major risk factors such as hypertension, diabetes, elevated serum cholesterol and lipids, lack of exercise, cigarette smoking, obesity, and stress.

AGE-RELATED VARIATIONS IN HEALTH PRACTICES
Health Practices in Young Adulthood

Young adulthood is a time when one searches for a place in society. Finding a mate, establishing a family, and initiating a career are major tasks to be accomplished. In all instances, the ability to integrate cognitive and socioemotional skills becomes critical. For some, their self-esteem and struggle for self-fulfillment will be decreased when certain expectations are not met. While physical health tends to be at a heightened period, certain health risk behaviors may develop, further affecting long-term health into middle adult-hood. Within this period of development, health care providers need to be aware of the individual's tendency and awareness for altering attitudes and behaviors that present major problems. Drug/alcohol abuse, automobile accidents, and stress-related illnesses present a major threat to the health of young adults.

Drug Abuse

It is estimated that 58% of young adults have some experience in the use of marijuana, whereas 20% have tried stronger drugs, such as cocaine or hallucinogens. Medically prescribed drugs are another source of experimentation. Used alone or together, barbiturates, amphetamines, or sedative-hypnotics reportedly bring about feelings of physical and psychologic well-being. In contrast to adolescents, the young adult tends to restrict drug use, to only a select few. Adolescents are more likely to experiment with a variety of drugs. Drug abuse continues to be associated with homicides, suicides, and inability to cope with adult responsibilities. Physical health problems account for more than 50% of the major acute and chronic problems of young adults who abuse drugs.[54]

Heroin users, for example, have a higher mortality rate because of overdosage or chronic disability associated with hepatitis, infections, contaminated supplies, and malnutrition.[54]

Alcohol Abuse

Alcohol is still considered by many as a nondrug. It is readily available, inexpensive, and considered socially acceptable. Although young adults may drink less regularly than older adults, they tend to consume larger amounts of alcohol at one time. Alcohol-related accidents among young adults continue to be the leading cause of death. Alcohol is a factor in more than 10% of all deaths in the United States and 60% of all highway fatalities involving young adults.[54]

Automobile Accidents

Despite the general good health in this period of life, auto accidents are a leading cause of death among young adults. In particular, they are responsible for more fatalities than all other causes of death combined. Most accidents occur in the late teenage years or early twenties, males are frequently involved in more accidents than females.[54]

Stress-Related Illnesses

Young adults encounter another type of risk to health—the pressure of achievement-oriented stress. This differs from stress in situational crises. The stress in an overachiever is brought about from internal pressures to succeed in relation to goals. Achievement stress often causes 'workaholic' habits, including lack of sleep and omission of meals. If this behavior becomes extreme, physical exhaustion, nutritional problems, and/or burnout may occur. Such behaviors may not be perceived by the individual and often go undetected until changes in bodily functions occur.[16]

Many young adults enjoy some sort of physical activity and are usually health conscious and willing to alter life-styles and patterns of behavior according to their concept of health. It becomes important for young adults to recognize stress as a risk factor and be able to recognize behaviors such as increased anxiety, nervousness, depression, or somatic complaints as indicators of a problem.[54]

IMPACT OF DIABETES MELLITUS ON NORMAL PHYSICAL CHANGES IN YOUNG ADULTHOOD

It has become increasingly clear that vascular disease is associated with diabetes mellitus. It is estimated to be 30 times more common in persons with diabetes as evidenced by the risk of gangrene which increases markedly among these persons.[10] The occurrence and progression of vascular disease may be directly related to prolonged elevation of blood glucose. Adults who have elevated blood glucoses over years appear to suffer the greatest impact with respect to vascular changes. However, some adults with diabetes never develop complications despite prolonged elevations.

Organ damage occurs in those tissues in which glucose transport across the cell membrane is not insulin-mediated or dependent. Thus, the vascular endothelium, the nerve sheath, the red blood cell, the lens of the eye, and other tissues are concentrated with amounts of glucose that are dependent on the degree of hyperglycemia. Such a situation can potentially lead to metabolic and functioning alterations within the cell structure.[4]

Although chronic or long-term complications of diabetes mellitus (degenerative cardiovascular changes, neuropathy, nephropathy, and retinopathy) occur in less than 20% of those between the ages of 20 to 35, the impact of prevention, early diagnosis, and treatment are of great importance to young adults with insulin-dependent type I diabetes mellitus (IDDM).[57]

Diagnosis

Adults with IDDM usually have an abrupt onset of signs and symptoms of insulinopenia before the age of 30. Individuals with IDDM produce little or no insulin, are dependent on exogenous insulin, and account for approximately 10% of all individuals with diabetes.[2] It may occur at any age, but usually is diagnosed before the age of 20. Commonly, adults experience an unexplained weight loss and test positive for urine ketones in conjunction with hyperglycemia.

Individuals with non–insulin-dependent type II diabetes (NIDDM) may at some point require insulin for persistent hyperglycemia. NIDDM can occur at any age, but usually is diagnosed after the age of 35 and is associated with obesity. The development of ketosis is not common, unless precipitated by such factors as infections, surgery, stress, or trauma.[2] Goals related to management of IDDM or NIDDM in the adult are presented in the accompanying box.

There are some instances in which NIDDM is present among children, adolescents, and young adults. This form of diabetes is referred to as maturity-onset diabetes of the young (MODY). MODY is a subtype of NIDDM that is inherited in an autosomal dominant fashion. It is found in early adolescence (9 to 14 years), particularly if sought on routine blood glucose testing in the younger generations of families with more than one generation of NIDDM. Intake of excessive calories leading to weight gain and obesity is probably an important factor in its pathogenesis. In general, principles of management are the same as those for NIDDM. Diet therapy alone may be sufficient for some, while others may require sulfonylurea drugs.[22]

Hyperglycemia and ketonemia are more common in young adults with IDDM. Specific aspects of treatment are presented elsewhere in this text. In general, to minimize wide fluctuations in blood glucose, individuals should balance medication, diet, and exercise. Many acute episodes can thus be anticipated and prevented. Diabetes education, which includes both the individual with diabetes and his or her significant others, will help to maintain a sense of well-being and prevent adverse stress and illness.

Physical Effects

The young adult with diabetes may be susceptible to developing complications associated with microvascular or macrovascular disease, depending on these predisposing factors.

MANAGEMENT GOALS OF DIABETES MANAGEMENT: IDDM VS NIDDM

IDDM

Eliminate and/or avoid ketoacidosis
Achieve metabolic control: minimize hyperglycemia while avoiding serious hypoglycemia
Maintain normal growth and development
Restoration of desirable body weight
Encourage physical and social activity appropriate to specific age group
Educate about pathophysiologic and psychologic aspects of diabetes mellitus

NIDDM

Achieve metabolic control
Institute a plan of diet modification
Increase physical activity appropriate to specific age group
Pharmacologic intervention with oral hypoglycemic agents or insulin

As previously noted, diabetic complications tend to be associated with degree and duration of hyperglycemia. In addition, genetic susceptibility may play a role (see Chapters 5-7). Much of the focus of diabetes management in young adulthood, then, is on modification of factors that discourage the development of long-term complications. With the advent of self-monitoring of blood glucose (SMBG), assessment of glycemic control allows individuals to note warning signs of hypoglycemia and hyperglycemia. SMBG provides the individual and health care provider with immediate and accurate clinical data. Following instruction, individuals are able to monitor and record their own blood glucose and make appropriate adjustments in diet, exercise, and medication. Such technology enables the adult to manage his or her diabetes in consultation with the health care team. In addition, newer technology has allowed health care providers to enter blood glucose values into computers for manipulation and interpretation.[13] Assessment of glycemic control requires a system that is interpretable by both the health care provider and individual. Compliance with SMBG is associated with understanding the results and how to appropriately respond. As such, adults with diabetes are prime candidates for learning SMBG as a tool for managing diabetes. However, careful education on how to monitor accurately and how to interpret and act upon results is critical if the benefits SMBG afford are to be realized.

Vascular Changes

The young adult with diabetes is more susceptible to developing microvascular or macrovascular disease then is his or her nondiabetic counterpart. As previously noted, diabetic complications tend to be associated with degree and duration of hyperglycemia. Much of the focus of diabetes management in young adulthood then, is on prevention and/or modification of factors that promote the development of long-term complications.

The impact of peripheral vascular disease (PVD) in young adults with diabetes is enormous. For the young adult with diabetes, the single most significant factor is prevention of PVD by educating and encouraging specific interventions for health maintenance such as those suggested in Chapter 16 of this text. In particular, studies have identified various risk factors associated with PVD: hypertension, elevated serum cholesterol and lipids, smoking, and obesity.[37]

First, hypertension in young adults with diabetes is of significant prognostic importance. By monitoring blood pressure values, early identification and treatment may decrease long-term complications. In addition to immediate impacts associated with PVD, hypertension in the young adult contributes substantially to the early cardiovascular morbidity and mortality of those with diabetes mellitus. Cardiovascular and renal mortality accounts for 50% to 60% of diabetic deaths and with advancing age and duration of the diabetes, the percentage is greater than 70%. Young adults with diabetes who present with hypertension need aggressive management and education to limit the likelihood of progression of disease.[46]

Life-style Changes

While genetic factors are a major component of the development of disease, life-style is also a major contributor. Young adults who exhibit modifiable risk factors should be targeted for extensive education and behavioral interventions to diminish the risk. Obesity is probably the major factor associated with hypertension and cardiovascular risk.[46] Young adults should be instructed to decrease their intake of salt and consider the high sodium content of commercially prepared foods, particularly the fast, convenient types that are so frequently used by this age group.

Second, elevated serum cholesterol and lipids are major components associated with atherosclerosis. Since atherosclerosis is commonly associated with diabetes, periodic evaluation of fasting lipids should be carried out. Studies have shown that elevated plasma LDL levels and suppressed HDL concentrations are frequently seen in adults with diabetes.[37] In young adults with IDDM, this appears in the presence of hyperglycemia. The diet recommended by the American Heart Association is integrated into the diabetes meal plan to lower the intake of saturated fat and thereby lower cholesterol levels.

Limiting the use of dietary fat and adding fiber to meals may have a positive influence on the management of diabetes. The typical diet contains approximately 10 to 15 g of dietary fiber. An increase to 25 to 35 grams of fiber per 1000 calories has been recommended by the ADA (see Chapter 2). There are two types of dietary fiber—water soluble and water insoluble. Water-soluble fibers include pectins and gums that are found in citrus fruits, oats, barley, and legumes. Water-insoluble fibers include cellulose and are found in leafy vegetables, wheat, cereal products, and most grains. Water-soluble fibers tend to form a gel with the GI tract, slowing absorption of glucose across the intestinal mucosa as well as lowering cholesterol. Water insoluble fibers increase bulk within the gastrointestinal tract and help to relieve constipation.[3]

Elimination of cigarette smoking is another means of preventing peripheral vascular disease. Smoking is one of the strongest risk factors for intermittent claudication. The fact that the risk of cardiovascular complications is enormously greater in those persons with diabetes should be an added deterrent to smoking. However, recent data suggest smoking remains a significant risk factor for adults with diabetes. Nicotine increases constriction of small blood vessels, further impeding an already diminishing circulation.[16,57]

Smoking tends to be initiated during adolescence. By young adulthood, the habit is well entrenched by several years. It is crucial that persons with diabetes who do smoke should be strongly encouraged to quit. Smoking cessation strategies by the diabetes health care team or referral to appropriate resources, such as those found through the American Lung Association or American Cancer Society, should be implemented. Careful and systematic follow-up should also be implemented.[11]

Finally, for young adults with diabetes, exercise is an important and essential component of diabetes management. Exercise provides an excellent means of maintaining ideal body weight and avoiding obesity commonly associated with PVD. While exercise alone is not an effective means of losing weight, since the caloric expenditure required to burn fat is enormous, exercise is an excellent method of "healthful stress" to the cardiovascular system. It will also promote a sense of well-being that is frequently needed when getting into shape. A more detailed discussion of exercise implications appear in Chapter 3 of this text.

NORMAL PHYSICAL TASKS OF DEVELOPMENT IN MIDDLE ADULTHOOD
Age and Physical Changes

While 40 years of age has significance in chronically demarcating the majority of persons with NIDDM from those with IDDM, it also signifies the beginning of middle adulthood or middlescence. This period of the life cycle connotes certain responsibilities and assumptions based on a normative system of age expectations. An age-graded system is socially defined and represents a means of rationalizing the life cycle and relevant life cycle events.

In contrast to the steady growth in adolescence, which peaks in young adulthood, physical changes among middle adults occur gradually and affect most body systems.[41,43] In general, the functional capacity of all systems begins to decrease. For example, in the gastrointestinal tract (GI), decreased metabolism leads to less enzyme production, resulting in lower hydrochloric acid levels decreasing the tone in the large intestines. As a result, middle adults seem to complain more of acid indigestion with increased belching.[16] Additionally, more middle adults will eat foods that are low in bulk that may contribute to the problem of constipation. That coupled with a sedentary life-style, diminishes motility through the GI tract.

Muscle size, strength, and reflex speed also begin a progressive decline. Size and strength that is lost from disuse, however, can be regained through rigorous exercise. Muscle strength of most men continues to be greater than that of most women throughout the life span.[41,43]

The bones lose further mass and density. As the cartilage between the vertebrae start to degenerate from normal wear, the vertebrae become compressed and the spinal column gradually begins to shorten. As adults age, they actually lose some of their height because of this compression of the spinal column. With increasing age the cartilage in all joints has a more limited ability to regenerate itself.[41,43]

In addition to muscular and skeletal changes, there are age-related changes in the endocrine glands. Both the basal metabolic rate and secretions of thyroid hormones decrease with age. Epinephrine and norepinephrine, the hormones of the sympathetic nervous system, are released more slowly in aging persons in response to stress. There is also evidence that the tissue response to these substances diminishes with age. Finally, there is a gradual decline of glucose tolerance and an increased prevalence of diabetes mellitus with age because of tissue resistance to insulin that occurs with progressive weight gain.[24] Skin also begins to lose its resilience and elasticity.

Between the ages of 25 and 70 there is a 35% loss of nephron units. The remaining nephrons increase in size and undergo degenerative changes. The entire weight of the kidney decreases. With blood supply also being diminished, the glomerular filtration rate is decreased by nearly one half.[16]

During middle adulthood the cardiovascular system undergoes several changes. The lungs and bronchi become increasingly less elastic, causing a progressive decrease in maximum breathing capacity. The ability of the heart muscle to contract decreases, leading to a lower cardiac index (the cardiac output per minute per square meter of body surface).[24]

Blood vessels lose elasticity and become thicker, further contributing to elevated blood pressure. Middle-aged adults are more prone to myocardial infarction, stroke, and hypertension, with heart disease being the leading cause of death for this age group.[54]

IMPACT OF DIABETES MELLITUS ON NORMAL PHYSICAL CHANGES IN MIDDLE ADULTHOOD
Age and Associated Changes

Sensoriperceptual decline related to aging, which begins in the fourth decade of life, involves changes in vision, hearing, and cutaneous sensitivity. As an individual approaches the sixth decade of life, sensoriperceptual changes begin to take place relative to taste, smell, balance, and motor processes. These functions are responsible for the reception, interpretation, processing, and translation of new information and skills.[19] Similarly, diabetes-related changes as a result of microvascular and neuropathic complications may be found in vision, cutaneous sensitivity, balance, proprioception, and motor function. It is important to note that the degree of decline and resultant alteration in function varies among individuals depending on age, type (IDDM versus NIDDM), and duration of diabetes.

Vision

Presbyopia, the farsightedness of aging, begins in the fourth decade of life causing most middle-aged adults to need corrective lenses. The lenses of the eyes gradually become less elastic with age, causing the eyes to lose their ability to bring near-point visual images into focus. At the same time, alterations in light perception begin to occur, which in turn affects night vision. These normal age-related changes in vision can be problematic for the individual with diabetes who is aware of and concerned with the potential for retinopathy. In addition, transient changes in lens refraction caused by fluctuations in blood glucose occur, which in turn affect visual acuity. Such refractive changes at high blood glucose levels result in myopia and at low blood glucose levels result in hyperopia.[36] These changes, whether age or diabetes related, represent a major source of stress in terms of the potential for visual impairment and loss of sight.

Diabetic retinopathy is the leading cause of new cases of blindness in the United States. The major source of stress related to the potential for loss of vision is made apparent by the fact that as compared with those individuals who do not have diabetes, individuals with diabetes are 29 times more likely to become blind.[55] When age is accounted for, the absolute risk of blindness caused by diabetic retinopathy increases with age, with the relative risk being greater for persons aged 30 to 50. In terms of risk related to duration of disease, 80% of all persons with diabetes have some form of retinopathy 15 years after diagnosis.

The goal of diabetes self-care is the attainment of optimal metabolic control in an effort to prevent or minimize both the acute and chronic complications of diabetes. When age and duration of disease are factored into the equation for potential visual impairment, good metabolic control alone is not the sole predictor of outcome. However, it has been shown that self-blame and guilt regarding metabolic control has been frequently expressed by visually impaired individuals.[42]

Cutaneous System

The cutaneous system is responsible for tactile, temperature, and pain reception or sensitivity. There are age-related changes that occur in thermal and vibratory sensitivity; however, evidence suggesting similar decline in pain sensitivity remains controversial. As an individual grows older and has increased duration of diabetes, the normal age-related changes are further compounded by the diabetes-related changes of peripheral neuropathy.

Diabetes associated changes in vibratory, thermal, and pain sensitivity are related to the existence of peripheral neuropathy. Sensory and motor nerve conduction have been shown to be impaired early in the course of diabetes without any clinical symptomatology.[20] With progression of disease this asymptomatic state turns into one of minimal symptomatology characterized by paresthesia of numbness and tingling. This in turn predisposes individuals to painless injuries that increase the potential for ulceration, infection, and amputation.

The implication of such physiologic changes related to visual acuity and cutaneous sensitivity is that individuals may encounter difficulty when performing self-care tasks such as insulin injection, self-monitoring of blood glucose, and foot care. Problems with manual dexterity may be further complicated by the presence of osteoarthritis, which is a common chronic illness in middle-aged adults.

Peripheral neuropathy affecting the lower extremities may interfere with one's ability to maintain a regular program of exercise and may also affect one's work role as well as involvement in social activities. Such impingements on activities of daily living can give rise to feelings of anxiety and depression, especially as one is confronted with the middlescent emotions of bodily decline and growing older.

Kidney Function

Age-related changes that occur in the urinary tract are associated with arteriosclerosis and a decrease in muscle tone, nephrons, and renal tissue growth. The glomerular filtration rate begins to decline in midlife as renal blood flow decreases. In addition to the age-related changes, the kidneys of individuals with diabetes undergo many functional and morphologic changes. These changes occur prior to the clinical appearance of proteinuria. However, the occurrence of proteinuria is usually first noted after 10 to 15 years of

Table 14-1   Age and Diabetes Changes that Affect Self-Care

Age-associated changes	Complications of diabetes	Responses
Vision	Retinopathy	Decrease in visual acuity
		Changes in light perception
		Changes in lens refraction
Cutaneous	Peripheral neuropathy	Altered tactile sensitivity
		Altered thermal sensitivity
		Altered vibratory sensitivity
		Decreased motor function
Renal	Nephropathy	Increased renal threshold
		Decreased renal clearance
		Increased drug half-life

SMBG, insulin injections, foot care—may be impaired by hypoglycemia/hyperglycemia

IDDM. In fact, after a 15-year duration of diabetes, approximately one third of people with IDDM and one fifth of those with NIDDM will develop diabetic nephropathy.[55]

Because the incidence of diabetic nephropathy is associated with duration of disease, middle-aged adults with diabetes feel vulnerable to its occurrence and perceive it as life threatening. The existence of hypertension may either precipitate or potentiate the progression of diabetic nephropathy. Many adults with diabetes develop hypertension that necessitates careful control.

Alterations in renal function related to aging and diabetes have implications for diabetes self-care. A decrease in renal excretion of drugs increases the half-life of drugs normally excreted by the kidneys. As a result, there is an increase propensity for frequent episodes of hypoglycemia caused by the increased half-life of oral sulfonylureas or insulin.

Various age-related changes that affect diabetes self-care activities are presented in Table 14-1.

Sexual Function

Sexual function is an important and integral part of middle adulthood as well as young adulthood. It is an essential component of a satisfying, intimate relationship with a significant other. Most individuals in young adulthood are concerned with the developmental task of child-bearing, whereas middle adults typically are not.

It is theorized that the sexual element is decreasingly significant in middle adulthood as individuals redefine men and women as companions and partners.[44] However, this notion of socializing versus sexualizing in relationships does not negate the importance of an individual's sexuality relative to sexual performance.

Normal age-related changes that occur in women are associated with the menopausal period (late forties to fifties). There are changes in vaginal elasticity with a reduction in vaginal lubrication. In males there are changes in the amount of time required for physical stimulation, for achieving an erection, and in the time and force of ejaculations. In both men and women there is no age-related decline associated with libido.

Sexual dysfunction related to diabetes, however, is of great concern to the individual with diabetes. Psychogenic and organic impotence are common findings among men with diabetes. The prevalence rate for impotency has been reported to be as high as 60%. Organic impotence is the result of diabetic neuropathy and therefore could occur at any time after adolescence, depending on duration of disease. Proximal vascular insufficiency can be detected by examining the femoral pulses. However, localized obstruction of the penile artery would need to be examined by measurements of the brachial/penile blood pressure ratio using Doppler flow studies. Normal erections on awakening or impotence only with a certain partner suggests a psychogenic cause.[40]

While sexual dysfunction has been widely studied in men, there is a lack of information regarding sexual function in women with diabetes. What has been described is that women are still functional and experience no decrease in libido or ability to achieve orgasm when compared with women without diabetes.[20]

For many cultural groups, the male holds the dominant sex role. Therefore, sexual dysfunction often causes disruption in the male self-image and self-esteem, which results in stress and conflict within significant intimate relationships. Individuals with a sexual dysfunction and their partners should be referred for sexual counseling. At that time, options for management can be discussed (e.g., alternative forms of mutual sexual gratification, penile prostheses).

Coronary Artery Disease

At least one third of all deaths occurring in individuals with diabetes after age 40 is caused by atherosclerotic heart disease.[35,43] Ischemic heart disease appears to be more prevalent among those individuals with NIDDM in whom coronary atherosclerosis has been accelerated. Likewise, those with IDDM who have aggressive premature macrovascular or microvascular complications are more prone to ischemic heart disease.[15] The risk for heart disease is two times greater for those with diabetes and is not necessarily associated with duration of diabetes.

Obesity and hypertension, as previously described, increase the risk of premature morbidity and mortality in individuals with diabetes and coronary artery disease. Modification and elimination of associated risk factors such as smoking, obesity, elevated cholesterol and lipids, and hypertension will reduce the risk of heart attack and stroke.

Because the majority of individuals with NIDDM are obese, the *importance of educational and behavioral interventions targeted at risk factor modification cannot be overemphasized.*

COGNITIVE PROCESSES IN YOUNG AND MIDDLE ADULTHOOD

Intellectual maturity continues throughout adulthood. Young adults begin to acquire knowledge and develop skills that improve performance abilities gained as adolescents.[31]

Piaget's stage of formal operational thought evolves from concrete operational thought in adolescence and extends into young adulthood.[45] During this developmental stage, young adults begin to analyze combinations of relations and construct hypotheses capable of being tested. It is a time when issues are approached realistically with important decisions being made. Young adults experiment with trial-and-error methodology and demonstrate use of problem-solving reasoning.

Piaget's stage of formal operational thought continues throughout middle adulthood with refinement in areas of spatial perception and problem-solving reasoning. Middle adults have the ability to deal more efficiently with complex problems of reasoning caused by life experiences and completion of adult developmental tasks.

IMPACT OF DIABETES MELLITUS ON COGNITIVE PROCESSES IN YOUNG AND MIDDLE ADULTHOOD

Fear of hypoglycemia is quite prevalent among individuals who have diabetes and may be a motivating factor in the maintenance of elevated blood glucose levels to avoid risk of hypoglycemic episodes.[12] The transient or permanent impairments of brain function that can occur with repeated episodes of hypoglycemia are rather serious. Central or peripheral nervous system dysfunction is the usual consequence of severe hypoglycemia. Individuals may exhibit symptoms of drowsiness or passivity; slow, confused thinking; impaired ability to judge the passage of time; impaired memory; impaired judgment; and slightly impaired auditory learning of declarative information.[9,14,23] In addition to memory and attention deficits, symptoms of hypoglycemia are unpleasant and often embarrassing.[27] Such episodes can undermine an individual's credibility and reliability within the context of work and family roles. Frequent episodes may cause family, friends, and work associates to cast an individual into a traditional sick role, thus relinquishing this person of certain responsibilities.

IMPACT OF DIABETES MELLITUS ON NORMAL PSYCHOSOCIAL DEVELOPMENT IN YOUNG ADULTHOOD

Erikson identified the development of self-esteem and self-satisfaction as major tasks during young adulthood. A sense of being open and capable of trusting others develops through the formation of intimate relationships. Erikson terms this period of psychosocial development as Intimacy vs. Isolation and Loneliness.[21] The concept of intimacy goes beyond sexual intimacy to a broader view of mutual psychosocial intimacy with peers, parents, and/or spouse. Intimacy requires mutual trust and involves reciprocal expression of affection. Young adults search for continuity and individuals in their lives who provide meaning. Those who are unsure of their identity may shy away from intimate contact with others that can result in loneliness. For those with diabetes, there may be concern about the quality of life and the impact of diabetes on establishing meaningful interpersonal relationships.

The strain faced by young adults dealing with newly diagnosed diabetes, or the focus

Table 14-2   Erikson's Psychosocial Development of Young and Middle Adulthood

Young adulthood		
Intimacy	vs	**Isolation**
Intimacy is expressed in psychosocial terms such as *affiliation* and *partnership*.		A lack of identity that leads to a defensiveness that could polarize relationships.
Affiliation indicates the meaning of intimacy as inclusive of friendships based on choice rather than family.		Unresolved identity questions lead to major problems with selecting a mate and finding a congenial social group.
Emotional intimacy refers to the capacity to perceive nondefensively the meaning of the emotion that the other person is expressing.		Expressive isolation is the self-protection of one's image. Individuals may function with societal roles, but have difficulties in close relationships.
Intellectual intimacy is the sharing of ideas without polarization of the relationship.		Receptive isolation is defensiveness expressed in the distortion of social and environmental stimuli.
Middle adulthood		
Generativity	vs	**Stagnation**
Characterized by a concern with the establishment and setting forth guidelines for future generations.		Characterized by an absorption with the self to the extent that it excludes the welfare of others.
The virtue of *care* develops. Expressed as one's concern for others by wanting to take care of others and share knowledge and expertise.		When generativity is weak the personality regresses and takes on a sense of impoverishment.

From Erickson EH: Adulthood, New York, 1978, WW Norton and Company, Inc.

on self-management issues associated with diabetes, may diminish or delay the accomplishment of developmental tasks as identified by Erikson. Other aspects of Erikson's psychosocial development of young and middle adulthood are discussed in Table 14-2.

Another psychosocial task of development during young adulthood is separation from parents. This task is usually accomplished by seeking education or pursuing a career away from home. Concerns about having diabetes may inhibit this developmental transition. It becomes critical to discuss with the young adult his or her perception of prognosis or quality of life in the context of long-term outcomes of diabetes. The health care team should also educate the young adult and his or her significant others as a means of encouraging optimal diabetes self-management.

Members of the health care team can assist young adults in being honest and realistic about the consequences of diabetes and the various options that are available. Employment can be a sensitive and critical issue for young adults with diabetes. Persons with diabetes may be restricted from pursuing certain jobs and should carefully consider career decisions in the light of their diagnosis. Federal and state legislation has been enacted in the last decade, limiting discriminatory practices. While nearly every job is now open to those with diabetes, certain positions that may negatively affect long-term health might be avoided. For example, the avoidance of those jobs requiring operation of heavy machinery, or working erratic schedules, should be recommended.[2,28] In some instances, adults with diabetes have been working when their diabetes was diagnosed, which suggests the need for job counseling or retraining.

The decision to marry and have a family represents another developmental task of young adulthood. Young adults may question entering into marriage when their life span may be shorter and additional economic burdens present. Their sense of self-worth and self-confidence may be decreased. Additionally, some may be ashamed of their condition and not willing to share various problems and/or complications with another individual in the context of a marriage and family. When entering into marriage, both the individual with diabetes and the spouse must learn what diabetes is, how to manage common crises, and what is involved with the treatment regimen. Discussion of long-term complications is also appropriate. Both should understand the risks of pregnancy for the woman with diabetes and the need for glycemia to be optimal at the time of conception so as to minimize the risk of congenital malformations.

For many women with diabetes, anxiety may surround the decision to have children or not. Specific management of diabetes during pregnancy is discussed in Chapter 9 and includes preconception metabolic control, rigid glycemic control throughout gestation, and close monitoring of mother and fetus all of which are essential components in the care of the pregnant woman with diabetes. Sensitive prepregnancy counseling for the woman with diabetes, along with her spouse, will provide an essential foundation for a healthy and successful pregnancy.[38]

Gestational diabetes, which is discussed in greater detail in Chapter 9 of this text, has been defined by the Second International Conference on Gestational Diabetes Mellitus as, "carbohydrate intolerance of variable severity with onset of first recognition during the present pregnancy." Estimates of the incidence of gestational diabetes have been as low as 3% to 20%. It becomes difficult to get a more accurate estimation because of the lack of population-based studies.[49] However, for many adult women (97%) this condition will rescind at the end of their pregnancy.[1] With increased technology (e.g., blood glucose monitoring, multiple-injection regimens, insulin pump therapy), many women with gestational diabetes are able to deliver healthy babies.

IMPACT OF DIABETES MELLITUS ON NORMAL PSYCHOSOCIAL DEVELOPMENT IN MIDDLE ADULTHOOD

In Erickson's theory of life span personality development, the middle adulthood period is characterized as a time of Generativity vs. Stagnation.[21] Generativity is defined by an expansion of ego interests, productivity, and creativity. It can likewise be conceptualized as a sense of having contributed to the future versus a sense of ego stagnation. This developmental period is a time of valuing wisdom versus valuing physical powers and socializing versus sexualizing in human relationships.[44]

Other expectations of middle adulthood include those of work, marriage, child rearing, caring for aging parents, and legal and social responsibility.[44] It is a period of time characterized by a sense of accomplishment as the individual views his or her life within the context of family and career. At the same time, however, there may also exist a sense of bodily decline, growing old, and recognizing one's mortality. Such feelings support the notion that individuals are aware of age norms and expectations in relation to their own patterns of timing, and that timing plays an important role with respect to self-concept and self-esteem.

During young and middle adulthood, various developmental tasks must be achieved and accomplished for the individual to continue successfully onto the next stage of development. A list of specific tasks for both young and middle adults are shown in the accompanying box.[41]

Because self-concept and self-esteem are developed through interactions between an individual's ego and society, chronic illness inherently can alter such interactions. This is caused by the ambiguous and often stigmatized nature of chronic illness, in which society considers an individual either sick or well.

Strauss and Glaser[52] call such a phenomenon "identity spread," when the symptoms of a chronic illness are intrusive. Society may then assume that the ill individual cannot work, act, or be like an ordinary, "normal" individual. In essence, chronic illness lacks normative definition with corresponding rights and responsibilities. As a result, an individual may become isolated and nonproductive contrary to a dominant cultural emphasis

---

_____ DEVELOPMENTAL TASKS OF YOUNG AND MIDDLE ADULTS _____

Young adults

Accepting and stabilizing self-concept and body image
Establishing independence from parental home
Becoming established in a vocation or profession that provides personal satisfaction, economic independence, and a feeling of making a contribution to society
Expressing love responsibly through more than sexual contacts
Establishing intimate bond with another individual
Finding a congenial social group
Formulating a meaningful philosophy of life

Middle adults

Accepting personal strengths and limits with a firm sense of identity
Striving for self-actualization; living up to highest potential
Assuring security for later years, financially and emotionally
Drawing emotionally closer as a couple
Maintaining contact with grown children and their families
Participating in community life beyond the family
Reaffirming the values of life that have real meaning

of active involvement and productivity. The potential for such is greatly increased among adults with diabetes-related complications. It is not uncommon for the central work role to be modified or lost because of disability or decreased capability for work role resumption. Similarly, the role within the family can be modified and altered.[17]

The coping responses of the chronically ill are affected by the characteristics of the illness and by reactions of members of the family and society. Cohen and Lazarus[34] define coping as the process of managing demands that are appraised as taxing or exceeding the resources of the person. This definition emphasizes management rather than mastery, which is important in understanding the nature of living with a chronic illness such as diabetes. Diabetes self-management facilitates coping and adaptation. Wood-Dauphinee and Williams[56] note that such adaptation can best be described by the concept of reintegration to normal living. It is the reorganization of physical, psychologic, and social characteristics of an individual in a way in which one can resume well-adjusted living after the diagnosis of chronic illness or an incapacitating complication of illness.

In consideration of the long-term complications of diabetes, such as peripheral and autonomic neuropathy, retinopathy, nephropathy, and cardiovascular complications, a redefining of role obligations may be necessary to facilitate an individual's adaptation. Haber and Smith[26] identify this process as normative adaptation that consists of three stages: (1) recognition of inadequacy, (2) attribution of responsibility, and (3) legitimacy of performance behavior. This process considers an individual's limitation, normalizing exceptional behavior within the framework of role obligations as a means of facilitating role maintenance. An individual's social and personal role obligations can be redefined so they are more in keeping with actual capabilities. An individual's performance can then be evaluated against redefined norms. Such an approach allows for a smoother transition into new roles while relinquishing old roles relative to both work and family. Normative adaptation to the complications of diabetes may mean the difference between productive adaptation or surviving in a state of discouragement and invalidism.

Whether the diagnosis of diabetes mellitus occurs during the middle adulthood period or at an earlier age, an individual is confronted with the issues of coping and adaptation within the context of negotiating middlescence. The diagnosis of diabetes-related complications during this time adds further to the conflict. The concerns of middle adulthood relative to bodily decline and a decreased sense of omnipotence are similar to the concerns and psychologic changes that can accompany illness. It is important, therefore, that members of the health care team understand the personal, familial, and social implications of living with a chronic illness such as diabetes mellitus.[30,32]

EDUCATIONAL AND BEHAVIORAL STRATEGIES

Diabetes education is a complex, multifaceted process that requires active participation on the part of the adult learner. Because learning capacity continues throughout the lifespan, both young and middle-aged adults are capable of learning new knowledge and skills. In designing various behavioral strategies for an educational intervention, members of the health care team must individualize care and educational goals according to young and middle adulthood. *An emphasis on preventive aspects of care and the importance of following a regular follow-up to monitor development or progression of complications are recommended.* The emphasis on changing behavior to eliminate modifiable risk factors (smoking, obesity) is important if the adult is to maintain an optimal level of health care.

Diabetes Care for Young Adults and Middle Adults

Effective education requires that all adults be well informed about aspects of diabetes. In young or middle adults who are newly diagnosed, reassurance is vital with initial discussion of diabetes focused on "survival knowledge." Such knowledge allows the individual to possess information and skills that have immediate applicability and allows participation in self-management. Adjusting to the diagnosis of diabetes may take weeks to months. Initially, the individual may be preoccupied with fears of death, use of needles, and implications of the diagnosis. Thus, it is unrealistic to expect adults to learn everything they need to know about their care in a few short days. As health care providers, highest educational priorities for newly diagnosed young and middle adults should include encouraging individuals to talk about their fears and offer reassurances that they are understandable and possibly under their control. Regular contact and availability of the health care provider for questions is important. Outlined in the accompanying box are basic diabetes concepts and survival skills.

Young adults who are most likely to be diagnosed with IDDM, and who have been diagnosed for at least 3 to 4 weeks, should receive more in-depth education, such as preventive aspects of care, exercise, prepregnancy counseling, complications, foot care, hygiene guidelines, career and job placement, travel guidelines, and driving a motor vehicle. Such information should be carefully documented and reviewed annually with the individual.[2] Information should be presented in small increments at a level the individual is

---

SURVIVAL SKILLS

Brief definition of and general information about diabetes

Basic principles of nutrition, essentials of food management, and basic meal planning

Maintaining balance: Food and stress increase blood sugar; insulin and activity lower blood sugar

Honeymoon (remission) phase for IDDM

Definition of hypoglycemia including basic treatment and prevention

Information regarding function of insulin and/or oral hypoglycemic agents; how to draw up, mix, and administer insulin.

Self-monitoring of blood glucose with an introduction to meters

Guidelines for sick day management including suggested foods and liquids

Urine ketone testing

Supplies and identification

Emergency telephone numbers

capable of accepting. Too much information too soon may be overwhelming. A typical example is the individual who is told his tests indicate diabetes, followed by approximately 20 minutes of instruction on injecting insulin and a standard preprinted diet sheet. Once the individual arrives home, he is confused, depressed, and overwhelmed. Adequate amounts of time are needed to allow young adults to ventilate their perceptions of the condition and discuss various coping and educational strategies.

Middle-aged adults with IDDM should be re-evaluated regularly in terms of diabetes knowledge and self-care skills. Although they have typically had diabetes for several years, these individuals need to be carefully evaluated as to their current knowledge, as well as receive regular physical examinations to screen for complications. Concerns related to additional health or financial problems or other concerns as related to tasks associated with growth and development previously described also need further evaluation by the health care team. Sample protocols for evaluation of diabetes status appear in the appendix.

Middle-aged adults newly diagnosed with NIDDM experience many of the same reactions associated with any individual newly diagnosed with a chronic disease.[2] Just as in the case of the young adult, information needs to be presented in frequent, small increments until such time as the individual is able to comprehend the tasks involved with self-care.

Adults with NIDDM are also prone to other health problems and financial concerns. Likewise, if diagnosed with diabetes during middle adulthood, there appears to be more vulnerability to sickness, loss of function, and possible disability when compared with those younger adults who have diabetes. For these reasons, middle adults need to seek continuing support and periodic re-education. It becomes essential that members of the health care team take the time to understand each individual's situation and problems, and be sensitive to these when designing a self-care plan. Care and education must be tailored to the individual's life-style if it is to be successful in promoting behavior change.

The success of care may in fact depend on an individualized education approach. Yet, many adults may be suffering from emotional aspects of the diabetes that create barriers to the therapeutic regimen, contributing to poor metabolic control. Improvement will ultimately depend on members of the health care team being able to identify and resolve underlying problems that interfere with self-management. Likewise, the individual's willingness to change is related to his or her perception of vulnerability to the complications of diabetes, sense of control over the condition, or the perceived benefits of adherence to delaying and/or preventing the long-term complications of diabetes. In particular, behavior-oriented education focusing on problem-solving and decision making, using small group strategies is effective.[5,36,53,51]

Adult Education

Effective diabetes education interventions utilize methods directed at the level of the learner. These methods are addressed in detail in Chapter 16 of this text. However, cer-

_____ **EDUCATIONAL FACTORS TO PROMOTE COMPREHENSION** _____

Primacy and organization of material
Brevity versus comprehensiveness
Repetition
Readability of material
Specificity

tain conditions must be met for adult learning to take place: (1) collaboration between teacher and learner, (2) learner identified needs and objectives, (3) methods for learning, and (4) learner self-evaluation of the teaching-learning process.[36] Educational strategies that promote comprehension, recall, and compliance include (1) primacy and organization: the most important information should be presented first, (2) brevity: amount of information given in a specific time frame should be short, and (3) specificity: information presented in specific terms as opposed to generalized terms is best understood and recalled.[25] The accompanying box summarizes educational factors that promote comprehension.

ADHERENCE ISSUES

One of the most significant issues in diabetes management is the inability or unwillingness of individuals with diabetes to adhere as closely to the recommended therapeutic program as is necessary to achieve control. Adequate knowledge does not guarantee that adults will adhere to the schedule that living with diabetes demands.[29,6,39]

In addition to readiness, willingness, and overall motivation, family support and cultural factors are critical determinants of patient motivation and adherence.[47] Satisfaction with members of the health care team and setting all have been shown to affect adherence behavior. Barriers to adherence and/or compliance, both perceived and actual, must be assessed as part of the educational process. For instance, if individuals believe and state that someone in their family has diabetes and is doing just fine, various consequences of diabetes need to be discussed. After correcting misconceptions, be sure adequate information and skills necessary to follow a prescribed plan is presented and tailored to the individual's lifestyle.

All health care providers involved in the care of individuals with diabetes should be sensitive to specific areas that can affect patient adherence. For example, financial resources is one factor that has an impact on compliance. Individuals who are unable to buy medications, certain types of food, and blood glucose monitoring equipment may not comply with recommended therapeutic interventions. Health care providers must be prepared for the realities of our society and possibly pursue avenues of financial assistance before educating individuals in basic survival knowledge. A list of commonly used strategies to promote adherence is shown in the box on p. 500.

_____ STRATEGIES TO PROMOTE ADHERENCE _____

Reminders
Tailoring regimen
Gradual regimen implementation
Active support of significant others
Contingency contracting
Self-monitoring

ROLE OF FAMILY AND SOCIAL SUPPORT

Social factors and family functioning play an important role in facilitating an individual's adaptive responses to diabetes and self-care management. Families and significant social networks can foster independence and self-reliance through active support. If at all possible, families should be included in teaching; however, if families are dysfunctional, careful assessment and subsequent decision making as to the level of involvement is needed. In an effort to maximize support, it is important to discuss with the individual the advantages of involving significant others in diabetes education and nutrition counseling.

Social and family support have been studied in relationship to adherence and diabetes control. These studies suggest that the perception of supportive behavior of family or significant others is predictive of compliance with the self-care regimen.[48,50] Similarly, studies of the influence of family function on diabetes control have demonstrated that individuals with diabetes in good metabolic control perceive family environment to be more achievement oriented as compared with those in poor control.[18] Good family function is predictive of good diabetic control.[8]

Social support network size and satisfaction are gender specific, serving different functions for both men and women. As such, the concept of social support may vary with individuals. In general, social support is believed to effect positive outcomes for the individual with diabetes.[29]

CASE STUDIES

The following vignettes will highlight some clinical concerns of diabetes management and relate them to issues of growth and development.

Case Study One

Ms. J is a 31-year-old white female who has had IDDM since her early twenties and is presently a graduate student. She came to your office with erratic dietary patterns, often "forgetting to take her insulin." She volunteered detailed information about her background. Two years earlier, she married a man somewhat older, which met with disapproval from her family. This caused some conflict, to the point where Ms. J doesn't talk with her mother. She also talked about having difficulties at work and wanting to quit and start a family. On her first two visits, Ms. J spoke very little about her diabetes and a recent episode of ketoacidosis that required hospitalization.

After several visits, Ms. J became more communicative about her diabetes and what frightened her the most. She began to verbalize how difficult it would be to go through a pregnancy without the support of her mother, mentioning her real concerns about having diabetes and wanting children. Ms. J received prepregnancy counseling and education. Months later, she became pregnant and started to become even more realistic about complications associated with pregnancy.

Discussion: Individuals with diabetes often use denial as a way to cope with their condition. In Ms. J's situation, her use of denial was notable when she elected not to initially talk about her diabetes. Likewise, denial can be used by family and friends and create a conflict-laden situation. Such was the case with Ms. J and her mother.

There was, however, an aspect of Ms. J's condition that possibly brought on her use of denial. As a young adult, Ms. J was faced with a great deal of cultural pressure to marry and have children. Americans so value a "family" that unmarried adults are sometimes treated as incomplete. Besides the developmental task of establishing an intimate bond with another individual, Ms. J was seriously troubled about having diabetes and wanting children.

In helping young adults who are in denial, health care providers need to begin by conducting a thorough assessment; gathering facts and information regarding behaviors and feelings. While gathering such information, it is critical to be a good listener and assess when is the best time to impart knowledge or information. In this case, the need for careful prepregnancy planning was identified. However, during periods of denial, individuals will not be receptive to the best teaching plan unless specific concerns and questions are addressed.

Case Study Two

Mrs. S is a 52-year-old recently widowed woman, with a 15-year history of NIDDM. She lives alone and works as an executive secretary for a busy law firm. Her two daughters live in the same city with their families. Mrs. S is 5'3" and weighs 151 pounds. She has a history of osteoarthritis and peripheral neuropathy. She has been on a regimen of Diabenese, 500 mg daily, for the past 4 years. Over the past 4 months she has had a 20-pound weight loss. Her glycated hemoglobin is 12.6%, and a random blood glucose was 297 mg/dL.

Two years ago she was taught to self-monitor blood glucose but found it difficult to read the visual strips and therefore lost her motivation for monitoring. Her poor control warrants initiation of insulin therapy. She states that she will have difficulty self-administering insulin and that she probably will not self-monitor for blood glucose.

Discussion: As a first step, it would be appropriate to consider Mrs. S's perception of her diabetes. How does she view her diabetes? Does she have an adequate and accurate understanding of NIDDM and the treatment regimen prescribed for her thus far? For some adults, they perceive that NIDDM is the "milder" form as opposed to IDDM and not as serious unless you take insulin. Assessing her beliefs and attitudes may also provide insight into how to structure further teaching.

In developing a teaching plan, it is essential to highlight the benefits of SMBG for adults with NIDDM. By using this information, Mrs. S would be able to modify meal plans and exercise programs and achieve normal blood glucose and glycated hemoglobin levels. One may approach Mrs. S by demonstrating a blood glucose monitoring meter that requires minimal manipulation. At the same time, show Mrs. S various finger-lancing devices that she could manipulate in order to find one that is easier to use. Once Mrs. S finds the meter and finger-lancing device that best suit her needs, proceed with patient teaching, which includes a return demonstration.

If the meter/lancing devices are too difficult to manipulate, explore to what extent her daughters would be able to provide active support and assistance. This would also be an opportunity to explore Mrs. S's feelings of ambivalence and dependency relative to her diabetes and need for insulin. It would also provide an opportunity to address issues related to her recent widowhood and other avenues of social support.

Problems of manual dexterity posed by peripheral neuropathy and osteoarthritis that interfere with SMBG may also impede self-administration of insulin. Considering Mrs. S's vision is good, there should be no problem in accurately drawing up the insulin if she is able to manipulate the insulin vial and syringe. If such manipulation is difficult, identify various aids for drawing-up and injecting insulin.

SUMMARY

Diabetes during young and middle adulthood presents a variety of challenges to the individual with diabetes, his or her family, and the health care team. An understanding of not only the physical changes that take place but also the psychosocial implications associated with diabetes management in this group need to be carefully assessed and individualized.

REFERENCES

1. American Diabetes Association, Inc: Summary and recommendations of the second international workshop—Conference on gestational diabetes mellitus, Diabetes 34:124, 1985.
2. American Diabetes Association: Physician's guide to insulin dependent (type I) diabetes: diagnosis and treatment, Alexandria, VA, 1988, American Diabetes Association.
3. Anderson J: Fiber and health: an overview, Am J Gastroenterol 81:892, 1986.
4. Bouchard BH: Hypoglycemia. In Travis LB, Bouchard BH, and Schreiner BJ, eds: Diabetes mellitus in children and adolescents, Philadelphia, 1987, WB Saunders.
5. Bouler MH and Morisky D: A small group strategy for improving compliance behavior and blood pressure control, Health Educ Q 10:57-69, 1983.
6. Brownlee-Duffeck M and others: The role of health beliefs in the regimen adherence and metabolic control of adolescents and adults with diabetes mellitus, J Consult Clin Psychol 55:139-144, 1987.
7. Burns KR and Johnson RJ: Health assessment in clinical practice, Englewood Cliffs, NJ, 1980, Prentice-Hall.
8. Cardenas L and others: Adult onset diabetes mellitus: glycemic control and family function, Am J Med Sci 293:28-33, 1987.
9. Casparie AF and Elving LD: Severe hypoglycemia in diabetic patients: frequency, causes, prevention, Diabetes Care 8:141-145, 1985.

10. Colvell JA: Peripheral vascular disease in diabetes. In Davidson JK, ed: Clinical diabetes mellitus: a problem oriented approach, New York, 1986, Thieme.
11. Concensus Statement: Role of cardiovascular risk factors in prevention and treatment of macrovascular disease in diabetes, Diabetes Care 13:53-59, 1989.
12. Cox DJ and others: Fear of hypoglycemia: quantification, validation and utilization, Diabetes Care 10:617-621, 1987.
13. Deebe LC: Computer-based monitoring in office-base practice, Practical Diabetology 7:10, 1988.
14. DosAnjos MN: "Locked-in" syndrome following prolonged hypoglycemia, Diabetes Care 7:613, 1984.
15. Draheim BB and Ashburn SS: Biophysical and cognitive development in young adulthood. In Schuster CS, and Ashburn SS, eds: The process of human development: a holistic approach, Boston, 1980, Little, Brown.
16. Edelman CL and Mandle, CL: Health promotion: throughout the lifespan, ed 2, St. Louis, 1990, Mosby–Year Book.
17. Entmacher PS: Employment and insurance for those with diabetes. In Davidson JK, ed: Clinical diabetes mellitus: a problem oriented approach, New York, 1986, Thieme.
18. Edelstein T and Linn M: The influence of family control of diabetes, Soc sci Med 21:541-544, 1985.
19. Eliopoulos C: Gerontological nursing, ed 2, Philadelphia, 1987, JB Lippincott.
20. Ellenberg M: Diabetic neuropathy. In Ellenberg M, and Rifkin H, eds: Diabetes mellitus: theory and practice, New York, 1983, Medical Examination Publishing.
21. Erikson EH: Adulthood, New York, 1978, WW Norton.
22. Fajans SS: Recognizing maturity-onset diabetes of the young (MODY), Practical Diabetol 9:1, 1990.
23. Franceschi M and others: Cognitive processes in insulin-dependent diabetes, Diabetes Care 7:228-231, 1984.
24. Freiberg KL: Human development: a life-span approach, ed 2, Monterey, CA, 1983, Wadsworth Health Sciences Division.
25. Green L: Evaluating health education programs. In Squyres W, ed: Patient compliance and patient education, New York, 1982, McGraw-Hill Book Co.
26. Haber L and Smith CT: Disability and deviance: normative adaptation of role behavior, J Am Psychiatr Assoc 15: 344, 1971.
27. Holmes DM: The person and diabetes in psychosocial context, Diabetes Care 9:194-206, 1986.
28. Holmes DM: Diabetes in its psychosocial context. In Marble A and others, eds: Joslin's diabetes mellitus, ed 12, Philadelphia, 1985, Lea & Febiger.
29. Kaplan RM and Hartwell SL: Differential effects of social support and social network on physiological and social outcomes in men and women with type II diabetes mellitus, Health Psychol 6:387-398, 1987.
30. Knowles M: The adult learner: a neglected species, Houston, 1973, Gulf Publishing.
31. Knox AV: Adult development and learning, New York, 1977, Jossey Bass Publishers.
32. Krall LP, Entmacher PS, and Drury TF: Life cycles in diabetes: socioeconomic aspects. In Marble A and others, eds: Joslin's diabetes mellitus, ed 12, Philadelphia, 1985, Lea & Febiger.
33. Kurtz SM: Adherence to diabetes regimens: empirical status and clinical applications, Diabetes Educ 16:50-59, 1990.
34. Lazarus RS and Cohen JB: Environmental stress. In Altman L and Wohlwill JF, eds: Human behavior and the environment: current theory and research, ed 2, New York, 1979, McGraw-Hill Book Co.
35. Leland OS and Maki PC: Heart disease and diabetes mellitus. In Marble A and others, eds: Joslin's diabetes mellitus, ed 12, Philadelphia, 1985, Lea & Febiger.
36. L'Eperance F and James W: The eye and diabetes mellitus. In Ellenberg M and Rifkin H, eds: Diabetes mellitus: theory and practice, New York, 1983, Medical Examination Publishing.
37. Lopes-Virella MLV and Colwell JA: Serum high density lipoproteins in diabetic patients, Diabetol 13:285-291, 1977.
38. Mann JI and Houston AC: Genetic factors in diabetes mellitus. In Davidson JK, ed: Clinical diabetes mellitus: a problem oriented approach, New York, 1986, Thieme.
39. McCaul KD, Glasgow RE, and Schafer LC: Diabetes regimen behaviors: predicting adherence, Medical Care 25(9):868-881, 1987.
40. Montague DK and others: Diagnostic evaluation, classification, and treatment of men with sexual dysfunction, Urology 14:545, 1979.
41. Murray RB and Zentner JP: Nursing assessment: health promotion through the life span, ed 2, Englewood Cliffs, NJ, 1979, Prentice-Hall.

42. Oehler-Giarratana J: Reactions to complications. In Hamburg B and others, eds: Behavioral and psychosocial issues in diabetes: proceedings of the national conference. NIH Publication no 80-1993, Washington, DC, 1980, US Goverment Printing Office.

43. Papalia DE and Olds SW: Human development, New York, 1978, McGraw-Hill.

44. Peck R: Psychological developments in the second half of life. In Neugarten B, ed: Middle age and aging, Chicago, 1968, Chicago University Press.

45. Piaget J: The theory of stages in congitive development. New York, 1969, McGraw-Hill.

46. Runyon JW: Co-existing hypertension and diabetes, Pract Diabetol 7:1-7, 1988.

47. Sackett DL and Haynes RB: Compliance with therapeutic regimens, Baltimore, 1976, John Hopkins University Press.

48. Schaefer LC, McCaul KD, and Glasgow RE: Supportive and non-supportive family behaviors: relationships to adherence and metabolic control in persons with type I diabetes, Diabetes Care 9:179-185, 1986.

49. Sepe SJ and others: Gestational diabetes: incidence, maternal characteristics and pernatal care, Diabetes 34:13, 1985.

50. Shenkel R and others: Importance of "significant others" in predicting cooperation with diabetic regimens, Int J Psychiatr Med 15:149-155, 1985.

51. Speers M and Turk D: Diabetes self-care: knowledge, beliefs motivation and action, Patient Counsel Health Educ 3:144-149, 1980.

52. Strauss A and Glaser B: Chronic illness and the quality of life, St. Louis, 1975, Mosby–Year Book.

53. Strowig S: Patient education: model for autonomous decision-making and deliberate action in diabetes self management, Med Clin North Am 66:1293-1304, 1982.

54. US Department of Health, Education, and Welfare (Public Health Service): Healthy people: the surgeon general's report on health promotion and disease prevention, pub no 79-55071, Washington, DC, 1979, US Goverment Printing Office.

55. US Department of Health, Education, and Welfare (Public Health Service): Diabetes in America, pub No 85-1468, Washington, DC, 1985, US Goverment Printing Office.

56. Wood-Dauphinee S and Williams JI: Reintegration to normal living as a proxy to quality of life, J Chronic Dis 40:491-499, 1987.

57. Younger D and others: Diabetes in youth. In Marble A and others: Joslin's diabetes mellitus, ed 12, Philadelphia, 1985, Lea & Febiger.

CHAPTER 15

Diabetes Mellitus and the Older Adult

MARTHA MITCHELL FUNNELL
AND
JENNIFER HAYDEN MERRITT

Diabetes is surprisingly common among older adults (60+ years of age), so much so that health professionals who specialize in diabetes care and education need to understand the specific physiologic and sociocultural challenges that elderly people encounter. In addition, health care providers who specialize in geriatric care and education need to keep abreast of advances in the treatment of diabetes. Diabetes is a serious disease, and its seriousness is often underestimated by the patient and, occasionally, by health care professionals, since its initial symptoms may make it appear harmless. But persons with all types of diabetes bear the risk of developing all of the complications.[71] Additionally, the detection, treatment, and ongoing care of diabetes in the elderly population meet with a unique set of challenges.

Who are the elderly with diabetes? How does diabetes differ from glucose intolerance of aging? How does diabetes present atypically in older adults? How do other concurrent diseases, polypharmacy, functional decline, and sensory loss, and the unique developmental and psychosocial issues of aging affect the care of diabetes in the elderly? What are the special considerations for the care of these persons? What are the special considerations for the education of these persons? This chapter will address these questions and describe the educational process for older adults with diabetes.

RELATIONSHIP BETWEEN DIABETES MELLITUS AND THE AGING PROCESS
Demographics

Currently 11% of the population is over age 65, and studies show that the number of people over 65 is increasing at a rate three times greater than that of the general population. It is expected that by the year 2020, over 20% of the population will be over age 65. Fur-

Table 15-1   Number of People with Diagnosed Diabetes and Percent of People Aged 45 Years and Older in the U.S. Population, 1986-1988

	Age (years)		
	45-64	**65-74**	**75+**
Number with diabetes (millions)			
Males	1.33	0.75	0.41
Females	1.30	0.90	0.65
Both sexes	2.62	1.65	1.06
Percent of U.S. population			
Males	6.2	9.8	10.3
Females	5.5	9.3	9.5
Both sexes	5.8	9.5	9.8

From the 1986-1988 National Health Interview Survey, National Center for Health Statistics. Harris MI: Epidemiology of diabetes mellitus among the elderly in the United States, Clin Geriatr Med 6:703-729, 1990.

thermore, persons over age 85 represent the fastest growing segment of the population.[46]

Diabetes is increasingly common with age. It is almost ten times as common among those over age 65 as those in the 20 to 44 age group.[7] Based on the National Health Interview Survey (NHIS) data, it was estimated that from 1986 to 1988, 9.6% of all people in the United States over age 65 were diagnosed with diabetes (Table 15-1). Alternately, roughly 43% of all people in the United States who were diagnosed with diabetes between 1986 and 1988 are over age 65.[29]

Prevalence of diabetes varies considerably by race. The NHIS data from 1980 to 1987 showed that the prevalence of diabetes is higher among blacks than whites, with black females showing a rate twice that of white females.[84] Among Hispanics the rate is even higher (Fig. 15-1).[29] African American women over age 75 had the highest rate, with almost one in four having diabetes (Fig. 15-2).

There have been multiple studies to determine the degree to which diabetes exists but is undiagnosed. The broadest study of this kind was the National Health and Nutrition Examination Survey II of 1976 to 1980 in which over 15,000 persons aged 20 to 74 participated in interviews, and almost 12,000 had a physical examination and an oral glucose tolerance test. The data revealed that by WHO criteria, undiagnosed diabetes existed at essentially the same rate as medical history of diabetes. In other words, half of all diabetes cases went undiagnosed. Table 15-2 shows the NHANES II data extrapolated to the U.S. population, 1986 to 1988.[29] Newer data will be available when the NHANES III is completed. An interim study in Finland revealed the prevalence of newly diagnosed NIDDM to be 7% compared with about 10% of previously diagnosed NIDDM.[60]

Because the NHIS has been conducted annually since 1958, one can see how prevalence of physician-diagnosed diabetes has changed over several decades and can make projections about future prevalence. In the three decades from 1960 to 1990 the rate of diagnosed diabetes increased 2.5-fold among people over 65 (Fig. 15-3). Harris noted

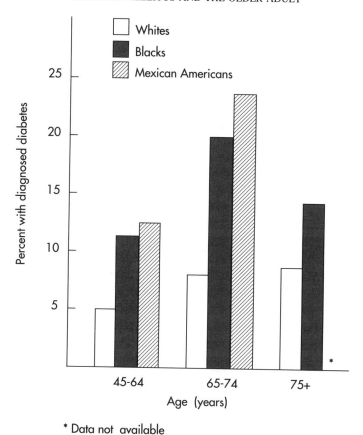

* Data not available

Fig. 15-1 Age-specific prevalence of physician-diagnosed diabetes among whites, blacks, and Mexican-Americans in the U.S. population aged 45 years and older, 1982-1984. (From the National Health and Hispanic Health Nutrition Examination Survey, National Center for Health Statistics. Harris MI: Epidemiology of diabetes mellitus among the elderly in the United States, Clin Geriatr Med 6:703-729, 1990.)

that this increase in prevalence is in addition to what can be expected as a result of the general aging of the population and projects that it will continue into the future.[29]

IDDM Versus NIDDM

Largely because of improved survival rates, there is an increasing percentage of older adults who have insulin-dependent diabetes mellitus (IDDM). To a lesser degree, IDDM may have its onset in late life, or older people with non–insulin dependent diabetes mellitus (NIDDM) may convert to IDDM in the course of the illness. The key diagnostic test is a C-peptide test performed both at fasting and at 90 minutes after glucose load. A very low serum C-peptide level at both times indicates minimal beta cell function and the pres-

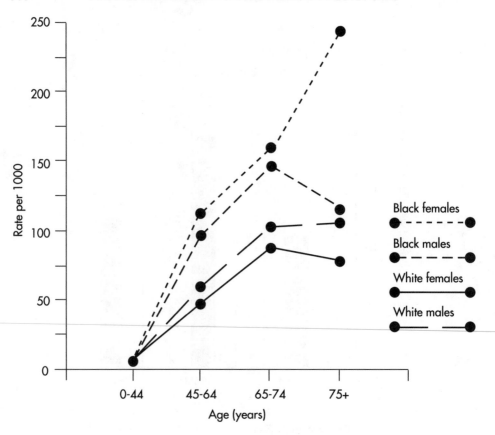

Fig. 15-2 Age-specific prevalence rate of diabetes, by race and sex, United States, 1987. (From Diabetes Surveillance 1980-1987, U.S. Department of Health and Human Services, 1990.)

ence of IDDM.[48] Since such tests are rarely done in routine outpatient care, there are limited data on the prevalence of IDDM among the elderly. However, the vast majority of elderly show characteristics of NIDDM, such as a strong association with obesity, positive family history and improved glycemia with diet, weight correction, and/or oral hypoglycemic agents. One study showed the prevalence of IDDM in the elderly to be only 0.3% [88]

Complications of Diabetes

Diabetes is not only common, it is serious, with long-term complications that are debilitating and demoralizing, especially as the person becomes more frail with advancing age. When compared with persons of the same age without diabetes, those with diabetes are 25 times more likely to become blind, 17 times more likely to develop kidney disease, 20 times more likely to develop gangrene, 15 times more likely to require an amputation, and twice as likely to have a cerebrovascular accident or myocardial infarction.[10] The risk

Table 15-2   Estimated Prevalence of Undiagnosed Diabetes and Impaired Glucose Tolerance Among People Aged 45-75 Years in the U.S. Population, 1986-1988

	Age (years)	
	45-64	65-74
Undiagnosed diabetes*		
Number of persons (millions)		
Males	0.8	0.8
Females	1.6	0.8
Both sexes	2.4	1.6
Percentage of the U.S. population		
Males	3.9	10.4
Females	6.8	8.5
Both sexes	5.4	9.3
Impaired glucose tolerance†		
Number of persons (millions)		
Males	3.2	1.7
Females	3.5	2.2
Both sexes	6.7	3.9
Percentage of the U.S. population		
Males	14.8	22.5
Females	14.7	22.9
Both sexes	14.8	22.7

From the 1976-1980 Second National Health and Nutrition Examination Survey, National Center for Health Statistics. Harris MI: Epidemiology of diabetes mellitus among the elderly in the United States, Clin Geriatr Med 6:703-729, 1990.
*Fasting plasma glucose ≥140 mg/dL and/or 2-hour plasma glucose after 75 g oral glucose ≥200 mg/dL.
†Fasting plasma glucose <140 mg/dL and 2-hour plasma glucose after 75 g oral glucose of 140-199 mg/dL. Number of people are computed by applying these rates to population estimates of the Bureau of the Census for 1986-1988.

for developing these long-term complications of diabetes increases with age. Hospitalization rates and the rates for nursing home admissions are noted to be significantly higher for people with diabetes when compared with those without diabetes. Older adults with diabetes show a hospitalization rate 70% higher than the general population (Fig. 15-4).[29] The rate of nursing home admissions is 1.2 times greater among people with diabetes.[67] Mortality is increased as well; diabetes is the fifth ranking cause of death and reduces the life expectancy of men by 9 years and women by 7 years.[68]

THE CHALLENGES OF GERIATRICS

Older adults experience common physical, cognitive, and psychosocial challenges as a result of the aging process and face similar developmental tasks as they near the end of their lives. Because of these inherent challenges, the needs of older people tend to be different from those of younger adults, including health care needs. This has led to rec-

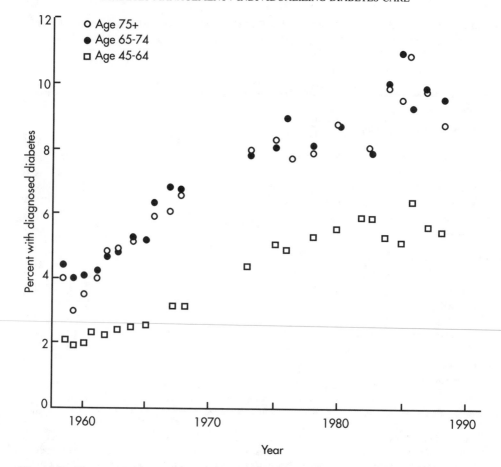

Fig. 15-3 Time trends in the percentage of the U.S. population aged 45 and older with physician-diagnosed diabetes, 1958-1988. (From the National Health Interview Survey, National Center for Health Statistics. Harris MI: Epidemiology of diabetes mellitus among the elderly in the United States, Clin Geriatr Med 6:703-729, 1990.)

ognition of the field of geriatrics as a distinct speciality, similar to the way that pediatrics is recognized as a speciality. The box on p. 512 outlines some of the common challenges of geriatrics. The ways that these challenges apply to diabetes care in older adults will be reviewed in this chapter.

Normal Physical Changes of Aging

Perhaps the first challenge of geriatrics is to understand what changes are "normal" aging and what changes represent disease process. Physical changes related to aging that are considered normal are best described as universal, progressive, and irreversible.[24] Table 15-3 outlines systems affected by aging and the potential consequences of these

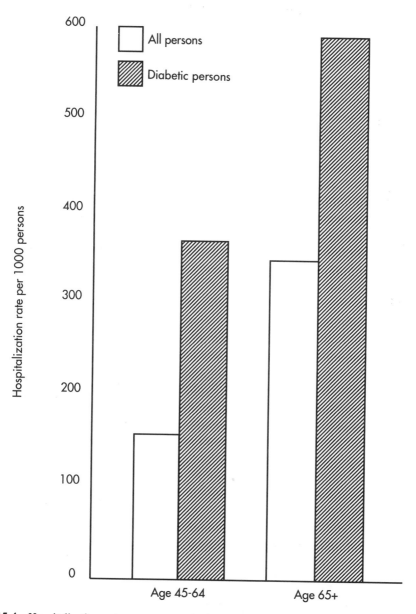

Fig. 15-4 Hospitalization rates among persons in the U.S. population aged 45 years and older, 1987. (From the National Hospital Discharge Survey, National Center for Health Statistics. Harris MI: Epidemiology of diabetes mellitus among the elderly in the United States, Clin Geriatr Med 6:703-729, 1990.)

_____ **CHALLENGES OF GERIATRICS** _____

Impaired homeostasis
Atypical presentations
Multiple concurrent disease interactions
Geriatric pharmacology
Iatrogenic disease
Physical and cognitive decline
Psychosocial and sociocultural issues
Educational and behavioral issues

Table 15-3   Physiologic Changes of Aging

System	Effect of aging	Consequences
Central nervous system	Decline in the number of neurons and the weight of the brain	Do not impair function
	Reduced short-term memory	
	Takes longer to learn new information	
	Slowing of reaction time	
Spinal cord/peripheral nerves	Decline in nerve conduction velocity	Slowness of "righting" reflexes
	Diminished sensation	Diminished sensory awareness
	Decline in the number of fibers in the nerve trunks	Reduced vibratory sensation
Cardiovascular system	Reduced cardiac output (normal?)	Reduced exercise tolerance
	Valvular sclerosis of the aortic valves common	
	Reduced ability to increase the heart rate in response to exercise	
Respiratory system	Decline in vital capacity	Diminished oxygen uptake during exercise
	Increased lung compliance	
	Reduced ciliary action	Reduced pulmonary ventilation on exercise
	Increased residual volume	
	Increased anteroposterior chest diameter	Increased risk of pulmonary infection
		Reduced exercise tolerance
Gastrointestinal tract	Decrease in number of taste buds	Reduced taste sensation
	Loss of dentition (normal?)	Possible difficulty in mastication
	Reduced gastric acid secretion	Potential cause of iron deficiency anemia
	Reduced motility of large intestine	Constipation if coupled with low fiber and fluid intake

Adapted form Gambert SR, ed: Handbook of geriatrics. New York, 1988, Plenum Publishing Corp.

Table 15-3   Physiologic Changes of Aging—cont'd.

System	Effect of aging	Consequences
Kidneys	Loss of nephrons	Decreased creatinine clearance
	Reduced glomerular filtration rate and tubular reabsorpton	
	Change in renal threshold	Reduced renal reserve may lead to reduced glycosuria in the presence of diabetes mellitus
	Decreased concentrating ability	
Musculoskeletal system	Decreased number of muscle fibers	Poor mobility; pain
	Shortening of tendons	Decreased vertical height
	Slower turnover of bone	May predispose to fractures
	Loss of bone density (normal?)	Change in posture
	Diminished lean muscle mass	Reduced strength
Endocrine/metabolism	Reduced basal metabolic rate (related to reduced muscle mass)	Reduced caloric requirements
	Impaired glucose tolerance	Must distinquish from true diabetes mellitus
Reproductive system	Men: Delayed penile erection, infrequent orgasm, increased refractory period, decreased sperm motility, and altered morphology	Dimished sexual response
		Decreased reproductive capacity
	Women: Decreased vasocongestion, delayed vaginal lubrication, diminished orgasm, overian atrophy	
Skin	Loss of elastic tissue	Increased wrinkling: senile purpura
	Atrophy of sweat glands	Difficulty in assessing dehydration
		Reduced sweating
	Hair loss	

changes.[23] It should be noted, however, that any changes or declines in ability should be evaluated for underlying pathology and not simply be dismissed as normal.

Impaired Homeostasis of Aging

In individuals without diabetes, glucose homeostasis, or euglycemia, is maintained by a complex of biochemical and hormonal mechanisms that balance glucose production with utilization. In the fasting state, the amount of glucose produced in the liver by gluconeogenesis and glycogenolysis is equal to the amount utilized by the body's cells. In the post-

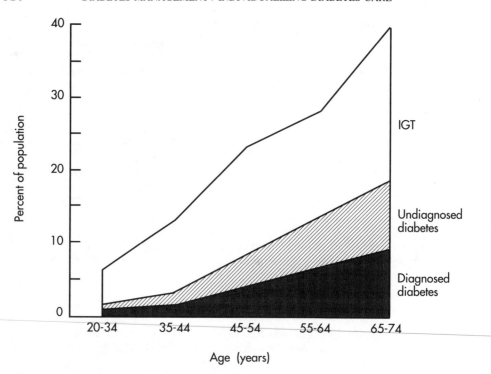

Fig. 15-5   Age-specific prevalence of diabetes and impaired glucose tolerance in the U.S. popula-tion, 1976-1980. (From the National Health and Nutrition Examination Survey, National Center for Health Statistics. Harris MI: Epidemiology of diabetes mellitus among the elderly in the United States, Clin Geriatr Med 6:703-729, 1990.)

prandial state when blood glucose levels are rising from digested food, the rise is limited by the release of insulin from the pancreas that acts quickly to suppress gluconeogenesis and glycogenolysis and transport of glucose into cells. As blood glucose then falls, so does the plasma concentration of insulin to maintain euglycemia. The counterregulatory hormones, including glucagon, epinephrine, growth hormone, and cortisol, work in con-cert to prevent hypoglycemia in this exquisite balancing act. With aging, there is often an impairment in this homeostatic mechanism called impaired glucose tolerance (IGT). With IGT, blood glucose ranges are above normal but below values diagnostic of diabetes. IGT is so common that controversy exists about whether it is a "normal" aging change or a common abnormality (Fig. 15-5). However, because it is not seen in a significant subset of elderly people, it is prudent to consider it an abnormality common among older adults, especially since increases in macrovascular disease (namely coronary and cerebrovascular disease) are associated with IGT.When detected, IGT warrants interventions such as weight reduction and exercise to decrease the risk of progression to NIDDM. In prospec-tive studies, roughly 20% of those with age-related IGT did develop overt diabetes at a rate of up to 5% per year.[9] In the past, persons with glucose levels in the IGT ranges

Table 15-4 Blood Glucose Values* Used to Differentiate Categories of Glucose Tolerance

	Normal	Diabetes mellitus	Impaired glucose tolerance
Fasting	<115	>140	<140
1 hour†	<200	>200	>200
2 hours	<140	>200	140-200

Adapted from the American Diabetes Association, Inc. From National Diabetes Data Group: Classification and diagnosis of diabetes mellitus and other categories of glucose intolerance, Diabetes 28:1039-1057, 1979.
*All figures refer to mg/dL venous plasma glucose levels in nonpregnant adults following a 75-g glucose load.
†Single reading at 30, 60 or 90 minutes.

Table 15-5 Comparison of Metabolic Abnormalities in Aging, Obesity, and NIDDM

	Aging	Obesity	NIDDM
Glucose			
Basal	NC	NC	NC or ↑
Glucose tolerance	↓	NC	↓↓↓
Insulin			
Basal	NC	↑	↓ NC ↑
Glucose loading			
Initial response	Delayed	↑	Delayed
Later response	↑	↑ ↑ ↑	Variable
Feedback inhibition of secretion	↓	↓	↓
Triglyceride	NC	↑	↑
Site of defect			
Insulin-receptor number	NC	↓	↓
Postreceptor defect	+	NC→+	+

Reproduced with permission of the American Diabetes Association, Inc. Adapted from Jackson RA: Mechanisms of age-related glucose intolerance, Diabetes Care 13(suppl 2):9-19, 1990.

were told that they had "borderline diabetes." This term has now been replaced by IGT, since the majority do not develop diabetes. Blood glucose values of persons with normal glucose tolerance and diabetes are compared with values of persons with IGT as now defined by the National Diabetes Data Group of the NIH in Table 15-4.[61]

Since serum insulin levels are higher among elderly persons with IGT (Fig. 15-6 on p. 516) and because insulin receptors are unchanged with aging alone, the belief has been that the primary defect that causes IGT is at the postreceptor site. However, this impairment is complex and not yet fully understood.[33] Research is currently underway to elucidate changes in insulin transport inside the cell that may be responsible for the defect. Nevertheless, the defects responsible for age-related IGT appear to be distinct from those associated with obesity and NIDDM (Table 15-5).[33]

Defects in the glucose homeostasis of NIDDM are even more intriguing, since it appears that the elevations in glucose further worsen insulin resistance, resulting in positive

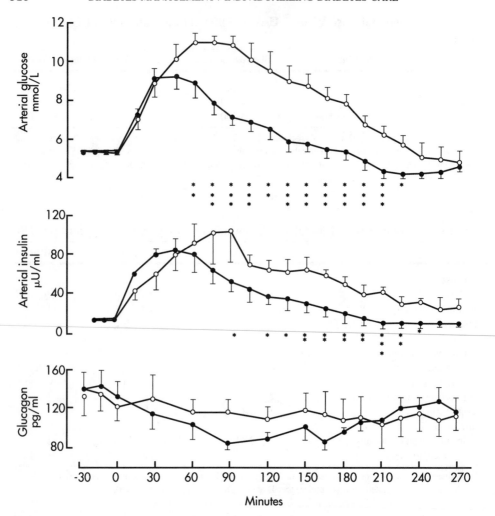

Fig. 15-6 Metabolic response to oral glucose loading in young (●) and elderly (o) subjects. *p <0.05; **p <0.01; ***p <0.001. (Reproduced with permission of the American Diabetes Association, Inc. From Jackson RA: Mechanisms of age-related glucose intolerance, Diabetes Care 13(suppl 2):9-19, 1990.)

feedback or self-perpetuation of the abnormality.[13] This phenomenon is detailed in Fig. 15-7.

Autonomic neuropathy, occurring as a complication of diabetes, can affect a multitude of other delicate homeostatic mechanisms. These include wider ranges in cardiac output, orthostatic hypotension, abnormalities in thermoregulation, and a tendency toward dehydration.[81] Impairments in the body's ability to maintain homeostasis with changing stresses significantly increases the person's overall "frailty" and therefore the quality of

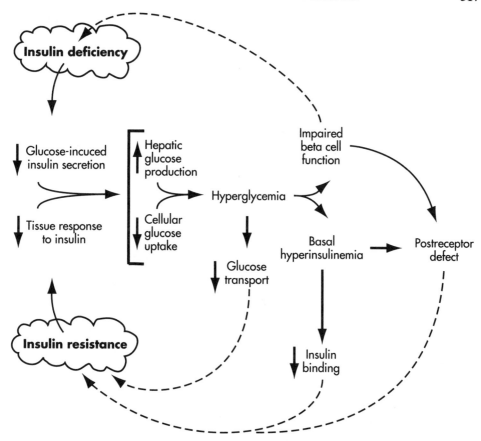

Fig. 15-7 Pathogenic sequence of events leading to development of insulin resistance in NIDDM. (Reproduced with permission of the American Diabetes Association, Inc. From Defronzo RA: The triumvirate: B-cell, muscle, liver: a collusion responsible for NIDDM, Diabetes 37:667-687, 1988.)

life. With orthostatic hypotension, for example, many people find it frustrating to have to get up slowly from a bed or chair to avoid dizziness, especially when they feel an urgency to urinate or answer the phone.

Atypical Presentations of Diabetes and its Complications

Diabetes can present atypically in older adults and so can its acute and chronic complications. Whereas the classic symptoms of hyperglycemia in younger adults are polyuria, polydipsia, and polyphagia, these symptoms may be masked by other illnesses or entirely absent in older adults. Detection of polyuria may be confounded by urinary incontinence. Thirst is commonly blunted in elderly people, increasing their chances of dehydration and electrolyte imbalance. Hunger may be blunted by the side effects of medication, depression, or gastrointestinal disease. Fatigue, also a common symptom of uncontrolled diabetes, may be discounted by the elderly person as "just part of getting old." Weight loss is sometimes profound but may be so gradual that it goes unnoticed for several years.

Acute complications of diabetes include hypoglycemia, hyperosmolar hyperglycemic nonketotic coma (HHNC), and diabetic ketoacidosis (DKA). These acute complications may present atypically in the older person, who may have a harder time physiologically coping with these challenges than a younger person. HHNC and DKA are relatively rare, especially DKA, since it occurs almost exclusively among patients with IDDM.[59] Efficient diagnosis and treatment is essential to reduce mortality but is often confounded by atypical presentations and the existence of other medical problems.

Hypoglycemia occurs almost exclusively in people taking insulin or sulfonylureas; thus, those who are diet controlled are not usually at risk. The adrenergic symptoms of hypoglycemia that result from the release of epinephrine (shaking, sweating, and nervousness), may be blunted or absent in older people. As a result, medications that block β-adrenergic receptors, such as propranolol, are not recommended. When hypoglycemia occurs without symptoms to prompt treatment, the reaction can progress to the point at which the patient requires the assistance of another person. This is called hypoglycemia unawareness. It is not only frightening, but may threaten the patient's level of independence in the eyes of others. It is precisely this issue that causes many health professionals to be concerned about avoiding hypoglycemia in the elderly, often to the point at which they are hesitant to treat asymptomatic *hyper*glycemia. Herein lies the basis of the debate about what glucose range is best, since many elderly adults have few symptoms of hyperglycemia, even when blood glucose levels average 350 to 400 mg/dL.

Generally, older adults have symptoms of chronic complications that are similar to those experienced by younger people. However, there are some caveats to note when working with the elderly. First, a chronic complication of diabetes such as peripheral sensory neuropathy or impotence may be the initial symptom of NIDDM that has actually been present for years. Second, the presentation of chronic complications may be atypical, may be misinterpreted, or may be overshadowed by other conditions. For example, a person may think the discomfort of peripheral neuropathy is "rheumatism" and try numerous over-the-counter arthritis preparations before consulting a health care professional. Small cerebral or myocardial infarcts may present "silently" and be diagnosed only when the patient's son or daughter brings them in "because Dad has really slowed down." Symptoms of peripheral vascular occlusive disease such as claudication may not occur in a person who does not exercise enough to induce the related ischemia. Last, retinopathy may go undiagnosed and untreated in an older adult who has dense cataracts.

Multiple Concurrent Disease Interactions

While some older adults have no chronic diseases or only one, the majority of elderly people suffer from more than one chronic illness. The prevalence of vascular, musculoskeletal, neurologic, ocular, urinary, foot, and gastrointestinal diseases is almost twice as great in patients 65 and over than in those in the 45 to 64 age range.[57] Progression of diabetes and other chronic diseases can lead to their long-term complications. Thus, the elderly are prone to multiple chronic conditions that may occur as primary disease entities or as secondary complications, and these may interact as previously described. The probability of disease interaction increases exponentially with age. Factors increasing this probability, including cultural, socioeconomic, and physical, need to be further examined.

Hypertension increases in incidence with age, particularly in the black population.[50] High blood pressure alone increases the incidence of renal, cardiovascular, and cerebrovascular disease; diabetes compounds the risk. Treatment of hypertension can be problematic in older adults with diabetes, since diuretics may further impair glucose tolerance and lead to electrolyte disturbances.

Coronary artery disease is the most common condition present among the elderly, and, despite improvements in related mortality with the advent of cardiac intensive care units, it remains the number one cause of death in people over age 65. Coronary artery disease is more common among older people with diabetes and has important implications for diabetes care. First, the avoidance of hypoglycemia is of particular importance for these patients. During a hypoglycemic reaction the counterregulatory hormones that raise blood glucose also raise the blood pressure and pulse. This increases myocardial oxygen demands and can cause angina. Second, some research studies suggest that silent myocardial infarctions are more common when diabetes is present, possibly as a component of autonomic neuropathy.[20] When a myocardial infarction occurs without the usual manifestations of angina (chest tightness or pain, often radiating to the left area or jaw), diagnosis and treatment are often delayed, increasing mortality. The prognosis is often poor for persons with diabetes who survive myocardial infarction; survival rates at 1 and 5 years following infarction are 82% and 58% respectively, compared with 94% and 82% for people without diabetes.[50]

Arthritic conditions are common in late life, and the older person may consider the related pain more serious than their diabetes. As an example, when an older woman with painful, debilitating osteoarthritis of the knees comes in for a routine appointment, advice about diet and blood glucose control may fall on deaf ears; she may only want pain medication and instruction in using a cane. Additionally, arthritis pain may lead to depression, overeating, and decreased activity that can worsen glycemic control in persons with NIDDM. Arthritis may hinder activities of diabetes self management.

Parkinson's disease, with its related tremors, muscular rigidity, and bradykinesia, can lead to difficulties with diabetes self-care practices. In its advanced stages, the fine motor skills needed for home glucose monitoring, insulin administration, and foot care may become impossible, causing frustration and an increased dependency on others.

HHNC is an important example of an interaction in which acute and chronic diseases overlap. In this syndrome, an older person with diabetes with compromised physiologic function usually suffers an acute insult such as pneumonia, myocardial infarction, or stroke (see box on p. 520).[59] The most common predisposing factor is infection.[85]

The stress response to the insult leads to the secretion of stress hormones including cortisol and epinephrine, which worsen hyperglycemia. As glucose is lost in the urine, dehydration and hyperosmolarity develop. The problem then becomes a self-perpetuating

_____ **RISK FACTORS FOR HHNC** _____

Events

Infection
Burn
Surgery
Cerebrovascular accident
Renal failure
Pancreatitis
Myocardial infarction

Drugs

Diuretics
β-blockers
Glucocorticoids
Anesthetic
Diphynylhydantoin

From Morrow L and Halter J: Diabetes mellitus in the older adult, Geriatrics 43(suppl):57-65, 1988.

positive feedback loop instead of a self-correcting negative feedback loop; the more the person secretes stress hormones in an effort to cope with the stress, the more dehydration and hyperglycemia develop because of relative insulin insufficiency. In addition, elderly persons have a lower total body water content ($\leq 60\%$) compared with a young adult (70%) and may therefore have as much as 8 liters of fluid less with which to buffer changes in osmolarity.[51] Ketogenesis does not develop in part because of the availability of some circulating insulin. However, the mechanism is not fully understood. HHNC usually develops over the course of 1 to 2 weeks and has a significant morality rate (similar to that of DKA), reportedly as high as 50%.[59] The mortality rate is particularly high among older persons and those with higher serum osmolarities and more severe concomittant illnesses. One third of all cases of HHNC are diagnosed in people with no prior history of diabetes.[85]

The person with HHNC may present with a lower level of consciousness such as acute confusion or lethargy but not necessarily coma. Because the chief problem is profound dehydration from hyperglycemic osmotic diuresis, signs of dehydration, such as orthostatic hypotension, tachycardia, and dry skin with poor turgor, are generally present. Serum osmolarity is greater than 320 mosm/L, indicating hypertonic dehydration. The plasma glucose value is typically more than 600 mg/dL and may be more than 1000 mg/dL.

The treatment of HHNC involves rehydration (which needs to be at a cautiously rapid rate in older adults), insulin, correction of electrolytes and pH, and diagnosis and treatment of the underlying cause. The signs, symptoms, and treatment of HHNC are summarized in Table 15-6. Health professionals need to be aware of the risk of HHNC in older

Table 15-6   Hyperglycemic Hyperosmolar Nonketotic Coma

History/symptoms	Signs	Treatment
Complains of fatigue, weakness	Orthostatic hypotension	Rehydration
	Tachycardia	Insulin
Caretakers note confusion, lethargy or unresponsiveness	Dry skin, tenting	Correct electrolytes and serum pH
	Poor skin turgor	
	Cold extremities	Treat underlying problem
Recent infection or other illness/injury	Glucose >600 mg/dL	
	Serum osmolarity >320 mOsm/L	
33% deny history of diabetes mellitus		

patients with NIDDM and encourage them to monitor blood glucose levels, report any trends in high readings, and drink plenty of noncaloric fluids. When a person with NIDDM is admitted to the hospital with infection or for surgery, blood glucose monitoring should be done frequently.

Geriatric Pharmacology

Persons over 65 have an average of three prescriptions to manage and take 5.6 medications per day.[56] Although the 25 million Americans over age 65 constitute about 11% of the population, they purchase 25% of drugs sold in the United States. Drug expenses may account for almost 20% of their personal budgets.[57] As a result, older people with chronic conditions are at risk for problems related to polypharmacy. Not only is there the possibility that a drug used to treat one illness may interact with another illness, there is also the possibility that the drugs can interact with each other. To compound this problem, older adults are often taking a broad variety of over-the-counter medications such as antacids, pain relievers, cold preparations, and laxatives.

Performance errors with medications occur in all age groups with alarming frequency, but there is no reason to believe that they occur with any greater magnitude among older adults than among younger persons.[2] However, because the elderly take more medications and because of their greater frailty, the risks for negative effects as a result of these errors are of greater concern. Older adults commonly experience other problems with medications, including receiving and sharing medications with peers and family members, and receiving medications from several care providers.[46] Health care providers may fail to provide clear instructions about the correct use, dosage, and timing of medications they prescribe. The fact that older patients are often taking several medications increases the potential for errors. Many pills look alike and one may be inadvertently substituted for the other. Discontinuing one drug to begin another is not always clearly explained, and patients may take both. Therefore, the use of both prescribed and over-the-counter medications needs to be carefully assessed, including how, when, and why the person decides to take them.

Use of alcohol should not be overlooked in the challenge of geriatric pharmacology. Older adults often continue to drink alcohol in later life, but may have a decreased tolerance for it. They are often unaware of the interactions between alcohol and other drugs, such as its synergistic effect with sedating medications, or that drinking alcohol may cause flushing in persons taking chlorpropamide. Depending on a broad array of factors, alcohol can promote hyperglycemia or hypoglycemia in the person with diabetes.[53]

The ingestion of alcohol, particularly for those with liver dysfunction, prolongs the hypoglycemic effect of many sulfonylurea agents (chlorpropamide, tolbutamide, acetohekamide, tolazamide, glipizide and glyburide).[81] Depression, not uncommon among older adults, may increase alcohol use. It is important that health care providers elicit information about alcohol use in a nonjudgmental way among all persons, especially those with diabetes.

Sulfonylureas can have interactions with other drugs and these interactions can affect glycemic control and are important considerations when working with older adults (see following box). The choice of an oral agent is especially important for the older adult who may have altered hepatic and renal function. Table 15-7 shows the daily dose, duration of action, and route of elimination for various oral sulfonylurea agents. Generally, drugs with a short duration of action and inactive metabolites are considered safer. Thus, chlorpropamide is not a drug of choice for older adults because of its long duration of action.

_____ IMPORTANT SULFONYLUREA INTERACTIONS _____

May diminish hypoglycemic efficacy

Diuretics
Diphenylhydantoin
Glucocorticoids
Lithium
Rifampin
Isoniazid
Nicotinic acid

May enhance or prolong hypoglycemic effect

Sulfonamides
Salicylates
Clofibrate
Dicumarol
Monoamine oxidase inhibitors
Nonsteroidal anti-inflammatory drugs
β-Adrenergic blocking agents
Alcohol

Reproduced with permission of the American Diabetes Association, Inc. From Halter JB and Morrow LA: Use of sulfonylurea drugs in elderly patients, Diabetes Care (Suppl 2):86-92, 1990.

Table 15-7   Comparison of Oral Sulfonylurea Drugs

Drug	Daily dosage range (mg)	Approximate duration of action (hours)	Route of elimination
Tolbutamide	500-3000	6-12	Hepatic metabolism; renal excretion of less active metabolites
Glipizide	2.5-40	8-12	Hepatic metabolism; renal excretion of inactive metabolites
Tolazamide	100-1000	12-16	Hepatic metabolism; renal excretion of less active metabolites
Acetohexamide	250-1500	12-24	Hepatic metabolism; active metabolism (hydroxyhexamide) has half-life of 5 hours and is excreted renally
Glyburide	2.5-20	24	Hepatic metabolism; renal excretion of less active metabolites
Chlorpropamide	100-750	40-72	80% hepatic metabolism, renal excretion of parent drug and less active metabolites

Reprinted with permission from Morrow LA, Halter JB: Carbohydrate metabolism in the elderly. In Sowers Jr, Felicetta JV, eds: The endocrinology of aging, New York, 1988, Raven Press.

Iatrogenic Disease

Iatrogenic disease is any adverse condition that results from the efforts of health care professionals to treat an illness or other kind of condition. These include the complications of immobility when a person is confined to bed in a hospital and nursing home, acute confusional states resulting from drugs and anesthesia, and nosocomial infections following surgeries and other procedures. The person with diabetes may be at increased risk for iatrogenic diseases because of compromised function and the worsening of blood glucose levels with stress hormones. For example, HHNC can be triggered iatrogenically by the use of certain medications, surgery, or infection secondary to procedures such as placement of an indwelling urinary catheter.

FUNCTIONAL ABILITY AND THE AGING PROCESS

This chapter has discussed normal aging changes, the prevalence of diabetes, and ways chronic conditions can interact. But what about function? Two older patients, both age 70 with diabetes, cataracts, cardiovascular disease, and arthritis, may be taking the same medications, yet one may be independent while the other is totally dependent on a spouse for help. Why is one person able to function independently while the other is not? Obviously one's functional capacity is not solely determined by age or health problems and medications.

Functional ability can be defined as the degree of independence with which a person is able to perform common activities of daily living. Each person's total functioning can be divided into four major areas: physical, cognitive, emotional, and psychosocial.[83] The body's organs and integrated physiologic function are essential for life. The mind's ability to learn, think, remember, communicate, and judge is essential for independence. Positive experiences and expression of emotion are essential for satisfaction. Contact with others and the fulfillment of vocational, leisure, social, financial, and cultural needs is essential for quality of life. Thus, the ability to function in all areas has an impact on total health and the ability to care for oneself. In addition, the significant happenings in a person's life, the demands of family and friends, the environment of daily living, and personal values related to daily living all serve to make up a person's total functional ability.[22]

Activities of daily living (ADL) can be divided into two areas, basic or personal ADLs and instrumental ADLs. Personal ADLs are those that have to do with basic self-care. Instrumental ADLs are those that relate to what is necessary for independent living. Examples of each are outlined in the box below. Both lists could be considerably longer. For example, basic ADLs could include shampooing hair and brushing teeth. Instrumental ADLs could include cutting food, lifting pots, and turning faucets.

The essence of geriatrics is to assist each person to attain and maintain his or her

---

_____ **EXAMPLES OF ACTIVITIES OF DAILY LIVING** _____

Basic activities of daily living

Eating
Bathing
Toileting
Dressing
Grooming
Transferring (to/from bed/chair/bath)
Ambulating (or other locomotion)
Communicating

Instrumental activities of daily living

Writing
Reading
Cooking
Cleaning
Shopping
Doing laundry
Climbing stairs
Using the telephone
Managing medications
Managing money
Traveling out of the home
Maintaining upkeep of home

optimal level of funtion, as cure of disease is often not possible.[64] In order for older persons to live as independently as possible for as long as possible, they require not only health care but often the care of many other people, both professional and nonprofessional.

Physical Changes with Aging

Older adults vary at the age and to the extent that the normal physical effects of aging occur. While there are generally declines in physical functioning, normal aging changes do not in and of themselves interfere with a person's ability to achieve and maintain a high level of independence and fulfillment.

Sensory declines that are common among the elderly have important implications for functioning. Among people over age 65, 18% to 20% have visual impairments, and there is an increased incidence of color blindness.[41] Cataracts and macular edema or degeneration are the most common visual problems among people over 65, but their symptoms are rarely reported. Early cataract development leads to a yellowing or browning of the lens and color distortions. Later cataracts lead to blurred vision. Macular edema may cause double vision while macular degeneration results in a loss of central vision, causing difficulty reading.[55] Presbycusis leading to hearing deficits is present in one fourth to one half of all older patients.[34,41] The number and size of taste buds may decrease and the sense of smell may be diminished, leading to a loss of interest in food.[23] Tactile sensation may also be decreased.[41]

Cognitive Changes with Aging

Healthy older adults vary greatly in the extent to which their cognitive abilities change with age, but research has shown that a significant decline in the elderly is not inevitable.[83] Cognitive impairment affects just about 5% to 10% of persons over age 65, and in only half of those patients is it severe.[46,86] Cognitive changes caused by normal aging include slowing but not elimination of the ability to create and retrieve memory; however, no normal aging change in and of itself has to be a threat to an older person's ability to function independently.[83]

Cognitive abilities, not surprisingly, are of paramount importance in an older person's ability to maintain independence. When an older person who has diabetes and cognitive deficits is challenged to coordinate a complicated treatment program, his or her independence is likely to be threatened.

In its early stages, cognitive impairment can cause problems such as inconsistently taking medication to manage diabetes and other health problems, but this may not be recognized. Erratic eating patterns may lead to erratic blood glucose levels, weight loss, malnutrition, and dehydration that may in turn further worsen cognitive function. Early detection of and intervention for cognitive deficits often leads to better health outcomes in older patients and can potentially help them stay in their own homes if appropriate community resources are used.

In more advanced dementia, such as later stages of Alzheimer's type dementia or severe multi-infarct dementia, the diabetes treatment program often needs to be redefined. For example, if an older person with diabetes develops Alzheimers disease with resultant weight loss, simply helping the patient obtain adequate nutrition may be more important than avoiding moderate hyperglycemia. In this situation most of the goal negotiation, education, and feedback needs to be between the health care team and the caretaker.

IMPACT OF DIABETES ON FUNCTIONAL ABILITY
Physical Considerations

Older persons with diabetes are at an increased risk for functional limitations. Diminished proprioception, peripheral vascular disease, peripheral neuropathy, postural hypotension, obesity, and cardiac disease may interfere with the ability to walk, climb stairs, and do other physical activities and increase the likelihood of falls and their debilitating results. Peripheral neuropathy and decreased circulation increase the risks for foot ulcers, infections, and resulting amputations. Carpal tunnel syndrome and diabetic amyotrophy may limit the ability to use one's hands for cooking, dressing, or other fine motor tasks.[83]

The prevalence of diabetic retinopathy increases with aging, from 10% at age 55 to over 30% by age 80.[58] There is also an increased prevalence of glaucoma and cataracts in older persons with diabetes. Visual impairment is a threat to independence because it affects activities of daily living, work or hobby activities, the ability to drive, and social relationships.

Diabetes-related problems increase both the likelihood that older adults will need surgery and their risk for complications during and after an operation. Frequent blood glucose monitoring is needed during all phases of the surgical process, and insulin may be needed until after the patient has fully recovered.

Elevated glucose levels are associated with other conditions that are likely to affect the lives of older adults. Hyperglycemia leads to poor red cell deformability that may worsen peripheral vascular disease. There is evidence that elevated gluocose levels increase platelet adherence. That increases the chances that a patient may have a myocardial infarction or cerbrovascular accident and may also impair recovery from strokes.[58]

Persons with diabetes report pain more frequently than other chronically ill patients. It has been suggested that hyperglycemia heightens pain perception.[58] Pain from other chronic conditions and neuropathies may therefore be more difficult to manage for the person with diabetes.

Loss of bladder control is generally devastating to the person's social and physical functioning. Hyperglycemia and the propensity for bladder infections among people with diabetes exacerbate difficulties with incontinence.[83]

Cognitive Considerations

It is fairly well established that persons with NIDDM perform more poorly on various cognitive tasks than those who do not have diabetes.[83] One recent study of older persons with NIDDM and age-matched persons who did not have NIDDM, all of whom were ambulatory, lived in the community and were capable of undergoing several hours of cognitive testing, showed greater cognitive deficits among those with NIDDM even when they perceived themselves to be in good health.[72] Poorer performance of relatively healthy older adults with NIDDM compared with the controls suggests that cognitive changes are related to the presence of NIDDM. Most of these differences parallel changes encountered with normal aging in that relatively minor differences are found for tests of immediate memory, and larger differences for more demanding tasks that require working memory.[83] No significant diabetes-related differences have consistently been revealed in the realms of attention, short-term memory, or semantic memory. While elevated glucose levels appear to contribute to cognitive deficits, the precise relationship is not clear. In addition, elevated triglycerides also appear to negatively affect cognition.[83] In one study, subjects with more severe diabetes, as evidenced by higher glycosylated hemoglobin levels and peripheral neuropathy, had a relatively greater impairment in cognitive function.[65] The presence of emotional problems such as anxiety and depression adversely affect cognitive measures in subjects with and without diabetes.

NORMAL PSYCHOSOCIAL DEVELOPMENT

The changes that occur during the aging process are not only biologic, but are also social and psychologic. As the developmental tasks of middle adulthood are completed, the tasks related to the end of the lifespan are begun.

Several theorists have proposed tasks that are specific to this stage of life. Erik Erickson described this phase, beginning at age 50, as integrity versus despair.[17] During this stage, an individual reviews his or her life for relevance and meaningfulness and develops a sense of integrity or acceptance versus a sense of despair or rejection of one's life.[3] Robert Havighurst theorized that individuals must learn to adapt to new roles, situations, and relationships throughout the life span. He defined the adaptations of later maturity, beginning at age 60, as adjusting to a decline in strength and health, retirement, death of one's spouse, difficulty affiliating with one's age group, and accepting death.[30] More recently, Levinson proposed a view of the life cycle as a series of eras, each lasting 20 to 25 years. The primary task of late adulthood, beginning at age 60, is to balance involvement with society with involvement with self.[44]

The developmental tasks for this stage represent major life adjustments and many losses. Therefore, this is one of the most stressful periods in the life span.[89] Depression is believed to be an extremely common response to these losses, although it is largely undetected and untreated. It is so common that it has been suggested that older adults go through a developmental depressive crisis, similar to the developmental crisis of adolescence.[22] The ability to make the many adjustments needed during this phase may be a function of what has occurred during the previous stages and whether earlier tasks were completed. This is not to say that growth and insight do not occur, because many older adults are able to review their lives, place events in perspective, and resolve lifelong conflicts.[38]

Older adults who are members of ethnic minorities appear to be at greatest risk for the negative impacts of the aging process on income, health, and some measures of life satisfaction. It is of interest, however, that on some measures of quality of life, differences in scores between whites and minority groups diminish with age.[38] Thus, aging appears to both enhance and level the problems associated with being part of a minority group. It is also important to note that members of every ethnic group are heterogenous and culturally reflect both personal and shared experiences.

Family Relationships

The family is one of the most basic institutions within our society. Most people are born into a family, live much of their lives within a family, and consider it to be a high priority in their value system.[3] However, the family structure, roles and relationships within the family, and its purpose and function change over time.[38]

The family has a dynamic life cycle that begins with marriage and ends with the death of one spouse. There are several models for the life cycle of a family, but the stages that generally occur among older adults begin when children start to leave home. The last four phases in a model adapted by Atchley are:

- Launching children (oldest child to youngest child leaving home)
- Middle years (children gone to retirement)
- Retirement (one spouse retired until start of disability)
- Old age (one spouse disabled until death of one spouse)[3]

The "empty-nest syndrome" is a relatively new phenomenon within the life of a family, as people live longer and healthier lives. It generally refers to the years a couple spends together between the launching of their last child and the death of one spouse. While the departure of the children is a disruption to the family and the parents, the majority of research indicates that this is a time many parents look forward to, prepare for, and do not find exclusively stressful.[5]

Family units often include more than one generation. Research into family forms and functions have not borne out the expectation that the isolated nuclear family would emerge as the norm. With the greater longevity of the current population, four-generational families are becoming more and more common, and the generations frequently share many links. The common thread that binds the generations in a system of shared beliefs, norms, values, and cultural traditions is the family.[8]

Ethnicity appears to play a strong role in family relationships. It is often assumed that minority persons have more extended family ties, including aunts, uncles, siblings, nieces, nephews, and cousins, than whites. This appears to be true for black elderly, with older black women playing an important role in this network. However, this does not appear to be true for older Hispanic adults. While extended family life is the tradition of this culture, it is rapidly becoming irrelevant with the increasing urbanization and assimilation of Hispanic families. While this has led to some tensions between generations, it does appear that the elderly are still respected and revered.[38] Many Asian-American and native

American elderly may be suffering from isolation for similar reasons. While members of the Asian-American minorities have generally been economically assimilated, the simultaneous accommodation to American values has left some older members isolated and alienated from their families. Native American elderly were traditionally held in high esteem by younger tribe members. While they still play an important role within the extended family, increased urbanization is also causing erosion in this family structure.[8]

The most important family relationship for many older adults is with their adult children. About 80% of older Americans have living children and most of them are not isolated from their offspring.[3] Most studies show that older adults and their children see each other quite often. Distance appears to be the strongest determinant for frequency of contact, and visitation is more frequent along the female line of the family.[38]

When asked, most parents and adult children report positive feelings for each other. Generally, older adults hold their children in high regard, and parents remain important to children throughout the lifespan.[3]

Despite these mutually strong feelings, almost all studies show that older adults prefer to live near, but not with, their children. Most appear to want "intimacy at a distance," citing the desire to preserve privacy and independence and to avoid conflict or interference with their children.[38] White elderly are more likely to move in with their adult children, while black and Hispanic elderly are more likely to have adult children move in with them.[8]

Mutual aid is also considered to be a crucial intergenerational dimension. Research indicates that there is a two-directional flow of assistance between parents and children. Financial and social support is provided by each generation to the other at different times over the years.[8] The assistance provided consists of both informal, nonessential services (e.g., babysitting, transportation) or highly organized, essential services (e.g. financial aid, housing). The type of assistance offered and received depends on the sex of the parents and children, ethnicity, and social class.[38] For example, compared with other ethnic groups, African-Americans are more likely to give or receive help across generations during difficult times, with the flow of assistance generally from old to young.[8]

The two-way flow of support may persist until the death of one spouse or extreme frailty in the elderly parent.[38] More attention is being given to the extent to which middle-aged people experience being in the middle between their children and their parents.[3] The expression "sandwich generation" identifies this dilemma. Many people believe that a role inversion or reversal occurs during this time. However, this should not be expected and may even be maladaptive. "Parentification" of the children and "infantalizing" the elderly not only leads to guilt, but is demeaning to everyone involved. Such behavior is often a reflection on the past relationship between parents and children and conflicts that have never been resolved.[79]

About 80% of older people have living brothers or sisters. With the advent of old age, the death of a spouse, and the leaving home of adult children, many older people seek to renew sibling relationships. Siblings are especially important in the lives of older adults who never married or had children.[3]

Marriage and Divorce

The number of older married couples is increasing because of the greater longevity of the population, particularly among men. The average couple can expect 15 years together after the departure of the last child.[38] Most older couples have grown old together, and their relationship is often the focal point in their lives.

Most studies have shown that the pattern of marital satisfaction is high in early adulthood, declines through middle age, and rises steadily again after child rearing. Happy couples provide great comfort and support to each other, show a high degree of interdependence, share many activities, and exhibit greater equity between partners than unhappy couples.[3]

Marital satisfaction is a primary factor for overall satisfaction with life. One of the functions of couplehood involves intimacy, including a sense of belonging, mutual affection, regard, trust, and sex. Sexuality is an important, but often neglected, component of intimacy among the elderly. Sexual activity reflects physical capacity, emotional needs, social norms, and means much the same to older people as it does to others. For couples who remain physically healthy, the later years generally reflect feelings of greater appreciation and affection for each other and an increase in the time and opportunity for companionship.[3]

Not all marriages become more satisfying over the years; a small proportion do not. The quality of the relationship and adjustments made in later life are probably a reflection of adjustments made earlier in life. Marriages among older couples reported as happy had generally been satisfying over the lifespan, whereas unhappy older couples reported difficulties from the beginning.[8]

The divorce rate is not high among older couples, but it has more than doubled since 1960. The difficulty of adjusting to divorce increases as age increases, making it more stressful. Compared with younger divorced persons, older adults report greater unhappiness, fewer positive emotional experiences, greater pessimism, and long-term dissatisfaction.[38]

Widowhood

The majority of older women are widows. The longevity gap between men and women has not been bridged completely, so the disproportion between the sexes increases with age.[79] The proportion of black and Hispanic widows is higher than that of whites because of decreased longevity found among black and Hispanic men.[8] There is considerable variation in the experiences of widowhood. Almost everyone is emotionally affected by the loss of a spouse, but some people are impacted more severely and for a longer period of time.

Lopata has proposed four stages in the adjustment to widowhood. First, there is the official recognition of the event that is a time of crisis and mourning. The second is the temporary disengagement stage, and the third is limbo, in which people confront their life without their spouse. The final phase is the re-engagement stage with the establishment of a new life style where one reorganizes one's life as a single person.[47]

While controversial, the adaptation process and difficulties encountered appear to be similar for men and women. The concurrent loss of a widower's occupational role may compound the loss of his wife, while widows often experience a loss in income.[8] It is clear that widowhood affects all family interactions, and widowed parents must adjust to different relationships with their adult children.[3] Having an effective social support network appears to soften the impact of a life event as stressful as widowhood.[8]

Grief is defined as a reaction to loss and bereavement refers to the state of having sustained a loss.[39] Grief can include physiologic, psychologic, and sociologic responses. People who experience a loss tend to go through predictable stages in the adjustment process. These include protest, despair, detachment, and reorganization.[8]

The elderly in our society are not always provided with an opportunity to express their grief. Many people believe that since older persons should expect loss as inevitable they should be able to "grin and bear it." The inability to express grief may lead to physical manifestations or symptoms that can be misinterpreted as dementia. Unresolved grief can also lead to increased risks for new illnesses, worsening of chronic illnesses, or even death.[66]

The person who becomes a widow is confronted with a variety of personal and familial problems. Widowed persons consistently show higher rates of mortality, mental disorders, and suicides. The death of a spouse is particularly difficult for persons who are heavily dependent on their marital partner.[8] For persons with diabetes, this may be a time of worsening in blood glucose control caused by stress, loss of support, or the gap left if the spouse was responsible for care activities or food preparation.

Remarriage

Remarriage may be desirable for many divorced or widowed older adults. However, the probability of remarriage decreases as age increases. This is partly a result of the smaller numbers of eligible men among the elderly population.

The primary reason for marriage among older adults tends to be companionship. Some older people remarry to allay their anxiety about poor health, for financial security, and to avoid dependency on their adult children.[3]

Marriages between the elderly appear to be generally successful, particularly when based on affection and mutual financial security. The approval of children also appears to contribute to success.[38] Having similar backgrounds and being well acquainted before marriage also increases the likelihood for success.[8] Impotence, which occurs frequently in men with diabetes, may hinder both the interest in and success of a late-life marriage.

Grandparenting

Increased life expectancy, earlier marriages, shorter child-rearing periods, and fewer children have exposed more middle-aged and older adults to grandparenthood than ever before.[8] About 75% of older adults are grandparents, but only a few adults over 65 have young grandchildren.

Neugarten and Weinstein identified five major styles of grandparenting:

1. Formal—maintain clearly defined lines between parenting and grandparenting and leave parenting exclusively to the mother and father.
2. Fun-seeking—informal and playful with an emphasis on mutual gratification.
3. Distant figure—contact is fleeting but benevolent.
4. Surrogate parent—cares for children while mother works; usually grandmother.
5. Reservoir of family wisdom—distinctly authoritative; usually grandfather.[62]

Older grandparents are more likely to have a more formal style of grandparenting, and women are more likely to look forward to the role of being a grandparent than men.[8]

More attention is now being paid to the growing number of great-grandparents in this country. There appears to be two styles of great-grandparenting: remote and close. There are many similarities between grandparenthood and great-grandparenthood, but increasing age, frailty, and distance have an impact on the relationship.[38]

Generally, grandchildren seem to have strong affection towards their grandparents.[38] Studies have shown that even as young adults, grandchildren rate relationships with their grandparents as very significant and keep in close contact.[3] While not meaningful to all older adults, most come to enjoy the role because it involves a minimum of responsibility and a great deal of personal fulfillment.[8]

Hispanics report the most frequent contact with their grandchildren, and African Americans have more contact than whites, except among the oldest groups.[38] More African American elderly persons appear to offer child-raising assistance with their grandchildren than do white elderly persons. Among elderly households headed by African American women, 41% include children under age 18, as compared with 9% headed by elderly white women.[8] Native Americans also appear to be influential in raising grandchildren, particularly those who live on reservations.[8] In cultures such as these, in which NIDDM is prevalent and the influence of grandparents is strong, one approach that may be helpful is to teach the importance of childhood nutrition to the grandparents in an effort to prevent obesity and the subsequent development of diabetes.

Retirement

Work and retirement are highly significant aspects in the lives of older adults. Work shapes an individual's daily activities and contributes to his or her self-concept and life satisfaction. Retirement is therefore a major event. It marks a change in daily activity, economic status, and is a symbolic transition to old age.[89]

Retirement is a process that involves withdrawing from work and taking on the roles of a retired person. Atchley describes four phases that persons go through when adjusting to retirement:

1. Preretirement—concerns about the financial aspects and activities during retirement begins. It includes a remote and near phase.
2. Honeymoon—immediately following retirement when freedom is enjoyed.
3. Disenchantment—a letdown during adjustment to a slower pace.

4. Reorientation—refocus of activities as people pull themselves together.[3]

Retirement is somewhat different for women and minorities than for white men. Most older women have had discontinuous work histories (or no employment history) at all. Gains that occurred during the Civil Rights movement of the 1960s occurred too late to have much impact on the educational level or economic conditions of today's elderly minorities. As a result, older African Americans fare worse than whites on a variety of economic indicators. The work histories of many African Americans, which include high levels of unemployment and overrepresentation in low-paying jobs, is reflected in their retirement incomes. Older African American women generally had higher educational levels than African American men, but have generally had lower-paying jobs. African American women are more likely to have worked steadily for all of their adult lives than white women, but are less likely to have retired.[38] Few Hispanics have had lengthy work careers to prepare for retirement. The combined problems of low-paying, unskilled jobs and questionable citizenship or residential status has led to Hispanic elderly persons staying in the work force longer than white elderly persons.[38] In general, lower educational levels among minorities and past discrimination in the work place has led to lower incomes, lower social security benefits available, and the postponement of retirement for as long as possible.

Despite the grim picture that is often painted of retirement, studies show that most people look forward to retirement and see it as a positive time. The adjustment to retirement is thought to be determined in part by the person's attitude toward it. Factors that impede the adjustment process include poor health, inadequate income, the inability to give up one's job gracefully, and any other situational changes that occur at the same time.[3] Research has shown that the health of retirees often improves, rather than worsening, as is generally believed. Because older African Americans were more likely to have been shut out of occupational positions of prestige, they are less likely to suffer a loss of status with retirement.[8]

Retirement before the age of 61 is considered early retirement. Very early retirees tend to be either in good health with high incomes or in poor health with very low incomes.[89] Unfortunately, early retirees among older adults with diabetes generally fall into the latter category.

Death and Dying

Death and the dying process are being looked at more and more as the terminal phase of the life cycle.[38] As people age and they are confronted with the deaths of friends and family members, they are less able to avoid thinking about this stage in their own lives and the inevitability of their own deaths.

The dying process is not conceptualized as an unbroken decline in health toward death. In the first or social stage, elderly persons are fighting the tendency of society to impose a premature social death. They may bargain to hold onto symbols that represent the future, such as a cane when they are no longer able to walk. In the second or terminal stage, death is more imminent and the person may bargain directly with God.[39]

The meanings that people give to death vary as a function of age. Studies indicate two meanings of death that are of particular significance for the elderly. One is death as an organizer of time. Anticipating the end of one's life may bring about a reorganization of time and priorities. The other is the meaning of death as loss. Facing death can make all possessions and other experiences appear to be transient and meaningless. The perception among the elderly of the finitude of life is reinforced both by people and institutions. American society appears to perceive older persons as not deserving of a major investment of resources.[39] At the same time, health care professionals sometimes appear to value preservation of life whenever possible, while older people who perceive their quality of life to be poor may want to avoid life-sustaining measures. The debate about how much societal values can supersede personal choice is increasingly an issue of concern among legislators and citizens.

The most common attitude toward death is fear, and the acceptance of death is viewed as true maturity. In general, studies have shown that older persons frequently are more accepting of death and have fewer anxieties about it. Among the aged population, those who report good health are most likely to be evasive about death, while those in poor health look forward to death in a more positive manner.[8] Scientific studies about the effect of religious beliefs on attitudes towards death are inconclusive.

IMPACT OF DIABETES ON PSYCHOSOCIAL DEVELOPMENT
Sociocultural Considerations

There is a complex interplay between the physical and sociocultural aspects of an illness among older persons.[8] Many of the negative things that happen to older adults are both physical and social and have an impact on total functional ability. For example, because of the dietary demands of diabetes, older people may isolate themselves from eating in restaurants or gatherings of family and friends, leading to loneliness and decreased support to cope with their illness. Impotence, which can occur as a complication of diabetes, may lead to isolation from one's spouse and marital difficulties.

Very little work has been done about the sociocultural impact of diabetes on older adults; however, it is believed that the impact is generally less severe than among the young. A study by Linn indicates that older adults are more likely to accept a chronic illness such as diabetes as a natural part of the aging process.[45] Jenny compared adaptation to diabetes among four age groups: younger (mean age, 19.7), middle (mean age, 35.9), older (mean age, 57.3), and aged (mean age, 71.7) adults. The older and aged adults identified the fewest barriers to adherence and the least number of special concerns about diabetes. However, they also identified the greatest number of health problems that interfered with diabetes management and the least amount of social support. Among the four age groups, diabetes was perceived as least severe by the aged patients.[34]

The issue of the sociocultural impact of diabetes is further complicated by differences in types of diabetes and treatment programs. One comparison of patients with IDDM (mean age, 34.8), NIDDM using insulin (mean age, 58.7), and NIDDM not using insulin (mean age, 62.3) showed that patients with NIDDM using insulin reported significantly more control problems, social problems, and barriers to adherence than patients with

NIDDM not using insulin. Persons with IDDM and NIDDM using insulin reported similar perceptions of their risk for complications of diabetes, while patients with NIDDM not using insulin reported a significantly lower perceived risk.[12] The perception of severity of diabetes as compared with other chronic illnesses in late life has been largely unexplored.

The emotional response to diabetes is probably similar to the responses of younger persons. The older adult's self-esteem, bodily integrity, self-worth, autonomy, independence, and control may all be challenged by a diagnosis of diabetes. The ability to deal with these feelings is probably affected by previous coping styles, social support, and economic factors.[83]

There has been little research on how chronic illness affects family relationships among older adults. Between husbands and wives, communication has been found to decrease and stress and loneliness increase. Many spouses (particularly wives) must accept care responsibilities and may find the demands overwhelming. The quality of the relationship between parents and adult children is also affected by a chronic illness. Negative feelings toward parents appear to increase as health declines and dependency increases.[43]

Very little is known about the impact of diabetes on the family members of older adults. The response to NIDDM may be complicated by the fact that it tends to run in families.[83] Two potential negative effects are increased dependency on family members caused by increased care needs related to diabetes or increased social isolation caused by dietary and other demands of daily diabetes care.

The incidence of chronic conditions and levels of physical limitations may give the impression that elderly people view themselves as being in poor health and unable to function. This is a false perception. In a large study of older adults, the majority viewed themselves as being in good to excellent health when compared with others their age.[38]

Socioeconomic Considerations

The importance of economic status among older adults cannot be overstated. Financial resources have a great impact on the ability to maintain control over one's life, participate in desired leisure activities, and adequately care for one's health.[38]

Although older adults have fewer expenses than those during their child raising years, they still have to pay for the same basic needs as other people. Additionally, declining health, increasing medical care costs, and the financial costs of a chronic illness such as diabetes raise the economic needs of older adults.[8]

Older Americans consistently have lower incomes, roughly two-thirds that of younger adults. The newly retired (the young-old) are more likely to have adequate incomes than those over 75 (old-old) years of age.[8] However, as a result of substantial improvements over the past 20 years, when noncash benefits are taken into account, a smaller percentage of the elderly are now below the poverty line when compared with the general population. Most elderly state that they are satisfied with their financial situation.[4]

Despite these gains, it is clear that economic status is of concern for many older adults. Hispanics, African Americans, those living alone, those with less than 8 years of education, those living in central cities, and African American women living alone are poorer than other older Americans. In the United States, elderly African Americans are the most economically disadvantaged of any group. Sixty-eight percent of rural, older African American women live in poverty, as compared with 21% of white women.[8] Because older adults spend proportionally more on health care, housing, and food than younger adults, these difficulties often manifest themselves in inadequate nutrition, housing, and medical care.[4]

Social Security is the major source of income for persons over age 65. Ninety percent of the elderly receive income from this source and it constitutes 40% of their income. Assets, pensions, and other earnings make up the rest of the income. More older Americans who have low incomes rely on Social Security than do those with high incomes.[4]

Health care costs

Health care costs have increased in this country at a rapid pace, particularly among older people. In 1981, the medical bill for the elderly population was three times that of other adults. One of the reasons medical costs are higher among the elderly is the prevalence of chronic illnesses such as diabetes. It was estimated that the inpatient and outpatient direct costs of diabetes in 1987 yielded a total of $9.6 billion.[67]

The largest health care expenditures among older adults are for hospitalizations, nursing home care, and medical care. Expenditures for medical care per person are 50% higher for those over 65 with diabetes than those without diabetes.[87] People with diabetes are twice as likely to be hospitalized as people without this illness and are prone to longer hospital stays.[38] The total amount spent on nursing home care for people with diabetes in 1987 was $941.5 million.[67]

Diabetes is also expensive on a daily basis. An estimate of the costs of medications, monitoring supplies, laboratory tests, hospitalizations, and doctor visits for patients with diabetes is about $4265 per year depending on the type of diabetes and intensity of treatment. For older adults, about $900, or 20% of this total, is an out-of-pocket expenditure.[87] Because per capita expenditures tend to increase with age, this is a conservative estimate of the cost for an older adult and can represent a substantial burden to patients with limited incomes.

Insurance

The principle funding mechanisms for health care among the elderly are Medicare and Medicaid.[38] Medicare was funded by Congress in 1966 to help alleviate medical costs incurred by older Americans. There are two parts to Medicare. Part A is compulsory hospital insurance and is provided at no cost to persons who receive Social Security, while Part B is optional and is available for a monthly fee. Part B partially covers doctor bills, medical supplies, and other outpatient services. The amount of money expended on Medicare increased eight times between 1970 and 1984.[35]

Medicare does not cover all medical costs. Medicare patients are still responsible for portions of their medical care costs through copayments (usually 20%), deductibles, and uncovered expenses.[38] On average, 22% of the total expenses are paid out-of-pocket, and these costs can quickly become prohibitive. Only 15% of older adults have just Medicare insurance, and most augment their coverage with a "Medigap" or supplemental policy.[87] These policies will generally cover the deductible and copayment portions of hospital care and doctor's services but may not provide coverage for medications and nursing home care. Such plans are not extensively used and have had little impact. Only about 5% of the total health care bill for older adults is covered by private insurance. Alternatives to Medigap policies include major medical insurance, health maintenance organizations, and hospital-indemnity policies.[35]

Medicaid is available to low-income elderly and pays for some services not provided through Medicare, such as eyeglasses and prescription drugs.[8]

Critics of Medicare and Medicaid maintain that it covers only acute problems and does not provide for many preventive services or for the daily needs of caring for a chronic illness. Coverage for diabetes-related supplies and equipment has improved a great deal in recent years, particularly for persons who take insulin. Despite these difficulties, Medicare and Medicaid do represent legal entitlement to medical care for older adults.[38]

TEACHING/LEARNING IMPLICATIONS

The daily care of diabetes is complex. Recommendations for diabetes treatment often initiate the need to incorporate meal planning, medications, exercise, and blood glucose monitoring into activities of daily living. While some older adults find these self-care practices difficult because of decreased physical abilities, memory loss, or other cognitive deficits, others are not only capable of performing these tasks but are very interested in doing so. It is important that health care professionals not be guilty of "agism" by assuming that older patients are unable to learn or unwilling to care for themselves. Most of the limits imposed by the effects of the aging process can be compensated for in some way through careful assessment, planning, and implementation of the teaching process.

Individualized Treatment of Goals for the Older Population

As with other age groups, it is important for all patients or the person primarily responsible for their daily care to establish individual goals and priorities in collaboration with the health care team. The individual's goals should then be used to consciously initiate a program of either basic diabetes care or more intensive diabetes care as the treatment strategy. The primary purpose of basic diabetes care is to prevent the acute complications of hyperglycemia by maintaining fasting blood glucose levels of less than 11 mm (200 mg/dL). This treatment program can be initiated by a physician with general training and includes meal planning, exercise, and an oral sulfonylurea when needed. In contrast, the primary purpose of intensive diabetes care is to prevent the long-term complications of diabetes through maintaining fasting blood glucose levels of less than 8 mm (140 mg/dL). Insulin is often recommended along with diet, exercise, and home blood glucose monitoring. While the link between hyperglycemia and the long-term complications of diabetes has not been firmly established for elderly patients, their prevalence among this population means that this is an issue that cannot be ignored.[27]

The implementation of more intensive treatment programs is often challenging but can be facilitated by using a team approach. The impact of such programs on older adults' quality of life is of concern, but this issue has not been studied. It is important to recognize that quality of life is a highly personal and individual perception, and health care professionals should not allow their own beliefs to influence the type of treatment recommended. As with all patients, older adults should be informed of treatment options, the costs and benefits of each option, and any other facts that they need to make a decision about their treatment programs.

The tools for the treatment of diabetes are the same for older adults as those for other individuals with IDDM and NIDDM. These include meal planning, weight control, exercise, and oral sulfonylureas or insulin. However, there are specific issues related to older adults that need to be taken into account with each of these tools.

Nutrition

Diet is generally considered to be the cornerstone of metabolic control in diabetes. Among older adults, current ADA dietary guidelines are probably reasonable, although there are no supporting data specific to this population.[74] The basis for individual dietary recommendations may include achievement of an ideal or reasonable body weight, blood glucose control, a decrease in the intake of saturated fats and cholesterol, and a nutritionally adequate and balanced diet. The dietary intervention can involve a specific meal pattern and calorie level or be more behaviorally focused. It is important to note, however, that radical dietary modifications are difficult at any age and may have a negative impact on quality of life.[69] The patient needs to first understand and then to weigh the potential advantages of any changes with their costs and potential disadvantages.

Weight control

Among patients with diabetes over 60 years of age, 40% are overweight, and an additional 15% are obese. These persons often achieve significant reductions in plasma glucose levels during periods of reduced calorie intake or with modest amount of weight loss.[74] The remainder of older persons with diabetes, particularly the very old, tend to have normal body weight or may actually be underweight. Eating similar amounts of food at regular times throughout the day may offer advantages to these patients in terms of blood glucose control. This can serve to smooth out blood glucose levels and prevent overtaxing a poorly functioning pancreas.[78]

Older persons with diabetes have the same problems related to nutrition as other older persons. Loss of appetite caused by lack of activity, other chronic illnesses, poor dentition, medication interactions, depression, and diminished senses of taste and smell are factors that can negatively affect nutritional status.[74] Skipping meals has been shown to correlate with poorer metabolic control of diabetes, perhaps because it leads to snacking or overeating later in the day.[78] This can also impede weight loss. Many older persons, particularly those who live alone, are socially isolated, or have functional impairments that make food shopping and cooking difficult, may actually eat very little and tend to be malnourished. Approximately 16% of white and 18% of African American elderly consume fewer than 1000 calories per day. Among the poor elderly, 27% of whites and 36% of African Americans consume less than 1000 calories per day.[74] Because eating patterns can be so variable among the elderly, it is particularly important, when insulin is required, that the dose is planned to fit the patient's usual eating habits, not the other way around.[70]

Exercise

Exercise is generally believed to be a component of the treatment for diabetes. There are few data that address the effects of exercise training on elderly persons with diabetes, but data on the positive effects of exercise among other groups of patients with NIDDM suggest that older adults could also receive the benefit of improved insulin action resulting from endurance training. Along with improved glucose utilization, the benefits of exercise for elderly people include improved cardiovascular status, preservation and maintenance of joint mobility and range of motion, toning, and an improved sense of well-being. Because the potential risks of exercise are greater for older patients, a thorough history and physical, assessment of diabetes control and complications, and an exercise stress test should be done before an exercise program is initiated. Aerobic exercises that do not cause excessive joint trauma, such as walking, swimming, or bicycling are generally recommended. Morning exercise may have the greatest benefit because that is the time of greatest insulin resistance; however, the timing of exercise needs to be individually planned, taking into account the person's treatment program and life-style.

Long-term adherence to exercise programs tends to be problematic for all ages, so every effort should be made for the exercise program to be a positive and enjoyable experience.[80] Walking with friends, a walking club, or exercise classes designed for senior citizens are strategies to increase the likelihood that patients will choose to exercise. Activity is often a neglected topic for the elderly because of assumptions that they are not able to exercise. It is important to ask about past exercise levels and what exercises patients are currently able and willing to do.

Oral sulfonylureas

Oral sulfonylureas are widely used in the management of older persons with NIDDM. In fact, 50% of the oral hypoglycemics prescribed are for persons over 65.[49] While there is very little data on their use specifically with older adults, it is reasonable to assume that they are safe and effective in lowering blood glucose levels. However, sulfonylureas may not be adequate to achieve euglycemia in many patients, and their ability to prevent long-term complications is controversial. Additionally, the interaction of these pills with other medications that potentiate their hypoglycemic effects needs to be considered, particularly among older persons who are frequently taking several medications for other chronic diseases.[28]

Hypoglycemia can occur with these medications, and older persons who tend to skip meals are particularly susceptible. These reactions are generally more severe, and because of their longer action time, are less amenable to treatment with a simple carbohydrate than those caused by insulin. Chlorpropramide can cause a mild antabuse-like reaction (flushing, sweating, headache) when alcohol is ingested. This drug is not recommended for persons who drink because of the likelihood that they will stop taking the medication or skip their dose on days when they will be drinking alcohol. Oral medications do offer the advantage of a medication in pill form, rather than injections, which makes them less costly and easier for patients to take. While individuals prefer oral medications over pills, studies have shown that compliance with pills is no better than with insulin.[41]

Insulin therapy

Insulin treatment offers some advantages in that it is usually possible to lower plasma glucose values, and dosages can be more precisely adjusted to avoid symptoms and achieve the patient's glucose goals. However, in order to avoid hypoglycemia, insulin does need to be implemented with an appropriate meal plan, may require frequent physician visits for dose adjustment, and generally increases the importance and frequency of home blood glucose monitoring. The functional ability of the patient to successfully draw-up and and administer insulin, carry out home blood glucose monitoring, follow a meal pattern, and manage hypoglycemic reactions needs to be taken into account before insulin therapy is initiated.[69] These factors are particularly important considerations when initiating insulin therapy on an outpatient basis, and the use of home care services may be a helpful and necessary resource during the initial phase.

The use of insulin along with oral agents has been proposed for the treatment of some persons, particularly those with insulin resistance. The benefits of using combination therapy remains controversial at this time.

Blood glucose monitoring is recommended for all persons taking insulin. It is used to provide longitudinal data related to blood glucose levels, as an aid in day-to-day decision making, recognizing emergency situations, and educating patients about the impact of food, activity, medication, and stress on their blood glucose levels.[1] However, it has been reported that only 6% of patients with NIDDM practiced blood glucose monitoring with some regularity, and of those only 20% used the information to make adjustments in insulin dosages.[31] There is evidence to support the value of home blood glucose monitoring for persons with NIDDM. In one study of patients with NIDDM (mean age, 56.3), less frequent blood glucose monitoring was significantly correlated with higher glycosylated hemoglobin values.[78] In another study of patients with insulin-requiring NIDDM (mean age, 55.6), patients who used daily fasting blood glucose measurements to make insulin dose adjustments based on an algorithm were able to bring their glycosylated hemoglobin values into the normal range.[18] Therefore, older adults need to be taught not only how to do home blood glucose monitoring but also how to use the information to make adjustments in meal planning, activity, and insulin doses. Blood glucose monitoring can also be a useful tool for persons taking oral medications and for those on diet only. It can provide concrete evidence to reinforce their behavior and needs to be presented as an appropriate option for them. Meters that are more user friendly and less technique-dependent are generally most appropriate for older adults.

Educational considerations

Older adults with diabetes appear to be a neglected population when it comes to education. Jenny found that aged adults (mean age, 71.7) received the least amount of diabetes instruction of any age group. Older adults (mean age, 57.3) had the highest level of motivation and the second lowest level of instruction.[34] Hiss found that in a study of 372 patients with NIDDM, 64% of those 64 years of age or less had attended a diabetes educational program within the past 2 years as compared with 55% of patients over 64 years of age. When specific areas of educational information were examined in this same study, it was found that patients 64 and older reported that they had been told to follow a diet less often (84% versus 92%), to exercise less often (22% versus 35%), and to take special care of their feet less often (52% versus 63%) than were patients 45 to 64 years of age.[31]

Perhaps one of the reasons diabetes education has been neglected among this population is because of the inherent difficulties of teaching older people. Difficulty in comprehension does increase with age, and other cognitive and sensory deficits may be present.[34] Yet this group deserves special attention and consideration because of the high incidence of diabetes in persons 65 and older and because they are at risk for developing its major complications.

Older persons can be taught and can learn more easily if providers adjust the teaching plan to meet their needs. Special considerations for teaching older adults include taking into account functional ability, particularly aspects that may be affected by the aging process, the treatment programs of any concomitant illnesses or diabetes-related complications, ethnic and cultural background, and the patients' personal strengths and goals related to their health and the treatment of diabetes.

Functional limitations

Functional limitations among the elderly have implications for both the educational approach and care practices. Visual or other sensory deficits may require the health care professional to make modifications in order to accommodate the needs of these patients. For example, if the teaching session involves using a chalkboard, white on black generally works best for patients with visual deficits. Glossy boards may create a glare and colored markers may be difficult to see, especially red, yellow, blue, and orange.[40] Patients with early cataracts or decreased ability to distinguish colors are not good candidates for visual methods of blood glucose monitoring. Insulin administration techniques may need to be modified to compensate for a decline in visual acuity or double vision. Magnifying glasses may be useful, particularly the types that attach to a syringe or can be worn around the neck, thus leaving the patient's hands free. In some cases, insulin may need to be prepared by a family member or home care nurse ahead of time to be administered by the patient.

Booklets, pamphlets, videotapes, and other visual aids are frequently used as adjuncts to an educational program. Materials that use a large amount of white space on each page, are written in a conversational style, use 10 or 11 point type, and are black type on white or yellow paper work best for older patients with visual deficits or impairments.[15] Glossy boards should not be used to project video images because of the potential for glare, and the sound needs to be carefully modulated. Video materials that can be played more than once may be especially helpful for older persons who need a longer time to process new information.[40] Choosing written and videotape materials that feature both older adults and appropriate ethnic groups will increase the elderly person's perception that the content is relevant to them.

Group classes may be less effective for persons with hearing deficits than one-to-one interactions in which the provider can assess whether the person is hearing what is said by asking him or her to repeat it. In these interactions, the provider should face the individual and enunciate words clearly. Eliminating background noises and providing education in a quiet room is also helpful. Because the inability to hear high-pitched tones is often lost, speaking loudly does not necessarily help the patient hear better.[40] Some types of hearing loss can be helped through the use of hearing aids, and it is recommended that all persons with hearing deficits be referred for testing.

Because of sensory and cognitive deficits, some older persons with diabetes respond more slowly to stimuli and may have a decreased ability to organize information. Adjustments in the teaching process need to reflect these changes in order to be effective. Content should be presented in a concrete, factual way so that it can be readily applied. Scheduling teaching sessions that are short, focused on a limited number of concepts, are paced to allow time to synthesize, and provide adequate time to request responses so that understanding can be checked, will increase the likelihood of success. Memory can be increased by helping the person "set the stage" for what is coming next by offering cues about the information that will be offered.[15] External cues to serve as a reminder are useful for patients with specific memory deficits. The cues should be specific and active, such as taping a syringe to the bathroom mirror.[83]

In order to care for diabetes, individuals require knowledge, skills, appropriate tools, and practice. Many areas of care require both knowledge and skills. For example, persons with diabetes need to not only hear about the importance of foot care but to also have the opportunity to practice the associated skills before they can carry it out at home.[21] When teaching skills to older adults, time must be given to process the instruction before the skill is performed. It is generally most effective to give the instructions one step at a time, allowing practice time between steps.[40] The opportunity to practice any required skills may become particularly important for older adults. The practice time not only allows the individual to enhance his/her skills but also provides the educator with the opportunity to observe the patient's ability to perform the skill. If physical limitations exist, the provider will need to suggest and teach alternative methods to carry out the skill. For example, persons with arthritis or tremors may find it easier to trigger a penlet device used to obtain the blood sample for monitoring by pressing the tigger down on a tabletop rather than trying to hold it steady and trigger the device.

The educational plan needs to take into account any concomitant acute or chronic illnesses and diabetes complications present. For example, for an individual who has a prosthetic leg, getting up, putting on the leg, getting to the bathroom, doing a blood glucose test, taking medications, and at last, getting to the kitchen and making a simple breakfast or having one that can be prepared ahead is an important consideration. The older person may also need assistance to manage several regimens, all of which may be complex and necessitate behavior change.

Ethnic and cultural considerations

Ethnicity is an important consideration in the educational process. Our ethnicity influences not only who we are, how we perceive ourselves, and our moral beliefs, but also our beliefs and perceptions about health and health care. Food, language, and health care practices are all symbols of ethnicity and cultural beliefs. When health professionals and persons with diabetes are from different ethnic and cultural backgrounds, they may have different beliefs and expectations about health behaviors, which can lead to conflict. For example, many cultures have active folk medicine systems that may be tried first or along with conventional methods.[75] Health care providers may not recognize some of the patients' self-care activities because they do not fit with the traditional medical model. Ethnic food preferences need to be incorporated into the meal pattern and folk medicine practices recognized as part of the diabetes care plan.

Incorrect health beliefs that stem from cultural influences need to be addressed. Many older patients' experiences with diabetes lead to the belief that its complications are inevitable. When combined with the fatalistic attitude toward illness and the strong sense of present common to many ethnic groups, education about preventative self-care practices may seem irrelevant and may lead to a lack of adherence.[32]

The educational program and materials need to be culturally sensitive and relevant to the persons for whom it is provided. The language and words used need to match the patient's language. Even among patients for whom English is the first language, words may be used differently or have a different meaning among some ethnic groups. Literal translations of English materials into other languages may not convey the actual message as appropriately as translating the material into words that express its meaning. Literacy in both the patient's native language and English needs to be taken into account. Some patients who speak more fluently in their native language may actually read better in English. The people depicted in print and video materials need to match the age group and ethnic mix of the intended audience.

Group classes

Group classes for diabetes education have become increasingly popular, in part because of reimbursement structures. Persons with limited social support may profit from the experiences of others, interaction with persons who face similar problems, and peer support. However, older persons may be intimidated by an educational program that is too formal or too much like school.[40] Group classes are probably most appropriate for patients who have basic knowledge about diabetes and no sensory or cognitive deficits.

Diabetes self-care does not occur in a vacuum and is carried out within the context of all aspects of a person's life. The educational program and choice of content needs to be selected based on jointly identified goals, interests, abilities, and needs.

One of the myths about aging is that older people cannot learn. Health professionals and older persons alike may believe that the elderly are not educable. This is a false perception. Learning continues throughout the life cycle, although some older adults may learn more slowly and be more discriminating about what is learned.[40] Education is an important part of the care of patients with diabetes, and older adults deserve the same opportunity to learn as their younger counterparts.

Behavioral strategies

The purpose of education is to provide new knowledge and understanding, and the purpose of health education is positive behavioral change.[16] While most behavioral intervention studies have not included age as a factor, it is reasonable to conclude that older adults living in the community are as amenable to behavioral strategies, such as contracting or goal setting, as their younger counterparts.[2] Teaching sessions that include a discussion of treatment benefits, techniques for making changes, specific information about ways to incorporate changes, and potential barriers may positively influence patient outcomes.[77] As an example, in the DIABEDS study, a sample of older, African American females, (mean age, 58.1) taught skill exercises and behavior modification techniques experienced significantly better self-care skills and adherence behaviors and improved metabolic control.[52] In addition, decreasing the complexity of the regimen and tailoring the intervention to the individual as much as possible are particularly relevent strategies for this age group.[2] It is likely that most older adults are just as capable of becoming active participants in their diabetes care as younger adults, and strategies that help to empower patients for that purpose are equally appropriate for both groups.

It is important to recognize any underlying social, functional, and psychologic changes related to the aging process when working with older adults. All aspects of functional states as well as all other acute and chronic illnesses must be taken into account when implementing any behavioral or life-style change programs.[2] If significant cognitive impairment exists, a complex regimen requiring extensive education, behavior change, and patient involvement is likely to fail.[42]

Assessment and Planning

As outlined in Table 15-8, patient assessment is the first step in the educational process for older adults. An example of an educational assessment for older adults is included in Appendix 15a. The assessment may appear to be lengthy and time consuming, but it is an essential beginning to education. Ultimately the assessment can save time by assisting the health professional to focus the teaching process and to plan for a more formal and extensive education program. Using information gleaned from the assessment prevents stereotyping of older patients into predetermined categories and allows the educational intervention to be tailored for individual needs. The assessment of newly diagnosed individuals is extensive and provides a baseline diabetes profile of each individual. However, the health status and functional abilities of older adults are not static and need frequent reevaluation.

Table 15-8 Educational Process for Older Adults

Assessment	Education	Follow-up/reassessment
Diabetes knowledge	Plan	Educational progress and adherence
Current health beliefs and practices		
Physical function/ability	Specific content	Coordinate home care and community resources
Sensory ability	Educational materials	
Cognitive ability	Use of appropriate teaching/behavioral strategies	
Social support		
Financial status		
Literacy		
Readiness to learn		

Reproduced with permission of the American Diabetes Association, Inc. Funnell MM: Role of the diabetes educator for older adults, Diabetes Care 13(suppl 2):60-65, 1990.

Thus, the assessment process needs to be ongoing and incorporated into each interaction.[21] Noting the individual's functional, sensory, cognitive, psychosocial, and educational status on the diabetes flow chart or patient education record is an effective strategy that not only helps the health care professional to follow the patient's progress but also serves as a reminder for reassessment.[63]

The initial assessment needs to include a review of the individual's existing functional abilities, including knowledge and beliefs about diabetes and its care, physical ability, sensory ability, cognitive ability, emotional status, social support system, financial status, literacy, and readiness to learn. During the assessment, older adults should be given the opportunity to express their own interests, beliefs, treatment goals, values, emotions, and attitudes about diabetes.[76]

Diabetes knowledge and beliefs

Even though newly diagnosed, older adults have frequently had experience with diabetes through spouses, family members, or friends. Some have seen the harmful effects of the complications of diabetes and believe that diabetes automatically means blindness or an amputation. Other individuals may view diabetes as a natural part of the aging process and do not take it very seriously. Still others have learned inaccurate information or have seen people with diabetes take poor care of themselves. These experiences and beliefs can have an impact on both the educational process and the individuals' willingness to care for their diabetes. Asking older adults if they have ever known anyone with diabetes and what effect it had on them is one way to obtain this information. Misconceptions about diabetes may need to be clarified and advancements in treatment options presented as the first step in the educational process. Written knowledge tests might also provide some of this information, but their usefulness has not been fully evaluated among older patients.[21]

Physical function

Age-related changes in physical function can affect diabetes self-care activities. These include anorexia leading to hypoglycemia and inadequate nutrition; arthritis or tremors interfering with insulin administration, home blood glucose monitoring, foot care, and food shopping and preparation; and concurrent illnesses with complex regimens that can interfere with the person's ability to do them.[58] Many of these physical impairments can be compensated for and strategies can be recommended to overcome deficits, if they are noted.

The older adult's ability to perform activities of daily living needs to be assessed. This assessment can range from informal questions to observing task performance to formal questionnaires. Because health professionals tend to overestimate functioning, a more systematic assessment is probably useful.[63] Many functional assessment tools that measure items related to physical function in various ways are available, but no single tool is appropriate for all patients.[22,36,63] Different tools uncover different problems to different degrees. The assessment instrument included in Appendix 15a includes questions related to overall physical functioning. Instruments specifically designed to test the functional capacity of older adults to perform self-management tasks, such as the Assessment of Diabetes Ability Performance Tool (ADAPT), may be useful.[11] This initial assessment needs to be followed-up with repeat administrations of the tool or direct observations of the patient's ability to carry out diabetes care tasks at each visit.

Pain from arthritis, peripheral neuropathy, or other problems may be present and more severe in older adults. The experience of pain has important implications for older adults and their ability to care for themselves, yet it is difficult to measure. Because pain is completely subjective, asking if older adults have pain and how much it limits their ability to perform ADLs should be part of the assessment process. Pain may not only lead to decreased activity, but also to sporadic intake of food and/or overeating, which can affect glycemic control. Treatment for any painful conditions is based on their causes.

Impotence occurs in 95% of the men with diabetes who are over the age of 70.[58] Because sexual functioning can play such an important role in total quality of life at any age, it needs to be addressed for both older men and older women.

Sensory ability

Altered vision can interfere with insulin administration and home blood glucose monitoring. Standardized visual acuity and color vision tests can be administered. In addition, asking patients to read standard news print, numbers on a syringe, or to repeat back what was said to them can provide information to assist the health professional in order to make adjustments in the teaching or care program. Annual ophthalmologic

Table 15-9   An Informal Hearing Test

Test words	Response in hearing-impaired
Fill	Fine
Catch	Cat
Thumb	Fun
Heap	Heat
Wise	Wives
Wedge	Red
Fish	Fifth
Snows	Phones
Bed	Bugs

Adapted with permission of the American Diabetes Association, Inc, from Miller LV: Managing the elderly patient with diabetes, Clin Diabetes 4:74-76, 90, 1985.

examinations are recommended for older adults with diabetes, just as they are for all adults with diabetes.

Diminished hearing can negatively affect an individual's ability to hear and understand the information that they need to care for themselves. Informal tests of hearing can be conducted by standing behind the person, saying a list of key words and asking the patient to repeat what you said.[56] An informal test of key words, and common responses that would indicate mild to moderate hearing impairments is listed in Table 15-9. Patients with any signs of hearing loss should be referred to an audiologist for further testing.

Cognitive ability

Cognitive abilities have an impact on the ability of the older person to both learn about diabetes care and carry out the treatment program. For example, choosing and measuring foods and deciding when to call a health care professional about a skin infection or blood glucose readings require both knowledge and judgment. Memory deficits are of particular concern for patients taking insulin. The ability to remember to take the insulin and whether a dose has been given or not has obvious safety implications for these patients. Principal areas of cognitive function that need to be assessed among older persons include orientation, attention, language, recall, calculation. and visuospatial ability.[57] All of these can be screened with standard mental status examinations such as the Folstein "Mini-Mental State" (see box on pp. 548-550) or other tests.[19,22] Subtle changes in cognitive function usually require formal neuropsychologic testing, which can also help to identify the degree to which depression is affecting cognitive impairment.

Emotional status

Depression is extremely common in older adults, but is not always recognized. Affective changes seen in younger persons may not be present in older adults. Signs and symptoms of depression such as an unkempt appearance, poor attention, reduced mem-

MINI-MENTAL STATE

Patient _____ Examiner _____ Date _____

Maximum	Actual score	Orientation
5	( )	What is the (year)(season) (date)(day) (month)?
5	( )	Where are we (state)(county) (town)(clinic) (floor)? Give 1 point for each correct.

		Registration
3	( )	Name 3 objects: 1 second to say each. Then ask the patient all 3 after you have said them. Give 1 point for each correct answer. This first repetition determines his score (0–3) but keep saying them until he can repeat all 3 up to 6 trials. Count trials and record. Trials: _____

Maximum	Actual score	Recall
3	( )	Ask for the 3 objects repeated above. Give 1 point for each correct.

		Language
2	( )	Name a pencil and a watch
1	( )	Repeat the following "No ifs, ands or buts"
3	( )	Follow a 3-stage command: "Take a paper in your right hand, fold it in half, and put in on the floor"
1	( )	Read and obey "CLOSE YOUR EYES" below
1	( )	Write a sentence on the line below
1	( )	Copy design below

Attention and calculation: serial 7's

5   ( )   Go back from 100 by 7's. 1 point for each correct. Stop after 5 answers. If the patient cannot or will not perform this task, ask him to spell the word "world" backwards. The score is the number of letters in correct order e.g. dlrow = 5, dlorw = 3

30

Total score _____

Indicate level of consciousness

Alert   Drowsy   Stupor   Coma

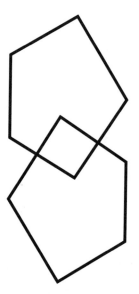

X _____

CLOSE YOUR EYES

INSTRUCTIONS FOR ADMINISTRATION OF MINIMENTAL STATE EXAMINATION

Orientation

(1) Ask for the date. Then ask specifically for parts omitted, e.g., "Can you also tell me what season it is?" One point for each correct.

(2) Ask in turn "Can you tell me the name of this hospital?" (town, county, etc.). One point for each correct.

Registration

Ask the patient if you may test his memory. Then say the names of 3 unrelated objects, clearly and slowly, about one second for each. After you have said all 3, ask him to repeat them. This first repetition determines his score (0-3) but keep saying them until he can repeat all three, up to 6 trials. If he does not eventually learn all 3, recall cannot be meaningfully tested.

Attention and calculation

Ask the patient to begin with 100 and count backwards by 7. Stop after 5 subtractions (93, 86, 79, 72, 65). Score the total number of correct answers.

If the patient cannot or will not perform this task, ask him to spell the word "world" backwards. The score is the number of letters in correct order. E.g. dlrow = 5, dlorw = 3.

Recall

Ask the patient if he can recall the 3 words you previously asked him to remember. Score 0-3.

Language

Naming: Show the patient a wrist watch and ask him what it is. Repeat for pencil. Score 0-2.

Repetition: Ask the patient to repeat the sentence after you. Allow only one trial. Score 0 or 1.

3-stage command: Give the patient a piece of blank paper and repeat the command. Score 1 point for each part correctly executed.

Reading: On a blank piece of paper print the sentence "Close your eyes," in letters large enough for the patient to see clearly. Ask him to read it and do what it says. Score 1 point only if he actually closes his eyes.

Writing: Give the patient a blank piece of paper and ask him to write a sentence for you. Do not dictate a sentence, it is to be written spontaneously. It must contain a subject and verb and be sensible. Correct grammar and punctuation are not necessary.

Copying: On a clean piece of paper, draw intersecting pentagons, each side about 1 inch, and ask him to copy it exactly as it is. All 10 angles must be present and 2 must intersect to score 1 point. Tremor and rotation are ignored.

Estimate the patient's level of sensorium along a continuum, from alert on the left to coma on the right.

From Folstein MF, Folstein SE, and McHugh PR: Mini-mental state: a practical method for grading the cognitive state of patients for the clinician, J Psychiatr Res 12:189-198, 1975, Pergamon Press.

ory, and lack of initiative are often mistaken for dementia. Standardized tests, such as the Geriatric Depression Scale, are available to assess levels of depression.[22, 90] In addition, asking older adults about their mood and feelings not only provides the health care provider with information, but lets the older adults know that these are important areas for discussion.

Older adults do experience strong feelings about having an illness such as diabetes, and these feelings need to be acknowledged and discussed. Because many older people were brought up to be stoic and not discuss their emotions, asking that they tell you their thoughts about their diabetes may elicit more of a response than asking how they feel about it.

Social support

The lack of social support identified by older patients has already been discussed. Asking older adults who helps them with their diabetes care and who they turn to in times of trouble can provide information about the amount of support patients perceive is available to them. In addition, asking who shops for and cooks most of the food is important when planning an educational intervention related to nutrition. Among minorities, extended families, friends, and church groups are likely sources of social support that need to be considered.

Financial status

As already noted, diabetes is an expensive disease. Because income and expenditures are often less clearly defined among older people, it is generally more useful to ask if their income is adequate or inadequate for their needs rather than to ask for the amount of the annual income. Information about insurance coverage for diabetes care and supplies is also important before recommendations are made for a particular care program. Additionally, individuals may not be aware of benefits to which they are entitled under changing Medicare and Medicaid guidelines, and they will benefit from this information.

Literacy

A survey of 105 patients over age 64 found that 21% read at less than eighth grade level, 30% at eighth to twelfth grade level, and 49% at above the 12th grade level.[31] Tests of frequently used diabetes patient education booklets revealed that the booklets were written at a mean grade level of 10.2, because the very nature of health-related information and terminology skews reading level toward the higher grades.[6,82] These studies demonstrate the importance of determining literacy and matching educational materials to the individual's reading and cognitive ability. Simple tools of reading ability are available and can be incorporated as part of the assessment.

Readiness to learn

Readiness to learn involves emotional and experiential readiness and is a reflection of the individual's background of experiences, skills, attitudes, and ability to learn. Readiness can be affected by both physical health and current emotional status and can reflect health beliefs.[73] For example, older adults who are experiencing strong emotions, such as shock or denial, are rarely ready to learn. The health care provider needs to be sensitive to the fact that these factors are subtle and may not be readily apparent in the assessment process.[76]

Ongoing care

The continuing assessment during ongoing care provides the opportunity to answer questions, reinforce previous learning, and give positive feedback on self-care strengths. Asking older adults to tell you what they are doing to care for their diabetes and observing their self-care skills, such as insulin administration and blood testing, are useful indicators of both changes from the initial assessment and current care practices. This information can be used to offer individualized recommendations and suggestions in areas of self-care declines or deficits. It is important, however, that the provider be nonjudgmental, be noncritical of the patient's self-care efforts, and reflect a positive and caring attitude.[76]

The ongoing assessment also includes continued follow-up with the patient to determine progress in meeting goals and to determine if other referrals or resources are needed.

Implementation and Evaluation

Specific diabetes content areas for the educational program are no different for older adults than other persons with diabetes. The content needs to be relevant to the type of diabetes that they have, stated interest, and treatment regimen and goals. Foot care is an often neglected topic that deserves particular emphasis for older adults because they are at risk for foot problems, gangrene, and amputations. It is generally recommended that, whenever possible, diabetes content be presented sequentially over a period of time at a pace that meets the individual's needs. This is particularly important for older patients who may need additional time to assimilate new information. Because of the amount of content needed for diabetes self-care, one approach that may be useful in working with older patients is to divide the content into manageable sections in an effort to make it less overwhelming to both older adults and health care providers.

One recommendation is to divide the content into three levels: initial, home management, and improvement in life-style. The initial management level includes only the survival skills needed for diabetes care. The person who is newly diagnosed, the person who has had diabetes for a while but has received limited formal education, or the person who is experiencing a major change in treatment such as starting insulin is generally at this level. The home management level contains information that patients can use in the daily care of diabetes and to enhance their ability to manage their illness in a more flexible, realistic, and appropriate way. This level includes the majority of the content areas. The improvement in life-style level contains information for persons who have learned to manage their diabetes successfully on a daily basis and who need information on specific topics.[26] An example of appropriate topics for each of these levels is listed in Table

Table 15-10   Sample Educational Program

Initial management	Home management	Lifestyle change
What is diabetes?	More facts about diabetes	Tips for changing your health
Feelings about diabetes	The balance of food, exercise,	habits
What foods should I eat?	and medicines	Coping with stress
Weight loss	Living with diabetes	Your exercise program
Diabetes pills	How families can help	Travel
Giving insulin	Why a "diet"?	What's in food?
Monitoring your diabetes	Healthy food choices	The exchange diet
Foot care	Practical tips for planning meals	What does the label say?
	Physical activity	Special diet food and
	Facts about insulin	sweeteners
	How to use monitoring	Eating away from home
	information	Fiber
	Low blood sugar	Alcohol and diabetes
	(hypoglycemia)	Taking charge of your diet
	High blood sugar	Sexual health
	(hyperglycemia)	Taking care of diabetes with
	Sick day care	other illnesses
	Personal care	The older person with diabetes
	Long-term problems and risk	Community resources
	factors	Being a smart shopper
	Complications of diabetes	Working with your health care
		team

15-10. It should be noted that the definition of each of these levels can vary according to individual needs and that some topics may need to be presented at more than one level in varying degrees of complexity.

Adherence issues

There is no clear-cut evidence that age is positively or negatively correlated with adherence. Issues that affect adherence among younger persons such as regimen complexity, patient-provider relationships, health beliefs, and social support appear to have similar effects on older adults' adherence behaviors.[2] In addition, the need to manage more than one complex regimen is more likely to negatively affect adherence among older patients, as are the physical limitations imposed by other chronic illnesses.

Older persons appear to accept diabetes as a natural part of the aging process and identify the least number of barriers to adherence.[34] However, the perception of diabetes as less threatening may also lead to decreased adherence with the treatment plan, particularly among those who do not use insulin.[12] Reinforcing that diabetes is a serious disease, without using scare tactics, may be appropriate when working with some patients. Assisting persons to cope with the demands and limitations of other illnesses and to organize self-care behaviors for all aspects of their health are also helpful to enhance adherence.

Role of the diabetes health care team

The health care team for older adults should include the same members as any other care team for adults with diabetes, with the addition of an expert in gerontology. Because most older adults strive to maintain their independence, social workers have a particularly important role to play. Appropriate referral to community resources can help patients to remain in their preferred environment as long as possible.

The role of the health care team is to first assess functional ability and put it into perspective along with the severity of diabetes and other health problems and total health status. Treatment goals should be established by the patient and those involved with their daily care. The role of the team is then to assist patients to carry out the diabetes care program, to meet their care goals, to maximize their self-care abilities, and to remain safe and independent for as long as is possible. The team's activities include diabetes care and education, coordination of community resources and referrals, and communication with other health care providers who are involved in the individual's total health care. This may include contact with pharmacists, podiatrists, neighbors, and extended family members, as well as community agencies.

For older adults who require foster care, nursing home, or other institutional care, the health care team needs to provide information and serve as a resource to the facility staff. If desired, inservice educational programs that are either targeted for the specific needs of that person or more general in nature can be provided.

Role of the older adult and family

Diabetes is a chronic illness that requires long-term active patient participation in order to maintain metabolic control. The need for the patient to carry out daily self-care behaviors is no less important simply because the patients are older. However, older adults do have unique difficulties and needs because of the physical limitations that may be imposed by the aging process and the increased likelihood of the presence of other chronic illnesses and complications. While these events do cause some difficulties, most can either be treated or be compensated for in some way.

Educational programs designed to meet the specific needs of older adults and their families need to be developed and provided. Including family members in the teaching process is of particular importance for older adults because of the likelihood that impairments related to the aging process will increase their need for assistance. Social support, or the lack of it, appears to have an impact on adherence behaviors. It may be beneficial to assist patients and family members to develop strategies to minimize the problems of social isolation related to diabetes, such as leaving insulin or monitoring supplies at a family member's house where they often eat dinner. In addition, it has been demonstrated that including spouses in diabetes education classes for older male adults (age 65 to 82) significantly improved metabolic outcomes, diabetes knowledge and family involvement, and reduced stress.[25]

While families can provide a great deal of assistance with and support for the diabetes care regimen, it is important to recognize that spouses may be frail or have chronic illnesses of their own and therefore be unable to adequately support or care for a spouse with diabetes. The daily nature of diabetes care may make it difficult for adult children with other family and work responsibilities to be involved in the routine aspects of care. In these situations, the patient may need referral to outside resources for assistance. Home care agencies, Visiting Nurse Associations, Meals-On-Wheels, or other community resources may be available to provide daily support. It may be helpful to suggest to family members that they can, however, recognize the patients' positive efforts to care for themselves and provide support and reinforcement even when daily assistance is not possible.

Outcome evaluation

A number of measures have been suggested as outcome evaluation criteria for diabetes care and education. These include metabolic control, adherence, knowledge, skills, behavior, patient attitudes, use of health services, days missed from work, hospitalizations, complications, and costs. None of these has been found to be entirely satisfactory criteria.[37] This is especially true for older adults who frequently have concomitant medical problems and other disabilities. Evaluation measures for older patients may best be based on maintenance or improvement in health status, quality of life, personal progress, goal attainment, and the ability of the patient or caregiver to effectively manage diabetes on a daily basis.[21]

RESEARCH IMPLICATIONS

Research about diabetes among older adults and its impact is a newer area of interest and a great deal of work still needs to be done. General areas include the physiologic impact of hyperglycemia on the elderly; appropriate treatment modalities for older adults; the concomitant physical and psychosocial effects of diabetes, its complications, and other illnesses among the elderly; the psychosocial impact of diabetes; and educational and behavioral strategies that are most effective with this population.

Specifically, the effects of metabolic control on the long-term health of older adults need to be explored further. Patients and health professionals often do not appear to consider diabetes to be a serious disease in older adults. Documentation of the effects of diabetes are needed to verify or alter this perception. Additionally, studies of the treatment methods to achieve the needed levels of glycemic control for this population are needed. Insulin use and particularly intensive insulin programs remain controversial for treating older patients and the efficacy, costs, and benefits of such programs need clarification. Because older adults frequently experience diabetes complications or have other chronic illnesses along with diabetes, both the physical and psychosocial impacts of multiple health problems in this population need to be explored.

The psychosocial impact of diabetes and the personal meaning that older patients and their families attach to it need further study. Strategies that can be used to increase the effectiveness of teaching efforts when working with older adults need to be tested and implemented. Educational materials specifically for older adults and methods that would enhance learning among this group of individuals need to be developed and tested. Another area in which more research is needed is in the field of adherence. Behavioral strategies that could be used to assist older patients to achieve their diabetes and other health care goals need to be designed and evaluated. In short, almost all components of diabetes care and treatment need further exploration for this special population.

REFERENCES

1. American Diabetes Association: Concensus statement—self-monitoring of blood glucose, Diabetes Care 13(suppl 1):41-46, 1990.
2. Anderson LA: Health-care communication and selected psychosocial correlates of adherence in diabetes management, Diabetes Care 13(suppl 2):66-76, 1990.
3. Atchley RC: Social faces and aging, ed 4, Belmont, CA, 1985, Wadsworth Publishing Co.
4. Bahr SJ: The economic well-being in aging families. In Bahr SJ and Peterson ET, eds: Aging and the family, Lexington, MA, 1989, DC Heath & Co.
5. Barber CE: Transition to the empty nest. In Bahr SJ and Peterson ET, eds: Aging and the family, Lexington, MA, 1989, DC Heath & Co.
6. Barr P, Hess G, and Frey ML: Relationships between reading levels and effective patient education, Diabetes 35(suppl):48A, 1986.
7. Barrett-Connor E: Commentary, Diabetes Spectrum 2:164-166, 1989.
8. Cox HG: Later life: the realities of aging, ed 2, Englewood Cliffs, NJ, 1988, Prentice-Hall, Inc.
9. Davidson MB: Diabetes in the elderly: diagnosis and treatment, Hosp Pract 17:113-120, 1982.
10. Davidson MB: The impact of diabetes in the elderly, Diabetes Educ 8:10, 1983.
11. Davis WK, Dedrick RF, and Anderson L: Assessing patients' functional capacity to perform diabetes self-management tasks, Diabetes 39(suppl 1):305A, 1990.
12. Davis WK and others: Psychosocial adjustment to and control of diabetes mellitus: differences by disease type and treatment, Health Psychol 6:1-14, 1987.
13. DeFronzo RA: The triumvirate: B-cell, muscle, liver: a collusion responsible for NIDDM, Diabetes 37:667-687, 1988.
14. Diehl AK, Sugarek NJ, and Bareer RL: Medication compliance in non–insulin-dependent diabetes: a randomized comparison of chlorpropamide and insulin, Diabetes Care 8:219-223, 1985.
15. Doak CC: Communicating with the elderly, Diabetes Educ 8:45-47,64, 1983.
16. Dudley J: Health education and perceived patient needs, Diabetes Educ 15:154-155, 1989.
17. Erickson E: Childhood & society, New York, 1963, WW Norton and Co.
18. Floyd JC Jr and others: Feasibility of adjustment of insulin dose by insulin-requiring type II diabetic patients, Diabetes Care 13:386-392, 1990.
19. Folstein MF, Folstein SE, and McHugh PR: Mini-mental state: a practical method for grading the cognitive state of patients for the clinician, J Psychiatr Res 12:189-98, 1975.
20. Funnell MM and McNitt PM: Autonomic neuropathy: diabetics' hidden foe, Am J Nurs 86:266-270, 1986.
21. Funnell MM: Role of the diabetes educator for older adults, Diabetes Care 13(suppl 2):60-65, 1990.
22. Gallo JJ, Reichel W, and Anderson L: Handbook of geriatric assessment, Rockville, MD, 1988, Aspen Publishers Inc.
23. Gambert SR, ed: Handbook of geriatrics, New York, 1988, Plenum Publishing.
24. Gambert SR: Atypical presentation of diabetes mellitus in the elderly, Geriatr Clin North Am 6:721-730, 1990.
25. Gilden JL and others: Diabetes education programs in elderly patients and their spouses, Diabetes 37(suppl):67A, 1988.
26. American Diabetes Association/American Association of Diabetes Educators: Guidelines for diabetes care, New York, 1981, American Diabetes Association.
27. Halter JB and Christensen NJ: Introduction: diabetes mellitus in elderly people, Diabetes Care 13(suppl 2):1-2, 1990.
28. Halter JB and Morrow LA: Use of sulfonylurea drugs in elderly patients, Diabetes Care 13(suppl 2):86-92, 1990.
29. Harris MI: Epidemiology of diabetes mellitus among the elderly in the United States, Clin Geriatr Med 6:703-729, 1990.
30. Havighurst RJ: Developmental tasks and education, ed 2, New York, 1972, McKay Publishers.

31. Hiss RG, ed: Diabetes in communities, Ann Arbor, 1986, University of Michigan, Diabetes Research and Training Center.
32. Hussey LC and Gilliland K: Compliance, low literacy and locus of control, Nurs Clin North Am 24:605-611, 1989.
33. Jackson RA: Mechanisms of age-related glucose intolerance, Diabetes Care 13(suppl 2):9-19, 1990.
34. Jenny JL: A comparison of four age groups' adaptation to diabetes, Can J Public Health 75:237-244, 1984.
35. Jewler D: A primer on medicare for people with diabetes, Diabetes Forecast 40:17-20, 1987.
36. Kane RA and Kane RL: Assessing the elderly: a practical guide to measurement, Lexington, MA, 1981, DC Heath and Co.
37. Kaplan RM and Davis WK: Evaluating the costs and benefits of outpatient diabetes education and nutrition counseling, Diabetes Care 9:81-88, 1986.
38. Kart CS: The realities of aging: an introduction to gerontology, ed 3, Boston, 1990, Allyn & Bacon.
39. Kart CS and Metress ES: Death and dying. In Kart CS, ed: The realities of aging: an introduction to aging, Boston, 1990, Allyn & Bacon.
40. Kick E: Patient teaching for elders, Nurs Clin North Am 24:681-686, 1989.
41. Knight PV and Kesson CM: Educating the elderly diabetic, Diabetic Med 3:170-172, 1986.
42. Laufer IJ: Diabetes in the elderly, Pract Diabetol 4:7-9, 1985.
43. Leifson J: Physical health of the elderly: impact on families. In Bahr SJ and Peterson ET, eds: Aging and the family, Lexington, MA, 1989, DC Heath & Co.
44. Levinson DJ and others: The seasons of a man's choice, New York, 1978, Alfred A. Knopf Inc.
45. Linn M, Linn BS, and Stein AR: Satisfaction with ambulatory care and compliance in older patients, Med Care 20:606-614, 1982.
46. Lipson LG: Diabetes in the elderly: diagnosis, pathogenesis and therapy, Am J Med 80:10-21, 1986.
47. Lopata H: Widowhood in an American city, Cambridge, MA, 1973, Schenkman Publishing Co.
48. Madsbad S: Classification of diabetes in older adults, Diabetes Care 13(suppl 2):93-95, 1990.
49. Martin DB and Quint AR: Therapy for diabetes. In Diabetes in America: Diabetes data compiled 1984. National Diabetes Data Group, US Department of Health and Human Services, NIH publication no 85-1468, 1985, Chapter XXIV.
50. Matz R: Diabetes mellitus in the elderly, Hosp Pract 21:195-218, 1986.
51. Matz R: Summaries and comments, Diabetes Spect 2:173-174, 1989.
52. Mazzuca SA and others: The diabetes education study: a controlled trial of the effects of diabetes patient education, Diabetes Care 9:1-10, 1986.
53. McDonald J: Alcohol and diabetes, Diabetes Care 3:629-637, 1980.
54. Meneilly GS and others: Counterregulatory responses to insulin-induced glucose reduction in the elderly, J Clin Endocrinol Metab 61:178-182, 1985.
55. Miller LV: Educating the elderly diabetic, Diabetes Ed 10(spec):67-69, 1984.
56. Miller LV: Managing the elderly patient with diabetes, Clin Diabetes 4:74-76, 90, 1985.
57. Minaker KL: What diabetologists should know about elderly patients, Diabetes Care 13(suppl 2):34-46, 1990.
58. Morley JE: Diabetes in elderly patients, Pract Diabetol 7:6-10, 1988.
59. Morrow L and Halter J: Diabetes mellitus in the older adult, Geriatrics 43(suppl):57-65, 1988.
60. Mykkanen L and others: Prevalence of diabetes and impaired glucose tolerance in elderly subjects and their association with obesity and family history of diabetes, Diabetes Care 13:1099-1105, 1990.
61. National Diabetes Data Group: Classification and diagnosis of diabetes mellitus and other categories of glucose intolerance, Diabetes 28:1039-1057, 1979.
62. Neugarten BL and Weinstein KK: The changing American grandparents, J Marriage Family 26:199-204, 1964.
63. O'Connor PJ and Jacobson AM: Functional status measurement in elderly diabetic patients, Clin Geriatr Med 6:865-882, 1990.
64. Pace WD: Geriatric assessment in the office setting, Geriatrics 44:29-35, 1989.
65. Perlmuter LC and others: Decreased cognitive function in aging non-insulin-dependent diabetic patients, Am J Med 77:1043-1048, 1984.
66. Pitcha BW and Larson DC: Elderly widowhood. In Bahr SJ and Peterson ET, eds: Aging and the family, Lexington, MA, 1989, DC Heath & Co.
67. Polin SS: Paying for health care: the high cost of diabetes, Clin Diabetes 3:108-116, 1985.

68. Poplin LE: Diabetes that first occurs in older people, Nutr Today 17:4-13, 1982.
69. Porte D Jr and Kahn SE: What geriatricians should know about diabetes mellitus, Diabetes Care 13(suppl 2):47-54, 1990.
70. Powers MA, Kohrs MB, and Raimondi MP: Diabetes nutrition and management for the elderly, Diabetes Educ 8:26-33, 1983.
71. Reaven GM: Clinician's guide to non–insulin-dependent diabetes mellitus, ed 2, New York, 1989, Marcel Dekker Inc.
72. Reaven G and others: Relationship between hyperglycemia and cognitive function in older NIDDM patients, Diabetes Care 13:16-21, 1990.
73. Redman BK: The process of patient teaching in nursing, ed 4, St. Louis, 1980, Mosby–Year Book Co.
74. Reed RL and Mooradian AD: Nutritional status and dietary management of elderly diabetic patients, Clin Geriatr Med 6:883-901, 1990.
75. Rempusheski VF: The role of ethnicity in elder care, Nurs Clin North Am 24:717-725, 1989.
76. Resler MM: Teaching strategies that promote adherence, Nurs Clin North Am 18:799-811, 1983.
77. Rosenstock IM: Understanding and enhancing patient compliance with diabetic regimens, Diabetes Care 8:610-615, 1985.
78. Rost FM and others: Self-care predictors of metabolic control in NIDDM patients, Diabetes Care 13:1111-1113, 1990.
79. Schwartz AN, Snyder CL, and Peterson JA: Aging and life: an introduction to gerentology, ed 2, New York, 1984, Holt, Rhinehart & Winston.
80. Schwartz RS: Exercise training in the treatment of diabetes mellitus in elderly patients, Diabetes Care 13(suppl 2):77-84, 1990.
81. Sherman RA: Diabetes and its complications, Diagnosis May, pp. 127-136, 1985.
82. Streif LD: Can clients understand our instructions? Image J Nurs Scholar 18:48-52, 1986.
83. Tun PA, Nathan DM, and Perlmuter LC: Cognitive and affective disorders in elderly diabetics, Clin Geriatr Med 6:731-746, 1990.
84. US Department of Health and Human Services: Diabetes surveillance 1980-1987, Atlanta, 1990, Centers for Disease Control.
85. Wachtel TJ: The diabetic hyperosmolar state, Clin Geriatr Med 6:797-806, 1990.
86. Weick HH and others: Senile dementia in geriatrics. In Platt D, ed: Geriatrics, New York, 1982, Springer Publishing Co.
87. Weinberger M and others: Economic impact of diabetes mellitus in the elderly, Clin Geriatr Med 6:959-970, 1990.
88. Wingard D and others: Community based study of prevalence of NIDDM in older adults, Diabetes Care 13(suppl 2):3-8, 1990.
89. Woodruff-Pak DS: Psychology and aging, Englewood Cliffs, NJ, 1988, Prentice-Hall, Inc.
90. Yesavage JA: Geriatric depression scale, Psychopharmacol Bull, 24:709-11, 1988.

Educational Assessment
of Older Adult With Diabetes
(Patient Form)*

To help us work with you, we would like you to fill out this form about yourself, the way you live, and the things you do at home to take care of yourself. Your answers to these questions are very important and help us to get to know you better. If you do not understand a question or are unsure of your answer, please leave it blank and we will review it with you.

1. Are you interested in learning more about diabetes and its care?
   ☐ No
   ☐ Yes

2. If you have been given information on the following topics, please check all that apply.

	Yes	If so, when	Would like more information
a. Feelings about diabetes			
b. Meal planning			
c. Exercise			
d. Insulin			
e. Blood sugar testing			
f. Low blood sugar			
g. High blood sugar			
h. Personal health habits			
i. Sick day care			
j. Complications of diabetes			
k. Risk factors (smoking, etc.)			
l. Other			

*Adapted from the Michigan Diabetes Research and Training Center: Diabetes care for older adults project, Ann Arbor, Mich, 1988.

3. Do you ever seek out information about diabetes?
   (e.g., TV programs, magazine articles, books)
   ☐ No
   ☐ Yes

4. How is your diabetes treated?
   ☐ Diet only
   ☐ Diabetes pills   Name of pill _____   Time taken _____
   Insulin: How many times a day _____
         Types of insulin _____
         Who gives your shot? _____

5. On the average, how many *days* out of a week do you:

   a. Eat breakfast?   None   1   2   3   4   5   6   7
   b. Eat lunch?   None   1   2   3   4   5   6   7
   c. Eat dinner?   None   1   2   3   4   5   6   7

6. Mark the times at which you *usually* eat by placing a B, L, D or S in the box below the time.

           B = breakfast
           L = lunch
           D = dinner
           S = snack

	AM						Noon								PM				
5	6	7	8	9	10	11	12	1	2	3	4	5	6	7	8	9	10	11	12

7. Do you eat your meals at the same time every day?
   ☐ Never
   ☐ 1 to 3 times/week
   ☐ 4 to 7 times/week
   ☐ More than 7 times/week

8. If you eat less than 3 meals a day, are you willing to eat more meals per day?
   ☐ No
   ☐ Yes

9. Do you follow any kind of special diet?
   ☐ No
   ☐ Yes   If yes, what? _____

10. Do you take any vitamin, mineral or other nutritional supplements?
    ☐ No
    ☐ Yes   If yes, what? _____

11. How long have you been at your current weight? _____

12. On the average, how often in a week do you eat sugar foods such as candy, cookies, pie, etc.?
    ☐ Never
    ☐ 1 to 3 times/week
    ☐ 4 to 7 times/week
    ☐ More than 7 times/week

13. Do you have a regular exercise plan?
    ☐ No   Why not? _____
    ☐ Yes   What is it? _____
            How many days of the week do you do it? _____
            How many minutes do you do it each time? _____

14. Would you like to have an exercise plan?
    ☐ No
    ☐ Yes   If yes, what would you be able to do? _____
    _____

15. Do you test for sugar at home?
    ☐ No
    ☐ Yes   How many days of the week do you test? _____
            On days you do tests, how often do you test? _____
            What times of the day? _____

16. Do you test your urine for ketones at home?
    ☐ No
    ☐ Yes   Who does the tests? _____

17. Do you change your diet, exercise, or medicine dose as a result of the tests?
    ☐ No
    ☐ Yes   What do you change? _____
            How do you change it? _____

18. Do you take special care of your feet?
    ☐ No
    ☐ Yes   What do you do? _____

19. a) Do you ever have **low** blood sugar?

☐ No

☐ Yes   If yes, about how often? _____

b) How do you feel when your blood sugar is **low?** _____

_____

c) What do you do if your blood sugar is **low?**

☐ Nothing

☐ Something, which is _____

_____

20. a) Do you ever have **high** blood sugar?

☐ No

☐ Yes   If yes, about how often? _____

b) How do you feel when your blood sugar is **high?** _____

_____

c) What do you do if your blood sugar is **high?**

☐ Nothing

☐ Something, which is _____

21. Most of the time, how well do you follow your treatment plan? (Circle one)

	No plan	Not well	Fairly well	Very well
a. diabetes medication	0	1	2	3
b. meal plan	0	1	2	3
c. testing for sugar	0	1	2	3
d. exercise plan	0	1	2	3

22. Do you wear/carry diabetes identification?

☐ No

☐ Yes

23. Place an X in the appropriate place to show whether or not you need help and whether or not you get help for each of the following:

	Do not need help	Need and get help	Need help but do not get it
a. Diabetes care (shots, tests, foot care)			
b. Care for other health problems			
c. Dressing			
d. Bathing			
e. Cooking			
f. Housework			
g. Yardwork			
h. Shopping			
i. Handling finances			
j. Transportation			
k. Seeing			
l. Hearing			
m. Walking			
n. Sleeping			
o. Eating			
p. Remembering			
q. Reading			
r. Writing			

24. If you get help, from whom?
    (Check all that apply.)   Specify from whom:
    a. ☐ Family   _____
    b. ☐ Friends   _____
    c. ☐ Visiting nurse   _____
    d. ☐ Hired help   _____
    e. ☐ Volunteer help   _____
    f. ☐ Community services   _____
    g. ☐ Other   _____

EDUCATIONAL ASSESSMENT OF OLDER ADULT WITH DIABETES (HEALTH PROFESSIONAL INTERVIEW FORM)

1. Do you have someone you can talk to about your diabetes?

    _____ No

    _____ Yes If yes, who? _____

2. How often do you see or talk to family or friends?

    _____ Daily

    _____ 1 to 3 times a week

    _____ 4 to 6 times a week

    _____ Less than once a week

    _____ Less than once a month

3. Do you see them as often as you like? _____

4. What makes it hard to live with your diabetes? _____

5. What would make it easier to live with diabetes? _____

6. a) How would you rate the stress you are currently under, using the following scale?

    ☐ Little or no stress

    ☐ Fair amount of stress

    ☐ Lot of stress

    b) What do you think causes stress in your life? _____

    c) What do you do about stress in your life? _____

7. a) What do you feel fear or anxiety about? _____

    b) What do you do about it?

8. a) Do you ever feel down or depressed?   _____ Yes   _____ No

    b) What do you feel down or depressed about? _____

    c) What do you do about it? _____

9. What do you do in your leisure time? (groups, friends, regular activities)

10. What good things are going on in your life?

11. Educational plan

    a) Areas of strength _____

    b) Areas of weakness _____

    c) Educational problem list

Problem	Plan	Date resolved Signature	Date identified Signature

    d) Other pertinent data (i.e., functional status, knowledge, test scores, psychosocial information, reading level)

CHAPTER **16**

Promoting Behavior Change: Teaching/Learning Strategies

DEBRA HAIRE-JOSHU AND CHERYL HOUSTON

Diabetes mellitus has biologic, psychologic, and social impacts. Consequently, the individual with diabetes must understand and act upon a variety of complicated clinical information to attain adequate self-management. To do this effectively, the patients with diabetes must interact with various members of the health care team, so as to solicit the knowledge and skills needed to successfully care for themselves. Effective diabetes education therefore involves all disciplines of the health care team (e.g., physicians, dietitians, nurses, physical therapists, social workers, and psychologists).[31,35]

The ultimate goal of our teaching, then, is to interact with the individual with diabetes and family so that he or she can obtain the skills needed to effectively modify his or her behavior.[46] The purpose of this chapter is to address the following questions from the perspective of the teaching/learning process: What do we teach a given individual about diabetes? How do we know whether or not our teaching has been effective? In terms of teaching skill, what are the characteristics associated with good teaching? How does a good teacher "get the point across"? To answer each of these questions, this chapter is divided into two sections. The first addresses the teaching/learning process and reviews in detail the seven steps of this process. The second section focuses on teaching skills and self-assessment practices associated with these skills.

THE TEACHING/LEARNING PROCESS

The development and application of a coordinated educational model is one means of promoting comprehensive diabetes education that draws upon the expertise of the various disciplines. There are several models of instruction based upon the educational, psychologic, and medical literature that depict the teaching/learning process.[19,40] In terms of diabetes education, any model of instruction needs to take into account the biologic, psy-

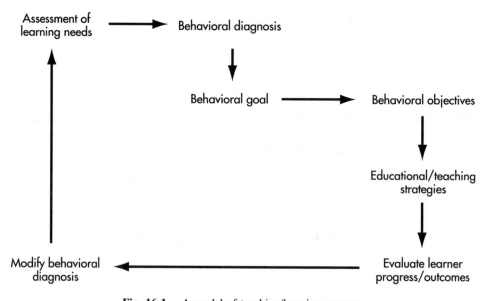

Fig. 16-1   A model of teaching/learning process.

chologic, and social components that influence that education. Without such comprehensiveness, there is a minimal bridge across the varying perspectives of different health disciplines, ideologies, and paradigms.

One model, which is depicted in Fig. 16-1, is suggested as an effective guide to the instructional process. The model depicts a systematic but cyclical procedure that includes several steps: (1) assessing the learning needs of the individual, (2) determining the behavioral diagnosis, (3) identifying appropriate behavioral goals and objectives, (4) organizing educational strategies for promoting behavior change, (5) evaluating learner outcomes, and (6) modifying the behavioral diagnosis.[19,52] Each of these steps is critical to achieving effective diabetes education, especially given that time constraints are often cited as a major deterrent to effective teaching.

Step 1: Assessing Learning Needs

Assessment represents the first step of gathering a variety of physical and psychosocial data that is necessary to determine an appropriate educational plan for diabetes self-management. The term learning assessment should not imply a review of diabetes knowledge or skill alone. Rather, a learning assessment results from the compilation of an accurate and thorough health history.[15] Such a history identifies strengths and weaknesses, or past and present susceptibility or resistance to psychologic as well as physical stresses. The history also identifies health risks such as heredity and environmental factors that may indicate potential or existing problems for diabetes care. As has been discussed in previous chapters, assessment of developmental stage is crucial to planning diabetes education. Just as a clinical determination is necessary prior to adjustment of insulin, so an educational assessment is necessary to determine the best strategies for incorporating diabetes management into the individual's life.

One issue that arises when conducting assessment is the lack of time. Assessment may prove to be very time consuming, with studies reporting up to 55% of an interaction reflecting the assessment phase.[15,44] However, the collection of comprehensive data lends itself to more effective translation of information to the individual with diabetes. As such, it should be carefully conducted with as much time devoted to careful completion as is needed. Examples of diabetes assessment forms can be found in Appendix E.

Information sources

The collection of data for the assessment of learning needs may come from a variety of sources, including the individual, medical records, family members, and other health care team members. For example, the physical aspects of the assessment generally come from the medical and/or nursing history, while a more detailed psychosocial/developmental history may be secured from a social worker's or psychologist's assessment. The ability to coordinate such findings makes for a very comprehensive picture of the individual and enables one to identify an appropriate learning diagnosis.[22,52]

Assessment variables

There are a variety of factors that may influence the learning assessment of the individual with diabetes. A brief discussion of each of these factors includes the following:

Demographic factors   Gender, age, and years of formal education are important variables in any assessment. Documentation of diabetes knowledge such as might be reflected on a knowledge test is also important.[38,43]

Cultural factors   Information regarding members of household, role and position in household, and position in extended family are important cultural variables.[4,42] The role in the household refers to the tasks and responsibilities assumed by the patient, while the position refers to placement in the structure of the household. For example, many women have the role of the breadwinner, mother, and homemaker. Position in the extended family makes reference to the individual with diabetes as grandparent, aunt, cousin, or sibling. In some situations, the grandparent assumes the role of primary caregiver for the child, not the parent. For a working parent without family support, the day-care worker assumes a major caregiver status. These assessment data describe the "actual" life situation of the individual and suggest other persons who may play a significant role in the diabetes education of the individual.

Environmental factors   A description of the neighborhood in which the individual lives, pattern of moving, description of home, and occupational health risks are helpful. A description of the neighborhood highlights the relationships with neighbors, location in reference to established health care facilities, and environmental risk, such as violence.[4,15] Persons who move frequently, such as may be found in lower socioeconomic groups, also tend to have less opportunity for establishing support systems and using community resources. They are therefore at higher risk for less than optimal care that further necessitates careful planning of educational interventions.

Economic profile   Is the individual with diabetes employed? If so, what type of occupation? Does this person have health insurance, and to what extent are the current health care costs impacting personal finances? How much does the individual spend on diabetes care in an average month? What percentage of this is monthly income? What other major economic expenditures does the individual and his or her significant others face?[15]

Activities of daily living   What are the usual activities of a given day? What are the normal sleep and activity patterns? Such information enables the health care provider to determine the amount of time devoted to leisure versus work and gives some sense of the extent to which diabetes is a focus of the person's life.[15] In the case of the child with diabetes, such information provides insight into parental fatigue and stress as is commonly associated with a "nonsleeping" child.

Current health practices   What is the patient's philosophy of health care? For example, does he or she exhibit a particular interest in preventive health care by seeking regular health care for diabetes management? In contrast, does he or she rely on the emergency room as a primary health care source? What is this individual's view on maintaining metabolic control? What is his or her attitude toward risky health behaviors such as obesity, alcohol, or drug abuse? Does he or she smoke and, if so, how many cigarettes per day?[22]

Psychosocial assessment   Diabetes causes a variety of emotional responses for the person with diabetes as well as for the significant others. These responses need to be clearly identified so they might be carefully assessed with regard to the teaching/learning process. Upon diagnosis of diabetes, patients move through various stages of acceptance in response to this diagnosis such as shock and disbelief, anger, guilt, depression, and acceptance (see Table 16-1).[22] In what stage is the person with diabetes? To what extent is the individual accepting of the diagnosis of diabetes? Is there a perception that parents, family, and friends assist with diabetes management? How would the patient describe the current level of emotional family support? How many close friends does he or she identify?

As is detailed in the previous chapters, developmental factors are an important component of a thorough psychosocial assessment and are important if the health care educator is to judge the extent to which diabetes has impacted normal developmental activities. An assessment of the individual's advancement through various developmental stages provides perspectives to life priorities as well as psychologic health. Developmental stages, summarized in Table 16-2, do not begin or end abruptly, rather they imply periods of transition.[15,16]

Each developmental stage is comprised of tasks that have been discussed in preceding chapters. Tasks refer to psychologic processes or behaviors and represent a "piece of psychologic work" that must proceed if progression is to occur. Table 16-2 reviews some of the developmental tasks associated with the life cycle critical to the teaching/learning process. Data related to learner needs are based, in part, on growth and development concerns. Variables of interest include: (1) family history, including descriptions of parents, relationships with parents or spouse; (2) school/occupational history, including level of

Table 16-1   Interactions in the Teaching/Learning Process

Stages of adaption	Patient	Diabetes educator	Facilitating the teaching/learning process
Disbelief	May refuse to accept diagnosis; claim to have something else; behave so as to avoid the issue.	Allow patient to deny disease if he needs to; function as noncritical listener.	Orient all teaching to the present and to the real-life situation of the patient. Explain all procedures and activities clearly and concisely.
Developing awareness	May use anger as a defense against being dependent.	Accept and support patient's expressions of anger and grief over loss.	Explain symptoms, care, and treatment in terms of their current necessity.
Reorganization	Can accept increased dependence and reorganizes relationships with significant others.	Encourage expression of feelings about patient's illness.	Use clear, concise explanations.
Resolution	Can identify with others with same condition.	Encourage expression of feelings.	Instigate group discussions, small group activities.
Identity change	Can define self as an individual that has undergone change.	Express confidence in person's ability to manage disease.	Realize more progressive needs will surface.
Successful adaptation	Can live comfortably with self as a person who has a specific condition.	Reinforce accomplishment of goals.	Develop a relationship in which the professional is a consultant to patient.

Adapted from Haire-Joshu D: Nursing care of adults with disorders of the pancreas. In Beare PG and Myer JL, eds: Principles and practice of adult health nursing, St. Louis, 1990, Mosby–Year Book, Inc.

achievement, satisfaction with work or school, career choices; (3) social history including peer relationships in childhood, adolescence, and adulthood; (4) sexual relationships, sexual identity, and marriage, including description of partners.

Physical status   This information is secured from laboratory or physical findings, typically found with the medical history. How long has the individual been diagnosed with diabetes, type of diabetes, physical and nutritional assessment, complication status, history, and current level of metabolic control.

Prescribed regimen   What is the current method of prescribed management of diabetes? To what extent is the individual following the regimen? Is the patient satisfied with the regimen? What is the most difficult part of the regimen for this person, or the most important problem?

Learner priorities   Documentation of what the individual sees as a priority of care is essential to a thorough educational assessment. What is the biggest overall concern for the

Table 16-2 Developmental Tasks Throughout the Life Cycle

Stage	Task	Examples of behavioral indications of stage
Preschool child		
Infancy/toddlerhood 0-3 years	Physical and psychologic separation from the primary care-giver.	Voluntarily leaves primary care-giver to play with another person or toy.
	Assumption of own individual characteristics.	Expresses specific food preferences.
Early childhood 3-7 years	Social interaction within the family.	Engages family members in play.
	Beginning of social interaction outside family.	Plays with other children.
Childhood 6-puberty	Formation of significant peer relationships.	Has close friends
	Development of new skills and interests.	Enjoys school, hobbies, sports.
Adolescence		
Puberty-20 years	Completion of physical and psychologic separation from parents.	Rebels against parental authority and forms new relationships.
	Completion of sexual maturity.	Develops secondary sex characteristics and experiments with sexual play.

Adapted from Fields WL, McGinn-Campbell KC: Introduction to health assessment, Reston, VA, 1983, Reston Publishing Co.

patient at this time in life? What is the major concern regarding diabetes management? Discussion with the individual as to how identified priorities compare with those noted by the diabetes health care team is important. Ultimately, it is the person with diabetes who will be asked to make any behavior changes, or carry out any regimen.[22,46,48] As such, it is necessary to determine the extent to which the changes are seen as important and to determine whether the individual possesses adequate skills and resources to complete the regimen.

Step 2: Determining the Behavioral Diagnosis

According to Bartlett, the behavioral diagnosis identifies barriers to the patient's ability to complete the diabetic regimen.[3] The behavioral diagnosis results from a synthesis of the data from the assessment resulting in the identification of a problem upon which the diabetes team and individual can focus their efforts.[27] As such, it is specifically worded in such a manner that barriers to the individual's diabetes management are cited.

Table 16-2   Developmental Tasks Throughout the Life Cycle—cont'd.

Stage	Task	Examples of behavioral indications of stage
Adulthood		
Early adulthood 18-40 years	Shift in commitment from family of origin to new partner.	Moves from parents' home.
	Establishment of occupation.	Completes education and makes career choice.
Middle adulthood 35-55 years	Adjustment to aging of own body.	Accepts beginning decline in physical abilities.
	Adjustment to illness and death of parents.	Mourns death of parent.
	Reordering of priorities and setting achievable goals in committed relationships and occupation.	Resolves problems in or leaves marriage; reevaluates occupational choice and decides to continue or change career.
	Consolidation of occupational identity.	Works toward maximum achievement in chosen occupation.
	Adjustment to adolescent children's physical and emotional independence.	Accepts children as adults.
Late adulthood 60 and over	Adjustment to personal illness and threat of death.	Accepts limitations of illness and adapts to altered life style.
	Adjustment to illness and death in significant others.	Mourns death of significant others and forms new attachments and interests.
	Adjustment to retirement.	Maintains active life by replacement of occupation with other interests.

As previously stated, the learning assessment is derived from a thorough health assessment. Since all factors (physical as well as developmental) influence learning and impact how effectively behavior change is initiated and maintained, it is imperative that a total view of the individual is obtained.[3,27] For example, nonadherence may be touted as the educational diagnosis when poor metabolic control is present in a young person with IDDM; in fact, further assessment reveals poor socioeconomic circumstances, and frequent mobility of residence results in a lack of regular diabetes care, the major contributing factor influencing metabolic control.

The behavioral diagnosis communicates consistent information to the individual with diabetes as well as other members of the health care team, so that an educational plan can be adequately developed and followed and appropriate learning strategies identified.

The behavioral diagnosis helps the health care provider to stage the learning of the

Table 16-3   Selection of Educational-Behavioral Strategies

Behavioral diagnosis	Stage	Educational-behavioral strategies
Confusion, lack of basic understanding	Survival	Teaching, instructional aids, repetition
Lack of basic skills	Survival	Explanation of skills, demonstration, and practice
Forgetfulness to perform SMBG	Ongoing	Simplify regimen, involve friend or family member
Lack of confidence to control condition	Ongoing	Reassurance, encouragement, referral to peer group discussion, practice self-management skills
Feeling of embarrassment with friends because regimen interferes with normal activities	Ongoing	Simplify regimen, schedule regimen so activities can be done at home
Competing values and priorities (e.g., job that demands shift work, travel)	In-depth	Identify salient values/goals of patient and explain how control of condition will allow fulfillment of goals
Sensory or physical handicaps (e.g., visual problems)	Ongoing	Provide instructional aids that can be comprehended with intact senses
Lack of support from family, friends	Ongoing	Invite significant other to accompany patient to next clinic visit
Inadequate money to purchase medications, foods	Ongoing	Give free medication samples, referral to social worker

Adapted from Bartlett EE: The stepped approach to patient education, Diabetes Educ 14(2):130-135, 1988.

patient, as is noted in Table 16-3. Staging determines whether the individual is ready for survival, ongoing, or in-depth education.[1,18,22]

Survival education

Survival education can be best defined as the critical information necessary if the individual is to be able to live on his or her own outside of the acute care environment. Typically, survival education refers to the content targeted to meet the immediate needs of the newly diagnosed person with diabetes, or those who are undergoing substantial stress and are unable to advance to more in-depth information. Survival information varies in content depending upon the age of the person but tends to focus on skills such as appropriate understanding of insulin management, treatment of hypoglycemia, monitoring, and basic dietary information.[4,18,22]

Ongoing education

Ongoing information is appropriate when the individual is comfortable with survival skills and verbalizes a readiness to learn additional skill related to diabetes management. Information associated with ongoing care focuses on skills associated with sick day management, intensive exercise therapy, or insulin adjustments based on the need to alternate working days and nights.[4,18,22]

In-depth education

This level of teaching falls into several categories. First, it might include those who are seeking alternative means of insulin delivery such as intensive or pump therapy. The correction of errors in learning, such as inadequate technique in monitoring blood glucose, might also be addressed. Much of this information is directed to what the individual perceives the most critical needs are, as well as a continuing assessment of the level of self-care.[4,18,22]

Step 3: Setting Behavioral Goals

Goals are broad statements of what will ultimately be accomplished by the person with diabetes.[19,46,52] For example, one goal might be that the patient will maintain ideal body weight by following a low-fat diet. The goal is generally a result of the behavioral diagnosis that identifies a specific problem area that has been recognized and needs modification.

Goal-setting focuses efforts on progression toward an ultimate accomplishment and should be established with the input of the person with diabetes. As previously noted, there is a need to involve individuals in a collaborative effort if long-term changes are to be realized. The health care provider works with this person in setting concrete, understandable goals that serve as positive reinforcers for self-management.

Specific guidelines for establishing treatment goals include negotiating individualized treatment goals designed to meet the patient's needs. If the necessary skills are not within the individual's repertoire, then easier goals should be employed until those skills are accomplished. Ultimately, the goals must lead to meaningful rewards for the individual.

Step 4: Developing Behavioral Objectives

Before one can teach or evaluate progress, the health care team must know *what* learning outcomes are expected. What behavior does the individual exhibit at the beginning of the educational intervention? How does this contrast with the expected behavior at the conclusion of the educational experience? What knowledge and understanding should the individual possess? What skills should be displayed?

In this section various types of behavioral objectives are defined and described. Behavioral objectives are learning outcomes that establish direction by stating expected changes in the individual's behavior. According to Mager, measurable objectives "are useful in pointing to the content and procedures that lead to successful instruction, help to manage the instructional process itself, and help to provide the means of finding out whether the instruction has been successful.[34] Without measurable behavioral objectives, learning cannot be successfully planned or evaluated. Behavioral objectives are stated below:

- Measure the behavior of the individual rather than health care educator duties/techniques.

- Establish the direction for learning.
- State the "ends" desired performance rather than the "means" of the performance of the individual.
- Indicate a specific rather than general goal for the individual to fulfill.
- Communicate to the individual his or her expected performance by identifying the performance itself, standard, or criterion by which the performance is to be judged, and the condition under which performance takes place.
- Contain only one specific action verb.
- Assist the health care provider in developing evaluation instruments.[19,34,40]

Taxonomies of learning

There are various "types" of objectives. Objectives typically are written using various action verbs. These action verbs imply a level of learning—some verbs imply a higher level of learning than others. These levels have been characterized as taxonomies of learning. This is a detailed classification system of objectives. It divides objectives into three major areas: cognitive, psychomotor, and the affective domain (see box on the opposite page).[20,52]

Each of these domains can be further divided into categories that "break down" each step of the learning process within the area described below. In other words, each domain has steps of difficulty (or performance levels) that help the health care provider plan for well rounded and comprehensive learning experiences. The taxonomy may be of value to the provider, since one can plan for the individual's growth in learning by presenting the individual with measurable performance objectives that range from "low" to "high" in level of difficulty. This is especially important when dealing with patients of varying ages. Fig. 16-2 depicts the taxonomy as well as an example of how verbs reflect the more advanced understanding associated with each domain. This list is not all inclusive but is meant only as an example.

The cognitive domain   This domain is concerned with knowledge outcomes and intellectual abilities and skills (e.g., understanding the difference between hypoglycemia and hyperglycemia) (see Fig. 16-2).[5] The cognitive domain classifies intellectual responses in a hierarchic order ranging from simple rote memory to complex problem solving thought processes. The cognitive processes are those processes whereby ". . . we organize, interrelate and respond to the data of the experience and is the range of intellectual activities one is capable of performing in order to sort, interpret, and respond to stimuli in the environment."[5,52] The cognitive domain comprises six levels that reflect simple to complex knowledge. These levels are:

1. *Knowledge.* This is the lowest level of performance in the cognitive domain, a measure of the person's ability to recall or recognize information in the same form it was presented. Before an individual can reach higher learning, he or she must have a basic "knowledge" of the material. For example, an individual with diabetes can list the symptoms of hypoglycemia.
2. *Comprehension.* This is defined as a measure of understanding at the most rudimentary level. This level takes the learner one step beyond knowledge or memo-

TAXONOMIES OF LEARNING MEASURABLE VERBS FOR USE _____ IN WRITING BEHAVIORAL OBJECTIVES _____

Cognitive (knowledge) domain

defines	applies
lists	illustrates
names	demonstrates
recalls	interprets
describes	differentiates
explains	debates
identifies	analyzes
discusses	compares

Psychomotor (skill) domain

imitates	adjusts
follows instructions	produces
manipulates	utilizes
return demonstrates	operates
skillfully demonstrates	incorporates
practices	computes
carries out	administers
performs	constructs

Affective (attitude) domain

acknowledges	accepts
shares	agrees
listens	cooperates
shows interest	values
seeks opportunities	argues
volunteers	defends
responds	judges
assumes responsibility	approves

From Istre SM: The art and science of successful teaching, Diabetes Educ 15:67-75, 1989.

rization. For example, the patient can explain why treatment of hypoglycemia is important to diabetes care.

3. *Application.* This is a measure of the person's ability to select and apply previously acquired information, requiring a higher understanding of material than the previous levels. The individual is expected to apply previously learned material to new situations or settings. For example, the patient recognizes the symptoms of hypoglycemia that dictate the use of glucagon versus less substantial treatment.

4. *Analysis.* This level is a measure of the person's ability to separate complex communication into its component parts and to recognize relationships among the common parts of a particular communication. For example, the individual is able

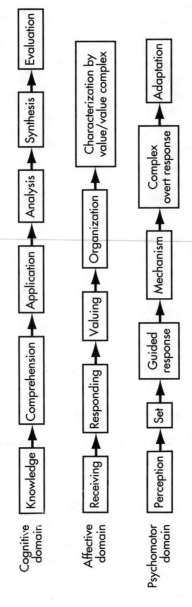

Fig. 16-2   Examples of verbs by learning taxonomy.

to discuss the components that interact to produce good control (e.g. diet, exercise, medication) and also is able to recognize that insulin is potentiated by exercise.

5. *Synthesis.* The individual should be able to "reorganize" the material that has been learned. For example, the patient with diabetes realizes that hypoglycemia may occur during exercise, realizes that exercise potentiates the impact of insulin, and arranges for additional snacks to cover activity during this time period.

6. *Evaluation.* The individual will be able to form judgments based upon agreed criteria concerning the values of ideas, plans, and so forth. For example, the patient recognizes the need to modify dietary activities further based on the occurrence of rebound hyperglycemia, caused by excessive treatment for low blood sugar during exercise.[5,46]

The affective domain   Affective objectives attempt to provide feedback to the health care educator concerning an individual's feelings or attitudes regarding a particular topic or situation. Affective objectives can be distinguished from cognitive objectives since affective objectives reflect a voluntary attitude or feeling, while cognitive objectives reflect a competency necessary for effective performance.[33,46] The five levels present in the affective domain, progressing from simple to more complex, are:

1. *Receiving.* This means the learner is aware and interested in the material being presented. For example, the individual with diabetes is interested in learning about multiple injections as a means of maintaining metabolic control.

2. *Responding.* The patient displays interest in the teaching/learning interaction by discussing pertinent information with the health care educator.

3. *Valuing.* The individual displays behaviors that suggest she/he has a degree of commitment or conviction to the accepted value. For example, great care is taken to follow a multiple daily injection routine in the belief that metabolic control will improve his or her quality of life.

4. *Organization.* The individual analyzes a concept and compares it with others with which he or she is familiar. For example, physical exercise is incorporated into weekly activities in the belief that such activities assist diabetes management.

5. *Characterization by a value or value complex.* This means that the individual responds in a consistent manner, based on his or her values. For example, the patient who values metabolic control as an outcome of personal behavior may exhibit a life-style that consistently promotes this as a goal.

The psychomotor domain   This domain deals with skill development, such as skills associated with diabetes management. There are six performance levels associated with this domain.[33,46,52] The components of this domain include:

1. *Perception.* This is a process of becoming aware of objects or qualities by way of auditory, visual, or other sensory organs. An example of this is when the individual recognizes the visual differences indicating blood glucose level on the strips.

2. *Set.* This implies the individual is prepared for the learning experience (e.g., has all the materials needed to perform blood glucose monitoring).

3. *Guided response*. The patient performs the activity (e.g., blood glucose monitoring) but under the guidance of the health educator.
4. *Mechanism*. At this point, the learned response becomes more habitual. Various aspects of trial and error may also take place with the patient finding a means of performing the task most appropriate to him or her.
5. *Complex overt response*. The patient now effectively and routinely can perform the skill. For example, the individual accurately performs blood glucose monitoring as validated by laboratory measures.
6. *Adaptation*. This implies an ability to alter motor activities pending the demands of new and problematic situations.

Writing objectives

Objectives should reflect the taxonomies of learning, encouraging learner progression. The structure for writing objectives always addresses the learner (e.g., parent of child with diabetes), the performance (plans a daily menu for a school age child using the exchange list), the standards for the performance (correctly 90% of the time), and the conditions under which the performance takes place (in the diabetes clinic).[25,34]

Objectives might also be written using the "who," "what," "when," "where," and "how" terms. The "who" is the learner or individual with diabetes. The "what" is the content or information the individual should acquire. The "how" is the measurable behavior the individual will exhibit, such as "will describe." The "when or where" describes the circumstances under which the learner will achieve the objective. For example, at the conclusion of the clinic/office visit (when/where), the individual with diabetes (who) will be able to demonstrate (how) the proper way to examine his or her feet (what).[2,25,34]

Step 5: Identifying Educational/Teaching Strategies

Once the behavioral objectives are readily defined, one can identify various teaching strategies that are available for use by the health care educator to enhance the patient's understanding and attainment of objectives. In general, learning is facilitated through reinforcement in an atmosphere in which persons with diabetes are given adequate time to assimilate information and skills at appropriate intervals. As importantly, patients are made aware of their progress at appropriate intervals through feedback.[41,51,56]

Although not meant to be all-inclusive, this next section identifies several techniques that have been found to be very effective in promoting learning.

Self-monitoring

This is a behavior modification technique based on the assumption that awareness of actions is a first step toward changing actions. The use of self-monitoring procedures in diabetes care are already an integral part of the regimen. The establishment of behavioral objectives and the self-monitoring of these objectives have a substantial impact since it is easier to monitor a behavior than a goal. Thus, it is easier for the individual with diabetes to realize what the behavioral objective is and to evaluate his or her effectiveness in achieving this objective.[51,56] To facilitate this process, it is helpful to have the individual identify positive aspects of monitoring. For example, how many times per week the patient *did* exercise as opposed to did not exercise.

Behavioral contracting

The contracting process is a technique that involves concrete discussions of specific behaviors that might be beneficial and how they might be carried out in order to fulfill the contract.[6,13] The critical ingredient in using behavioral contracting is the negotiation of the contract by the individual and the provider.

Specific guidelines for formulating a contract appear in the box on p. 580 and include:

- A clear and detailed description of the required instrumental behavior be set *(the individual with diabetes will walk 30 minutes a day, 3 times per week)*.
- Some criterion should be set for the time or frequency limitation constituting the goal of the contract *(for 2 weeks)*.
- Specific positive reinforcements contingent upon fulfillment of the criterion *(after which she will buy a new dress)*.
- Bonus clauses should indicate the additional positive reinforcements obtainable if the persons exceeds the minimal demands of the contract *(and go out to eat if she walks 5 days a week)*.
- Specify means by which contract response is observed, measured, and recorded *(to be documented by her spouse)*.
- Timing for delivery of reinforcement contingencies *(with the rewards to be received within 2 weeks of completion of the contract)*.[26,28]

Skills training

In order for an individual to manage diabetes, he or she must have component skills, such as planning, stress management, and assertiveness. Enhancement of problem-solving skills is a critical skill and may also benefit the individual with diabetes. Problem solving is a form of skills training. Problem solving forces the focus on one specific aspect associated with diabetes care and also identifies any solutions. Such strategies are especially effective when one considers findings that patients need less information on pathophysiology and more on ways of integrating information into their regimen. Knowledge about one's regimen, not about one's disease, is predictive of clinical outcome. Problem solving encourages a critical look at specific problems and also collaborative efforts toward solutions, further demanding the involvement of the patient in the process. Problem solving relies on oral questioning to generate strategies for resolving the problem. Via oral questioning, the health educator helps the patient to:

- Recall what has been learned.
- Think critically.
- Apply concepts.
- Become more actively involved in diabetes care.
- Learn more on his or her own.

GUIDELINES TO FOLLOW IN FORMULATING A BEHAVIORAL CONTRACT

1. A clear and detailed description of the required instrumental behavior be stated.
2. Some criterion should be set for the time or frequency limitations constituting the goal of the contract.
3. The contract should specify positive reinforcements contingent upon fulfillment of the criterion.
4. Provisions should be made for some aversive consequences contingent upon nonfulfillment of the contract within a specified time or with a specified frequency.
5. A bonus clause should indicate the additional positive reinforcements obtainable if the person exceeds the minimal demands of the contract.
6. The contract should specify the means by which the contract response is observed, measured, and recorded: a procedure is stated for informing the patient of his or her achievements over the duration of the contract.
7. The timing for delivery of reinforcement contingencies should be arranged to follow the response as quickly as possible.

An example of a behavioral contract

Health-care contract

Contract goal: (specific outcome to be attained)

I, (client's name), agree to (detailed description of required behaviors, time and frequency limitations)

in return for (positive reinforcements contingent upon completion of required behaviors; timing and mode of delivery of reinforcements)

I, (provider's name), agree to (detailed description of required behaviors, time and frequency limitations)

(Optional) I, (significant other's name), agree to (detailed description of required behaviors, time and frequency limitations)

(Optional) Aversive consequences: (Negative reinforcements for failure to meet minimum behavioral requirements)

(Optional) Bonuses: (Additional positive reinforcements for exceeding minimum contract requirements)

We will review the terms of this agreement, and will make any desired modification, on (date). We hereby agree to abide by the terms of the contract described above.

Signed: (Client)

Signed: (Significant other, if relevant)

Signed: (Provider)

Contract effective from (Date)

to

(Date)

Adapted from Kanfer FH and Gaelick L: Self-management methods. In Kanfer FH and Goldstein AP, eds: Helping people change, ed 2, New York, 1986, Pergamon Press.

- Become more interested in diabetes care.
- Develop a positive self-concept.
- Become motivated to take greater responsibility for care.[26]

Evaluation of the adequate use of problem-solving techniques and/or skill development demands an assessment of the process. Some steps one might evaluate to assure proper use of this technique include those listed in the box below.

Follow-up

There is substantial evidence that persons with diabetes forget or do not recall the specifics of what they have been told by the physician/health care educator once they have left the office. Consistent follow-up is an important mechanism to include in any educational experience as a means of promoting learning. Follow-up in the form of mailings or telephone contacts, as well as additional appointments or memory aids (refrigerator stickers), may be important to those who are learning new information and may be anxious regarding the new expectations.[28,47]

Selecting educational materials

Carefully selected educational materials can contribute substantially to the learning of the individual. There are a variety of materials available (audiovisual aids, pamphlets, brochures) that are pertinent to various groups, meaning availability of materials is not typically a problem. However, a major concern prior to using any material is whether the material is appropriate to the reading level of the individual, or group, who is to receive the material.

Issues concerning literacy are of major concern regarding diabetes care. Hosey and associates found that a large majority of diabetes materials are devised for people with at least a tenth grade reading level. However, illiteracy is common in our country, with high school graduates exhibiting poor reading skills.[12,14,39,53] This is especially true in the low income groups.[8]

Concerns for literacy suggest a need to carefully evaluate both materials and reading skills of the population. One of the most common methods for assessing reading skills is

---

_____ **PROBLEM-SOLVING SKILLS** _____

Assist the patient to:

Define the problem clearly in behavioral terms (give examples).

Analyze what one cannot do and why.

Generate possible solutions to each problem to solve.

Evaluate the pros and cons of each proposed solution.

Rank the solutions from least to most practical and desirable.

Try out the most acceptable and feasible solution.

Reconsider the original problem in light of this attempt at problem solving.

the Wide Range Achievement Test (WRAT). This test measures a person's availability to pronounce a graded list of words. The resulting raw score converts to a school grade equivalent. While the WRAT was designed for use in the classroom setting, it has previously been modified for use as a screening tool in a clinic setting. This was effectively done so that the test can be completed in less than 5 to 10 minutes.[24,55]

There are various means of assessing the readability of materials. In general, such methods attempt to "grade" an individual in terms of reading skills based upon sentence length, number of syllables or word length, number of words per page, and number of illustrations per number of words.[17,21,29,37,54] The SMOG formula is one of the most common methods of measuring readability and is described in the box below. As with other methods, the use of several as opposed to only one method, provides the most reli-

---

―――――――――― **SMOG READABILITY FORMULA** ――――――――――

1. Count 10 consecutive sentences near the beginning of the text to be assessed, 10 in the middle, and 10 near the end. Count as a sentence any string of words ending with a period, question mark, or exclamation point.
2. In the 30 selected sentences count every word of three or more syllables. Any string of letters or numerals beginning and ending with a space or punctuation mark should be counted if you can distinguish at least three syllables when you read it aloud in context. If a polysyllabic word is repeated, count each repetition.
3. Estimate the square root of the number of polysyllabic words counted. This is done by taking the square root of the nearest perfect square. For example, if the count is 95, the nearest perfect is square 100, which yields a square root of 10. If the count lies roughly between two perfect squares, choose the lower number. For instance, if the count is 110, take the square root of 100 rather than that of 121.
4. Add 3 to the approximate square root. This gives the SMOG Grade, which is the reading grade that a person must have reached if he or she is to understand fully the text assessed.

SMOG score and interpretation

Grade level (score)	Level of style	Typical magazine example
6-7	Very easy	Comics
8	Easy	Pulp fiction
9-10	Average	*Reader's Digest*
11-13	Fairly difficult	*Atlantic Monthly*
14-16	Difficult	Academic magazines; *Psychoanalytic Review, Child Welfare*
17+	Very difficult	Scientific, professional magazines; *Music Educator Journal*

Numbered list reprinted with permission of the International Reading Association. McLaughlin G: SMOG grading—a new readability formula, J Read 639, May 1969.

Table adapted from Powers, RD, Sumner, WA, and Kearl BE: A recalculation of four adult readability formulas, J Educ Psychol 49:99-105, 1958.

Table 16-4   Variables Used in Selected Readability Formulas

Formula name	Variables used in each formula
SMOG	Average number of words of 3 syllables or more per 30 sentences
Flesch-Kincaid	Average number of words per sentence
	Average number of syllables per word
Gunning's FOG	Average number of words per sentence
	Average number of words of 3 syllables or more per 100 words
Flesch Reading Ease	Average number of words per sentence
	Average number of syllables per 100 words
Fry Graph	Average number of syllables per 100 words
	Average number of sentences per 100 words

Adapted from Hosey GM, et al: Designing and evaluating diabetes education material for American Indians, Diabetes Educ 16(5):407-14, 1990.

able means of assessing material readability. Table 16-4 depicts some of the more commonly used formulas.

Many health care providers find it useful to systematically review teaching materials by means of a standard evaluation form before including them in their diabetes education program. These forms should be kept on file for subsequent use by other members of the health care team. The form can vary in length depending on the needs of the program. At the very least, general information (title, distributor, cost), format (video, slides, pamphlet), target audience (children, adults, type of diabetes), and content (accuracy, adequacy) should be included. An example of a teaching-material evaluation form can be found in the box on p. 584.

Step 6: Evaluating Individual Outcomes

Evaluation results provide the answer to the question: How effectively has the individual progressed toward meeting the behavioral goal/objectives? Evaluation is discussed in greater detail in Chapter 17 of this text.

Three major principles that are of concern include, first, matching evaluation instruments to behavioral objectives. This is basic to effective evaluation and should receive considerable attention. Properly used, evaluation procedures can contribute directly to improved individual learning by clarifying the nature of the intended learning outcomes; providing short-term goals; providing feedback concerning learning progress; providing information for overcoming learning difficulties and for selecting future learning experiences.

Second, measurable objectives also allow for a quick assessment as to whether or not an individual has accomplished learning (e.g., conducting accurate blood glucose monitoring). The behavioral objectives will clearly specify the desired changes in behavior and will provide a relevant measure or description of the same behavior. However, follow-up evaluation needs to be conducted to determine whether long-term learning has been accomplished.

_____ **EDUCATIONAL MATERIALS REVIEW** _____

Title: _____

Author: _____

Where available:

    (Company name) _____

    (Street address) _____

    (City) _____ (State) _____ (Zip) _____

(Phone number) (_____) _____

Purchase price _____ Rental charge _____

Description (circle):   movie   video   (1/2" VHS, 3/4")   slide/tape

                      slides only   print   other _____

Length _____

Target audience (sex, age, group) _____

Educational level (circle):   Survival   Ongoing   In-depth

Comments: _____

Readability rating

A. Formula/method used: _____

B. Score: _____

C. Comments: _____

Content

A. Technical accuracy _____

_____

B. Logical sequencing _____

_____

C. Amount of information presented (too much/too little)_____

_____

Sound and picture quality/attractiveness (if applicable): _____

_____

Summary

A. Strengths _____

B. Weaknesses _____

Overall rating (circle):   excellent   very good   good   fair   poor

Reviewed by: _____

Date: _____

Finally, the use of a *variety* of evaluation instruments is the most effective means of evaluating learning. This is particularly important since an individual may be hesitant to provide accurate information if he has not met the behavioral objective (e.g., maintain a low-fat diet).[49,50] Some of the means of collecting data are diary format versus asking for verbal recall; reporting to an independent source as opposed to the health care professional; return by mail versus in-person reporting, measures that request specific information as opposed to global outcomes.

Step 7: Modifying Behavioral Diagnosis

Careful documentation of teaching/learning activities and progress during the teaching session is necessary if communication among diabetes team members is to be clear. Plans for follow-up and securing of additional information are also required. Documentation should occur at the time of the teaching and not be postponed until a later date. Following documentation, team discussion of modifications of the behavioral diagnosis is not only appropriate, but critical to good education as well as to the instructional plan.

TEACHING SKILLS

While the process for learning is dependent in great part on following a systematic procedure for educating the individual with diabetes, it is also dependent on a health educator who can effectively teach. We have all been exposed to individuals who are excellent teachers, while we might also have identified those who are not skilled in such a manner. What is good teaching? What factors make a person such a good teacher?

DR. FIRM

Certain skills, which can be summarized below by use of the mnemonic of DR. FIRM, are considered essential teaching functions because they appear to be present in the most effective educational programs.[10,45]

- *D*emonstrations, presentations, problem solving.
- *R*ehearsal of content.
- *F*eedback and correctives given to individuals.
- *I*ndependent practice of new learning by individuals on their own.
- *R*eview and reassessment at periodic intervals.
- *M*otivation to persevere with new behaviors.

Reflecting these same skills, Shea and associates suggest good health care educators must possess, at minimum, the following characteristics.[49,50]

Recognize Individual Differences

Everyone learns a little differently and has his or her learning affected by a variety of stimuli (e.g., environmental stimuli, emotional, physical). A good teacher recognizes these individual differences or styles and plans the teaching so that it effectively deals with these styles. A very good example of this is how health care educators deal with adults versus children. Strategies for teaching children are addressed in Chapters 11 through 13. What is clear is that adult learners have unique learning needs that *differ* from those of the child. According to Knowles there are four basic principles to adult learning:[30]

As a person matures, his or her self-concept moves from dependency to a self-directed position. Children are in a constant state of flux, from dependence to independence. Adults have achieved a sense of independence and have a deep psychologic need to be self-directing. An adult receiving a diagnosis of diabetes may experience tension since she or he may now have to rely on others (health professionals, family, friends) for information and care, something that has not been necessary, possibly since childhood. The normal reaction can be one of resentment and resistance. However, a health educator who takes the time to do a careful assessment actively involves the individual in the teaching process, provides adequate feedback, and facilitates the person's movement back toward a position of independence.

Adults accumulate many experiences over a life-time, and these experiences are rich resources for learning. Children reflect an eagerness to learn and try new activities with which they have no previous experience. For the adult learner, past experiences provide a broadened world view with which to relate new learning experiences. Health care educators should decrease their emphasis on traditional teaching methods such as lecture or prepared audiovisual presentations in favor of discussion, group projects, and other action-learning techniques that allow the learner to tap, analyze, and build on his or her experiences.

Adults tend to have a problem-centered orientation to learning, and the information should have immediate application. Adults often enter an educational experience because they are experiencing difficulty with a current problem. This is in contrast to children, who have incorporated learning and school as a major part of their life. This may mean that the focus of an educational intervention for the adult be simply how to adjust diet while traveling for the business trip planned for next week, as opposed to general, nice-to-know information such as the pathophysiology of diabetes.

The readiness to learn in an adult is often related to developmental tasks required for a social role. Children are naturally curious and seek learning experiences. Adult learning theory assumes that adults are ready to learn those things they *need* to because of an event or change in a given situation.

In comparison with children, adult learners are more heterogeneous in experience and background, more sensitive about themselves, and fearful of failure. Adults tend to be reluctant to adapt to new ways, a critical problem when one considers the changes demanded by the diabetic regimen. This is in contrast to children who tend to adapt much more readily to change in their life-styles. Finally, adults are busy with outside responsibilities that compete for time and commitment with their learning. This means that changes must be carefully thought out so as to minimally impact an already very busy life-style no more than is absolutely necessary. Consideration of these aspects of learner differences are critical to successful teaching and should be reflected in the diabetes teaching curriculum.

Motivation

Another component of good teaching is *how* motivation is encouraged. Does the health care provider reiterate what is to be learned or assist the individual in understanding the personal significance of learning the specified knowledge, skills, and attitudes? Is the instruction presented in a stimulating manner, as opposed to some way that is boring or routine, so persons feel respected and accepted? Does the health educator build the patient's self-confidence and reassure the individual of his or her skills to maintain the regimen? All these factors encourage motivation.

Motivation is also facilitated through interaction in an atmosphere in which the teaching process provides for active participant involvement by including cooperative experiences, differing opinions, and other means of participant-instructor discussion. Such a climate also supports the individual's right to make mistakes and varies procedures to prevent boredom. While the physical environment may be predetermined (e.g., clinic, doctor's office), the health educator establishes the environment within which motivation to learn is either fostered or inhibited. Various types of environments, encouraged by teaching style, can be described as authoritarian, democratic, and laissez-faire (see Table 16-5).[6] In most instances individuals respond better in a democratic climate. This is especially true if the individual with diabetes is to effectively assume responsibility for managing his illness.[11,23]

Table 16-5 Facilitating Motivation: The Instructional Climate

Authoritarian climate	Democratic climate	Laissez-faire climate
1. All determination of teaching content by the diabetes educator.	All content is a matter of patient/family/educator discussion and decision, encouraged by the educator.	Complete freedom for group or individual decision, without any educator participation.
2. Techniques and activity steps dictated by the educator, one at a time, so that future steps are uncertain to the patient.	General steps to the goal are identified. Where technical advice is needed, the diabetes educator suggests two or three procedures from which choices can be made.	Various materials supplied by the diabetes educator, who makes it clear that information is supplied when asked.
3. The diabetes educator is "personal" in praise and criticism of the activities of the patient.	The diabetes educator is "objective" or "fact-minded" in his or her praise and criticism.	Very infrequent comments on patient activities unless questioned.

Demonstrate Good Interactional Skills

A number of interactional skills are empirically related to an individual's learning, making such skills a necessary and important component of clinical competence and education. Teaching is ineffective when the individual does not believe or have confidence in the expertise of the provider. It seems obvious that the establishment of rapport and trust with an individual is critical to teaching. However, it is sometimes difficult to characterize the skills needed to accomplish this.

There are several major sets of interpersonal skills that are cited as imperative if a teaching relationship is to be successfully established.[10,30] These skills are empathy, or the ability to understand others' emotions; genuineness, the ability to disclose personal feelings; immediacy, the ability to elicit the current feelings of the individual; confrontation, the ability to tactfully identify inconsistencies in an individual's communication; and concreteness, the ability to translate information into specific examples.[7,31,36]

The use of good interactional skills implies the health care team:[7,31,41]

- Addresses concerns raised by the individual, and ensures that the objectives of the visit, even if different from that of the clinician, are consistently being met. Find out what the patient wants to know. Ask the individual directly "What are your concerns?" Respond directly to the patient regarding the identified concerns.
- Encourages questions. The individual probably has numerous questions related to health care or diabetes concerns. An effective teacher encourages the individual to ask questions. The health educator frequently reinforces asking questions by responding with statements such as "That's a good question" to further support question asking.
- Presents treatment instructions in a clear and simple manner. The medical language is often complex and technical without realization that individuals may have little understanding of terms such as insulin, etc. When a patient uses such terms, the health educator checks to make sure he or she understands the meaning and is not simply repeating jargon.
- Uses concrete advice. The health educator gives detailed, specific advice. For example, the individual should walk for 25 minutes after supper, as opposed to the individual should take a daily walk. Sensitivity to the timing of the information is noted with care taken not to overload the learner with information.
- Repeats and stresses the importance of critical components of the advice. Reinforce the advice whenever possible with written materials.
- Provides advanced organizers of what is to be said. Explicit categorization is demonstrated when the provider divides the instructions into content categories and announces these before giving the individual with diabetes information pertaining to each area. (First I will talk and describe the procedure for foot care, then I will demonstrate, with your assistance).
- Checks the individual's understanding. Persons with diabetes can be asked to demonstrate what they have been shown, or asked to restate treatment recommendations.

- Uses a variety of communication channels. Whenever possible, diagrams and models are used. Oral and written materials are also provided, perhaps with simple written instructions that can be taken home.
- Reduces the complexity of the regimen. A substantive amount of evidence indicates that learning, as well as adherence, is more likely when the complexity of the regimen is reduced.[41] The health educator may ask the individual to make relatively small changes in the beginning. The regimen is then graduated so the treatment is divided into a series of behaviors in order of difficulty. As the individual achieves behavioral change, components are gradually added, building toward the final regimen. The treatment is tailored to the person's life-style. For example, specific events are anchored around existing routines (SMBG prior to brushing teeth).
- Provides feedback. Critical to the feedback process is *how* feedback is provided to the individual. Deci and Ryan suggest there are two ways in which feedback is most likely given: informational and controlling.[11] Informational feedback is perceived by the individual as promoting choice and self-determination while providing information that is useful for a person attempting to interact effectively with the environment. Informational feedback is critical to the goal-setting process in that it implies a mutual agreement for the goal being set and employs the aspect of choice throughout the communication process.

  Controlling feedback, in contrast, implies pressure to achieve a behavioral outcome, often set by the health care team, as opposed to a mutually agreed upon goal. Controlling feedback also implies a deadline (e.g., you should lose 10 pounds by the next clinic visit, or your glycosylated hemoglobin should be below 9 mg/100 ml). The perception from such communication is that one will feel guilty or incompetent if the goal is unmet by the next visit. Such feedback encourages extrinsic motivation, which is less likely to maintain a behavior change.
- Involves significant others whenever possible. Social support is a helpful prerequisite to optimal diabetes care. The involvement of family and significant others in the learning process facilitates environmental adaptations that must frequently be made to accommodate the diabetic regimen.

Self-Assessment

In order to improve effectiveness in dealing with persons with diabetes, the health educator should periodically evaluate his or her teaching skills. One approach that can be implemented on a regular basis is self-assessment. Self-assessment enables the instructor to "self-monitor" teaching skills. A format for self assessment includes:[9]

1. *Planning.* Before conducting the educational intervention, ask yourself several questions. What impact will the session have on the individual with diabetes? What should the patient be able to do as a result of the session? What teaching strategies will be used? How will success be measured? What behaviors will the learner exhibit that demonstrate that the teaching experience was successful?
2. *Conduct the session.* Audio or videotape the session.

3. *Assessment.* Before reviewing the tape, and as soon after the session as possible, answer the following questions:
   - What is your overall impression of the experience?
   - How do you think the patient felt? Write down some examples that support your interpretation.
   - What went easily? What gave you more difficulty?
   - What, if anything, had you planned or hoped to have happen that did not? Explain.
   - If your session did not go as you planned, if the behavioral objective was not achieved to your satisfaction, try to account for the difference between what you planned and what happened? Focus only on those components that are within your control.
4. *Review the tape.* How similar is what you believed happened to what actually happened? What is different from what you might have expected? Perhaps the individual is being directed by the use of closed instead of open-ended questions or some verbal or nonverbal communication is being used that interferes with the establishment of rapport. Maybe the patient is not allowed to express his or her own goals for the session. Finally, what are the problems that are most important to address in improving current teaching skills? Focus on those items first.
5. *Have a colleague review the tape.* To what extent does the colleague validate your assessment?
6. *Identify a strategy for improving your teaching.* Work on one behavior/skill at a time. Schedule additional periods of self-assessment.

SUMMARY

Good diabetes education does not occur by accident. It is the result of time, practice, innovation, and energy on the part of the diabetes team and the individual with diabetes. The teaching skills of each of the disciplines, the systematic instruction of the individual, along with regular follow-up and evaluation of educational progress is critical to good diabetes education.

REFERENCES

1. American Diabetes Association Committee on Youth Education: Curriculum for youth education, Alexandria, VA, 1988, American Diabetes Association, Inc.
2. American Diabetes Association Task Group of Goals for Diabetes Education: Goals for diabetes education, Alexandria, VA, 1986, American Diabetes Association, Inc.
3. Bartlett EE: How can patient education contribute to improved health care, Health Policy 6:282-294, 1986.
4. Baver-Stein T: Reflections on diabetes education and culture, Diabetes Educ 13:269, 1987.
5. Bloom BS, ed: Taxonomy of educational objectives: handbook I: cognitive domain, New York, 1956, David McKay Co, Inc.
6. Boehm Steckel S: Patient contracting, Norwalk, 1982, Appleton-Century-Crofts.
7. Brookfield SD: Understanding and facilitating adult learning, San Francisco, 1986, Jossey-Bass Publishers.
8. Center for Disease Control: Diabetes surveillance policy program research, Atlanta, GA, 1990, The Division of Diabetes Translation.

9. Connell K: Problem solving assessment tool, Chicago, 1984, Institute for Inquiry in Education, Inc. Unpublished hand-out.

10. Cruickshank D and Armaline WD: On becoming clear: a research review with clues to instructors, Diabetes Educ 13:394-397, 1987.

11. Deci EL and Ryan RM: Intrinsic motivation and self-determination in human behavior, Rochester, NY, 1985, Plenum Press.

12. Doak L and Doak C: Patient comprehension profiles: recent findings and strategies, Patient Counsel Health Educ 2:101-106, 1980.

13. Dobson T, Nord W, and Haire-Joshu D: The use of goal setting by physicians in the treatment of diabetes, Diabetes Educ 15:62-65, 1989.

14. Drury T, Danchik K, and Haris M: Sociodemographic characteristics of adult diabetics. In National Diabetes Data Group: Diabetes in America: diabetes data compiled 1984. DHHS publication no (NIH)85-1468, Bethesda, MD, 1985, Public Health Service, National Institutes of Health.

15. Fields WL and McGinn-Campbell KC: The health history. In Fields WL and McGinn-Campbell KC, eds: Introduction to health assessment, Reston, VA, 1983, Reston Publishing Co.

16. Freiberg, KL: Human development: a lifespan approach, Monterey, CA, 1983, Wadsworth Health Sciences.

17. Fry EB: Fry's readability graph: clarifications, validity and extension to level 17, J Read 21:242-52, 1977.

18. Gallaway JA, ed: Diabetes mellitus, Indianapolis, 1988, Eli Lilly Co.

19. Gronlund NE: Measurement and evaluation in teaching, ed 3, New York, 1976, MacMillan Publishing Co., Inc.

20. Gronlund NE: Stating behavioral objectives for classroom instruction, New York, 1970, Macmillan Publishing Co, Inc.

21. Hafner L: Cloze procedure, J Read 9:415-21, 1966.

22. Haire-Joshu D: Nursing care of adults with disorders of the pancreas. In Beare PG and Meyer JL, eds: Medical surgical nursing, St. Louis, 1990, Mosby–Year Book, Inc.

23. Haire-Joshu D: Motivation and diabetes self-care, Diabet Spect 1:279-282, 1990.

24. Hosey GM and others: Designing and evaluating diabetes education material for American Indians, Diabetes Educ 16:407-14, 1990.

25. Istre SM: The art and science of successful teaching, Diabetes Educ 15:67-75, 1989.

26. Janz NK, Becker MH, and Hartman PA: Contingency contracting to enhance patient compliance: a review, Patient Educ Counsel 5:165-178, 1984.

27. Jenny J: Knowledge deficit: instructional or behavioral diagnosis? Patient Educ and Counsel 11:91-93, 1988.

28. Kanfer FH and Gaelick L: Self-management methods. In Kanfer FH and Goldstein AP, eds: Helping people change, ed 2, New York, 1986, Pergamon Press.

29. Klare GR: Assessing readability, Reading Res Q 10:62-102, 1974.

30. Knowles M: The adult learner: a neglected species, Houston, 1980, Gulf Publishing.

31. Knox AB: Teaching adults effectively: new directions for continuing education, San Francisco, 1980, Jossey-Bass Publishers.

32. Krall L: Education: a treatment for diabetes. In Marble A and others, eds: Joslin's diabetes mellitus, ed 12, Philadelphia, 1985, Lea and Febiger.

33. Krathwohl DR, Bloom BS, and Masia BB: Taxonomy of educational objectives: handbook II, affective domain, New York, 1964, David McKay Co.

34. Mager RF: Preparing instructional objectives, Belmont Ca, 1962, Fearon Publishers.

35. Mazzuca SA and others: The diabetes education study: a controlled trial of the effects of diabetes patient education, Diabetes Care 9:1-01, 1986.

36. Mazzuca SA and Weinberger M: How clinician communication patterns affect patients' comprehension and satisfaction, Diabetes Educ 12:370, 1986.

37. McLaughlin GH: SMOG grading: a new readability formula, J Read 12:639-46, 1969.

38. McNeal B and others: Comprehension assessment of diabetes education program participants, Diabetes Care 7:232-235, 1984.

39. Meade CD and Byrd JC: Patient literacy and the readability of smoking education literature, Am J Public Health 79:204-206, 1989.

40. Mehrens WA and Lehmann IJ: Measurement and evaluation in education and psychology, New York, 1973, Holt, Rinehart and Winston, Inc.

41. Meichenbaum D and Turk DC: Enhancing the relationship between the patient and health care provider. In Meichenbaum D and Turk DC, eds: Facilitating treatment adherence: a practitioner's guidebook, New York, 1987, Plenum Press.

42. Mellor L and Hoskins P: Problems of diabetes education in different cultures, Diabetes Educ 12:384-386, 1986.

43. Miller LV, Goldstein J, and Nicholaisen G: Evaluation of patients' knowledge of diabetes self-care, Diabetes Care 1:275-280, 1978.

44. Pichert JW: Teaching strategies for effective nutrition. In Powers MA, ed: Handbook of diabetes nutritional management, Rockville, MD, 1987, Aspen Publishers.

45. Pichert JW: Effective patient teaching, Pitman, NJ, 1984, American Association of Diabetes Educators Continuing Education Self-Study Program (Module 3).

46. Redman BK: The process of patient education, ed 5, St. Louis, 1989, Mosby–Year Book, Inc.

47. Richardson JL: Perspectives on compliance with drug regimen among the elderly, J Compl Health 1:33-44, 1986.

48. Roter DL, Hall JA, and Katz NR: Patient-physician communication: a descriptive summary of the literature, Patient Educ Counsel 12:99-119, 1988.

49. Shea ML, Boyum PG, and Spanke MM: Health occupations clinical teacher education series for secondary and post-secondary educators. Clinical evaluation: theory and practice in health occupations, Springfield, IL, 1985, Illinois State Board of Education.

50. Shea ML, Boyum PG, and Spanke MM: Health occupation clinical teacher education series for secondary and post-secondary educators. Clinical evaluation: the use of appropriate evaluation instruments, Springfield, IL, 1985 Illinois State Board of Education.

51. Southam MA and Dunbar JM: Facilitating patient compliance with medical interventions. In Holroyd K and Creer T, eds: Self-management of chronic disease, New York, 1986, Academic Press.

52. Staropoli CJ and Waltz CF: Developing and evaluating educational programs for health care providers, Philadelphia, 1978, FA Davis Co.

53. Streiff LD: Can clients understand our instructions? Image: J Nurs Scholar 18:48-52, 1986.

54. Taylor WS: Cloze procedure. A new test for measuring readability, Journalism Q 30:415-33, 1953.

55. Wide range achievement test (WRAT): Wilmington, Del, 1984, Jastek Association.

56. Wing RL and others: Behavioral self-regulation in the treatment of patients with diabetes mellitus, Psychol Bull, 99:78-89, 1986.

CHAPTER 17

The Process of Evaluation in Diabetes Education

DEBRA HAIRE-JOSHU

Evaluation is a critical component of diabetes practice that can be defined as a continuous process that underlies all good teaching and learning; delineates, obtains, and provides useful information for defining decision alternatives; and determines congruence between performance and objectives.[12,21] Evaluation is the process of determining the degree of success in achieving a predetermined objective and comparing an objective of interest against a level of acceptability.[10,28]

One measures or evaluates characteristics or properties of people such as their knowledge of diabetes, their willingness to perform certain aspects of the regimen, etc. Or one might measure properties of programs, such as content, materials, and effectiveness. Carefully collected evaluation data assist the health care provider in understanding the learner, planning the learning experiences, and determining the extent to which the instruction and objectives are being achieved. The need for such data is critical to the quality assurance of diabetes education, as dictated by the National Standards for Diabetes Patient Education and the American Diabetes Association. (See Appendix G.)[3,24,25] The evaluation process provides a more dependable basis for making judgments about the teaching/learning process and the effectiveness of the educational program.[17] It also produces an educational experience/program that is flexible enough to meet the needs of the learner. Educational decisions are more likely to be sound when they are based on information that is accurate, relevant, and comprehensive.

The purpose of this chapter is to describe in greater detail the evaluation *process* and its relationship to diabetes education. This process is critical to any educational intervention at the level of the individual with diabetes, health care provider, or program. The focus of this chapter will be primarily on programmatic evaluation. Evaluation of the individual and professional will be addressed only in relation to programmatic evaluation. Therefore, the content of this chapter will define evaluation; discuss the principles of evaluation; differentiate among the three levels of evaluation; identify the categories of evaluation; describe the steps of a systematic evaluation; explain the various components of evaluation; analyze various data collection techniques; compare the concepts of reliability and validity; contrast experimental and nonexperimental designs; and summarize the components associated with the evaluation process.

GENERAL PRINCIPLES OF EVALUATION

There are several critical principles associated with evaluation that have been identified by numerous sources.[12] In general, Gronlund summarizes these principles as follows:

1. *"Evaluation is the process of delineating, obtaining, and providing useful information for judging decision alternatives that underlie all good teaching and learning."*[12] The critical ingredient in any educational intervention is to be able to adapt to changing requirements. Without evaluation, the educator must rely on anecdotal data, making it difficult to empirically establish the level at which our interventions work.[12] Data from evaluations are thus necessary if one is to validate the effectiveness of teaching/learning strategies and methodologies[8,29] as well as programmatic impacts.[14,31]

2. *"Evaluation techniques should be selected in terms of the purposes to be served."*[12] Evaluation techniques are too frequently selected on the basis of how *convenient* they are to use. The more critical question should be whether the evaluation technique is the most effective method for determining what we want to know about the learner or program. For example, a diabetes knowledge test may be used because it is brief and easily scored. However, such a test does not measure learner attitudes toward diabetes care, which may provide more valuable information to the educator. In fact, a person with diabetes may have already obtained the knowledge needed to care for his or her diabetes but may have a negative attitude toward conducting the self-management regimen. The knowledge test will not provide accurate data regarding this aspect of care and, ultimately, requires more time than if an appropriate measure of attitude had initially been used.

The process of selecting appropriate evaluation instruments is critical to evaluation and is addressed with considerable expertise by diabetes health care providers.[14] Without such care, we cannot be sure we are measuring, with any certainty, the variable that we wish to measure.

3. *"Comprehensive evaluation requires a variety of evaluation techniques."*[12] The use of multiple measures in evaluating all aspects of diabetes education (e.g., teaching skills or educational materials), assures the first principle of evaluation, the delineation of useful information, is met. No single evaluation technique is adequate for appraising the patient's progress towards all of the important outcomes of instruction.[7,33] Most evaluation techniques are rather limited in scope, providing unique but limited evidence on some aspect of the behavior of the patient with diabetes. An objective test of factual knowledge regarding diabetes, as was described in the previous example, provides important evidence concerning a patient's knowledge but little evidence concerning how attitudes are changing, how she or he would perform in an actual situation requiring applica-

tion of knowledge, or what influence knowledge might have on personal adjustment. Another example might be the use of glycated hemoglobin as a means of documenting metabolic control. This is an accurate laboratory measure of metabolic control but, of course, provides us little direct information about such subjects as the patient's knowledge, self-management techniques, or attitudes toward diabetes.

4. *"An understanding of evaluation techniques implies an awareness of their limitations as well as their strengths."* [12] Even the best evaluation methods fall far short of the precision one would like them to have.[32,33] The care with which the health care provider assures the reliability of laboratory measures and the accuracy of results, is justified as well in any use of educational/behavioral measures. Without such information one cannot be sure of what is measured or that the findings accurate in our findings.

5. *"Evaluation is a means to an end, not an end in itself."* [12] The use of evaluation techniques implies there is a purpose for the evaluation and that the health care provider is aware of the purpose. Too frequently, the purpose of the evaluation is lost while extensive amounts of data are gathered. Ultimately, these data are probably filed away with the hope that someday this information will prove worthwhile. Such evaluation activities are wasteful of both the professional's and patient's time and effort. One means of avoiding the trap of collecting "everything" and using "nothing" is to view evaluation as a process of obtaining information upon which to base *educational* decisions.[33] This implies that the types of decisions to be made will be identified *before* the evaluation procedures are selected and that no evaluation procedure will be used unless it contributes to improved decisions of an instructional nature.[12,35]

Levels of Evaluation

There are three levels at which a diabetes education program can be evaluated: process, impact, and outcome. In a process evaluation, the objective of interest is focused more toward professional practice and the standard of acceptability for appropriate practice.[10] In contrast, the impact evaluation focuses on the immediate impact of the program or some aspect of it. Have short-term goals been met? Is a risk to the person with diabetes reduced? Is the program cost-effective?

The third level of evaluation is outcome. The focus is on the extent to which the program has impacted the health status of the person with diabetes. Has detection or treatment changed as a result of this program?[10]

As an example, a process evaluation would be conducted if one wanted to know how many individuals had seen a film of foot care that is being shown in the waiting room of all public health clinics. The impact evaluation would be a measure of how many individuals with diabetes who were sitting in the waiting room can recall the specifics of the film demonstration and can themselves demonstrate foot care. The outcome evaluation would focus on increased self-report of foot examinations and verification of diminished clinic visits for foot problems among individuals who viewed the film.

Categories of Evaluation

While levels of evaluation characterize its focus, categories of evaluation characterize when the evaluation takes place. The evaluation categories are helpful in characterizing the general philosophy as to why the evaluation is being conducted. The categories clarify purpose and lend further guidance to the selection of materials and techniques for conducting the evaluation.[12,21]

Formative evaluation

When information is needed to provide immediate feedback to improve diabetes care and program efficiency, a formative evaluation is conducted. Formative evaluations are a systematic collection of data used to construct a profile of the learning program and to obtain feedback that allows ongoing modification of the program.[12,21]

Health care providers may use the formative approach as part of the decision-making process during routine education. Patient progress is assessed so a determination can be made as to the immediate learning/clinical needs. Feedback to the individual provides reinforcement for successful learning and identifies the specific learning errors that need correction (e.g., accurate injection procedures). Feedback to the team provides information for modifying diabetes information and/or for providing additional assistance in the form of referrals to community programs. Formative evaluation depends heavily on specifically prepared evaluative procedures for each segment of instruction.

Summative evaluation

This form of evaluation typically comes at the end of a period of instruction.[12,21] It determines the extent to which the instructional objectives have been achieved and is used primarily for determining whether the learning outcomes have been mastered. Summative evaluation also provides guidelines for determining the appropriateness of learning objectives. Typical examples of summative evaluations include a postprogram evaluation that generally occurs immediately following a formal program, or at 6- and 12-month intervals, to assess impact.

Placement evaluation

This category of evaluation is less associated with diabetes education and is more frequently referred to in the school setting. Placement evaluation is defined as the extent to which an individual has mastered certain learning objectives or possesses appropriate skills so that additional information would be appropriate.[12,21] Placement evaluation is concerned with the person's initial behavior (e.g., newly diagnosed persons with diabetes) and typically focuses on questions such as the following: (1) Does the individual with diabetes possess the knowledge and skills needed to begin more in-depth instruction? (2) To what extent do the individual's learning style and personality characteristics indicate that one mode of instruction might be better than another (group versus individual)? An example of placement evaluation might be the decision of whether an individual with

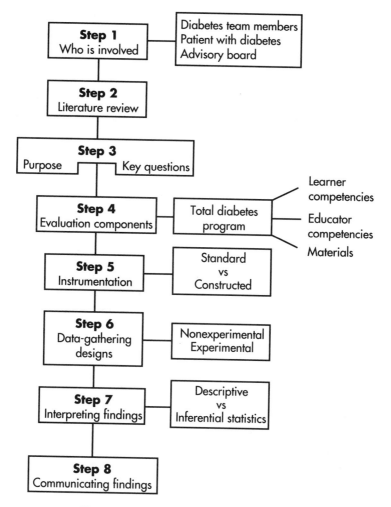

Fig. 17-1 A model of systematic evaluation.

diabetes is in need of "survival" versus "in-depth" education, as is discussed in other chapters. It is also a critical component when considering the needs of the patient with diabetes as differentiated by age.

A MODEL OF SYSTEMATIC EVALUATION

Any evaluation will generally include the formulation of the objective(s), identification of the criteria to be used in measuring success, and determination and explanation of the degree of success.[11,31,35] More detailed steps, as are depicted in Fig. 17-1, are guided by these general characteristics.

Step 1—Who Is Involved

Relevant persons who are involved with and impacted by the diabetes education program should participate in the evaluation.[9,16] When conducting a program evaluation, one would include members of the diabetes education team as well as members of the organizational staff not associated directly with the program such as nurses, dietitians, and other staff who have contact with the diabetes education program only peripherally. In addition, it is often appropriate to involve administration personnel in the evaluation process. Finally, individuals with diabetes who are affected by the program should be represented in any evaluative procedure as they are the ones most affected by any changes. The formation of an advisory committee is an effective strategy for incorporating multiple views.

Step 2—Literature Review

An examination of previous evaluations that have been conducted will assist in determining the most effective means for conducting the current evaluation, as well as familiarizing the evaluation team with the state of the literature in their area.[9,32] The literature review identifies the measures developed or used, how reliable these measures were, the findings, the issues that were or were not addressed, and potential resources for consulting assistance with the current planned evaluation.

Step 3—Purpose and Key Questions

A major initial task of any evaluation is to identify the purpose and key evaluation questions that are to be answered. The purpose of the evaluation can most succinctly be defined as "who wants to know what and why." The answer to this question clarifies for the provider and any other members of the evaluation team what is being undertaken.[31,35]

The purpose statement gives direction to the evaluation process.[14,35] Examples of an evaluation purpose might be:
- To determine the effectiveness of the outpatient diabetes education curriculum.
- To determine the availability of community resources.
- To determine the cost effectiveness of a program.

The key evaluation questions are drawn from the evaluation purpose. The key questions serve to specifically focus the evaluation from the purpose statement down to the individual parts or segment of the component being evaluated.[35] Some examples of key questions are:
- Is the learning module aspect of the dietary education component more efficient than the traditional, didactic approach?
- Is there a comprehensive listing of community resources that are used by the diabetes program?
- What is the average cost spent on educational materials for the diabetes program?

Step 4—Evaluation Components

The evaluation can be organized to focus on four general content areas that can be assessed either individually, or together, depending upon the purpose of the evaluation. [14,33]

Learner competencies

Systematic diabetes education has demonstrated significant improvements in learner knowledge, skills, and self-care behaviors across the life-span.[4,19,30] Evaluation of diabetes education includes information specific to what one wants the learner to know by program conclusion. What can a learner and/or the learner's family expect to get from the diabetes education program? Are there a list of behavioral objectives that guide the learning experience for the individual with diabetes. Are educational assessment techniques thorough and conducted with regularity?[22] How are basic and more complex skills assessed?[20] What are the strengths and weaknesses of the individual with diabetes with regard to learning and how can the diabetes health care team meet these needs? Is there a documented learning plan to assist in meeting the needs of the patient?

Educator competencies

The role of the health care provider is critical to diabetes education.[2,5] The patient with diabetes cannot readily learn without effective teaching. There has been extensive work identifying the key skills associated with good teaching as is described in the previous chapter.[26,27] Evaluation of these skills is critical to determine how well an educator displays teaching competence and to identify ways in which the educator might improve upon teaching.

The diabetes educator needs to be carefully and regularly evaluated as to teaching skills and or competency. As previously addressed in Chapter 16, self-assessment is one means of evaluating teaching. Other methods include peer or learner evaluation of the educator. Evaluation forms should assess six aspects of diabetes teaching including:[36]

1. *Planning.* The planning of programs, course content, and lessons is an essential activity. Information secured from the learner can contribute to planning.
2. *Individual differences.* The patients who have participated in the diabetes education program can best indicate whether they were served as individual learners by that program.
3. *Motivation.* How "interested," "excited," are patients by the course/program as contrasted with other activities? Such information provides data about educator effectiveness and rapport with the learners.
4. *Command of subject.* The patient's assessment of educator knowledge provides critical data as to receptivity of instruction.
5. *Teaching techniques.* Individuals with diabetes (and/or their parents/family) experience a variety of teaching techniques and are excellent judges of appropriateness of each technique.

6. *Environment*. The patient can evaluate the area in which teaching occurs and whether or not it is conducive to learning. For example, is there adequate privacy and space allotted for the interaction with the educator?

Other questions related to the evaluation process include: How frequently has the health care provider been evaluated by a peer or person with diabetes regarding teaching skills? Does the educator effectively implement the teaching/learning process? How thoroughly does the educator assess the learner? How recently has the educator attended continuing education courses or sought additional formal instruction? What evidence is there that the professional alters practice based on new information?[18]

Educational materials

Instructional materials are tools or aids that facilitate the learning process. These include both print and nonprint products such as films, transparencies, brochures, or pamphlets. These materials should meet standards for use that are appropriate to the individual with diabetes to whom they are distributed. In order to determine appropriateness, one must assess the means of identifying seldom-used media, outdated or inadequate media, or new materials.[6,13,23] Frequently, the review of such material is completed by the instructor. To secure consistent and objective data, information as to effectiveness of the materials should be carefully documented on evaluation forms, an example of which appears in the box on the opposite page. Such a form can be modified to reflect the particular specifics of other educational materials.

There are other questions that should be considered when evaluating materials. Is the learner involved in the evaluation of the instructional aids? What measures are used to evaluate the materials? How is this information analyzed and summarized? How is the diabetes team made aware of current materials? Is there an ongoing procedure for discarding inappropriate materials, as well as piloting new materials? How are decisions made to purchase materials?

Program evaluation

Program evaluation is a comprehensive assessment of program effectiveness; that is, the extent to which established program objectives are attained as a result of the program activities and efficiency and the resources used in the actual attainment of objectives relative to the total resources expended.[28,31,35] Typically, the person with diabetes, educator, and material evaluations are individual components that are assessed at some point in a program evaluation. In addition, however, the programmatic evaluation seeks to answer a variety of additional questions.[35] Following is a list, not intended to be all-inclusive, that identifies some of the core components critical to any program evaluation.

Program curriculum—How is the curriculum sequenced? How is it determined that the goals of the individual with diabetes were or were not achieved? What is the impact of the program on persons other than the individual with diabetes (e.g., family members)? Is there accurate compilation of formative as well as summative evaluation data?

Evaluation of facilities—What data are available regarding adequacy of existing facilities? Is there a need for renovation of facilities or modernization. What are the priori-

— PROGRAMMED INSTRUCTIONAL MATERIALS EVALUATION FORM —

Reviewer's Name _____

Review Date _____

Title _____

Source _____

Date of Publication _____ Programming ____ Adjunct ____ Branching ____ Linear

Medium (Check all applicable banks)

____ Recorded instruction	____ Teaching machine	____ Simulator	____ Computer keyed	____ Slides
____ 8mm single concept	____ Programmed text	____ Filmstrip	____ Printed matter	____ Record
____ Television	____ Book	____ Tape	____ Film	

General Criteria

	YES	NO
Is this material congruent with course or program objectives?	☐	☐
Is the material technologically accurate?	☐	☐
Is the material up-to-date?	☐	☐
Is the material free from racial and sexual bias?	☐	☐
Is the reading level appropriate to grade level of users?	☐	☐

What is the cost of the materials? _____ (A NO on any of the above five questions

(Purchase or Rent)   may disqualifty this material)

Appraisal of Content and Organization	Poor		Average		Excellent
Clarity of instructions to learner 0		1	2	3	4
Sequence of information .0		1	2	3	4
Step size of information 0		1	2	3	4
Continuous involvement of learner 0		1	2	3	4
Allows response from learner 0		1	2	3	4
Provides for help from instructor 0		1	2	3	4
Material can be easily pretested 0		1	2	3	4
Material is relevant to subject 0		1	2	3	4
Program sets desired goal for learner 0		1	2	3	4
Repetition of material 0		1	2	3	4
Availability of cues 0		1	2	3	4
Technical Quality					
Printing 0		1	2	3	4
Photography 0		1	2	3	4
Sound 0		1	2	3	4
Hardware 0		1	2	3	4

Composite Rating _____

Evaluation comments:

Adapted from Wentling T, et al: Locally directed evaluation, Springfield, IL, 1978, Illinois State Board of Education.

ties for space? More specifically, is there available space to adequately conduct diabetes education classes?

Referral and use of community resources—Are there adequate and available community resources to facilitate additional diabetes education? Is there a comprehensive listing of available resources for use by individuals with diabetes? How are the resources evaluated and is this evaluation ongoing? How much communication is there between the community resources and the diabetes program?

Cost outcome evaluation—The cost outcome analysis is crucial to making resource allocation decisions, providing accountability indices, and determining the advisability of financing the development of new programs.[1,16,34] It also provides information as to ways of decreasing the costs of the program and provides assistance in choosing among instructional alternatives.[35] A major area of concern includes how frequently the provider collects cost data on all aspects of the program (e.g., salary, instructional materials expenditure, equipment, travel, administrative costs, community service costs, capital outlay including fixed building costs). A sample of a cost summary data sheet that might be used to record pertinent information is included in Fig. 17-2.

Step 5—Instrumentation

Instrumentation is the process of selecting or developing devices and methods appropriate for measuring the criteria established for making decisions in relation to an evaluation

General course information		Cost information							
1	2	3	4	5	6	7	8	9	10
Diabetes education program components	Number of patients	Equipment	Supplies	Books	Media	Travel	Other		Total

Fig. 17-2   Educator/cost data instrument.

problem.[7,31] One of the most challenging, yet vulnerable, aspects of the evaluation process is the measurement of the variables. Multimodal measurement provides more assurances that the measures are accurately quantifying the variable in question. The health care team might use a variety of techniques to determine the type of information the learner should receive including pretests on diabetes information, self-report inventories, and observational techniques, etc. Other techniques of data collection are listed in the box on p. 604.

What is measured?

Just as objectives can be classified according to a taxonomy of behavioral outcomes, so can measurement devices of the learner's ability to meet these objectives.[12,21,29] Cognitive instruments are tests of a participant's knowledge or achievement in a specific content area. They are used to assess the accomplishment of objectives before and after an educational program or to assess participant's knowledge and understanding of content as they progress through a learning experience. Cognitive measures are the most frequently used types of instruments and are frequently written tests (e.g., Diabetes Patient Knowledge Tests).[31]

Affective measures seek to determine interests, values, and attitudes. Since these attributes are difficult to distinguish, one might describe them as acquired behavioral disposition or tendencies to respond in consistent manners to certain stimuli. The most direct approach to determining affect is to ask the individual with diabetes directly what his or her attitudes or interests are. Self-report inventories are designed to yield measures of adjustment, appreciation, attitudes, interest, temperament, and the like and may provide an indicator of change in affective behavior. Another means of determining affective change is to conduct interviews or engage in role-playing activities. [31]

Psychomotor measures, since they are generally focused toward performance of a skill, typically reflect task analysis procedures. [31] The particular task is broken down into individual steps, with an observer evaluating the individual's performance at each step. An example of this would be evaluation of the individual with diabetes performing an insulin injection.

Who constructs the instrument?

Standardized measures are developed for wide use.[12,21] Norms regarding various knowledge tests are also established and generally available. These types of tests probably have been used little in terms of cognitive measures for persons with diabetes but have implications regarding psychologic aspects of the disease process.

Informal or educator-made tests are common in diabetes education and are usually written by the educator for personal use. There are a variety of sources available that detail the methods for constructing measures.[32,33] In general, however, the process includes developing items that adequately assess the attainment of the given behavioral or programmatic objectives. The objectives and their proposed measurement techniques should be reviewed carefully by other educators and members of the health care team to assure comprehensive inclusion of all data needed for accurate measurement. The instrument is

---

_____ **SAMPLE DATA-COLLECTION TECHNIQUES** _____

INTERVIEWS

Interviews can be structured with a form or interview schedule that specifies the questions to be asked of each respondent. Interviews can also be open-ended, with the use of a topical outline that guides the interviewer in knowing what areas should be probed. The interview can be conducted face to face or by telephone.

QUESTIONNAIRES

Questionnaires are printed forms designed to collect information and judgments from respondents. They can include many different item types, including checklists, graphic rating scales, multiple-choice items, numerical rating scales, matching items, etc. Questionnaires can be administered by mail or distributed personally. In either case, a strong follow-up effort is essential in order to secure an adequate, representative response.

CHART REVIEW

Chart review/audit involves the analysis of already existing information that may be of secondary use. It can be done in a very formal way using checklists or other structured instruments.

TESTING

The administration of patient tests can provide valuable information. Testing can focus on cognitive, affective, and/or psychomotor behaviors. Instruments used in testing can include paper-and-pencil tests, inventories, simulation tests and performance tests.

OBSERVATION

Observation can provide descriptive information regarding the way something is constructed or behaves. Observation can be unstructured, or it can be structured through a special recording form. Observation can be either open, secret, or visually recorded.

Adapted from Shea ML, Boyum PG, and Spanke MM: Health occupations clinical teacher education series for secondary and post-secondary educators. Clinical evaluation: theory and practice in health occupations, Springfield, IL, 1985, Illinois State Board of Education.

then revised based on suggestions by the reviewers. Following revision, the educator should pilot the instrument on a small group of individuals closely related to the ones who will be using the measure on a regular basis. Feedback from these groups is very helpful in further refining the measure. Determination of reliability and validity of the measure, as is subsequently described, is also needed.

How reliable is the measure?

Reliability refers to consistency in measurement.[21,28,32] Factors that affect this consistency include the manner in which the measure is coded, characteristics of the measure

Table 17-1 Methods of Estimating Reliability

Type	Reliability measure	Procedure
Test-retest method	Measure of stability	Give the same test twice to the same group with any time interval between tests from several minutes to several years.
Alternate-forms method	Measure of equivalence	Give two forms of the test to the same group in close succession.
Test-retest with equivalent forms	Measure of stability and equivalence	Give two forms of the test to the same group with increased time interval between forms.

Adapted from Gronlund NE: Measurement and evaluation in teaching, ed 3, New York, 1976, MacMillan Publishing Co.

itself, the physical state of the learner at measurement time, and properties of the situation in which the measure is administered, such as the room. For example, one would expect that glycated hemoglobin reflects an accurate reading of metabolic control from one time of measurement to another. A paper and pencil measure of diabetes knowledge should also reflect an accurate measure of knowledge from one time to another.

Reliability refers to *results* obtained with an instrument and not to the instrument itself. Reliability is primarily statistical in nature with analysis of test results providing information as to how reliable the measure is. All measures should undergo testing for reliability. Some of the more common tests are noted in Table 17-1.

The degree of reliability required depends upon what we plan to use the measure for. How confident do we need to be in our results? If we are measuring blood glucose level, we would like a reliability of *at least* 95% since we need to be very confident in how the individual with diabetes is progressing physically in terms of his or her diabetes. If we are measuring attitudes toward diabetes care, we may be willing to accept a reliability of 80%. The most important consideration is that, *if reliability is low, we must not treat the scores as highly accurate.*[21,32] Factors that may also influence decisions regarding reliability include the ease of administration, the time required for administration, and the ease of scoring and interpretation.

How valid is the measure?

Validity refers to the extent to which the results of an evaluation serve the uses for which they are intended. If the results are to ensure the individual's attitude toward diabetes, then we need to be sure we are not measuring knowledge instead. As we previously noted, reliability refers to the consistency of evaluation results. If we obtain similar scores over time, we are somewhat confident that our measure is reliable. However, validity indicates that we do in fact measure what we say we are measuring. In short, we can have a very reliable measure, but it may have low validity.[10,21,28]

There are several characteristics associated with validity. First, validity pertains to the results of a test and not to the instrument itself. Second, validity is a matter of degree.

Table 17-2   Types of Validity

Type	Meaning	Procedure
Content validity	How well the test measures the subject matter content and behaviors under consideration.	Compare test content to the universe of content and behaviors to be measured.
Criterion-related validity	How well test performance predicts future performance or estimates current performance on some valued measure other than the test itself.	Compare test scores with another measure of performance obtained at a later date (for prediction) or with another measure of performance obtained concurrently (for estimating present status).
Construct validity	How test performance can be described psychologically.	Experimentally determine what factors influence scores on the test.

Adapted from Gronlund NE: Measurement and evaluation in teaching, ed 3, New York, 1976, MacMillan Publishing Co.

It is not present on an *all or none* basis. And finally, validity is always specific to some particular use and is not a general quality. For example, a test may be a valid measure of cognitive knowledge of diabetes but not of psychomotor knowledge.

There are three basic types of validity: content, criterion-related, and construct validity. [12,21] These are defined in Table 17-2.

Step 6—Data-Gathering Designs

The data-gathering option selected will depend in large part on the purpose of your evaluation. If the purpose is to evaluate teaching, or materials, very simple designs can be implemented to answer questions necessary to improve teaching practice. If the concern involves research evaluation, the approach is much more complex.

There are several research designs that lend themselves well to the evaluation of both the program components as well as the entire diabetes education program. In most instances, the criteria guiding the selection of the design reflects procedures aimed at reducing the ambiguity of results. In addition, there are a number of factors that should be examined prior to embarking on an evaluative program. These include:

Who is available to conduct or coordinate the evaluation.

The amount of money available for consultation time, computer time, and instrument development.

The effort of the individual required to obtain the needed data.

The size of the problem/program to be studied.

The availability of a large enough sample to serve as an adequate study population.

The answers to such questions will enable the health care provider to better plan a realistic evaluation. An evaluation plan, documenting roles and target dates, is a helpful strategy when working with various individuals or when the evaluation will involve only one person. A sample of one such form appears in the accompanying box.

For the purposes of this chapter, the various designs will be only generally discussed and characterized as to major differences and/or feasibility with regard to the health care provider. More detailed information, as is appropriate for the evaluation researcher, can be attained by reviewing various resources cited in the references.

Two of the major differences between designs are whether they are experimental or nonexperimental designs.[10,14,32] Nonexperimental designs provide an accurate description of what exists in the particular program or how one factor corresponds with another in the program (e.g., counseling is related positively to lower glycated hemoglobin). Experimental designs are generally conducted as a part of evaluation research and are usually reserved for those situations in which it is possible to randomize subjects to treatment, a control group is desirable or necessary, or in which cause and effect relationships are of interest.

Nonexperimental designs

The simplest and in many cases most practical evaluation designs, which are frequently used by health educators, are nonexperimental designs.

Single group posttest design The single group posttest design (see Fig. 17-3) identifies a single point during which program participants complete the selected measure. For example, if this design were used at the conclusion of a diabetes education program, one

---

———— SAMPLE EVALUATION PLAN ————

Purpose	To determine the effectiveness of community resources.
Key questions	What are the current community resources most frequently used for referral purposes?
	How effective is the referral system?
	How satisfied are patients with referral services?
Resources	Patients
	Patient charts
	Social work department
Constraints	No central file of referral resources
	Time limitations for staff

Activities	*Participants*	*Target Dates*	
		Begin	*End*
1. Assess patients regarding referral recommendations, use, satisfaction	Nurse educator	Week 1	Week 12
2. Compile list of formal referral recommendations	Social worker	Week 1	Week 4

Single Group Posttest Design

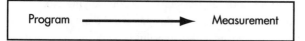

Single Group Pretest—Posttest Design

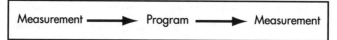

Nonequivalent Control Group Design

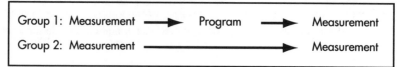

Nonequivalent Comparison Group Design

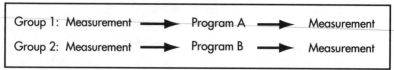

Fig. 17-3   Nonexperimental designs.

could characterize the knowledge, attitudes, or beliefs of the participants regarding diabetes care. However, it would be impossible to state how much change there had been in these variables as a result of the program since only a one-time postmeasure was used.[9,20]

Single group/pretest-posttest design   The addition of a pretest prior to the initiation of a program lends strength to findings by providing data as to what changes have occurred. However, while this design is stronger then only the single-group design, it does not enable the investigator to attribute the change to the program.[14,32] While such a design provides evidence of some type of relationship between the program and behavior change, one cannot say this relationship is causal, only that it is present. The best example of this is the maturation that occurs in children during a given time period. In the case of a diabetes program, such maturation may be the factor that most impacts attitudes toward diabetes. While this design has some risks, it is also a very simple and effective design to use and may prove to be very appropriate to the needs of the program, especially if the evaluator tries carefully to account for any rival explanations for the findings.[10,35]

Nonequivalent control group design   One way of accounting for rival explanations that may limit the strength of findings in the single/group pre-postdesign is to add a control group to the design.[14] The control group comprises patients who have not received the program that is being offered. In other words, the control group is untreated. An example of this would be if the provider measured knowledge of individuals who have received diabetes education with those who have not yet received the education. The advantage to such a design is that it enables the evaluator to say, with more confidence, what the impact of the program is on a specific group of subjects.

Nonequivalent comparison group design. This design allows the investigator to compare one program to another (see Fig. 17-3).[14] Such a comparison may assist in determining which program components are more effective. For example, if a provider is comparing the impact of group versus individual education, one might use this design.

Controlled experimental designs

Research designs that require randomization of subjects to either a control or intervention/experimental condition promote equivalence between groups, facilitating the likelihood that any significant differences between groups will be related to the program being offered. Such designs include randomization as a component and are most frequently used as a component of research studies.[14,32]

Randomization procedures allow the generalization of findings to other programs or to a larger population and are therefore an important aspect of evaluation research. This is by far the preferred method for selecting samples. In simple random sampling, each and every unit of the study (e.g., all persons with diabetes), has an equal and independent chance of being selected for study. Thus, by chance one can assume persons with diabetes selected to be evaluated are representative of the entire group of persons with diabetes.

Experimental designs depicted in Fig. 17-4 include the following:

Pretest-posttest control group design In this design randomization occurs, ensuring that each patient could have been assigned to either the experimental or control group (see Fig. 17-4).[14,32] Final assignment to a group depends on chance alone. For example, 100 patients with diabetes attending a program have an equal chance of being assigned to a control group receiving the usual brochure information on diet and diabetes, or an experimental group in which they receive information from a dietitian. Any differences between groups, as established by comparing the pretest and posttest scores, have a significant chance of being caused by the intervention.

Pretest-posttest comparison group design Instead of a control group, patients are randomized to a comparison group program (see Fig. 17-4).[14,32] For example, in this case, the investigator is interested in whether a group-oriented diabetes program is more effective than a modular self-study program given over the same length of time. Since patients are randomized to one of the two conditions, any changes would most likely be a result of the intervention.

Step 7 — Interpreting Findings

Interpretation of findings can range from a simple task, when only a few measures and subjects are involved, to a very complicated task requiring extensive data analysis.[9,15] Any statistical analysis that might be conducted is concerned with the collection, organi-

Pretest—Posttest Control Group Design

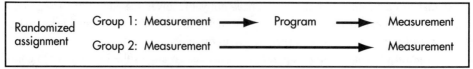

Pretest—Posttest Comparison Group Design

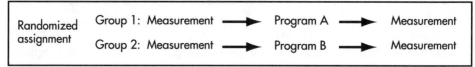

Posttest-only Control Group Design

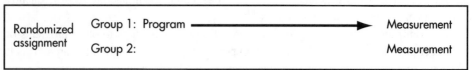

Fig. 17-4 Experimental designs.

zation, and interpretation of data according to well-defined procedures. The objective of statistical analysis is to then draw conclusions and understand more about the sources of the data.

There are two general types of statistics: descriptive and inferential.[15] Descriptive or correlational relationships suggest whether or not a relationship exists, not that one factor causes another.[10] For example, an individual has a perfect score on a diabetes knowledge test and excellent metabolic control as determined by glycosylated hemoglobin levels. One cannot say that high knowledge causes excellent metabolic control, only that there is a positive relationship between knowledge and control. The practical value of descriptive statistics is such that it allows for characterization or description of the data. Percentages, means, and chi-square are examples of descriptive statistics. Descriptive statistics allow for the direct measurement of an entire population (e.g., all members attending a diabetes education program) and allow the investigation to make inferences only about that group of patients and not about all the patients with diabetes attending an education course.[14,15]

Inferential statistics allow us to examine relationships in terms of causality.[14,15] These are experimental relationships that allow the researcher to manipulate the levels of one variable and observe changes in another. Inferential statistics also allow us to randomly sample a member of a population and infer that the characteristics of our sample are representative of the entire population. We may infer, from a random sample of persons with diabetes who attend a diabetes education class, what the average level of knowledge for the entire population of persons attending diabetes education classes. This done **without** sampling each and every one. This is in contrast to the descriptive or correlational relationships that are simply observed as they occur in the natural environment.

The design of the program will often determine the type of analysis to be used. It is important to recognize that statistical analysis assists in understanding the environment and can aid the educator in improving the educational programs. As such, care should be taken to use available expertise and resources to effectively and accurately draw conclusions from the data collected during the evaluation process.

Step 8—Communicating Findings

Effective writing and presentation of an evaluation report are critical if the findings are to result in improvements or necessary changes. A clear and concise report enhances the possibility of effective impact and represents the first step in having findings effectively used.

The evaluation report should contain five sections:[28,31] (1) purpose and key questions; (2) description of the program or program component being evaluated; (3) description of the evaluation methodology used, (4) evaluative findings, (5) conclusion and recommendations.

Purpose and key questions should open with "Who wants to know what and why?" The key questions of the evaluation are presented. An introductory paragraph is also helpful, such as providing a description of the program, including demographic information such as who is in charge, how long has the program been operational, and the major characteristics of the setting.[35]

The program/program component description provides an overview of what is being evaluated. For example, in a program evaluation, the reader should be able to determine the context of the program, resources, and problems. This section might also include program goals, educational objectives, available program staff, and other characteristics.[35]

A detailed description of the evaluation methods and instruments used (e.g., chart audit, questionnaire) should be included. The Procedures section should address with sufficient detail, the actual method of collection. Included should be discussion of subject protection, including guarantees of confidentiality and anonymity. A copy of the questionnaire might also be included for the reader.[35]

Findings or outcomes of the evaluation activities, including a display of information collected should be presented. Data should be presented in as clear a manner as is possible. This section should clearly present findings from the evaluation with tables being a very effective way of presenting the data. This section can range from very brief, if only one question was examined during the evaluation, to very lengthy. Typically, the results are presented without interpretation of their findings.[35]

The most important section of the report is that which contains the interpretations, conclusions, and recommendations based on the evaluation results.[35] There are general areas in which information might be used including changing the diabetes curricula to better meet the needs of the learners, informing administrators of activities and needs, staff

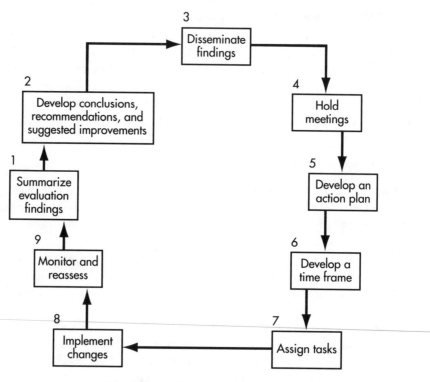

Fig. 17-5   Evaluation results model.

development supporting equipment requests, recruiting persons with diabetes to the program, discontinuing programs or program components. However, the evaluation is not complete until a plan is in place to act upon any results. What if any action is needed based on the evaluation process? How will the results be used?

To facilitate constructive change based on the findings, a plan for how the results are to be used should be included. A model for such a plan appears in Fig. 17-5. The inclusion of a plan ensures that change and improvement become an acceptable, common process that is a logical extension of any evaluation activity associated with diabetes care and education.

SUMMARY

Evaluation should be incorporated into every activity associated with diabetes education. It is a critical ingredient whereby the educator has objective and concrete feedback upon which to address future educational decisions. It is also critical to the ultimate validation that without such education, diabetes care and management will not achieve the quality standards that are necessary to promote optimal care.

REFERENCES

1. American Diabetes Association: Third-party reimbursement for outpatient education and nutritional counseling, Diabetes Care 7:505-506,1984.
2. Anderson RM and others: The diabetes care and education provided by nurses working in physicians' offices, Diabetes Educ 14:532-536, 1988.
3. Berlin N and others: National standards for diabetes education programs: pilot study results and implementation plan, Diabetes Educ 12:292-297, 1986.
4. Bloomfield S and others (Department of Child Life and Health, University of Edinburgh, UK): A project in diabetes education for children, Diabetic Med 7:137-142,1990.
5. Davis ED: Role of the diabetes nurse educator in improving patient education, Diabetes Educ 16:36-38,1990.
6. Farrell-Miller P and Gentry P: How effective are your patient education materials? Guideline for developing and evaluating written educational materials (Professional Development), Diabetes Educ 15:418-422,1989.
7. Fitz-Gibbon CT and Morris LL: How to design a program evaluation, Newbury Park, CA, 1987, Sage Publication.
8. French DG, Wittman JK, and Gallagher PJ: Evaluation of diabetes education programs: getting the answers you need, Diabetes Educ 15:176-180, 1989.
9. Garrard J and others: Clinical evaluation of the impact of a patient education program, Diabetes Educ 16:394-400,1990.
10. Green LW and others: Health education planning: a diagnostic approach, Palo Alto, CA, 1980, Mayfield Publishing Co.
11. Green LW and Lew FM: Measurement and evaluation in health education and health promotion, Palo Alto, CA, 1986, Mayfield Publishing Co.
12. Gronlund NE: Measurement and evaluation in teaching, ed 3, New York, 1976, MacMillan Publishing Co.
13. Hosey GM and others: Designing and evaluating diabetes education material for American Indians, Diabetes Educ 16:407-414, 1990.
14. IOX Assessment Associates: Diabetes education: program evaluation handbook, Los Angeles, 1988, IOX Assessment Associates.
15. Kachigan SK: Statistical analysis: an interdisciplinary introduction to univariate and multivariate methods, 1986, Radius Press.
16. Kaplan RM and Davis WK: Evaluating the costs and benefits of outpatient diabetes education and nutrition counseling, Diabetes Care 9:81-86,1986.
17. Lorenz RA and Pichert JW: Evaluation of education program developments: illustration of the research and development cycle, Diabetes Educ 25:253-257.
18. Mazze R, Deeb L, and Palumbo PJ: Altering physicians' practice patterns—a nationwide educational experiment: evaluation of the Clinical Education Program of the American Diabetes Association, Diabetes Care 9:420-425, 1986.
19. Mazzuca SA and others: The diabetes education study: a controlled trial of the effects of diabetes patient education, Diabetes Care 9:1-10, 1986.
20. McNeal B and others: Comprehension assessment of diabetes education program participants, Diabetes Care 7:232-235, 1984.
21. Mehrens WA and Lehmann IJ: Measurement and evaluation in education and psychology, New York, 1973, Holt, Rinehart and Winston, Inc.
22. Miller LV, Goldstein J, and Nicholaisen G: Evaluation of patients' knowledge of diabetes self-care, Diabetes Care 1:275-280,1978.
23. Mulrow C and others: Evaluation of an Audiovisual Diabetes Education Program: negative results of a randomized trial of patients with non-insulin-dependent diabetes mellitus, J Gen Intern Med 2:215-219,1987.
24. National Diabetes Advisory Board: National standards and review criteria for diabetes education programs, Diabetes Educ 12:286-291, 1986.
25. National Diabetes Advisory Board: Quality recognition for diabetes patient education programs: review criteria for national standards from the American Diabetes Association, Diabetes Care 9:XXXVI-XL, 1986.
26. Pichert JW: Effective patient teaching. In Pitman NJ: American Association of Diabetes Educators Continuing Education self-study program (module no 3), Chicago, 1984, American Association of Diabetes.
27. Pichert JW: Teaching strategies for effective nutrition. In Powers MA, ed: Handbook of diabetes nutritional management, Rockville, MD, 1987, Aspen Publications.

28. Posavac EJ and Carey RG: Program evaluation: methods and case studies, Englewood Cliffs, NJ, 1985, Prentice-Hall, Inc.
29. Redman BK: The process of patient education, ed 5, St. Louis, 1989, Mosby–Year Book, Inc.
30. Rosenqvist U, Carlson A, and Luft R: Stockholm Council Teaching Centre for Diabetes, Landstingets Undervisningscentrum for Diabetes, Sweden: Evaluation of comprehensive program for diabetes care at primary health-care level, Diabetes Care 11:269-274,1988.
31. Shea ML, Boyum PG, and Spanke MM: Health occupations clinical teacher education series for secondary and post-secondary educators. Clinical evaluation: theory and practice in health occupations, Springfield, IL, 1985, Illinois State Board of Education.
32. Shelley SI: Research methods in nursing and health, Boston/Toronto, 1984, Little Brown Co.
33. Staropoli CJ and Waltz CF: Developing and evaluating educational programs for health care providers, Philadelphia, 1978, FA Davis Co.
34. Third-party reimbursement for outpatient diabetes education and counseling, Diabetes Care 13(suppl 1):36,1990.
35. Wentling J, and others: Locally directed evaluation handbook, Springfield, IL, 1978, Illinois State Board of Education.
36. Wentling T and others: Student evaluation of instruction, Springfield, IL, 1978, Illinois Office of Education.

Diabetes Resources*

PUBLICATIONS

A complete listing of diabetes-related materials can be obtained from:
National Diabetes Information Clearinghouse
Box NDIC
Bethesda, MD 20892
1-301-468-2162

Selected resources/publications include the following:
Diabetes Forecast is a magazine for people with diabetes. For information contact:
American Diabetes Association, Inc.
1660 Duke Street
Alexandria, VA 22314
1-800-ADA-DISC (1-800-232-3472)

Diabetes in the News
Ames Company
Division, Mills Laboratory, Inc.
P.O. Box 3105
Elkhart, IN 46515

Diabetes Self-Management is published six times a year and has information on diabetes care and research. To subscribe, contact:
Diabetes Self-Management
P.O. Box 52890
Boulder, CO 80322-2890

Adapted from Funnell MM: Resources for you: life with diabetes, 2/e, Ann Arbor, 1988, Michigan Diabetes Research & Training Center, University of Michigan Press.

Health-O-Gram is published by the Sugarfree Center and includes information about living with diabetes, recipes and products. For more information contact:
Sugarfree Center for Diabetes
P.O. Box 114
Van Nuys, CA 91408
1-800-972-2323

If Your Child Has Diabetes. By Joan Elliott. A Perigee Book.
Publishing Group
200 Madison Ave.
New York, NY 10016

You Can't Catch Diabetes from a Friend. By Lynne Fipnis and Susan Adler.
Triad Publishers
P.O. Box 13096
Gainesville, FL 32601

Exercise and Diabetes. A Workbook for Better Health! By J. Kapetanios.
Central Massachusetts Area Health Education Center
900 Main Street
Worcester, MA 01546

EXCHANGE LISTS AND COMPANION MATERIALS

These publications are available from:

American Dietetic Association	**American Diabetes Association**
216 W. Jackson Blvd., Suite 800	National Service Center
Chicago, IL 60606-6995	1660 Duke Street
(312) 899-0400	Alexandria, VA 22314

Family Cookbook: Volume 1, Volume 2, Volume 3.
Goals for Diabetes Education
Month of Meals Menu Planner I and II
Meal Planning Approaches in the Nutrition Management of Diabetes
Nutrition Guide for Professionals: Diabetes Education and Meal Planning
Exchange Lists for Meal Planning, 1986
Eating Healthy Foods (pictures with brief text)
Large Print Exchange Lists for Meal Planning

Ethnic and Regional Food Practices—A Series
*Mexican American Food Practices, Customs and Holidays (professional manual)
*Meal Planning with Mexican Foods (client piece)
*Planificacion de Comidos con Alimartos Mexicanoamericanos (client piece in Spanish)
*Jewish Food Practices, Customs, and Holidays (professional manual)
*Meal Planning with Jewish Foods (client piece)

*Chinese American Food Practices, Customs, and Holidays (professional manual)
*Navajo Food Practices, Customs and Holidays (professional manual)
(Additional publications for Alaska Native, Vietnamese, and Traditional Southern Cooking are scheduled for 1991).

Modified Diets Based on the Exchange Lists for Meal Planning
*Guidelines for use of the Exchange Lists for Low-Sodium Meal Planning
*Guidelines for use of the Exchange Lists for Low-Fat Meal Planning
*Guidelines for use of the Exchange Lists for Low-Sodium, Low-Fat Meal Planning
 Healthy Food Choices
*Como Escoger Alimentos Saludables (Spanish version of Healthy Food Choices)

These publications are available from:
The International Diabetes Center
 Diabetes Center, Inc.
 P.O. Box 739
 Wayzata, MN 55391
 *Convenience Food Facts
 *Exchanges for All Occasions
 *Eating with Food Choices
 *Fast Food Facts
 *The Guiltless Gourmet
 *The Joy of Snacks

ORGANIZATIONS

American Diabetes Association (ADA) is a nonprofit, voluntary health agency supported by donations. The ADA offers funding for research, free screening programs, doctor referrals, written materials, support groups, education, and recognition of education programs that meet certain standards. The national office address is:
 American Diabetes Association, Inc.
 1660 Duke Street Alexandria, VA 22314
 1-800-ADA-DISC (1-800-232-3472)

Juvenile Diabetes Foundation (JDF) is a nonprofit voluntary health agency supported by donations. Money is used for educational programs, camping programs, and support groups. The national office address is:
 Juvenile Diabetes Foundation International
 432 Park Avenue South
 New York, NY 10016
 1-212-889-7575
 1-800-223-1138

American Association of Diabetes Educators:
American Association of Diabetes Educators
500 North Michigan Avenue
Suite 1400
Chicago, IL 60611
1-312-661-1700

The Diabetes Care and Education Practice Group of the American Dietetic Association
216 West Jackson Blvd., Suite 800
Chicago, IL 60606-6995
312/899-0040

Diabetes Research and Training Centers
National Diabetes Information Clearinghouse
Box NDIC
Bethesda, MD 20892
1-301-468-2162

International Diabetic Athletes Association. The purpose of the IDA is to promote healthful participation in sports and vigorous exercise by diabetic persons. Membership includes a subscription to *The Challenge: Newsletter of the International Diabetic Athletes Association.*
International Diabetic Athletes Association
P.O. Box 10010
Phoenix, AZ 85064

SPECIAL GROUPS
Visually Impaired

American Council for the Blind
1211 Connecticut Avenue, NW
Washington, DC 20036
1-800-424-8666

American Foundation for the Blind
15 West 16th Street
New York, NY 10011
1-212-620-2000

National Association for the Visually Handicapped
221 West 21st Street
New York, NY 10010

National Society to Prevent Blindness, Inc.
79 Madison Avenue
New York, NY 10016

The National Library Service for the Blind and Physically Handicapped of the Library of Congress provides a lending service. The collection of Braille and talking books and magazines. For more information contact:
National Library Service for the Blind and Physically Handicapped
Library of Congress
1291 Taylor Street, NW
Washington, DC 20542
1-202-287-5100

Other source for reading material on tape or records is:
American Printing House for the Blind
1839 Frankfort Avenue
Louisville, KY 40206
1-502-895-2405

The LIONS Clubs also offer services for blind persons. Contact your local group or:
LIONS Club International
300 Twenty-Second Street
Oakbrook, IL 60570
1-312-571-5466

Kidney Disease

National Kidney Foundation
2 Park Avenue
New York, NY 10016
1-212-889-2210

National Association of Patients on Hemodialysis and Transplantation
150 Nassau Street
New York, NY 10038
1-212-619-2727

Heart Disease

American Heart Association
7320 Greenville Avenue
Dallas, TX 75231
1-214-750-5300

Amputations

National Amputation Foundation, Inc.

12-45 150th Street
Whitestone, NY 11357
1-718-767-8400

Impotence

Impotents Anonymous

5119 Bradley Avenue
Chevy Chase, MD 20815
1-301-656-3649

Smoking

American Cancer Society

Call the local ACS unit listed in your telephone book for more information about publications and services. Programs include:

Fresh Start: a group smoking sessation program consisting of multiple sessions.

Smart Move! a single session smoking cessation program. Both programs are offered to the public free of charge by trained volunteers in ACS Units nationwide. ACS also provides materials for youth of all age groups from preschool through high school.

50 Questions...Smoking and Health...and Answers. Brochure that compiles questions most frequently asked about smoking.

National Cancer Institute (NCI)

Office of Cancer Communications
Building 31, Room 1OA24
Bethesda, MD 20893
Cancer Information Service: 1-800-4-CANCER

American Lung Association (ALA)

Call the local lung association for more information about publications and services. Some selected information includes:

Freedom from Smoking: A 7-week behavior modification program for people who want to quit, offered to the public by trained members of local lung associations nation wide.

A Healthy Beginning: The Smoke Free Family Guide for New Parents. A handbook for health care professionals on counseling new parents to quit.

A Lifetime of Freedom from Smoking. A 28-page self-help booklet that includes many coping strategies for relapse prevention.

Freedom from Smoking for You and Your Family. A 56-page self-help manual.

Growing Healthy. A comprehensive school health education program that includes smoking information for kindergarten through 7th grade.

National Heart, Lung, and Blood Institute (NHLBI)
Information Center
4733 Bethesda Avenue, Suite 530
Bethesda, MD 20814
(301) 951-3260

Office on Smoking and Health (OSH)
Parklawn Building, Room 1-16
5600 Fishers Lane
Rockville, MD 29857
Patient Education: (301) 443-5287
OSH continually develops new patient, public, and professional education materials that are available while supplies last. Some materials are produced in both English and Spanish.

HEALTH AND LIFE INSURANCE

The Diabetes Insurance Program offers life insurance to people with diabetes between the ages of 6 and 40. For more information contact:

Diabetes Insurance Program
P.O. Box 72
Westport, CT 06881
1-203-226-9911

SOCIAL SECURITY

The **Social Security Administration** is a government agency which may provide income when family earnings are stopped or reduced because of retirement, disability, or death.

MEDICARE

Medicare provides hospital and medical insurance for those age 65 and over, or for persons of any age who are blind or disabled and who have received Social Security disability checks for 24 months in a row.

Disability benefits—These benefits provide monthly checks to workers who are disabled.

Survivor's benefits—Monthly checks or a one-time payment may be made to some family members when a person becomes disabled or dies.

Supplemental security income (SSI)—Monthly checks may be provided to people in need who are over age 65, or to blind and disabled persons of any age.

DEPARTMENT OF SOCIAL SERVICES

The **Department of Social Services** is the agency that makes financial and medical help, food stamps, and social services available to people who qualify. Those most useful for people with diabetes are:

Medicaid—This is a medical assistance program for persons who have a low income.

Aid to Families with Dependent Children (ADC)—This is a program of financial aid for families with children under 18 years where either 1 or both parents are missing or 1 or both parents are disabled for 90 days or more.

Food stamps—The food stamp program enables low-income families to buy more food for the same amount of money.

Social services—This agency provides a broad range of social and other services.

Veterans' Administration—Veterans of the Armed Forces can call their local Veterans' Administration (VA) for information about benefits.

COMMUNITY HEALTH CARE RESOURCES

Planned Parenthood—Planned Parenthood provides birth control advice and services for men and women, pregnancy tests, and problem pregnancy counseling. It is listed in the white pages of the phone book under "Planned Parenthood," and in the yellow pages under "Clinics" and "Birth Control Information Centers."

County public health departments—Health departments generally offer a wide range of services for people who live in that county. They offer education about diet, health problems, sex, birth control, and alcohol abuse. Public health departments are usually listed in the white pages of the phone book under "County government."

Visiting nurse associations—Visiting nurses provide nursing care and education in your home. Third-party payment (Medicare, Medicaid, Blue Cross, other insurance) will often pay for these services. Look in the white pages under "Visiting Nurse Association" or in the yellow pages under "Nurses."

Home health care—Many home health agencies are available. The types of services, expertise, and requirements vary from agency to agency. Some services may be covered by insurance.

Meals on Wheels—Meals on Wheels provides one meal a day for homebound or invalid people who qualify. Look under "Meals on Wheels" in the white pages of the phone book, or contact the Department of Social Services for information.

Lawyer Referral Service—The Lawyer Referral Service will provide a list of lawyers available in your area. The service can be reached at 1-800-292-7850.

RESOURCES FOR OLDER ADULTS

Senior Citizens' Centers—Senior Citizens' Centers provide activities, classes, and programs for those age 55 and older. Call your local city recreation department for details.

The American Association of Retired Persons (AARP)—The AARP is a nonprofit organization for older persons. Persons age 50 and older, retired or not, are eligible to belong for a small fee. The AARP offers information, publications, discount coupons, help with tax forms, a prescription and nonprescription drug service, and insurance plans. For more information, contact:
American Association of Retired Persons
 National Headquarters
1909 K Street NW
Washington, DC 20049
1-202-872-4700
1-800-441-7575

National Council of Senior Citizens—The National Council of Senior Citizens offers low-cost insurance, support groups, and other kinds of help. For more information, contact:
National Council of Senior Citizens
925 Fifteenth Street NW
Washington, DC 20005
1-202-347-8800

National Association of Area Agencies on Aging (NAAAA)—The NAAAA represents agencies that offer services to older adults. For information about agencies in your area, contact:
NAAAA
600 Maryland Avenue SW
Washington, DC 20024
1-202-484-7520

Advocate—The Advocate offers information about local resources. It was founded to enhance the lifestyle of older adults.
 Advocate
29 Wellington Road
North Syracuse, NY 13212
1-315-458-2780

Children of Aging Parents—Children of Aging Parents is a national group for information and referral services. They also offer support groups for caregivers of their parents.
 Children of Aging Parents
2761 Trenton Road
Levittown, PA 19056
1-215-945-6900

SPECIAL CONCERNS

Weight loss programs—The American Dietetic Association can provide information about meal planning and weight loss programs. They can be reached by calling or writing:

American Dietetic Association
430 N. Michigan Avenue
Chicago, IL 60611
1-312-280-5000

Overeaters Anonymous (OA)—OA is a nonprofit, self-help fellowship group. If Overeaters Anonymous is not listed in the white pages of your phone book, you can contact the national office at:

Overeaters Anonymous World Service Office
P.O. Box 92870
Los Angeles, CA 90009
1-213-542-8363

Weight Watchers—Weight Watchers is a weight control group that offers diet information and support. Weight Watchers is listed in the yellow pages of the phone book, or contact:

Weight Watchers International
The Jericho Atrium
500 N. Broadway
New York, NY 11753-2196
1-516-939-0400

TOPS (Take Off Pounds Sensibly)—TOPS is a program of nutrition information, weight loss, and support. TOPS is listed in the yellow pages of the phone book, or you can contact them at:

TOPS
4574 So. Fifth Street
Milwaukee, WI 53207
1-414-482-4620

Other groups are available for eating disorders. These groups offer information about the disorders.

ANAD (Anorexia Nervosa and Associated Disorders)
Box 271
Highland Park, IL 60035
1-312-831-3438

AANA (American Anorexia Nervosa Association)
133 Cedar Lane
Teaneck, NJ 07666
1-201-836-1800

SUBSTANCE ABUSE PROGRAMS

Alcoholics Anonymous (AA)— AA is a self-help group for people who want to stop drinking or using drugs. Look in the white pages of the phone book for local groups, or contact:

Alcoholics Anonymous
P.O. Box 459
Grand Central Station
New York, NY 10163
1-212-686-1100

DIABETES IDENTIFICATION

Medic Alert Foundation is a charitable, nonprofit organization that provides identification through the Medic Alert emblem. This tag is worn as a bracelet or necklace.

Medic Alert Foundation
Turlock, CA 95381
1-209-632-2371
1-800-344-3226

EMPLOYMENT

Vocational Rehabilitation is a federally funded program for the vocationally handicapped. People with diabetes are eligible for their services, which include:

* medical and psychologic services
* vocational testing
* job counseling
* job training and placement
* help with employer problems

TRAVEL

Resources are available to help people with diabetes plan ahead for traveling.

The Diabetic Traveler is published four times a year and is designed to help people with diabetes to plan trips. It offers advice on where to visit and say, restaurants, airlines, and cruise lines. It is available from:

The Diabetic Traveler
P.O. Box 8223
Stamford, CT 06905

Intermedic informs travelers about doctors and specialists in over 60 countries. If you are traveling out of the United States, you will want to contact this group before you leave so that you are ready in case of a problem.

Intermedic, Inc.
777 Third Avenue
New York, NY 10017

Types of Diabetes Mellitus and Other Categories of Glucose Intolerance

Clinical classes	Distinguishing characteristics
Diabetes mellitus (DM)	
Type I Insulin-dependent diabetes mellitus (IDDM)	Patients may be of any age, are usually thin, and usually have abrupt onset of signs and symptoms with insulinopenia before age 40. These patients often have strongly positive urine glucose and ketone tests and are dependent upon insulin to prevent ketoacidosis and to sustain life.
Type II Non–insulin-dependent diabetes mellitus (NIDDM) (obese or nonobese)	Patients usually are older than 40 years at diagnosis, obese, and have relatively few classic symptoms. They are not prone to ketoacidosis except during periods of stress. Although not dependent upon exogenous insulin for survival, they may require it for stress-induced hyperglycemia and hyperglycemia that persists in spite of other therapy.
Other types of diabetes mellitus	Patients with other types of diabetes mellitus have certain associated conditions or syndromes.
Impaired glucose tolerance (IGT) (obese or nonobese)	Patients with impaired glucose tolerance have plasma glucose levels that are higher than normal but not diagnostic for diabetes mellitus.
Other types of impaired glucose tolerance	Patients with other types of impaired glucose tolerance have certain associated conditions or syndromes.
Gestational diabetes mellitus (GDM)	Patients with gestational diabetes mellitus have onset or discovery of glucose intolerance *during* pregnancy.
Statistical risk classes*	
Previous abnormality of glucose tolerance (PrevAGT)	Persons in this category have normal glucose tolerance and a history of transient diabetes mellitus or impaired glucose tolerance.
Potential abnormality of glucose tolerance (PotAGT)	Persons in this category have never experienced abnormal glucose tolerance but have a greater-than-normal risk of developing diabetes mellitus or impaired glucose tolerance.

*Used for epidemiologic and research purposes.
Adapted from classification developed by an international workgroup sponsored by the National Diabetes Data Group, National Institutes of Health. National Diabetes Data Group: Classification and diagnosis of diabetes mellitus and other categories of glucose intolerance, Diabetes 28:1039, 1979.

Comparison of Insulin-Dependent Type I Diabetes Mellitus (IDDM) and Noninsulin-Dependent Type II Diabetes Mellitus (NIDDM)

	IDDM	NIDDM
Clinical features		
Age at onset	Usually <30, but can occur at any age	Usually >35, but can occur at any age
Onset	Often rapid	Insidious
Weight	Nonobese, thin	Often obese, may be normal
Ketosis	Common	Rare
Symptoms	Polydipsia, polyphagia, polyuria	Frequently not recognized or less acute in presentation
Complications	Frequent	Frequent
Epidemiology		
Occurrence	10-20% of all diabetes	80-90% of all diabetes
Sex	Slight male prevalence	Female prevalence
Seasonal variation	Present	Unknown
Genetics		
Concordance in identical twins	<50%	>90%
HLA association	Present	Absent
Environmental factors	Virus, toxins, autoimmune stimulus	Obesity, nutrition
Pathology		
Control of diabetes	Often difficult with wide fluctuations of glucose	Variable; helped by dietary measures
Functioning islet cell	Severely reduced	Moderately reduced
Dietary management	Essential	Essential, may suffice for glucose control
Medication		
Insulin	Required for all	Required for 20% to 30%
Sulfonylurea	Not efficacious	Efficacious

Modified from Galloway JA et al: Diabetes mellitus, ed 9, Indianapolis, 1988, Eli Lilly Co, Inc.

Sample Diabetes Care Protocol

INITIAL VISIT
Medical History

Medical history components to be assessed in patients with diabetes include:
- Symptoms and laboratory test results related to the diagnosis of diabetes
- Dietary habits, nutritional status, and weight history; growth and development in children
- Details of previous treatment programs
- Current treatment of diabetes
- Exercise history
- Frequency, severity, and cause of acute complications (e.g., ketacidosis and hypoglycemia)
- Prior or current infections
- Symptoms and treatment of chronic complications associated with diabetes
- Risk factors for atherosclerosis: smoking, hypertension, obesity, hyperlipidemia, and family history
- Psychosocial and economic factors
- Gestational history

Physical Examination

A complete physical examination should be performed during the initial evaluation. Specific components of the examination should include:
- Height and weight measurement (and comparison to norms in children)
- Sexual maturation staging
- Blood pressure determination (with orthostatic measurements)
- Ophthalmoscopic examination, if possible with dilation
- Thyroid palpation
- Cardiac examination
- Evaluation of pulses (with auscultation)
- Foot examination

- Skin examination (including insulin-injection sites)
- Neurologic examination
- Dental and periodontal examination

Laboratory Evaluation

Each patient should undergo laboratory tests that are appropriate to the evaluation of the individual's general medical condition. These include:
- Fasting plasma glucose
- Glycated hemoglobin (HbA_1 or HbA_{1c})
- Fasting lipid profile
- Serum creatinine
- Urinalysis
- Urine culture
- Thyroid function tests
- ECG (in adults)

Management Plan

The management plan should include:
- Statement of goals
- Medications
- Individualized nutrition recommendations and instructions
- Recommendations for life-style changes
- Patient and family education
- Monitoring instructions
- Referral to an eye doctor for a comprehensive eye and visual examination
- Consultation for specialized services as indicated
- Agreement on ongoing support and follow-up
- Birth control information for women of childbearing age

VISIT FREQUENCY

The frequency of patient visits depends on the type of diabetes, degree of blood glucose control achieved, changes in the treatment regimen, and presence of complications of diabetes or other medical conditions.
- Patients beginning treatment by diet or oral glucose-lowering agents may need to be contacted weekly until reasonable glucose control is achieved and the patient is competent to conduct the treatment program.
- Major modifications of the treatment plan should include patient follow-up no more than 1 month following the modification.
- Regular visits should be scheduled for insulin-treated patients at least quarterly and for other patients at least semiannually.

- Patients must be taught to recognize problems with their glucose control and to report problems to the health-care team.
- Patients should be taught to recognize early signs and symptoms of acute and chronic complications and to report these promptly.

CONTINUING CARE
Physical Examination

- A comprehensive physical examination should be performed annually.
- A complete eye and visual examination by an ophthalmologist should be performed at least annually in all patients > 30 years old and in patients between 12 and 30 years of age with a diagnosis of diabetes of at least 5 years' duration.
- The feet should be examined routinely.

Laboratory

- A glycated hemoglobin determination should be performed at least semiannually in all patients and preferably quarterly in insulin-treated patients and in non–insulin-treated patients with poor metabolic control.
- Triglycerides, total cholesterol, and HDL cholesterol should be tested annually in adults and every 2 years in children.
- Routine urinalysis should be performed yearly. After 5 years duration of diabetes, or after puberty, total urinary protein excretion should be measured yearly, by a microalbuminuria method if possible.

Management Plan

The plan should be reviewed at each regular visit. Assessment should include:
- Nutritional evaluation and weight control
- The exercise regimen
- The control of blood glucose
- Frequency of hypoglycemia
- Assessment of complication
- Psychologic adjustment

BIOCHEMICAL INDICES OF METABOLIC CONTROL: TOP LIMITS

	Normal	Acceptable	Fair	Poor
Fasting plasma glucose	115 mg/dL	150 mg/dL	200 mg/dL	>200 mg/dL
Postprandial plasma glucose	140 mg/dL	175 mg/dL	235 mg/dL	>235 mg/dL
Glycosylated hemoglobin	6%	8%	10%	10%
Fasting plasma cholesterol	200 mg/dL	225 mg/dL	250 mg/dL	>250 mg/dL
Fasting plasma triglyceride	150 mg/dL	175 mg/dL	200 mg/dL	>200 mg/dL

Adapted from American Diabetes Association: Clinical practice recommendations, American Diabetes Association 1990-1991, Diabetes Care, 14(suppl 2):10-13, 1991.

Diabetes Health Assessment Form

———————— DIABETES HEALTH ASSESSMENT FORM ————————

Patient Name ————————————   Today's Date ————————————

I. Background information

1. Sex   ————— Male   ————— Female
2. Age   ————— (years)
3. Marital status (circle):
   Never married   Married   Separated/divorced   Widowed
4. Highest level of school completed
   1   2   3   4   5   6   7   8   9   10   11   12   13   14   15   16+
5. a. Number of people living in household (excluding patient)
   ————— Adults (18 years and over)
   ————— Children
   b. Location of primary household ————————————————
   c. Length of time at current address ————————————————
6. Occupational status
   ————— Employed (occupation: —————————————————)
             How satisfied are you with your current position?
             ————————————————————————————

   ————— Homemaker
   ————— Student
             Do you like school? —————————————————
             Favorite part? —————————————————————
   ————— Retired
   ————— Unemployed
   ————— Disabled
7. Describe your average activities in a 24-hour day. —————————
——
——

———————— **DIABETES HEALTH ASSESSMENT FORM** *(continued)* ————————

II. Diabetes regimen

  A. *Medication (insulin)*

    1. What type of insulin do you take? How much? When?

	Type	*Units*	*Time taken*
Morning dose	————	————	————
Afternoon dose	————	————	————
Evening dose	————	————	————
Night Time dose	————	————	————

    2. Where are injections given? (check all that apply)

    ———————— Arm   ———————— Leg   ———————— Buttocks

    ———————— Abdomen   ———————— Other

    3. Do you rotate injection sites? ———————— Yes   ———————— No

    4. Do you inject your own insulin?————————Yes   ————————No

    If no, who does? ————————————

    5. How many injections have you missed in the past 2 weeks? ————————

    6. Do you have any trouble drawing up the correct amount of your insulin?

    ———————— Yes   ———————— No

    If yes, describe: ————————————————————————————

    ————————————————————————————————————

    7. Do you have any trouble injecting your insulin?

    ———————— Yes   ———————— No

    If yes, describe: ————————————————————————————

    ————————————————————————————————————

    8. Please show me how you draw up and inject your insulin.

    Comments: ————————————————————————————————

    ————————————————————————————————————

    ————————————————————————————————————

  B. *Medication (pills)*

    1. How many pills have you been told to take each day? ————————

    2. How many pills do you take each day? ————————

    3. How many times in the past 2 weeks have you missed taking your diabetes pills? ————————

    4. What are the names/dosages of your diabetes pills?

Name of pill	*Strength (mg)*	*Time(s) of day taken*
————	————	————
————	————	————
————	————	————

————— **DIABETES HEALTH ASSESSMENT FORM** (*continued*) —————

C. *Diet history*
   1. Has your doctor recommended you follow a diet or meal plan to:
      a. Control your diabetes? _____ Yes   _____ No   _____ Not sure
      b. To lose weight?   _____ Yes   _____ No   _____ Not sure
   2. How many calories a day are included in your diet?
      _____ Calories   _____ Not sure
   3. How many calories a day do you usually eat?
      _____ Calories   _____ Not sure
   4. What times do you usually eat?
      Breakfast _____
      Lunch   _____
      Dinner   _____
      Snacks   _____
   5. How many meals have you skipped in the past 2 weeks? _____
      (circle meal times)
      Missed: Breakfast   Lunch   Dinner   Snacks
   6. Who shops for your food? _____
   7. Who prepares your food? _____
   8. What part(s) of the diet are hardest to follow?
      _____ Cutting down on sweets
      _____ Cutting down of fats
      _____ Cutting down on the amount of food
      _____ Too much food
      _____ I don't like _____ (example: milk)
      _____ Other _____
   9. What is your height? _____ inches
  10. What is your weight? _____ pounds
  11. How has your weight changed in the past year?
      _____ Stayed the same
      _____ Lost intentionally (_____ pounds)
      _____ Lost unintentionally (_____ pounds)
      _____ Gained (_____ pounds)
  12. What would you like to weigh ? _____ pounds
  13. What questions do you have about following your diet/meal plan?
      _____
      _____
      _____

_____ **DIABETES HEALTH ASSESSMENT FORM** (continued) _____

D. *Exercise*

1. Is exercise a part of your diabetes regimen? _____ Yes   _____ No

   If yes, describe the type, frequency, and duration of exercise.

	Type	*Number of times per week*	*Duration*
example:	brisk walking	3	40 minutes each time
	_____	_____	_____
	_____	_____	_____

2. What questions do you have regarding exercise and diabetes? _____

   _____

   _____

   _____

E. *Monitoring*

1. How do you test your diabetes control?

   _____ I don't test

   _____ Urine glucose checks

   _____ Urine ketones

   _____ Blood sugar (visual check)

   _____ Blood sugar (using meter) Type of meter _____

2. How often have you checked urine or blood sugar in the last month?

Urine sugar	*Blood sugar*
_____ times per day, week, month	_____ times per day, week, month
_____ no urine sugar checks	_____ no blood sugar checks

3. Have you had any of the following in the past 2 weeks?

   _____ Tired, very thirsty

   _____ Confusion

   _____ Feelings of being shaky

   _____ Up to bathroom two or more times during the night

   _____ Nightmare or bad dreams during the night

4. How do you feel when you have a low blood sugar reaction?

   _____

   _____

   _____

5. How often have you felt this way in the past 2 weeks? _____

6. How do you treat a low blood sugar reaction? _____

   _____

7. What is the cost of your diabetes supplies per month? _____

8. Is paying for diabetes supplies a problem? _____ Yes _____ No

9. What is the most difficult part of your diabetes regimen to follow? _____

   _____

   _____

10. (If test blood glucose) Please show me how you check your blood sugars.

11. Glycated hemoglobin (if applicable) _____ % Date measured: _____

—————— **DIABETES HEALTH ASSESSMENT FORM** *(continued)* ——————

III. Complications

Do you have any of the following conditions along with your diabetes?

_____ Cataracts	_____ Skin problems
_____ Eyesight worsened by diabetes	_____ Pain or numbness in feet or legs
_____ Heart problems	_____ Foot problems
_____ High blood pressure	_____ Sexual problems
_____ Kidney problems	

IV. Current health practices

1. Do you have a primary care physician? _____ Yes _____ No
   If yes, what is his or her name? _____
2. How frequently do you see a physician regarding your diabetes care? _____
3. Who do you contact for routine questions regarding diabetes care? _____
4. Have you been seen in an emergency room for your diabetes in the past 12 months?
   _____ Yes _____ No
   If yes, how many times? _____
5. Do you smoke cigarettes? _____ Yes _____ No
   If yes, how many packs per day? _____
6. Do you drink alcohol? _____ Yes _____ No
   If yes, a. What do you drink? _____
   b. How often? _____
   c. How many drinks do you have at one time? _____
7. Do you smoke, inhale, or inject any recreational drugs?
   _____ Yes _____ No
   If yes, what type of drugs and how often do you use? _____
   _____
   _____

V. Psychosocial

1. When were you first told you had diabetes? _____
2. How did you feel when you were told you had diabetes? _____
   _____
   _____
3. How do you feel now? _____
   _____
   _____
4. Does your family/friends help you manage your diabetes?
   _____ Yes _____ No
   If yes how? _____
   _____

   If no, what would you like them to do? _____
   _____

———————— **DIABETES HEALTH ASSESSMENT FORM** *(continued)* ————————

VI. Summary

1. What is your major concern (e.g., job, family) you have at this time? ————
   _____
   _____

2. What is your major concern regarding your diabetes care at this time? ————
   _____
   _____

3. What questions or concerns do you have about your diabetes? ————————
   _____
   _____
   _____
   _____

VII. Learner priorities   **Diabetes health care team priorities**

1. ———————————   1. ———————————————
2. ———————————   2. ———————————————
3. ———————————   3. ———————————————
4. ———————————   4. ———————————————

Education Modules for Children with Diabetes Mellitus

**EDUCATION MODULES FOR CHILDREN WITH
_____ DIABETES MELLITUS _____**

Session I: Initial Family Assessment

Date   Initial

____   ____ Introduce self, unit staff, dietitian, and social worker.

____   ____ Basic explanation of treatment and length of hospitalization.

____   ____ Interview family in regard to support systems: other family members, main caretakers, babysitters, working parents, religious beliefs, other diabetic relatives, educational background, daily family routines of parents and child, when parents can be present for education.

____   ____ Assess financial status and medical insurance benefits.

____   ____ Assess signs and symptoms of hyperglycemia experienced in the last 2 months.

____   ____ Assess diabetic ketoacidosis experienced in last 2 months.

____   ____ Assess for signs and symptoms of hypoglycemia experienced; if so, when and which ones occurred.

                 If diagnosed with diabetes before this hospitalization assess:

____   ____ Meals and snacks (exchanges).

____   ____ Use of waiting times.

____   ____ Relationship of exercise to blood glucose levels.

____   ____ Blood glucose testing times.

____   ____ Knowledge of insulin times.

____   ____ Knowledge of insulin dosage adjustments.

EDUCATION MODULES FOR CHILDREN WITH
_____ **DIABETES MELLITUS** (*continued*) _____

Basic physiology and ketoacidosis

Date reviewed	Initial	Date reinforced	Initial	
_____	_____	_____	_____	IDDM vs. NIDDM.
_____	_____	_____	_____	Genetics and triggers that stimulate diabetes in children.
_____	_____	_____	_____	Basic physiology of pancreas, insulin, and cells.
_____	_____	_____	_____	Why insulin cannot be given as a pill.
_____	_____	_____	_____	Importance of insulin.
_____	_____	_____	_____	Honeymoon—explanation of and presence of unexplained hypoglycemia.
_____	_____	_____	_____	Signs of hyperglycemia (thirsty, ↑ urinating, exhausted, headache) and reasons for their appearance.
_____	_____	_____	_____	Signs of ketoacidosis (nausea, vomiting, stomachache, Kussmahl respirations, acidotic breath) and reasons for their appearance.

Session II: Hypoclycemia/Insulin Reactions

Date reviewed	Initial	Date reinforced	Initial	
_____	_____	_____	_____	Signs and symptoms of insulin reactions (shaky, sweaty, sleepy, *very* hungry, pale, dizzy, combative) during the day and reasons why.
_____	_____	_____	_____	Signs, symptoms, and causes of hypoglycemia (restless, sleepwalk, sleeptalk) at night and reasons why.
_____	_____	_____	_____	Causes of insulin reaction (miss meal or snack, ↑ exercise, too much insulin).
_____	_____	_____	_____	Treatment of low blood sugar.
_____	_____	_____	_____	Role of epinephrine (adrenalin) and glucagon in ↑ blood sugar.
_____	_____	_____	_____	Glucagon use and storage in cool place required; not to exceed 85° F and not to freeze.
_____	_____	_____	_____	If child passes out or has seizure, give glucagon IM.

EDUCATION MODULES FOR CHILDREN WITH
_____ **DIABETES MELLITUS** (continued) _____

Insulin actions

Date reviewed	Initial	Date reinforced	Initial	
_____	_____	_____	_____	Types of insulin (beef, pork, human).
_____	_____	_____	_____	Time actions of regular insulin begins ½°; peaks 2-3.°
_____	_____	_____	_____	Time actions of NPH insulin begins 1°; peaks 6-8.°
_____	_____	_____	_____	Time actions of ultralente insulin.
_____	_____	_____	_____	Importance of peak insulin times to hypoglycemia.
_____	_____	_____	_____	Effect of circardian rhythms on night-time blood glucose levels, especially ↓ hormones and ↓ blood sugar and especially with NPH peak 2 to 4 AM and ↑ hormones and ↑ blood sugar and ↓ insulin 5 to 8 AM.
_____	_____	_____	_____	Relationship of blood glucose and ketone testing to time and actions of insulin; (i.e., need to test for ↓ blood sugar <60 mg/dL and when insulins are peaking).
_____	_____	_____	_____	Relationship of food, exercise and insulin injections to blood glucose levels (food ↑ blood sugar; exercise ↓ blood sugar; insulin ↓ blood sugar).
_____	_____	_____	_____	Times and reasons for blood glucose testing and urine ketone testing at home.
_____	_____	_____	_____	Determination of individualized diabetic regimen schedule for both usual school and weekend home schedule.
_____	_____	_____	_____	Determination of individualized diabetic regimen for summer (i.e., changes in exercise schedule and increased need to check for ↓ glucose sugars, possibility of need to ↑ snacks).

EDUCATION MODULES FOR CHILDREN WITH
——————————— DIABETES MELLITUS *(continued)* ———————

Session III: Diabetic Skills—Mixing and Injecting Insulin and Demonstration of Blood Glucose Monitoring Machines

Date reviewed	Initial	Date reinforced	Initial	
———	——	———	——	Explanation of insulin syringe parts— plunger, barrel, unit markings, 3/10cc syringe, 5/10cc syringe, 1cc syringe, needle, bevel.
———	——	———	——	Differences in types of insulin syringes: BD, terumo, monoject.
———	——	———	——	Demonstration of mixing regular and NPH insulin by nurse.
———	——	———	——	Demonstration of insulin injection technique by nurse, including pinching up skin and fat, insert at a 90-degree angle, aspirate to check for blood, rotate syringe before removing needle.
———	——	———	——	Injection sites and importance of rotating sites (from arms to abdomen one week to legs and abdomen the next week).
———	——	———	——	Return demonstration of mixing and injecting insulin by parents.
———	——	———	——	Return demonstration of mixing and injecting insulin by child.
———	——	———	——	Return demonstration of mixing and injecting insulin by significant others.
———	——	———	——	Demonstration of urine ketone testing using ketostix.
———	——	———	——	Return demonstration of urine ketone testing.
———	——	———	——	Storage of insulin (environmental temperature not to exceed 85° F).
———	——	———	——	Demonstration of the usage of two to three blood glucose monitoring meters.
———	——	———	——	Demonstration of two to three different types of blood glucose strips.
				Return demonstration on meter and blood glucose strips of choice:
———	——	———	——	By child.
———	——	———	——	By parents.
———	——	———	——	By significant other(s).

EDUCATION MODULES FOR CHILDREN WITH
_____ **DIABETES MELLITUS** (continued) _____

Session IV: Insulin Dose Adjustments

Date reviewed	Initial	Date reinforced	Initial	
_____	____	_____	_____	Explanation of times that dose will need to be increased or decreased—illness, puberty, growth spurts, increased or decreased activity, menses, times of stress.
_____	____	_____	_____	Need to keep accurate daily records of blood sugar tests.
_____	____	_____	_____	Explanation of what and how necessary information needs to be recorded in relation to insulin dosages and blood glucose values, exercise, dose adjustments, and other notes.
_____	____	_____	_____	Discuss principles of dose adjustments.
				Explanation of how much the dose will need to be increased of decreased:
_____	____	_____	_____	Change by ½ units with preschoolers.
_____	____	_____	_____	Change by 1 unit with school-age children.
_____	____	_____	_____	Change by 1-2 units with adolescents
				Practice making dose adjustments by role playing with blood glucose diary.
_____	____	_____	_____	Mother
_____	____	_____	_____	Father
_____	____	_____	_____	Child
_____	____	_____	_____	Significant other(s)
_____	____	_____	_____	Identification of patterns of blood glucose levels and when to call for insulin dose changes.
_____	____	_____	_____	Meaning of glycated hemoglobin/AIC.

EDUCATION MODULES FOR CHILDREN WITH
_____ **DIABETES MELLITUS** (*continued*) _____

Date reviewed	Initial	Date reinforced	Initial	
				Problem solving with concrete age-appropriate situations.
				Hypoglycemia
_____	___	_____	___	Shopping mall
_____	___	_____	___	Park
_____	___	_____	___	Float trip
_____	___	_____	___	Camping
_____	___	_____	___	Skiing
_____	___	_____	___	Sport events
_____	___	_____	___	Movie theater
_____	___	_____	___	Night-time
				Hyperglycemia
_____	___	_____	___	Before sport events/activities
_____	___	_____	___	After sport events/activities
_____	___	_____	___	During infections, growth
				Ketoacidosis (before and after)
_____	___	_____	___	Sports events
_____	___	_____	___	Infection
_____	___	_____	___	Exercise
_____	___	_____	___	With normal blood glucose values
_____	___	_____	___	With low-blood glucose values
_____	___	_____	___	With high-blood glucose values
				Snacks:
_____	___	_____	___	In relation to low bedtime blood glucose
_____	___	_____	___	In relation to bedtime glucose of 150 to 250
_____	___	_____	___	In relation to high bedtime blood glucose
_____	___	_____	___	Whether or not to include AM and PM snack
				When you need to increase/decrease a snack
_____	___	_____	___	Morning
_____	___	_____	___	Afternoon
_____	___	_____	___	Bedtime
_____	___	_____	___	With exercise
_____	___	_____	___	Use of waiting times to keep blood glucose levels even

EDUCATION MODULES FOR CHILDREN WITH
_____ **DIABETES MELLITUS** (*continued*) _____

Session V: Sick-Day Management

Date reviewed	Initial	Date reinforced	Initial	
_____	____	_____	____	What to do:
_____	____	_____	____	If blood glucose value is greater than 250, then check for ketones in urine.
_____	____	_____	____	If have stomach/abdominal pain, then call endocrine doctor on call.
_____	____	_____	____	If ketones present, drink 8 to 12 oz. fluid × 2 hours and retest, and if ketones still present call endocrine doctor on call.
_____	____	_____	____	If child vomits × 2 or more, then call endocrine doctor on call.
_____	____	_____	____	If blood glucose value in range and has ketones, then call for insulin dose.
_____	____	_____	____	If night-time hypoglycemia occurs, then give ½ glass orange juice.
_____	____	_____	____	How to handle emergencies:
				When to call _____
				Who to call _____
				If no one answers, call _____ ask for diabetes doctor on call immediately.
_____	____	_____	____	If child can't eat, then use full and/or clear liquid diet.

Discharge Planning

Date reviewed	Initial	Date reinforced	Initial	
_____	____	_____	____	Diabetes Quiz taken and passed with 80% accuracy.
_____	____	_____	____	Discharge prescriptions given—insulin, glucagon, and blood testing supplies.
_____	____	_____	____	Follow-up appointment made to outpatient endocrine offices (call _____ to make this).
_____	____	_____	____	Family instructed to call the endocrine doctor or nurse daily for dose adjustment.

EDUCATION MODULES FOR CHILDREN WITH
_____ **DIABETES MELLITUS** (continued) _____

Nutrition Checklist

Day 1
___ Nutritional history taken and compared with hospital-ordered meal pattern.
___ Change ordered hospital diet to reflect child's usual eating pattern.
___ Provide family, and patient, if age-appropriate, rationale of meal pattern, focusing on need for balance, timing of meals, and consistency required.
___ Give exchange booklet and begin explanation of content.

Day 2
___ Explanation of ADA exchanges and guidelines.
___ Importance of CHO distribution throughout day.
___ Need for balance of 20% protein, 30% fat, and 50% CHO (approximate balance).
___ Instruction on exchanges with booklet.
___ Explain how various foods affect the blood glucose level differently.
___ Provide rationale for keeping fat less than 30% of kcals.
___ Discuss "diet," "lite," and "dietetic" foods.
___ Fills out hospital menu according to exchanges allowed and writes appropriate amounts of each item. Child should do this with parent, if appropriate cognitive development present.
___ Assignment to write out a typical menu for use at home.

Day 3
___ Review explanation of diet.
___ Review menu and discuss corrections if needed.
___ Give "Eats and Treats" booklet and discuss.
___ Sick-day management and basic explanation of replacement CHO.
___ Prepare sick-day menu to replace CHO at each meal.
___ Explanation of exercise guidelines.
___ Discuss holiday or special day's menus.
___ Discuss importance of label reading.
___ Discuss how to convert a product with an appropriate label to exchanges.

Day 4
___ Discuss use of "fast foods."
___ Prepare one meal of "fast foods" into allotted exchanges.
___ Provide phone number for questions, encourage family to contact if any questions should arise.

_____
Dietitian

_____
Date

EDUCATION MODULES FOR CHILDREN WITH
_____ DIABETES MELLITUS *(continued)* _____

Psychosocial/Family/Child Assessment

Initial

_____ Assess parents' emotional response to diagnosis, family structure and supportiveness, ability to communicate with each other, lifestyle including daily routine, ability to learn, problem-solving ability, financial status, cultural or religious considerations.

_____ Assess parent/child relationship.

_____ Assess child's reaction to diagnosis and medical procedures, behavior at home and school, grades, possible learning problems, attendance record.

_____ Identify family factors or stresses that might interfere with adjustment and adherence to the regimen (i.e., single-parent family, other health problems in the family, financial problems). Did family respond appropriately to child's symptoms before diagnosis?

Education/Support

Initial

_____ Discuss emotional reactions to diagnosis. Explain grief process.

_____ Discuss previous knowledge of diabetes/parents fears. Correct misconceptions.

_____ Reassure patient and family of competence and support of medical staff. Familiarize with diabetes program and functions of diabetes team.

_____ Discuss reactions of parents and child to medical procedures (e.g., testing, injections). Suggest ways to ease trauma and reinforce child's efforts. Teach parents behavioral reinforcement techniques.

_____ Discuss possible effects of diabetes on child's behavior, home life, social life, and school performance. Discuss importance of maintaining appropriate discipline.

_____ Discuss possible effects of diabetes on parents and siblings.

_____ Discuss patient's return to school. Provide teacher literature. Discuss ways to keep diabetes from interference with school experience.

_____ Help child anticipate return to school, including telling friends, sticking to the diet, parties, outings. Discuss child's feelings, fears, and concerns.

_____ Help family plan diabetes care task assignments (i.e., who will do what at home). Be sure father is included and child is assigned age-appropriate tasks.

_____ Discuss problem-solving approach to diabetes care and realistic expectations of diabetes control.

_____ Familiarize patient and family with community supports, support groups.

_____ Give family opportunity to discuss their concerns. What problems do they anticipate? Help with beginning problem-solving efforts or refer to appropriate staff for assistance.

_____ Help shape effective parenting behaviors by reinforcing parents' efforts to utilize learnings from diabetes classes and counseling.

Adapted from St. Louis Children's Hospital, 1991, St. Louis, Missouri.

National Standards for Diabetes Patient Education and American Diabetes Association Review Criteria*

NEEDS ASSESSMENT

A successful program is the product of a flexible policy based on the needs of the community it is intended to serve. Because the diabetes caseload varies from one institution to another, each institution should assess its own needs and match its resources to the needs of its caseload. The needs assessment should be performed initially to guide the management of the program and to form the basis for program planning. It should be a continuing process that will allow the program to adapt to changing service requirements. In addition to the needs of the program, the needs of the individual patient should be assessed to provide the basis for the instructional program offered to each patient. The person with diabetes is recognized to be an equal partner in all aspects of the educational process.

Facility

Standard 1. The facility shall assess its diabetes caseload to determine the allocation of personnel and resources to serve the instructional needs of the caseload.
  Review criterion
  1. The applicant annually determines the case mix of diabetes patients to be educated.

Standard 2. There shall be a reasonable match between caseload requirements and resources allocated.

---

*Reprinted with permission from American Diabetes Association: Diabetes Care 9:36, 1986.

Review criteria

2. For lectures, resources are provided to support the appropriate caseload.
3. Demonstration class size is limited to 16 people (including patient and family members) per instructor.
4. Return demonstration session is limited to 4 people per instructor.

Program

Standard 1. An individualized and documented ongoing assessment of needs shall be developed with the patient's participation. This shall include medical history, present health status, previous diabetes education, health services utilization, associated medical conditions or risk factors, diabetes knowledge, skills, attitudes, self-assessment, identification of support system, barriers to learning, and financial status.

Review criteria

5. On enrollment of each patient into the program, a needs assessment is conducted that includes the items specified above.
6. Each patient's needs assessment is a permanent part of his or her written education record or is included in the medical record.

Standard 2. The needs assessment shall be the basis for the education program delivered to each patient.

Review criterion

7. A written individualized education plan based on the needs assessment is developed. The person with diabetes is a participant in this process, and the written plan is shared with him or her before instruction.

PLANNING

Planning is an essential component of a diabetes patient education program. The planning process should describe the program's goals and objectives, target audience, setting (inpatient, outpatient), patient-referral mechanisms, procedures, and evaluation methods. This process should be a cooperative effort involving people with diabetes and health professionals.

Facility

Standard. The facility shall have a written policy that affirms patient education as an integral component of quality diabetes care.

Review criterion

8. The applicant has a written statement concerning diabetes patient education that is consistent with the goals and intentions of the standards.

Program

Standard 1. The planning participants shall include health professionals involved in the care and education of people with diabetes and their families.

> **Review criterion**
>
> 9. An advisory committee is formed to oversee the diabetes patient education program. Members of the committee must include at least one physician, nurse (or qualified diabetes health educator), dietitian, and consumer.

Standard 2. The planning process shall define, in the following order, program goals and objectives, target audience, patient access mechanisms, instructional methods, resource requirements, patient follow-up mechanisms, and evaluation.

> **Review criteria**
>
> 10. Program goals and objectives: The applicant provides goals and measurable objectives of the diabetes patient education program. These should be consistent with the goals and intentions of the standards.
> 11. Target audience: The applicant specifies the age range of the patients, the types of diabetes patients the program serves, or any unique characteristic of the patients (e.g., language barriers, learning disabilities).
> 12. Patient access mechanisms: The applicant defines how a patient gains access to the patient education program. Methods of access include health-care professional referral, health-care agency referral, or patient self-referral.
> 13. Instructional methods: The applicant identifies the instructional format (i.e., one-to-one, classroom, group, self-instruction modules, etc., or any combination of these) for each of the curricular areas.
> 14. Resource requirements: The applicant identifies the space, staffing, budget, and instructional materials that are part of the patient education program.
> 15. Patient follow-up mechanisms: The applicant identifies its patient follow-up methods.
> 16. Evaluation: The applicant identifies the program evaluation mechanisms.

PROGRAM MANAGEMENT

Effective management is required to implement a patient education program successfully. Various health-care professionals are involved in the total care of people with diabetes. Clear lines of authority and efficient systems for communication should be established among everyone involved in the program. The ultimate responsibility for all aspects of program management should rest with one person designated the *program coordinator*. In addition, an advisory committee should be established to assist the coordinator and other members of the program staff in setting policy and managing the program.

Facility

Standard 1. The facility shall designate a coordinator responsible for all aspects of the program.

Review criterion

17. It is desirable that the coordinator be a health care professional who holds either a valid license or registration. In addition, certification or a health-related degree from an accredited educational institution is desirable.
18. The coordinator completes an education program (minimum 24 hrs) that includes instruction in the 15 content areas listed under the CONTENT/CURRICULUM program standard as well as in educational principles.
19. The coordinator annually completes a minimum of 6 hrs of continuing education in diabetes and educational principles.
    a. If the program coordinator is not a health-care professional, he or she must complete a basic 24-hrs education program (as above), maintain 6 annual continuing education hours (as above), and not function as a program instructor.
20. The coordinator is responsible for
    a. liaison between the advisory committee and facility administration
    b. planning and participating in orientation of diabetes patient education personnel
    c. providing and/or coordinating in-service education for diabetes patient education personnel
    d. participating in the preparation of the program budget
    e. evaluating program content and effectiveness
    f. coordinating program curriculum

Standard 2. The organizational relationships, lines of authority, staffing, and operational policies shall be defined.

Review criteria

21. The placement of the diabetes patient program within the organizational structure of the institution is defined.
22. The line of authority of the program coordinator is defined.
23. The approval mechanisms for both policy and program changes within the facility are defined.

Program

Standard. A standing advisory committee with both medical and community/consumer representation shall be established.

Review criteria

24. The advisory committee's responsibility is to recommend policy, review curriculum, and provide advice concerning the diabetes patient education program.
25. Advisory committee members attend at least two meetings a year.

COMMUNICATION/COORDINATION

Several levels of communication are essential to the effective coordination of the program. Physician or nurse educator leadership and participation are necessary to ensure the integration of patient education into the treatment regimen. A physician should be identified to serve as liaison between the education program coordinator and the medical staff. In addition, the institution should maintain regular channels of communication with its staff and the community it serves to inform diabetes patients and their families about the availability of the program. All information on the patient's educational experience should be incorporated into the permanent medical or educational record.

Facility

Standard 1. The facility shall select a physician to serve as liaison between the program coordinator and the medical staff.

Review criterion

26. The physician's liaison activities include
    a. attendance at advisory committee meetings.
    b. communication of new developments and activities of the program to medical staff, administration, and the medical community.
    c. communication of input from medical staff, administration, or the medical community to the program coordinator and advisory committee.

Standard 2. The facility shall regularly inform its staff and the diabetes patients (and potential diabetes patients) it serves of the availability of its diabetes patient education program.

Review criteria

27. The applicant informs its staff twice yearly of the availability of the program, its content, and the referral process.
28. Newly employed health-care professionals are informed of the institution's diabetes patient education program during orientation.
29. The applicant identifies a communication system that informs the target population of available patient education services. For inpatient programs, the target audience is all patients with diagnosed diabetes at the time of admission. For outpatient programs, the target audience is the general public, physicians, and referral agencies in the service area.

Program

Standard 1. All information about the patient's educational experience shall be incorporated into the patient's permanent medical or educational record maintained by the institution.

    Review criteria

    30. The program establishes a diabetes education record that documents the educational experience and becomes a part of the patient's permanent medical or educational record.

    31. The documentation of the educational experience includes:

        a. preprogram assessment

        b. patient education plan

        c. content, dates delivered, instructors identified

        d. postprogram assessment

        e. plan for follow-up

Standard 2. The role of each education team member shall be clearly defined, and the intercommunication between each shall be documented in the patient's record.

    Review criteria

    32. Members of the diabetes patient education staff have written job descriptions that state their responsibilities for patient care and patient instruction.

    33. Education team members use the patient's permanent record to communicate about the patient's diabetes education.

Standard 3. There shall be written evidence of coordination between different care settings.

    Review criterion

    34. On completion of the education program, and with the patient's permission, the patient's permanent medical or educational record is made available to other health-care settings. On request, a copy of the educational record is also given to the patient.

PATIENT ACCESS TO TEACHING

It should be the policy of the institution to facilitate access to patient education for the target audience specified in the plan. This is promoted by a commitment to inform patients and staff routinely about the availability and benefits of patient self-care programs. Diabetes patient education should be regularly and conveniently accessible, and the instructional program should be able to respond to patient-initiated requests for information. The program permits referral by health-care professionals, health-care agencies, or individual patients. The instructional design encourages active patient participation.

Facility

Standard. The facility shall have a policy to inform patients routinely about the benefits and availability of patient education.
Review criterion
35. See criterion 29.

Program

Standard 1. The program shall be regularly and conveniently available.
Review criteria
36. For health-care institutions, individualized education services at diagnosis or times of crisis are available.
37. Diabetes patient education programs are offered at least quarterly or as the case-load warrants.

Standard 2. The program shall be responsive to patient-initiated requests for information and/or participation in the program's activities.
Review criterion
38. A person is designated within the program to be responsible for receiving and answering patient-initiated requests during business hours.

CONTENT/CURRICULUM

The individual needs assessment provides the basis for the instructional program offered to each patient. The assessment should be documented and should include all relevant information regarding the patient's treatment, education, and support systems. Responsibility for various facets of the assessment can be divided among the instructional team members. Curriculum and instructional materials should be appropriate for the specified target audience, taking into consideration the type and duration of diabetes and the age and learning ability of the individual. Both curriculum and available community resources should be reviewed and updated periodically. The institution should provide the program with adequate space, personnel, budget, and materials.

Facility

Standard 1. The facility shall provide space, personnel, budget, and instructional materials adequate for the program.

Review criterion

39. Space, personnel, budget, and instructional materials are available in the institution to support each content item identified in the CONTENT/CURRICULUM program.

Standard 2. The facility shall periodically assess the availability of community resources.

Review criterion

40. The applicant, at least once every 3 years, assesses public, private, and nonprofit health agencies within the service area for their potential contribution toward improving diabetes education. This assessment includes the name, address, and telephone number of each identified resource.

Program

Standard 1. The program shall be capable of offering information on the following content items as needed:

a. general facts
b. psychologic adjustment
c. family involvement
d. nutrition
e. exercise
f. medications
g. relationship between nutrition, exercise, and medication
h. monitoring
i. hyperglycemia and hypoglycemia
j. illness
k. complications (prevent, treat, rehabilitate)
l. hygiene
m. benefits and responsibilities of care
n. use of health-care systems
o. community resources

Review criterion

41. Each program content area has written and measurable behavioral objectives, a content outline, a designated instructional method, instructional materials, and a means of evaluating the achievement of objectives.

Standard 2. The applicant shall specify the mechanism by which the curriculum shall be reviewed, approved, and updated.

Review criterion

42. The curriculum is annually reviewed and approved by the advisory committee and modified accordingly.

INSTRUCTOR

Qualified personnel are essential to the success of a diabetes patient education program. Each institution should be responsible for identifying and evaluating its instructors. Instructors should be skilled professionals with recent experience and training in both diabetes and educational principles. The number of instructors should be proportional to the caseload requirements.

Facility

Standard 1. The facility shall identify appropriate instructional personnel and ascertain their competence.

Review criteria

43. Instructors are health-care professionals who hold either a valid license or registration. In addition, certification or a health-related degree from an accredited educational institution is desirable.
44. Primary instructional personnel must complete a diabetes education program (minimum of 24 hrs) that includes educational principles.

Standard 2. The number of personnel identified shall be suitable for the diabetic caseload within the institution.

Review criterion

45. Appropriate resources are provided to support the case mix. See criteria 2-4.

Standard 3. Instructors shall be allotted sufficient time to accomplish the educational objectives.

Review criterion

46. The number and type of instructors are appropriate to the case mix, with adequate time for teaching provided. The teaching process must include program planning, implementation and instruction, documentation of the patient educational experience, and participation in program development and evaluation.

Program

Standard. A comprehensive diabetes patient education program has instructors skilled in teaching the curriculum of the program.

Review criteria

47. See criterion 32.
48. Instructors annually complete a minimum of 6 hrs of continuing education in diabetes and educational principles.

FOLLOW-UP

Follow-up services are important because diabetes requires a lifetime of proper care. The facility should provide follow-up services that include periodic reassessment of the patient's knowledge and skills and should offer supplementary educational services when warranted. Written communication between the program staff and the primary-care physician is essential for ongoing identification of the patient's needs. This is especially appropriate in regard to referral for early diagnosis and treatment of the complications of diabetes.

Referral to community resources may also provide ongoing support for long-term psychosocial needs and behavior modification skills. If a patient changes care settings, the institution should request the patient's permission to send his or her records to the new setting.

Facility

Standard. The facility shall transmit the educational record to other appropriate health-care settings when a patient transfers his or her care responsibilities.

Review criterion
49. See criterion 34.

Program

Standard. The program shall provide follow-up services for patients who want to maintain continuity of education within the institution. These services shall include:
  a. periodic reassessment of knowledge and skills
  b. timely reeducation based on reassessment
  c. communication with the primary-care provider about the need for professional and nonprofessional services.

Review criteria
50. The applicant informs and encourages the patient to utilize education follow-up services.
51. Patients who return for follow-up receive knowledge and skill reassessment
52. Follow-up services/education needs are communicated to the primary-care provider.

EVALUATION

The facility should review the educational program periodically to ascertain that it continues to meet the national standards. This review should be conducted by the advisory committee. The results of this review should be used in subsequent program planning and modification. An assessment of each patient's needs and progress should also be conducted at regular intervals.

Facility

Standard. The applicant shall periodically review the performance of the instructional program and ascertain that it continues to meet national standards.

Review criterion

53. The advisory committee and appropriate institutional officials conduct and record a yearly internal review of the program.

Program

Standard 1. The program shall conduct and record an individualized assessment of each patient's original needs and progress at regular intervals.

Review criteria

54. See criteria 5, 6, 30, and 31.

Standard 2. The program shall be reviewed continually for both process and outcome, and the results of this evaluation shall be used in subsequent planning and program modification.

Review criteria

55. Program process measures used for ongoing evaluation include but are not limited to
    a. yearly review of the curriculum
    b. program description
    c. target population
    d. number of participants
56. Program outcome measures of patient knowledge and skills are based on the program's stated objectives.
57. Results of process and outcome evaluations are utilized in program modifications.

DOCUMENTATION

Program planning and evaluation should be documented to provide the basis for future program development and modification. All information about the patient's educational experience should be documented in the patient's permanent medical or educational record, as should communication among treatment and education professionals.

Facility

Standard. All aspects of the evaluation program shall be recorded by the facility and reviewed periodically to ascertain that national standards are being maintained.

Review criterion

58. See criterion 53.

Program

Standard. All aspects of the educational program offered to each patient shall be recorded in that patient's permanent medical or educational record as maintained by the facility.

Review criteria

59. See criteria 6, 7, 30, and 31.

Index

Page numbers in italics indicate illustrations and boxed material; *t* indicates tables.

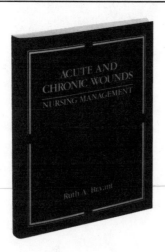
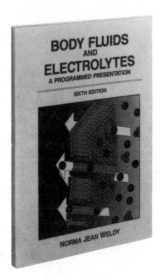
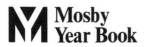